Melanocytic Tumors of the Skin

AFIP Atlas
of
Tumor Pathology

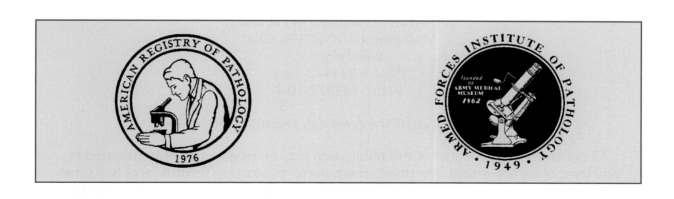

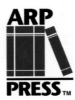

ARP
PRESS™

Silver Spring, Maryland

Editorial & Production Manager: Mirlinda Q. Caton
Production Editor: Dian S. Thomas
Editorial Assistant: Magdalena C. Silva
Editorial Assistant. Alana N. Black
Copyeditor: Audrey Kahn

Available from the American Registry of Pathology
Armed Forces Institute of Pathology
Washington, DC 20306-6000
www.afip.org
ISBN 1-933477-10-5
978-1-933477-10-7

AFIP ATLAS OF TUMOR PATHOLOGY

Fourth Series
Fascicle 12

MELANOCYTIC TUMORS OF THE SKIN

by

David E. Elder, MB, ChB, FRCPA
Professor of Pathology & Laboratory Medicine
University of Pennsylvania School of Medicine
Vice Chair for Anatomic Pathology
Hospital of the University of Pennsylvania
Philadelphia, Pennsylvania

George F. Murphy, MD
Professor of Pathology
Harvard Medical School
Director of Dermatopathology
Brigham & Women's Hospital, Department of Pathology
Boston, Massachusetts

Published by the
American Registry of Pathology
Washington, DC
in collaboration with the
Armed Forces Institute of Pathology
Washington, DC
2010

AFIP ATLAS OF TUMOR PATHOLOGY

EDITOR
Steven G. Silverberg, MD
Department of Pathology
University of Maryland School of Medicine
Baltimore, Maryland

ASSOCIATE EDITOR
William A. Gardner, MD
American Registry of Pathology
Washington, DC

ASSOCIATE EDITOR
Leslie H. Sobin, MD
Armed Forces Institute of Pathology
Washington, DC

EDITORIAL ADVISORY BOARD

Manuscript Reviewed by:
Ralph J. Tuthill, MD
Mark R. Wick, MD

EDITORS' NOTE

The Atlas of Tumor Pathology has a long and distinguished history. It was first conceived at a cancer research meeting held in St. Louis in September 1947 as an attempt to standardize the nomenclature of neoplastic diseases. The first series was sponsored by the National Academy of Sciences-National Research Council. The organization of this Sisyphean effort was entrusted to the Subcommittee on Oncology of the Committee on Pathology, and Dr. Arthur Purdy Stout was the first editor-in-chief. Many of the illustrations were provided by the Medical Illustration Service of the Armed Forces Institute of Pathology (AFIP), the type was set by the Government Printing Office, and the final printing was done at the Armed Forces Institute of Pathology (hence the colloquial appellation "AFIP Fascicles"). The American Registry of Pathology (ARP) purchased the Fascicles from the Government Printing Office and sold them virtually at cost. Over a period of 20 years, approximately 15,000 copies each of nearly 40 Fascicles were produced. The worldwide impact of these publications over the years has largely surpassed the original goal. They quickly became among the most influential publications on tumor pathology, primarily because of their overall high quality, but also because their low cost made them easily accessible the world over to pathologists and other students of oncology.

Upon completion of the first series, the National Academy of Sciences-National Research Council handed further pursuit of the project over to the newly created Universities Associated for Research and Education in Pathology (UAREP). A second series was started, generously supported by grants from the AFIP, the National Cancer Institute, and the American Cancer Society. Dr. Harlan I. Firminger became the editor-in-chief and was succeeded by Dr. William H. Hartmann. The second series' Fascicles were produced as bound volumes instead of loose leaflets. They featured a more comprehensive coverage of the subjects, to the extent that the Fascicles could no longer be regarded as "atlases" but rather as monographs describing and illustrating in detail the tumors and tumor-like conditions of the various organs and systems.

Once the second series was completed, with a success that matched that of the first, ARP, UAREP, and AFIP decided to embark on a third series. Dr. Juan Rosai was appointed as editor-in-chief, and Dr. Leslie H. Sobin became associate editor. A distinguished Editorial Advisory Board was also convened, and these outstanding pathologists and educators played a major role in the success of this series, the first publication of which appeared in 1991 and the last (number 32) in 2003.

The same organizational framework applies to the current fourth series, but with UAREP no longer in existence, ARP plays the major role. New features include a hardbound cover, illustrations almost exclusively in color, and an accompanying electronic version of each Fascicle. There is also an increased emphasis (wherever appropriate) on the cytopathologic (intraoperative, exfoliative, and/or fine needle aspiration) and molecular features that are important in diagnosis and prognosis. What does not change from the three previous series, however, is the goal of providing the practicing pathologist with thorough, concise, and up-to-date information on the nomenclature and classification; epidemiologic, clinical, and pathogenetic features; and, most importantly, guidance in the diagnosis of the tumors and tumorlike lesions of all major organ systems and body sites.

As in the third series, a continuous attempt is made to correlate, whenever possible, the nomenclature used in the Fascicles with that proposed by the World Health Organization's Classification of Tumors, as well as to ensure a consistency of style throughout. Close cooperation between the various authors and their respective liaisons from the Editorial Board continues to be emphasized in order to minimize unnecessary repetition and discrepancies in the text and illustrations.

Particular thanks are due to the members of the Editorial Advisory Board, the reviewers (at least two for each Fascicle), the editorial and production staff, and—first and foremost—the individual Fascicle authors for their ongoing efforts to ensure that this series is a worthy successor to the previous three.

Steven G. Silverberg, MD
William A. Gardner, MD
Leslie H. Sobin, MD

ACKNOWLEDGEMENTS

The development and completion of this Fascicle was dependent upon a diverse array of people, whose expertise, devotion, and support made it all possible. We remember with gratitude Dr. Herbert Z. Lund, whose fascicles on skin tumors written almost half a century ago provided a solid base for the formulation of this work and its predecessor. Dr. Martin C. Mihm, Jr., and the late Dr. Wallace H. Clark, Jr. provided us with much of the training, knowledge, and analytical sense that enabled us to undertake this challenge. For these critical tools and training, we thank them.

A host of other great teachers, mentors, textbook authors, and scholars have provided the foundation upon which we have tried to build. Among these are Drs. Bruce Howie, Jim Gwynne, Ian Aarons, John Blennerhasset, and Vincent McGovern, as well as Ramzi Cotran, Piero Paci, and Thomas B. Fitzpatrick from our respective earlier training years, whose legacies we are proud to be counted among. The editors and reviewers, including Drs. Ralph Tuthill and Mark Wick, provided valuable and constructive criticism, for which we thank them. Our Editorial and Production Manager, Ms. Mirlinda Q. Caton, has worked closely, patiently and expertly with us to develop this superbly finished product. We are also most grateful for the proofreading and editing assistance provided by Drs. Sookjung Yun and Ryan Hick, and Ms. Robin Schanche. Finally, we thank our wives, Peggy and Sharon, and our children, Kate, Kenneth, Erin, and Emily, for their love, patience, faith, forbearance, and encouragement.

David E. Elder, MB ChB, FRCPA
George F. Murphy, MD

CONTENTS

INTRODUCTION: MELANOCYTES AND THEIR TUMORS

The biologic significance of melanocytic tumors, and of pigmented lesions in general, depends on their relationship to malignant melanoma. Most benign melanocytic lesions are biologically unimportant, but others have significance as benign simulants of melanoma, as potential precursors of melanoma, or as markers of risk for melanoma. In addition, some pigmented lesions, such as giant congenital nevi, have major cosmetic and psychosocial significance for affected patients.

Malignant melanoma is the most common potentially fatal neoplasm of the skin. Based on a comparison of primary metastasizing tumors, melanoma is arguably the most virulent human malignancy. Its incidence, controlling for factors related to early detection and diagnostic thresholds, has increased more rapidly over the last several decades than that of any other cancer except for those related to smoking. In young adults, melanoma is now among the leading causes of cancer mortality. Melanoma (this term is synonymous with "malignant melanoma" in our usage) is still uncommon when compared to the major killers, such as lung, colon, or breast cancer. The lifetime risk for melanoma in a white child born today in the United States is about 1 percent, compared to 7 to 9 percent for these more common cancers (1).

The rising incidence and mortality from melanoma, however, have led to greater interest and awareness in physicians and patients, resulting in the presentation and diagnosis of the disease at earlier stages in its evolution. The pigmented lesions submitted to pathologists for interpretation today are less likely to be the large, ulcerated, pigmented masses that were the rule 50 years ago, and are more likely to be smaller patch lesions or papules in which the changes are much more difficult to interpret accurately and reproducibly. This tendency toward more subtle histopathologic presentations of smaller, earlier lesions may be expected to increase in the future.

This Fascicle discusses tumors of melanocytes as well as some selected tumor-like lesions that are significant as melanoma simulants or risk markers. In classic pathology, the term "tumor" means no more than a mass or a swelling. Tumor formation, for example, is one of the classic signs of inflammation. In modern usage, however, the term is almost exclusively applied to lesions that are considered to be neoplastic. According to Nowell's definition (2), neoplastic cells have a "selective growth advantage" compared to normal cells. In general, neoplastic cells proliferate to form a tumor mass, but this is not always so: leukemic cells are considered to be neoplastic but it is unusual for them to proliferate in contiguity to form a mass. Similarly, there is a stage of development of nevi and melanomas when the neoplastic melanocytes proliferate in the epidermis alone or along with single cells within the papillary dermis. The clinical lesion that is formed is a macule, a patch, or a plaque, not a tumor, but the lesion is a neoplasm. In the later evolution of nevi and melanomas, the cells may extend into the papillary dermis and reticular dermis, where a true tumor forms. This property of migration from epidermis to dermis seems to be inherent in benign as well as malignant neoplastic melanocytes, complicating the recognition of "invasion" in melanomas.

The diagnosis of melanocytic neoplasms, especially those early lesions that are confined to the epidermis and superficial dermis, requires some appreciation of the morphology and function of the normal melanocyte. Melanocytes are cells originally derived from the neural crest, and defined in terms of their capacity to produce melanin pigment, for which purpose they possess characteristic organelles termed melanosomes. Ultrastructurally, melanocytes demonstrate no intercellular junctions or desmosomes, and contain variable numbers of melanosomes in various stages of melanization. Early (nonmelanized) premelanosomes appear as small, membranous, elliptical cytoplasmic vacuoles, often with internal lamellae exhibiting fine periodicity. After melanization, these

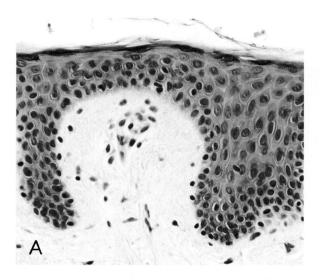

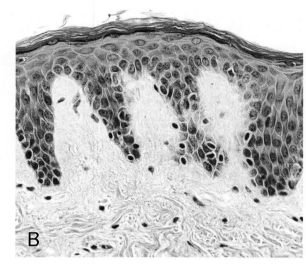

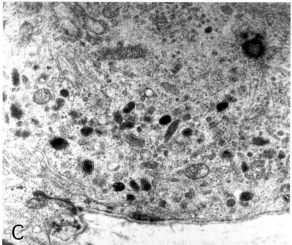

Figure I-1

NORMAL MELANOCYTES

Normal melanocytes tend to hang down slightly from the basement membrane zone into the papillary dermis. They are surrounded by a clear halo in hematoxylin and eosin (H&E)-stained sections. The cell bodies of the melanocytes are separated from each other by a variable number of intervening keratinocytes (A). In type V skin (e.g., African-American), the arrangement of the melanocytes is essentially the same, with differences in the amount and packaging of melanin pigment, most of which, as in Caucasian skin, is in the keratinocytes (B). An electron micrograph shows melanosomes in different stages of maturation (C)

structures become dense, opacified bodies. These mature melanosomes are, in the normal situation, transferred to epidermal keratinocytes via elongated dendritic processes that extend from the melanocyte cell body and insinuate between adjacent keratinocytes. Nonmelanocytic tumor cells (basal cell carcinoma cells, for example) may phagocytize melanized mature melanosomes from benign melanocytes, and thus the detection of early melanosomes (premelanosomes) is necessary for the ultrastructural confirmation of true melanocytic or closely related differentiation.

Histologically, melanocytes are dendritic cells that are normally restricted to the basal layer of the epidermis. For most body sites, melanocytes appear to be separated from neighboring melanocytes by up to 10 basal keratinocytes, although their dendrites, which ramify among the surrounding and overlying keratinocytes, may be in contact with one another at their extremities (fig. I-1). A single melanocyte, together with the surrounding keratinocytes, constitutes the "epidermal melanin unit." Although normal melanocytes are capable of proliferation (3), especially in response to stimuli such as ultraviolet light (fig. I-2), it is rare to see two or more normal melanocytes lying together in contiguity with one another, perhaps because there is a molecular mechanism of mutual repulsion (4). In chronically sun-damaged skin, the ratio of melanocytes to keratinocytes in the basal layer often is increased (from 1:10 to 1:5), and occasional isolated melanocytes have enlarged

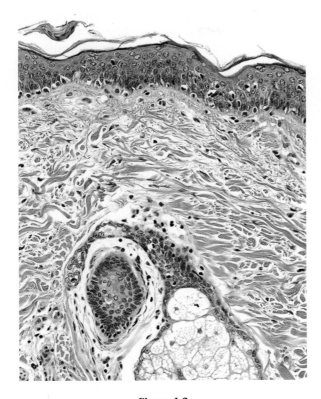

Figure I-2

**MELANOCYTIC HYPERPLASIA IN
CHRONICALLY SUN-DAMAGED SKIN**

The number of melanocytes is variable in skin areas, particularly in chronically sun-damaged skin, where they may be increased. This image is from skin in a region where a melanoma was excised. Some of the cells may represent "field cells," cells with genetic alterations that preceded the development of the melanoma.

hyperchromatic nuclei (fig. I-3). Normal melanocytes synthesize and then promptly transfer pigment to keratinocytes, probably through active phagocytosis of melanosome-containing dendrite fragments by the keratinocytes (5). Thus, melanocytes are not conspicuously pigmented cells in fair-skinned people and most melanin pigment in such skin actually resides in epidermal keratinocytes (6).

One useful way to categorize melanocytic lesions, and pigmented lesions in general, is to divide them into two broad categories of neoplastic and non-neoplastic lesions. *Neoplastic pigmented lesions* are true melanocytic neoplasms characterized by a contiguous proliferation of transformed melanocytes and by related alterations of their normal properties.

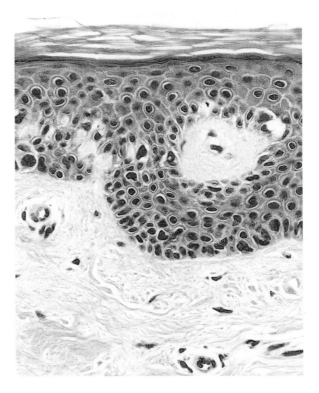

Figure I-3

ISOLATED ATYPICAL MELANOCYTE

An occasional enlarged atypical melanocyte is seen, especially in chronically sun-damaged skin. It is uncertain whether these cells contain genetic alterations.

For example, the "nevus cells" of a melanocytic nevus are increased in number, lie in contiguity with one another, characteristically migrate from the basal epidermis into the papillary dermis, and at earlier evolutionary stages tend to retain pigment in the cytoplasm (7). In all of these properties, they differ from normal melanocytes which, as noted above, are separated from each other by 5 to 10 keratinocytes, do not in general migrate into the dermis, and freely transfer pigment to adjacent keratinocytes. The cells of melanomas exhibit similar properties to those of nevus cells, but in addition, tend to proliferate inexorably and ultimately to acquire metastatic capabilities. The tendency of nevus cells to form localized clusters, associated with an apparent ability to proliferate for a limited time independent of a clearcut stimulus, suggests that nevi, like melanomas, should be regarded as true neoplasms. The fundamental difference that separates nevus and melanoma cells from reactive proliferations and from hyperpigmentations, such as freckles, is the phenomenon of contiguous melanocytic proliferation, which we consider to be an expression of their neoplastic status.

Non-neoplastic pigmented lesions are characterized by increased pigment synthesis and by transfer of this pigment by noncontiguous melanocytes to keratinocytes or other cells such as dermal melanophages in a local region of the skin, but with little or no proliferation of melanocytes. Even when the melanocytes are increased in number, they retain a normal relationship to other melanocytes, so that, like normal melanocytes, they are rarely seen in direct apposition to one another. These lesions, which may be characterized by noncontiguous melanocytic proliferations (or by hyperpigmentation without proliferation), are probably not true melanocytic neoplasms. It is possible that the primary abnormality in some of these lesions (freckles, for example) lies in the keratinocytic component of the epidermal melanin unit. Certainly, keratinocytic neoplasms such as basal cell carcinomas or seborrheic keratoses may be associated with noncontiguous proliferation of morphologically unremarkable melanocytes, and with hyperpigmentation. The cells in these keratinocytic neoplasms, like normal keratinocytes, appear to be capable of "accepting" the pigment presented to them by hyperplastic melanocytes. In the same way, one may speculate that the keratinocytes of a freckle somehow stimulate the regional melanocytes to synthesize and transfer an increased amount of melanin pigment.

There are several categories of lesions that present as focal hyperpigmentations but are not considered to be neoplastic proliferations of melanocytes. These are described in the next chapter.

REFERENCES

1. Silverberg E, Boring CC, Squires TS. Cancer Statistics, 1990. CA Cancer J Clin 1990;40:9-26.
2. Nowell PC. The clonal evolution of tumor cell populations. Science 1976;194:23.
3. Jimbow K, Roth SI, Fitzpatrick TB, Szabo G. Mitotic activity in non-neoplastic melanocytes in vivo as determined by histochemical, autoradiographic, and electron microscopic studies. J Cell Biol 1975;66:663-670.
4. Lindstrom S, Rosdahl I. Mutual repulsion between epidermal melanocytes. Pigment Cell 1981. In: Seiji M, ed. Phenotypic expression in pigment cells. Tokyo: Univ. Tokyo Press; 1982:225-231.
5. Valyi-Nagy IT, Murphy GF, Mancianti ML, Whitaker D, Herlyn M. Phenotypes and interactions of human melanocytes and keratinocytes in an epidermal reconstruction model. Lab Invest 1990;62:314-323.
6. Hu F. Melanocyte cytology in normal skin, melanocytic nevi, and malignant melanomas: a review. In: Ackerman AB, ed. Pathology of malignant melanoma. New York: Masson; 1981:1-22.
7. Elder DE, Greene MH, Bondi EE, Clark WH Jr. Acquired melanocytic nevi and melanoma: the dysplastic nevus syndrome. In: Ackerman AB, ed. Pathology of malignant melanoma. New York: Masson; 1981:185-216.

1 NON-NEOPLASTIC HYPERPIGMENTATIONS

EPHELIDES (FRECKLES)

Ephelides are small, circumscribed, focally pigmented lesions in which, despite their increased and persistent pigment synthesis, the constituent melanocytes have not acquired the neoplastic characteristics of nevus cells. The hyperpigmentation that characterizes these lesions is observed histologically as an increased content of melanin in the keratinocytes, with little or no evidence of melanocytic proliferation. These lesions may represent acquired functional derangements in the epidermal melanin unit involving keratinocytes as well as melanocytes. Although these lesions are not generally of great clinical importance, it is occasionally necessary to distinguish them clinically from nevi, and some also may simulate melanoma, thus prompting biopsy.

SIMPLE EPHELIS (FRECKLE)

Definition. *Simple ephelis* is a circumscribed area of hyperpigmentation typically located on sun-exposed skin, less than about 4 mm in size, and not associated with significant melanocytic proliferation.

Clinical Features. Simple ephelides are light tan, fairly uniform, pigmented lesions with slightly irregular and indefinite borders. They are usually approximately 2 mm in diameter, almost always less than 4 mm, and are distributed on light-exposed areas of skin, especially on the shoulders and upper limbs. There is no alteration of skin surface marking patterns, and the lesions are not palpable. In susceptible individuals (those with skin that can burn in the sun and that tans poorly), freckles begin to appear in childhood, while their numbers generally remain fairly constant in adulthood unless heavy exposure continues. They often darken with sunlight exposure and fade in winter. The freckle appears to represent a localized area of skin in which the epidermal melanin unit has become more or less permanently altered, resulting in more abundant pigment synthesis

and donation compared with the surrounding skin. Since freckles occur preferentially in individuals with fair skin that is easily damaged by the sun, they may be viewed as a localized, albeit incomplete, protective response induced by ultraviolet (UV) light.

Microscopic Findings. At scanning magnification, there is a small circumscribed area of epidermal hyperpigmentation without obvious melanocytic proliferation. The epidermal architecture is normal, with perhaps slight rete ridge elongation. The excess pigment may be recognizable only by careful comparison with adjacent, normally pigmented "internal control" skin. Although confirmation that melanocytes are not increased in number may require immunohistochemical confirmation in occasional cases, normal basal melanocytes generally are distinguished from adjacent keratinocytes by their slightly smaller cell bodies, which often bulge downward into the basement membrane zone (fig. 1-1), their round to ovoid uniformly hyperchromatic nuclei, and a thin clear mantle devoid of intercellular junctions that envelops the cell. There are no large epithelioid melanocytes, no rows of contiguous melanocytes, and no nests of melanocytes in the dermis or epidermis. Simple ephelis are most often seen in melanoma or other skin resection specimens as an incidental finding.

Higher magnification reveals only coarse pigment granules in keratinocytes that are increased by comparison with adjacent skin, but are otherwise unremarkable. There is no obvious morphologic abnormality of melanocytes, which, if anything, tend to be reduced in number by comparison with surrounding skin (1).

Differential Diagnosis. Clinically, ephelides overlap with simple lentigines, but histologic distinction is easy, based on the absence of evidence of melanocytic proliferation. There is also considerable overlap with the lesion described next, the actinic (solar) lentigo.

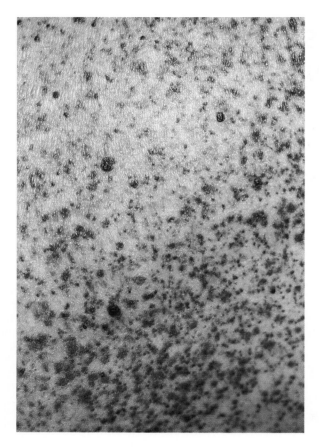

Figure 1-1

LENTIGINES, FRECKLES, AND SMALL JUNCTIONAL NEVI IN CHRONICALLY SUN-DAMAGED SKIN

The multiple lesions are clinically consistent with lentigines, freckles, and small junctional nevi. These small macular lesions are indistinguishable from one another clinically. Together, they constitute risk factors for the development of cutaneous melanoma.

ACTINIC (SOLAR) LENTIGO

Definition. Variously known as *actinic lentigo, solar lentigo, sunburn freckle, age spot, liver spot,* and so on, these common lesions present, especially in middle age and beyond, as poorly circumscribed focal areas of hyperpigmentation that are larger and more irregular than most simple ephelides (fig. 1-1). Although morphometric studies have revealed a subtle increase in melanocytic number compared to control skin, this proliferation is subtle and noncontiguous, unlike that of a true lentigo. Strictly speaking, the term "lentigo" may be inappropriate, but it is hallowed by tradition.

Clinical Features. Actinic lentigines are poorly circumscribed, tan or brown, slightly variegated pigmented lesions, usually measuring about 4 to 10 mm in diameter. Larger lesions, especially those with marked pigmentary variation or dark colors, may overlap with lentigo maligna, occasionally prompting biopsy. The lesions are distributed on sun-exposed skin in individuals with fair (type I) skin, especially on the shoulders, and there is sometimes a history of their relatively sudden appearance after a blistering sunburn. Some lesions have a slight scale, or a scale can be elicited by light rubbing or scratching.

Actinic lentigines are probably representatives of a heterogeneous and poorly characterized group of conditions that are all associated with epidermal hyperplasia with or without atypia, with hyperkeratosis, and with hyperpigmentation. There is a spectrum of morphologic overlap with pigmented actinic keratoses, pigmented seborrheic keratoses, and the freckles induced by psoralen and UV therapy (PUVA freckles) (2). Because they are indicators not only of exposure to UV light, but also of sensitivity to its effects, the presence of moderate to many actinic lentigines on the skin is associated with an increased relative risk for melanoma in case-control studies (3,4).

Microscopic Findings. The keratinocytic epithelium shows elongation and variable thinning of the rete ridges in association with a slightly noncontiguous lentiginous melanocytic proliferation (figs. 1-2, 1-3). There is usually obviously increased pigment, mainly in the basilar keratinocytes. The papillary dermis may contain a few patchy lymphocytes and melanophages, or be unremarkable. Often, there is obvious actinic elastosis. Although melanocytes in the basal layer may be normal in number or slightly increased, as assessed by morphometry, this may or may not be recognizable histologically when compared with the surrounding skin, and in any case, there is never any florid evidence of melanocytic proliferation. The melanocytes are neither contiguous nor nested, and show no atypia. Pigment in keratinocytes is increased by comparison with the surrounding epidermis. Moreover, these keratinocytes may appear somewhat enlarged and demonstrate incomplete or slightly disordered maturation, at times

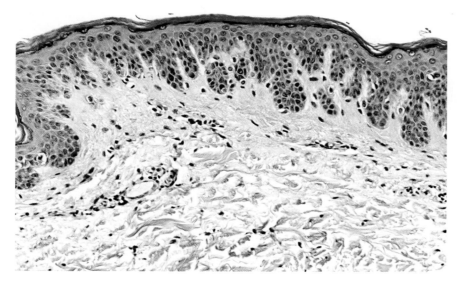

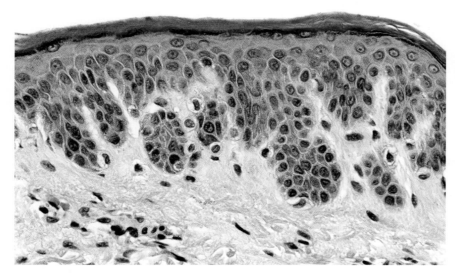

Figure 1-2

ACTINIC LENTIGO

Top: In a region of chronically sun-damaged skin, there is an area where the rete ridges are elongated.

Bottom: Hyperpigmentation of basal keratinocytes is seen in the region of elongated rete ridges. In this region, the number of melanocytes is measurably increased compared to adjacent skin, leading to the use of the term "lentigo" rather than "freckle."

suggesting some overlap with the pigmented variants of actinic keratosis (fig. 1-4).

Differential Diagnosis. A darkly pigmented variant, which we term the *reticulated lentigo* in our clinic, occasionally leads to patient or physician concern because it presents as a variegated jet black patch with a finely reticulated pattern that may suggest melanoma. The lesion occurs on intermittently sun-exposed skin, especially the shoulders, and may appear suddenly after a sunburn. The affected patient usually has skin type I (always burns, never tans). The lesions, which are sometimes multiple, are about 4 to 10 mm in diameter, poorly circumscribed, and impalpable, and have highly irregular,

strikingly jet black borders with a reticulated surface pattern (fig. 1-5). Once formed, they are stable. The clinical appearance occasionally leads to some clinical concern, but the lesions histologically are quite banal and not at all alarming. The keratinocytic epithelium shows lentiginous elongation of rete ridges without obvious melanocytic hyperplasia. There is markedly increased pigment in the basilar keratinocytes, distributed in a patchy pattern. The dermis may be normal or show a few patchy lymphocytes and/or melanophages. The melanocytes in the basal layer are unremarkable in number or morphology, with pigment in keratinocytes increased by comparison with the

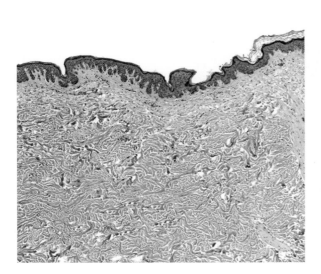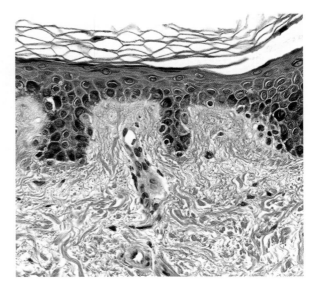

Figure 1-3

ACTINIC LENTIGO

Left: Rete ridge elongation, basal hyperpigmentation, and an increased number of melanocytes (right) are seen in a localized area along the dermal-epidermal junction.

Right: The greater increase in number of melanocytes is unusual for an actinic lentigo, bordering on the appearance of a lentigo simplex; however, the melanocytes are not in contiguity, which is consistent with the diagnosis of actinic lentigo.

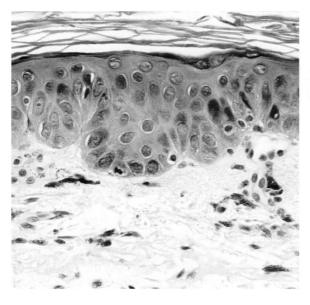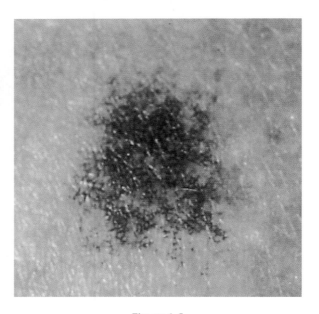

Figure 1-4

ACTINIC LENTIGO

Hyperpigmentation of basal keratinocytes, without notably increased melanocytes. There is a slight variation in nuclear size. Some degree of melanocytic or keratinocytic cytologic atypia is common in solar lentigines, and also in otherwise unremarkable skin from sun-exposed sites. There is also overlap with pigmented actinic keratoses.

Figure 1-5

RETICULATED LENTIGO

This highly characteristic lesion appears to be a variant of a solar lentigo. (Fig. E from Plate I, Fascicle 2, Third Series.)

surrounding epidermis. There is no melanocytic or keratinocytic atypia in terms of dysplastic nuclear changes. These clinically interesting lesions are probably variants of actinic lentigo, from which they are often histologically indistinguishable.

In syndromes characterized by multiple macular hyperpigmentations, such as the *multiple lentiginosis syndrome*, the lesions tend to be characterized by the lentiginous proliferation of single melanocytes without the formation of nevus cell nests. In larger macules, however, there may be junctional nevus cell nests, and there may even be nevus cell nests in the upper dermis. Thus, these syndromes overlap with lentiginous junctional nevi (5).

The presence of occasional giant melanin granules has been described in various forms of lentigines and lentiginous nevi, as well as in other conditions associated with hyperpigmentation, including the café au lait spots of neurofibromatosis and, less commonly, in café au lait spots without neurofibromatosis and even in normal skin (6,7). They have no diagnostic specificity (fig. 1-6).

MISCELLANEOUS HYPERPIGMENTATIONS

A miscellaneous group of lesions may present as relatively broad patches of hyperpigmentation, and may occasionally be significant either as a cosmetic problem or as a clinical simulant of melanoma. Histologically, the hyperpigmentation is usually associated with only a slight melanocytic proliferation. If melanocytes are increased in number, they retain normal characteristics, including the properties of pigment transfer to the keratinocyte and contact inhibition, so that the proliferation is noncontiguous and the lesional melanocytes are typically separated by intervening hyperpigmented keratinocytes. When these lesions are broad, and especially when there is pigmentary incontinence with melanophages in the dermis imparting a blue-black color, the resemblance to melanoma may be alarming. The histologic distinction is usually easy, however, because of the lack of melanocytic proliferation or atypia.

Mucosal Melanosis (Genital Lentiginosis)

Definition. *Mucosal melanosis* is a pigmented patch on a mucous membrane (commonly af-

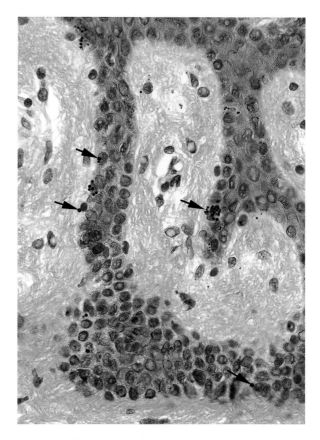

Figure 1-6

LENTIGO WITH MACROMELANOSOMES

Actinic elastosis in the dermis is not prominent. There is elongation of the rete ridges, hyperpigmentation of basal keratinocytes, and an increased number of solitary melanocytes, all consistent with a lentigo. This lesion could represent a form of nonactinic lentigo, such as those seen in Albright syndrome, however, the presence of macromelanosomes (arrows) is not specific for a particular entity.

fecting the vulva but also described on the penis and on the lip) that may simulate melanoma clinically but is histologically represented by keratinocytic hyperpigmentation with incontinence of pigment. There is no marked melanocytic proliferation and no significant atypia. Because there may be a slight increase in number of melanocytes, although there is no nest formation, the term *genital lentiginosis* has recently been proposed for these lesions (8).

Clinical Features. In the common location on the vulva, this process may appear quite alarming clinically, presenting as a broad, irregular and asymmetric patch of brown to blue-black

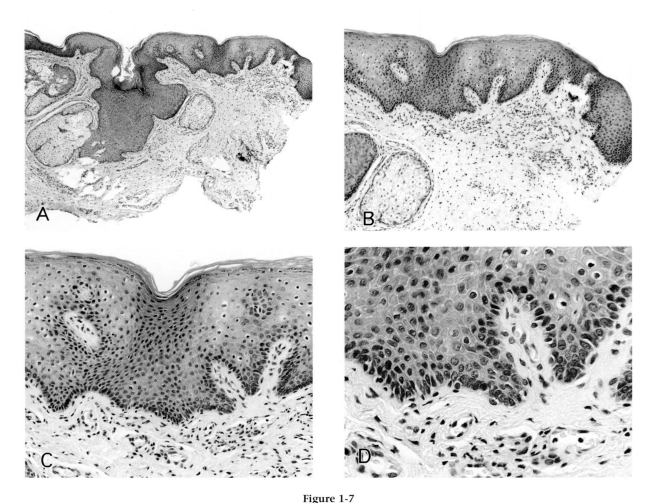

Figure 1-7

MUCOSAL MELANOSIS OF VULVA

A: There is variable hyperpigmentation of basal keratinocytes. This may give rise to a highly variegated, clinically alarming lesion.

B–D: At increasing magnification, melanocytes appear normal or slightly increased in number. There is no contiguous proliferation, no atypia, and no mitotic activity.

hyperpigmentation, easily meeting the "ABCD" criteria for melanoma discussed in chapter 9 (9). The lesion may appear to be multicentric, with alternating areas of normal and pigmented mucosa resembling the areas of regression of a radial growth phase melanoma. It is clinically reassuring to note that the lesion is entirely macular, unusual in an invasive melanoma.

Microscopic Findings. At first glance, a biopsy specimen may appear normal. The major finding is the presence of hyperpigmentation of basal keratinocytes, which can be recognized only in comparison with the surrounding normal

epithelium. The key feature is the absence of a neoplastic melanocytic proliferation. Although the melanocytes may be normal in number, in most instances, they are slightly increased (fig. 1-7). In contrast to true melanocytic neoplasms (nevi or melanomas), the cell bodies of the lesional melanocytes are separated by keratinocytes. Occasionally, especially in penile lesions, there are prominent dendritic melanocytes with their dendrites ramifying among the hyperpigmented keratinocytes. There may be associated mild keratinocytic hyperplasia, and melanophages are often scattered in the papillary dermis (responsible for the blue-black color that may simulate melanoma clinically). Thus, the process appears to be one of reactive hyperplasia with some features of postinflammatory hyperpigmentation, rather than of neoplasia. The phenomenon appears to be benign.

Differential Diagnosis. The histologic differentiation from the radial growth phase of malignant melanoma is easily made, and is greatly reassuring to clinicians and their patients. Similar lesions occur on the male genitalia and in the oral cavity, where they appear to be equally innocuous. The so-called labial lentigo (labial melanotic macule), a hyperpigmented macule of the lip, appears to be a related but distinguishable clinicopathologic entity. It is rarely biopsied because the clinical appearance is characteristic and does not suggest malignancy. These lesions are uniformly pigmented light brown, usually completely macular, and usually less than about 6 mm in diameter. Histologically, there is keratinocytic hyperpigmentation (by comparison with the surrounding epithelium). Melanocytic hyperplasia is not conspicuous by routine microscopy, although formal counts have revealed a slight increase in the number of melanocytes without atypia (10).

Café Au Lait Spot

Definition. *Café au lait spot* is a congenital or acquired hyperpigmented patch of variable size, occurring anywhere on the skin, and completely impalpable, with sharply defined borders and a uniform pale brown-tan color.

Clinical Features. The uniform pale brown or tan "coffee with milk" color gives the lesion its name (fig. 1-8). Café au lait spots are usually fairly symmetric, but may be irregular in outline, with a sharply defined border. They vary in size from a few millimeters to many centimeters, and in number from single to many. The lesions are either present at birth or appear in early life, so they are usually considered to be "birthmarks" by patients and their parents. Café au lait spots are only rarely a cause of concern to patients because of cosmetic considerations, but usually they are well tolerated. They should be distinguished from congenital nevi, which unlike café au lait spots may require excision or follow-up. A single café au lait spot is very common in the population, occurring in perhaps 10 percent or more of newborns. Two

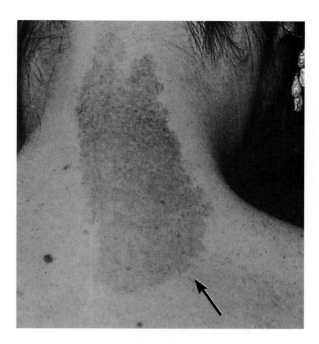

Figure 1-8

CAFÉ AU LAIT SPOT

There is a macular area of hyperpigmentation with a somewhat "jagged coastline." *(Fig. F from Plate I, Fascicle 2, Third Series.)*

or more spots are unusual in normal individuals, and more than six such lesions is usually associated with von Recklinghausen neurofibromatosis (11). The axillary freckles that are characteristic of neurofibromatosis are said to be histologically identical to café au lait spots (1).

Microscopic Findings. Although the diagnosis is almost always clinical, occasionally a biopsy may be indicated to rule out a congenital nevus. At scanning magnification, the epidermal architecture is normal. There may be a slight increase in melanin pigment in the keratinocytes, but this may be difficult to perceive if a portion of normal skin is not included. At higher magnification, giant melanosomes may be present. These so-called "macromelanosomes" represent membrane-bound condensations of melanosomes within melanocytes and have characteristic ultrastructural features. These were once thought to be specific for neurofibromatosis, but they are seen in many other conditions including, most commonly, dysplastic nevi, lentigines and common nevi, congenital nevi, and the melanotic patches of Albright syndrome (which are closely related to café au lait spots and morphologically indistinguishable) (1).

Becker Nevus

Definition. *Becker nevus* is a benign acquired hamartomatous condition of the epidermis and hair follicles associated with focal hyperpigmentation and hypertrichosis. It measures several centimeters in diameter.

Clinical Features. Becker nevi characteristically occur on the shoulder, chest, or scapular region of a man, but they may occur almost anywhere. They are usually first noted in childhood or adolescence, beginning as patches of irregular pigmentation which coalesce and spread at the periphery. Later, large dark hairs develop in the lesion. The outline of the lesion is irregular and islands of pigment may be present in the surrounding skin. The lesions are impalpable or there may be slight thickening of the skin in the center. The color is stable, or may darken with sun exposure. The lesions are not often a source of concern to patients, but may be confused by clinicians with melanocytic neoplasms or with congenital nevi. The pigmentation and hair distribution are highly variable, and subtle lesions may be difficult to distinguish from a café au lait spot.

Microscopic Findings. Biopsy is occasionally performed to distinguish a lesion from a melanoma or a congenital nevus. At scanning magnification, the architecture of the epidermis is normal or there may be a slight elongation of the rete ridges. There is a fairly obvious increase in melanin in the keratinocytes, with a few melanophages in the dermis. Large terminal hairs are prominent in some lesions. Melanocytes may be increased in number, but there are no nests of nevus cells, readily distinguishing the lesion from congenital nevus (12,13). Ultrastructurally, the number and size of the melanosome complexes may be increased (14).

Dermal Melanocytoses

The *dermal melanocytoses* are defined clinicopathologically as purple-blue-brown macular lesions that are composed histologically of dendritic and/or spindle-shaped pigmented melanocytes placed among collagen bundles in the reticular dermis (fig. 1-9). There are several variants, including the common (but not often biopsied) *Mongolian spots* and the rarer *nevi of Ota*

and *Ito*. These lesions are defined chiefly by their clinical distribution. Mongolian spots are most commonly seen in the sacrococcygeal region and they seem to be common in infants of Asian and African origin. They are of no clinical consequence, and usually disappear by adolescence. Nevus of Ito involves the skin of the shoulder region and is rare in Caucasian populations, while nevus of Ota will be described in more detail because of its association with cutaneous and leptomeningeal melanoma as well as its distinctive clinical features. In the last few years, the use of Q-switched lasers has revolutionized the treatment of these conditions (15).

Nevus of Ota

Definition. *Nevus of Ota* is a congenital or acquired hyperpigmentation of the skin of the face and ocular mucous membranes in the distribution of the branches of the trigeminal nerve. It is also known as *oculodermal melanocytosis* and *nevus fuscoceruleus ophthalmomaxillaris* (15).

Clinical Features. Nevi of Ota are classified into various types based on extent, ranging from mild ocular involvement only to ocular, periocular, zygomatic, cheek, and temple involvement, unilateral or bilateral (16). The lesions present as macular, completely nonpalpable speckled cutaneous pigmentations of various hues: black, purple, blue-black, blue, slate blue, brown. The intensity of the pigmentation may appear to vary from day to day. The skin lesions are occasionally associated with melanosis of the optic tract and meninges. The occurrence of malignant melanoma (either involving the skin or the meninges) has been reported in nevus of Ota in Caucasians (17–19) but, curiously, rarely if ever in Japan where the lesion is common (20).

The lesions most often present in early childhood, and they persist indefinitely once formed. They are generally asymptomatic, except for cosmetic concerns. Because the intensity of pigmentation is generally moderate, they are amenable to cosmetic concealment. Biopsy is generally not indicated unless there is a suspicion of malignancy, such as the appearance of a mass lesion or the occurrence of focal color or topographic changes.

Microscopic Findings. At scanning magnification, increased cellularity of the reticular dermis may be apparent. At higher magnification,

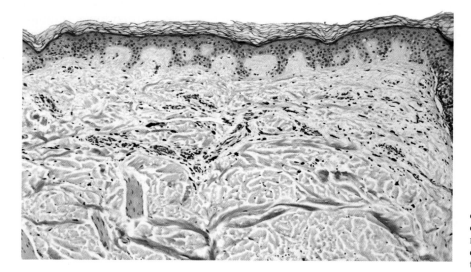

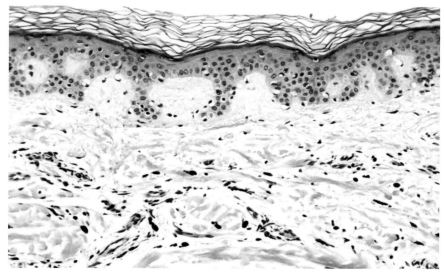

Figure 1-9

DERMAL MELANOCYTOSIS

There is an increased number of pigmented, somewhat dendritic, elongated spindle-shaped melanocytes among the reticular dermis collagen bundles. They tend to be completely separate from one another, unlike in blue nevi, where they tend to be in contact. These features are seen in dermal melanocyte hamartoma, nevus of Ota, nevus of Ito, and related conditions.

pigmented stellate and dendritic melanocytes are scattered, often sparsely, in the reticular dermis. The cells may be situated about appendages, and often are oriented parallel to the surface of the epidermis. There is no epidermal component, and there are no associated ordinary nevus cells. Compared to Mongolian spots, where the pigmented cells tend to be in the deep reticular dermis, the cells of nevus of Ota are more superficial, larger, and more numerous. Nevus of Ota is indistinguishable histologically from nevus of Ito.

The few malignant tumors that we have seen in association with nevus of Ota have not presented any difficulty in diagnosis. They have consisted of bulky tumor masses, composed of cytologically atypical cells with frequent mitoses and obvious pigment synthesis. We have observed these malignancies in the meninges and in the orbit, and have classified them as *malignant melanomas arising in nevus of Ota*. Malignancies that have been described in the skin in association with nevus of Ota include dermal and subcutaneous masses that should not be mistaken for metastases.

Although the histogenesis of dermal melanocytoses is incompletely studied, it is possible that such lesions arise in association with intradermal rests of dendritic melanoblasts that are prematurely arrested during migration from neural crest to their normal intraepithelial microenvironments.

Variants and Differential Diagnosis. Nevus of Ito is histologically similar to nevus of Ota, but involves the area of innervation of the lateral supraclavicular and lateral brachial nerves on the shoulder. The lesions may be distinguished from common blue nevi by their lower cellularity, the lack of associated thickening of collagen bundles as is seen in blue nevi, and their much greater size, as well as the characteristic clinical and gross features.

REFERENCES

1. Breathnach AS. Melanocyte distribution in forearm epidermis of freckled human subjects. J Invest Dermatol 1957;29:253-261.
2. Rhodes AR, Stern RS, Melski JW. The PUVA lentigo: an analysis of predisposing factors. J Invest Dermatol 1983;81:459-463.
3. MacKie RM, Freudenberger T, Aitchison TC. Personal risk-factor chart for cutaneous melanoma. Lancet 1989;2:487-490.
4. Garbe C, Kruger S, Stadler R, Guggenmoos-Holzmann I, Orfanos CE. Markers and relative risk in a German population for developing malignant melanoma. Int J Dermatol 1989;28:517-523.
5. Selmanowitz VJ, Orentreich N, Felsenstein JM. Lentiginosis profusa syndrome (multiple lentigines syndrome). Arch Dermatol 1971;104:393-401.
6. Jimbow K, Horikoshi T. The nature and significance of macromelanosomes in pigmented skin lesions: their morphological characteristics, specificity for their occurrence, and possible mechanisms for their formation. Am J Dermatopathol 1982;4:413-420.
7. Konrad K, Wolff K, Honigsmann H. The giant melanosome: a model of deranged melanosome-morphogenesis. J Ultrastruct Res 1974;48:102-123.
8. Barnhill RL, Albert LS, Shama SK, Goldenhersh MA, Rhodes AR, Sober AJ. Genital lentiginosis: a clinical and histopathologic study. J Am Acad Dermatol 1990;22:453-460.
9. Maize JC. Mucosal melanosis. Dermatol Clin 1988;6:283-293.
10. Sexton FM, Maize JC. Melanotic macules and melanoacanthomas of the lip. A comparative study with census of the basal melanocyte population. Am J Dermatopathol 1987;9:438-444.
11. Whitehouse D. Diagnostic value of the cafe au lait spot in children. Arch Dis Child 1966;41:316-319.
12. Copeman PW, Jones EW. Pigmented hairy epidermal nevus (Becker). Arch Dermatol 1965;92:249-251.
13. Tate PR, Hodge SJ, Owen LG. A quantitative study of melanocytes in Becker's nevus. J Cutan Pathol 1980;7:404-409.
14. Lever WF, Schaumburg-Lever G. Histopathology of the skin, 6th ed. Philadelphia: Lippincott; 1983.
15. Chan HH, Kono T. Nevus of Ota: clinical aspects and management. Skinmed 2003;2:89-96.
16. Hori Y, Takayama O. Circumscribed dermal melanoses. Classification and histologic features. Dermatol Clin 1988;6:315-326.
17. Piercecchi-Marti MD, Mohamed H, Liprandi A, Gambarelli D, Grisoli F, Pellissier JF. Intracranial meningeal melanocytoma associated with ipsilateral nevus of Ota. Case report. J Neurosurg 2002;96:619-623.
18. Rivers JK, Bhayana S, Martinka M. Dural melanoma associated with ocular melanosis and multiple blue nevi. J Cutan Med Surg 2001;5:381-385.
19. Patel BC, Egan CA, Lucius RW, Gerwels JW, Mamalis N, Anderson RL. Cutaneous malignant melanoma and oculodermal melanocytosis (nevus of Ota): report of a case and review of the literature. J Am Acad Dermatol 1998;38:862-865.
20. Hidano A, Kajima H, Ikeda S, Mizutani H, Miyasato H, Niimura M. Natural history of nevus of Ota. Arch Dermatol 1967;95:187-195.

2 COMMON ACQUIRED MELANOCYTIC NEVI

BENIGN MELANOCYTIC TUMORS

Most benign melanocytic tumors fall into the category of lesions termed *melanocytic nevi*. Melanocytic nevi are proliferative lesions of melanocytes; the altered melanocytes that comprise a melanocytic nevus are termed nevus cells. Although the term "nevus" strictly connotes a hamartomatous malformation of any cutaneous tissue (nevus verrucosus, for example, is a malformation primarily of keratinocytes), the unqualified term nevus is generally used synonymously with the more precise and self-explanatory terms *melanocytic nevus*, *nevus cell nevus*, or *nevocytic nevus*. We use the term "nevus cell" to describe the lesional cells (also known as nevomelanocytes or melanocytes of nevi) that constitute the parenchymal cell type of nevi.

Four major characteristics distinguish nevus cells from normal melanocytes. First is a loss of the normal dendritic shape and adoption of a more compact, rounded contour (so-called nevus cell transformation). Next is an apparent loss of normal contact inhibition (the nevus cell bodies lie in contiguity with one another, often in small clusters or nests). Third is a tendency to retain pigment in the cytoplasm. Fourth is a tendency to migrate from the basal epidermis into the papillary dermis (1,2). This last property of benign nevus cells complicates the interpretation of invasion in dysplastic nevi and radial growth phase melanomas. Ultrastructurally, Golgi vesicles and rough endoplasmic reticulum are reduced in nevus cells compared to melanocytes. In nevus cells melanosomes are predominantly arranged in groups as melanosome complexes, while in melanocytes they occur as single melanosomes and as premelanosomes in all stages of maturation (3). Melanocytic nevi may be congenital or acquired, usually during childhood.

There is one category of predominantly benign melanocytic tumors first described in 1947 by Sophie Spitz as *juvenile melanomas* (4) in which the use of the term "nevus" has been recently called into question (5,6). Nevus generally implies an unequivocally benign lesion, whereas the tumors described by Spitz are distinguished from other nevoid melanocytic lesions because they share certain histologic attributes with melanomas. Although these lesions generally have an excellent prognosis, especially in young children, there is a degree of uncertainty about their biologic behavior such that the term "Spitz tumor" now seems to us to be more appropriate than the generally synonymous term "Spitz nevus," particularly when lesions develop in adulthood.

A classification of melanocytic tumors, based on the work of an international committee convened by the World Health Organization (WHO), was recently published (7). The benign melanocytic tumors in this WHO classification are listed in Table 2-1 and follows in the present text. The WHO classification of malignant melanoma is presented in chapter 8.

COMMON ACQUIRED MELANOCYTIC NEVI

Although nevi are sometimes considered hamartomatous malformations (and this may well be true of the congenital varieties), *acquired nevi* meet important criteria for a benign neoplasm since their constituent cells appear to have a selective, although temporary, growth advantage compared to adjacent normal melanocytes and keratinocytes (8). Recent molecular studies have confirmed that nevi, in many if not all instances, are clonal (9–11), and a high percentage of nevi contain activating mutations of the oncogenes *BRAF* or (less commonly) *NRAS* (12–15). The growth of nevi differs from that of melanomas in that it is not inexorable, but this should not be considered inconsistent with their essential neoplastic nature, or with the notion that some nevi may be induced by the same etiologic agent(s) that also induces some melanomas.

Although the activation of the oncogenes *BRAF* and *NRAS* might suggest that there should be a tendency to the activation of the mitogen-activated protein (MAP) kinase pathway leading

Table 2-1

WHO CLASSIFICATION OF BENIGN MELANOCYTIC TUMORS

Congenital melanocytic nevi
    Superficial type

Proliferative nodules in congenital melanocytic nevi

Dermal melanocytic lesions
    Mongolian spot
    Nevi of Ito and Ota

Blue Nevus
    Cellular blue nevus

Combined nevus

Melanotic macules, simple lentigo, and lentiginous nevus

Dysplastic nevus

Site-specific nevi
    Acral nevus
    Genital nevus
    Meyerson nevus

Persistent (recurrent) melanocytic nevus

Spitz nevus

Pigmented spindle cell nevus (Reed)

Halo nevus

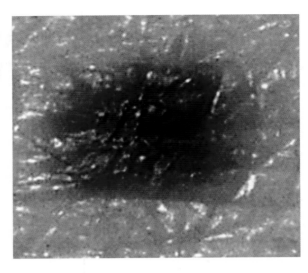

Figure 2-1

LENTIGO SIMPLEX/JUNCTIONAL NEVUS ("JENTIGO")

This lesion is small, well circumscribed, and uniformly colored in a tan/brown shade of pigment. The border is slightly raised. Histologically, this lesion may be a lentigo simplex or a lentiginous junctional nevus, or may even have a few cells in the dermis and be a lentiginous compound nevus.

to proliferation of the nevus cells (16), this is not the case as nevi are stable lesions. It appears that the proliferative stimulus is held in check in benign nevi by high levels of tumor suppressors such as p16 (CDKN2A) (17) or the recently described IGFBP7 (18), which act through autocrine/paracrine pathways to inhibit BRAF-MEK-ERK proliferation pathway signaling and induce senescence and apoptosis. Immunohistochemical analysis of human skin, nevus, and melanoma samples has recently implicated loss of IGFBP7 expression as a critical step in melanoma genesis, representing the phenomenon known as "oncogene-induced senescence" (18–20). Expression of the cell cycle inhibitors p16 and p27 also tends to be lost with the progression from nevus to melanoma (21). It has been aptly suggested that nevi represent senescent clones of neoplastic melanocytes (20).

Because of their melanin retention, particularly within the more superficial cellular components, early evolutionary stages of acquired nevi are recognized clinically as small pigmented lesions when they are only a millimeter or so wide. An early nevus, because of its superficial, highly visible location and its pigment, consti-

tutes one of the smallest neoplasms that can be recognized clinically.

Acquired nevi are such ubiquitous lesions that they are often regarded as normal phenotypic characteristics, like fair skin or dark hair; however, they do not appear to represent a genetically programmed constitutional trait. They appear first in early childhood and reach a maximum number in adolescence (22). In later life, nevi progressively decline in number, undergoing a characteristic continuous evolution followed by involution, which may result in the disappearance of the nevus after many years.

When it first becomes visible as a pigmented macule about 1 to 2 mm in diameter, a nevus is often termed a *lentigo simplex* (fig. 2-1) (1). Histologically, a lentigo is a proliferative lesion in which melanocytes are increased in number, are somewhat enlarged and rounded, and are arranged in a linear pattern in the basal epidermis, often associated with elongation of the rete ridges (fig. 2-2). This pattern or arrangement of melanocytes, whether seen in a lentigo or in another class of melanocytic lesion, is termed "lentiginous" because the lentigo is its prototypic expression. The lentiginous pattern, because it

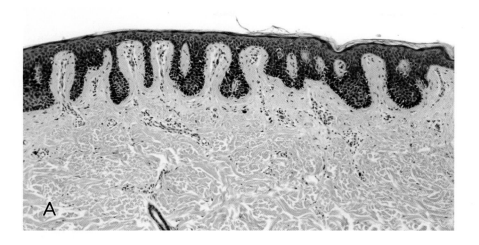

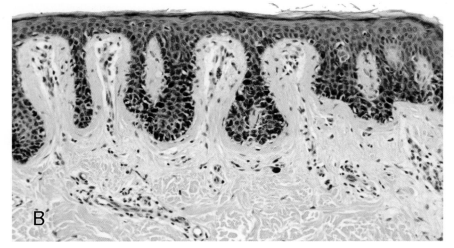

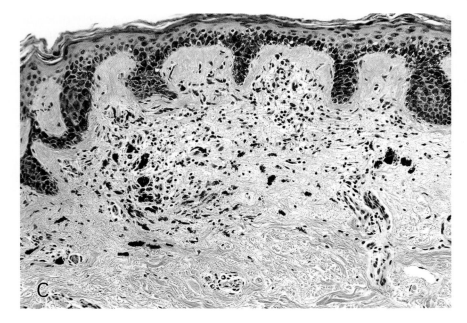

Figure 2-2

LENTIGO SIMPLEX

A: The rete ridges are uniformly elongated, with hyperpigmentation of basal keratinocytes, which is more prominent here than is usual in most simple lentigines. There is an increased number of nevoid melanocytes, mainly around the tips and sides of the elongated rete ridges, without nest formation.

B: Focally at least, the melanocytes are in contiguity with one another.

C: An area of pigmentary incontinence, with lymphocytic inflammation and slight fibroplasia in the dermis, is an unusual finding in a simple lentigo.

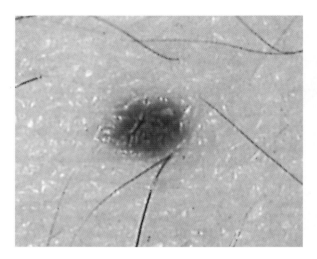 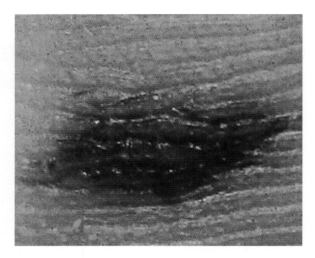

Figure 2-3

JUNCTIONAL NEVUS

Junctional nevus of glabrous (left) and acral (right) skin. Note the preservation of dermatoglyphs (A and B from Plate I, Fascicle 2, Third Series).

is seen in a newly evolving, presumably recently induced and promoted melanocytic lesion that has not been remodeled by the differentiation pathway to be described below, might be termed a "primitive" pattern of growth. There are no nests, by definition, in a lentigo simplex. The lesional cells and associated keratinocytes usually contain abundant pigment, making the lesions darker than most normal nevi, and sometimes rendering them even black.

In the next phase of the ontogeny of a common acquired nevus, a few clusters or nests of enlarged, rounded melanocytes, similar to those that comprise the lentiginous proliferation, appear at the dermal-epidermal junction, most often near the tips of epidermal rete ridges. By strict definition, the presence of nests is a requirement for the designation of a "nevus cell" (1). A nest of melanocytes consists of five or more cells in a single cluster as viewed in two-dimensional sections. A lesion that contains a few nests but is otherwise indistinguishable from a lentigo simplex may be termed a *junctional nevus* (figs. 2-3, 2-4). In reality, it is likely that there is a continuous evolution from a lentigo to a junctional nevus, and this hypothesis is reflected in the term *nevoid lentigo*, or the whimsical term "jentigo," applicable to either lesion (23). A few junctional nevi are composed entirely of nests, without a lentiginous component (fig.

2-5). Pigmentation in junctional nevi begins to fade over time compared to lentigines; most lesions are brown or tan, not black. Since there is nothing in the dermis other than perhaps a few lymphocytes and melanophages, junctional nevi are either macular or only slightly raised to side-lighting; they are almost always impalpable. They may remain small, or may grow laterally in a radially symmetric manner, but rarely become larger than about 7 mm and are usually less than 5 mm in diameter. Nevi greater than 5 mm in diameter that are completely macular may be banal junctional nevi, especially on the palms and soles, but the diagnosis of dysplastic nevus (see chapter 6) also should be considered for such large macular nevi.

In the next phase of this evolutionary process, some of the nests migrate from the epidermis into the papillary dermis to form a papular *compound nevus*. This migration takes place as nests of nevus cells protrude downward into the dermis while still surrounded by the basement membrane (24). Gradually, the connection with the epidermis becomes more attenuated until it is lost, and the basement membrane now completely surrounds the nest. With continued migration of nested melanocytes, the dermal component of the nevus is built up like a brick wall and the epidermis is elevated above the young nevus to form the clinical manifestation

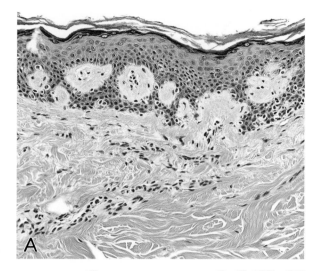

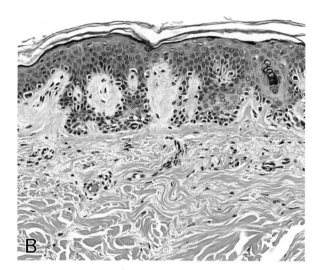

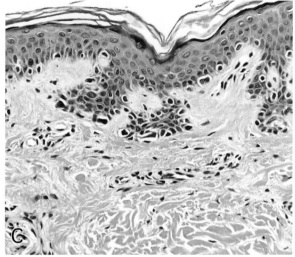

Figure 2-4

LENTIGINOUS JUNCTIONAL NEVUS

Single melanocytes are predominantly near the tips and sides of uniformly elongated rete ridges, with a continuous proliferation between the rete (A–C). There are a few nests, some of which bridge adjacent rete ridges (B,C). There is slight nuclear enlargement and irregularity, insufficient in degree for a diagnosis of melanocytic dysplasia.

of a compound nevus. The compound nevus is entirely papular, since migration of cells from the epidermis into the dermis occurs across the entire breadth of the nevus.

Finally, often after several years, the cells in the epidermis complete their migration into the dermis or involute, and the lesion becomes a purely *dermal nevus*. The dermal nevus, over many years or decades, then enters a phase of involution or senescence. As clinical pigmentation fades and the lesion becomes pink or flesh colored, the dermal component becomes "neurotized" (resembling the Schwann cells of a neurofibroma). This process begins deep within the dermal component, although nevi with advanced neurotization may be difficult to distinguish from neurofibromas. The dermal

stroma of other involuting nevi may become dominated by mature adipocytes, presumably via stromal metaplasia, or show angiofibromatous changes akin to fibrous papules.

Architecturally, involuting nevi may become polypoid, and eventually slough as a consequence of torsion and ischemia. Other "normal" nevi slowly disappear over time, perhaps by remodeling into normal-looking skin. The process of senescence in nevi may be related to low telomerase activity and to activation of the p16/Rb pathway (20,25–27).

While the evolutionary scenario provided above appears to hold true for most common acquired melanocytic nevi, it remains an open question as to whether all ordinary nevi exhibit this behavior. We have occasionally seen

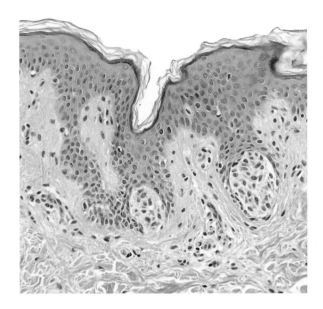

Figure 2-5

JUNCTIONAL NEVUS: NESTED PATTERN

The nests are present mainly at the tips of the elongated rete ridges. There are few single cells; a mixed lentiginous and nested pattern is common in small benign nevi.

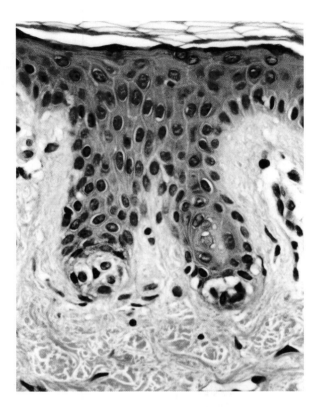

microscopic foci of small (restricted to one or two nests) dermal nevi as incidental, presumably subclinical findings in skin surrounding non-melanocytic lesions in excision specimens. It is possible that such small intradermal lesions do not evolve from junctional and compound nevi, but rather arise from embryonic rests of rare intradermal melanocytes or from dermal stem cells capable of melanocytic differentiation.

Numerous epidemiologic studies have demonstrated that the finding of excessive numbers of nevi on the skin constitutes a risk marker for the development of cutaneous melanoma, especially when the nevi are large or have other atypical features, such as pigment variegation or irregular borders (28–32). Modern case-control studies of the relationship between nevus pattern or phenotype and melanoma incidence have found an approximate 40-fold excess risk for melanoma in patients with increased and atypical nevi compared to members of the general population (33–35). This suggests that nevi and melanoma may have a common pathogenesis. Indeed, as is believed to be true for many melanomas, the evidence suggests that nevi are somehow induced by sunlight. In

Western Australia, the number of nevi on the forearms of immigrants correlated with age of arrival in Australia. Immigrants who arrived in this sunny climate before the age of 10 had more nevi than those who arrived at an older age. They also had a higher risk of melanoma (36). Nevi are most numerous on areas of the skin that are intermittently exposed to sunlight, as is also true for melanoma (22). These observations, coupled with the fact that most nevi make their appearance in childhood and adolescence, are consistent with the hypothesis that the "carcinogen" for nevi is sunlight, and that the human skin is most vulnerable to solar nevogenesis in the first decades of life.

Lentigo Simplex

Definition. *Lentigo simplex* is a small, impalpable localized area of hyperpigmentation associated histologically with a focally contiguous melanocytic proliferation (distinguishing it from a freckle, see chapter 1), but without nest formation (in contrast to a junctional nevus). Although not meeting the strictest definition of a nevus, a lentigo simplex may be regarded as an immature form of junctional nevus.

Clinical Features. A typical lesion is a 1- to 3-mm (up to perhaps 4- to 5-mm), well-circumscribed, flat, pigmented region of skin that is generally completely impalpable (see fig. 2-1). The pigment is dark brown or even black, a feature that in a larger lesion should prompt serious consideration of melanoma. Some larger lesions deviate from the bilateral symmetry expected for benign junctional nevi, also a potential cause for biopsy. The lesions may be slightly raised to side-lighting, or may be perfect macules. In the latter case, it may be impossible to distinguish a lentigo from an ephelis clinically. There is complete clinical overlap between lentigines and small junctional nevi. This phenotypic ambiguity complicates the epidemiologic exercise of determining the prevalence of nevi, but is of little or no clinical importance. Similar to acquired nevi, lentigines appear first in early childhood and continue to develop into early adult life. They tend to be distributed preferentially on sunlight-exposed areas, especially on the forearms. Lentigines may be stable for long periods or for life, or may evolve into junctional and then compound nevi. Probably some lesions also involute or differentiate, losing their pigment and disappearing (1).

Microscopic Findings. The epidermis at scanning magnification shows the characteristic elongation and thinning of the rete ridges in a pattern similar to that seen in dysplastic nevi (see fig. 2-2). There may be abundant pigment within basal keratinocytes, often extending to the stratum corneum, but the lesional melanocytes always remain confined to the basal layers. In the dermis, there are patchy collections of lymphocytes, often with melanophages, and sometimes with compressed collagen bundles about the elongated rete (eosinophilic fibroplasia, which is also seen in dysplastic nevi and is discussed later).

The key feature that defines this lesion is the presence of a single layer of enlarged, rounded, nondendritic melanocytes in the basal layer of the epidermis, many of them lying in contiguity with one another. These melanocytes are not continuous between the rete, and are often most heavily concentrated at or near the tips of the rete ridges, where melanin within keratinocytes may also be more prominent. This pattern of proliferation of melanocytes has been termed *lentiginous hyperplasia* because of its association

with lentigines. Since we now believe that simple lentigines are likely to be small melanocytic neoplasms, the term *lentiginous proliferation* may be more appropriate than hyperplasia. There is often an associated proliferation of keratinocytes, resulting in the rete ridge elongation that is a highly characteristic feature of lentigines as well as some other lentiginous lesions such as dysplastic nevi. There are no nests, by definition, in a lentigo, and thus no "nevus cells," if these cells are defined by the classic criterion of nested growth patterns. However, the contiguous melanocytes exhibit the other key features of nevus cells: temporally limited proliferation with loss of contact inhibition resulting in the formation of a focal lesion, a compact rounded shape, and a tendency to retain pigment in their cytoplasm (although there is also considerable transfer to keratinocytes). Furthermore, lesions indistinguishable from lentigines by any other criteria may be found to have occasional nests, especially if serial sections are done. Thus, we are in agreement with Maize and Ackerman (37) that lentigines represent immature, evolving nevi, at least in some instances, although this evolution is not inevitable.

Junctional Melanocytic Nevus

Definition. *Junctional melanocytic nevus* is a focal pigmented lesion characterized by an increased number of neoplastically altered, aggregated melanocytes in the epidermis. By definition, at least some of these lesional cells (nevus cells, or nevomelanocytes) are arranged in nests or theques. Cytologically, junctional nevus cells tend to be larger and more rounded than melanocytes, with lesser degrees of cytoplasmic retraction artifact and without evident dendrites. By definition, there are no nevus cells in the dermis in a junctional nevus (1).

Clinical Features. Junctional nevi are generally small lesions (1 to 4 mm); larger lesions should lead to a consideration of dysplastic nevus. They are symmetric, well circumscribed, and uniformly pigmented (see figs. 2-3–2-5). Like simple lentigines, smaller lesions (1 to 2 mm size range) may be jet black, but larger lesions are almost always brown. Their preferential distribution on sun-exposed surfaces is similar to that of lentigines, from which they are not readily distinguishable on clinical grounds. Classically impalpable, they may be slightly raised to side-lighting. The lesions are clinically stable, but over a period of years may evolve into a compound nevus, and they probably undergo some undescribed form of involution, since their numbers appear to decline in later life. These changes are usually imperceptible to patients, but some of them have been documented with serial photography beginning in childhood.

Microscopic Findings. The histologic features in most lesions are identical to those of the simple lentigo, except that, by definition, at least one nest of melanocytes is present (and usually there are multiple nests), accounting for the synonymous term *nevoid lentigo* (lentigo with nests) and the whimsical term *jentigo* (see figs. 2-2, 2-4) (37). In many lesions, there is lentiginous proliferation of melanocytes, with uniformly elongated rete ridges as seen in lentigines. The lesional cell population is arranged, similar to that of the lentigo, predominantly as a row of enlarged, rounded, contiguous single cells within the epidermal basal cell layer among which are a few to numerous nests of similar cells. Sometimes spindle cells are prominent, and in either case, the nevus cells typically have clear, unstained cytoplasm that tends to retract from the surrounding keratinocytes. This "retraction artifact" is usually less prominent in melanoma cells than in nevus cells (38). In many lesions, especially small ones, the nests are inconspicuous, and the predominant pattern is that of the simple lentigo.

The nested and single nevus cells are located at the dermal-epidermal junction, usually concentrated at the tips of elongated rete ridges, and often protruding downward toward the papillary dermis above an intact basement membrane (38). There are no nests in the dermis by definition. A few lesions, rare in common practice, are composed almost entirely of nested melanocytes. Generally, junctional nevi are less heavily pigmented than lentigines, and they are less likely to be associated with a brisk dermal host response of lymphocytes and melanophages.

At higher magnification, the nested or single nevus cells are somewhat enlarged compared to normal melanocytes. They have more abundant cytoplasm, which usually contains moderate quantities of relatively coarse pigment. In heavily pigmented lesions, however, much of the pigment is in the keratinocytes.

The black color of some heavily pigmented small lentigines and junctional nevi is associated histologically with pigment in the stratum corneum, which has been carried there in the normal process of keratinocytic maturation and shedding. The spread of benign nevus cells into the epidermis is unusual, but may be seen as a focal phenomenon in some lesions of childhood (38), perhaps representing a process of transepidermal elimination (39). In such cases, nests predominate over single cells, and other features of melanoma are lacking.

The cells in the epidermis of junctional nevi tend to be somewhat larger than their dermal counterparts seen in compound and dermal nevi, and they are more likely to have relatively small, blue nucleoli or "chromocenters." Although there may be slight random variation in nuclear size and shape in junctional nevi (40), there is no high-grade atypia, large eosinophilic nucleoli are absent, and mitotic figures are only rarely seen in acquired nevi of any kind.

Compound Melanocytic Nevus

Definition. A *compound melanocytic nevus* is a melanocytic nevus in which the nevus cells are found in both the dermis and the epidermis.

Clinical Features. Most lesions range in size from about 1 to 7 mm. Compound nevi larger than 10 mm are rare, while lesions smaller than 2 to 3 mm are more likely to be junctional nevi or lentigines. The smallest lesions may be impalpable although slightly raised to side-lighting, and these lesions are indistinguishable from junctional nevi or lentigines. Lesions larger than this are papules. The prototypic common acquired compound nevus is an entirely raised papule, circumscribed and symmetric, tan or brown, almost as tall as it is broad, with a smooth regular border and a fairly uniform pigment pattern (figs. 2-6–2-9). Like other nevi, compound nevi are located preferentially on sun-exposed areas of skin, especially on the face and trunk. Nevi on the limbs are more likely to be small and flat, resembling junctional nevi.

After an initial period of evolution in childhood or adolescence, compound nevi are stable for several decades. After many years, they subsequently evolve ("differentiate") into dermal nevi, progressively losing pigment and becoming flatter, and ultimately fading into

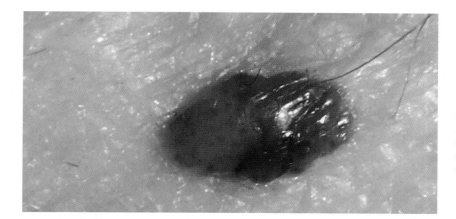

Figure 2-6

COMPOUND NEVUS

A papular compound nevus is entirely raised above the surface of the skin, without an adjacent macular component, as would be seen in a dysplastic nevus. It is uniformly colored, smoothly bordered, and symmetric in outline.

Figure 2-7

LENTIGINOUS COMPOUND NEVUS

There is an extensive, largely lentiginous junctional component, with only a few nests of mature nevus cells in the dermis. There is no substantial cytologic atypia.

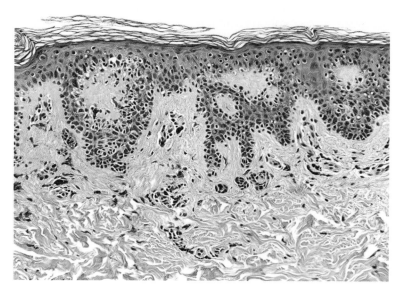

normal skin. Thus, papular pigmented compound nevi are uncommon in older people, and such lesions should lead to a heightened suspicion for melanoma in this age group. Like most nevi, compound nevi are usually asymptomatic, but occasionally a lesion becomes pruritic. Protruding lesions are vulnerable to trauma, occasionally leading to a history of bleeding.

There is considerable clinical variation in size, elevation, and surface texture of the lesion. The configuration of the lesions ranges from a barely raised plaque, to a nodule, to a pedunculated polyp (fig. 2-6). The surface ranges from smooth (although rarely shiny as it may be in nodules of melanoma), to mammillated, to verrucoid. The color ranges from brown to pink or flesh colored (more characteristic of dermal or Spitz nevi). Common nevi are rarely black, and this

is a finding that should suggest melanoma or pigmented spindle cell nevus (if the lesion is small and symmetric).

Microscopic Findings. At scanning magnification, most compound nevi are small, well-circumscribed, symmetric lesions. The pigment is variable in amount, and is located both in the keratinocytes and particularly in superficial dermal and intraepidermal nevus cells. By definition, nevus cells are present in the dermis as well as in the epidermis. In some lesions, only a few cells are present in the dermis and the lesion is otherwise indistinguishable (both clinically and histologically) from a lentiginous junctional nevus or lentigo (fig. 2-7). Larger lesions are distinctly papular, with confluent nests and sheets of nevus cells usually confined to the papillary dermis or extending slightly into the reticular dermis in some acquired lesions. Nests that often dominate the more superficial dermal layers tend to give rise to cords as smaller and less pigmented or amelanotic nevus cells descend symmetrically into deeper layers. In a typical compound nevus, the epidermal component does not extend to form a "shoulder," defined as the region of epidermis beyond the lateral border of the dermal component. The keratinocytic epithelium typically shows some rete ridge elongation, occasionally markedly exaggerated in a papillomatous pattern that may resemble seborrheic keratosis.

Ackerman (41) has described two distinct patterns for dermal and compound nevi at the interface of the papillary and reticular dermis. In one of these patterns, attributed to Unna (42), the lesion is exophytic, like an acrochordon (fibroepithelial polyp), and the deepest dermal nevus cells lie above the interface of the papillary and reticular dermis. This is a common pattern in nevi of the trunk and limbs. In the second pattern, attributed to Miescher (43) and seen especially in lesions of the head and neck, nevus cells permeate the reticular dermis in a wedge-shaped pattern with the base toward the epidermis. A detailed study of these patterns has been presented and it has been proposed that the histogenesis of these two forms of nevi may differ (44). Whatever the significance, if any, of this distinction, when the dermal component of a nevus extends far into the reticular dermis, the possibility of a small congenital nevus may be considered (see Congenital Melanocytic Nevi). However, most of these "small deep" nevi cannot be documented to have been present at birth (45), particularly when this pattern involves the skin of the head and neck.

At low-power magnification, the dermal collections of nevus cells appear to be arranged in sheets of confluent cells, without any suggestion of a "capsule" or other induced host stromal response. There are basement membranes and reticulin fibers between each cell, as can be demonstrated with appropriate special stains. Especially when the reticular dermis is involved, the borders of these collections of nevus cells may be jagged and irregular, sometimes giving rise to an impression of infiltrative growth (figs. 2-8, 2-9). Some of these features occasionally suggest a malignancy, especially to the neo-phyte observer. An unusual pattern occasionally seen in the dermal component of nevi is the formation of cavernous or slit-like spaces among the nevus cells. This pattern of growth has no known clinical significance except that the appearance can be mistaken histologically for that of an angioma (38) or may falsely suggest the possibility of lymphatic invasion (46) (see next section, Dermal Melanocytic Nevus).

At higher magnification, the cells are arranged in nests and anastomosing cords separated by delicate stroma. This stroma, in a typical banal nevus, surrounds individual cells or small groups of cells and is demonstrated with a reticulin stain. Melanoma cells, by contrast, tend to reside in larger true sheets or in clusters many cells wide, with little or no reticulin framework between the individual cells. Despite the morphologic suggestion that the dermal nevus cells may have had some capacity to permeate the reticular dermis during the development of some lesions, there is no evidence of progressive expansile growth in a common acquired nevus; for example, nodules of cells compressing adjacent lesional components are not observed, as is typically seen with reticular dermal involvement of vertical growth phase melanoma. This, however, does not invariably hold for certain less common nevus variants (see Cellular Blue Nevus and Deep Penetrating Nevus).

Severe cellular atypia, large eosinophilic nucleoli, and mitoses are usually absent in common acquired compound nevi. Their presence should lead to a serious consideration of melanoma unless the lesion can be placed into the category of spindle and epithelioid nevi (see below). In most compound nevi, the lesional cells have small nuclei without prominent nucleoli or with small to intermediate blue nucleoli. The nuclear membranes may be regular or somewhat convoluted, especially in the larger superficial nevus cells, and there may be considerable variation in nuclear size and shape. Nuclear membranes tend to be uniformly thin and generally smooth in contour, and nuclear chromatin is delicate and evenly dispersed. Individual nevus cells within the dermis often develop multinucleation, a poorly understood phenomenon without biologic significance. When multiple nuclei coalesce or

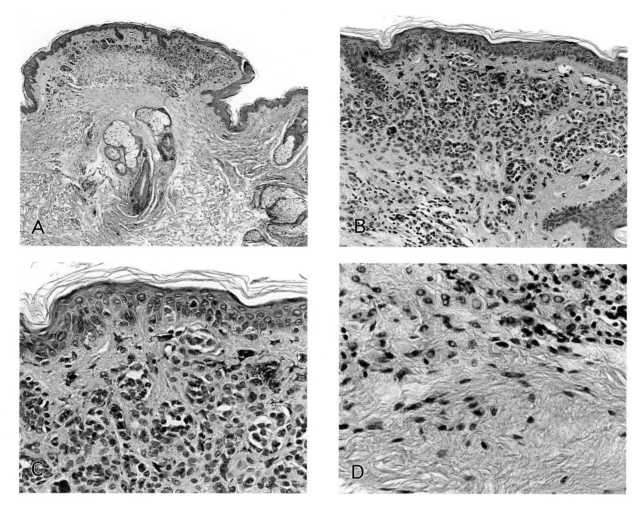

Figure 2-8

COMPOUND NEVUS

This papular compound nevus in a 48-year-old patient is composed of orderly nevus cells which mature from larger cells superficially to smaller cells at the base. At the base of the lesion, single cells permeate among collagen fibers of the superficial reticular dermis. This pattern of "dispersion," although seemingly infiltrative, is more characteristic of nevi than of melanomas, except for desmoplastic melanomas. Although the lesion is mostly dermal, a few junctional nests are present. Note the presence of cytoplasmic invaginations with the appearance of "inclusions" in D.

become superimposed, however, there may be an impression of profound nuclear atypia upon cursory inspection.

Although most nevi are composed of a single cell type, there is a characteristic pattern of "maturation" from superficial type A, large round pigmented nevus cells forming nests, to a deeper type B, smaller round nonpigmented cells forming cords. In some older lesions, a third type C spindle cell is seen at the base of the lesion (illustrated in the next section on dermal nevi). Accompanying this process of maturation or senescence is a subtle increase in eosinophilic stromal substance between the individual nevus cells, so that the type C cells may be quite widely separated from one another. These type C cells are arranged in a characteristic fascicular and bundled pattern that may suggest a neurofibroma and is consistent with schwannian differentiation. Occasionally, these cells form structures that mimic Wagner-Meissner corpuscles. Type C, but not type A or B, nevus cells

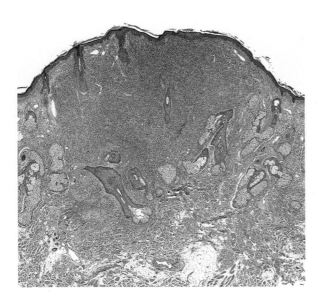 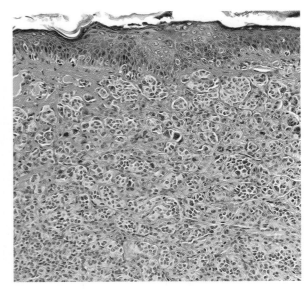

Figure 2-9

COMPOUND NEVUS: CONGENITAL PATTERN

In this lesion of the face, orderly nevus cells extend down from near the epidermis and into the reticular dermis, placed among reticular dermis collagen bundles and around the skin appendages. This congenital pattern is not diagnostic of a true congenital origin.

react with the Schwann cell–associated antigen AHMY1 (47). The type A cells conversely tend to express S-100 protein (and also the pigmentation apparatus–associated markers HMB45 and to a lesser extent Melan-A) more strongly than the spindle cells (48–50). This pattern of neurotization is more common in dermal than in compound nevi.

In summary, the process of maturation in the dermal component of a nevus is characterized by transition from the superficial to deep component, which involves the evolution of 1) nests into cords; 2) larger cells into smaller cells; 3) rounded cells into spindled, neuroid cells; and 4) pigmented cells into nonpigmented cells. It is possible that as nevi progressively involute and disappear, the schwannian spindle cells are replaced by cells indistinguishable from fibroblasts.

Differential Diagnosis. Both junctional and compound ordinary acquired nevi may retain some degree of lentiginous melanocytic proliferation with associated thinning and elongation of involved rete ridges and residual lamellar fibrosis within the underlying papillary dermis. Such lesions, however, are usually small and lack cytologic atypia, intraepidermal nests that deviate from rete tip localization, a junc-

tional shoulder that extends beyond the dermal component, and other criteria for classification as dysplastic nevi (see chapter 7). These lentiginous nevi should, therefore, not be classified as or confused with authentic dysplastic nevi.

Most compound nevi are composed of relatively large epithelioid type A cells with coarse melanin pigment superficially, and smaller type B cells with little or no pigment at the base of the lesion near the interface of the papillary and reticular dermis. If a nevus is built up like a brick wall by the migration of nests from the epidermis that pile up on nests that are already in the dermis, the cells at the base of the lesion represent the oldest and presumably the most mature cells. This pattern of maturation from the larger pigmented cell to the smaller non-pigmented cell is an important distinguishing characteristic from nodular and vertical growth phase malignant melanoma. In melanomas, the cells are less likely to become smaller and more likely to retain their pigment with descent into the dermis, perhaps because proliferation occurs more randomly and diffusely in dermal tumors or nodules of melanoma, so that the deeper cells are no more likely to be mature than the superficial ones. In common acquired nevi, there is no evidence of a cellular population in the dermis with the characteristics of a selective growth advantage (expansile, mitotically active nodule) compared to the neighboring cells.

McGovern (38) wrote that lesions are usually benign when the superficial but not the deeper cells have pigment, while lesions tend to be malignant when occasional isolated cells are pigmented or when there are irregularly and deeply situated small groups of pigmented cells. Although we would agree that the presence of pigment in the deep portion of a nodule of melanocytes is one of several suggestive features of malignancy, there are occasional nevi in which a so-called "inverted type A pattern" is seen, with pigment increasing to the base of the lesion in a paradoxical but benign pattern (fig. 2-10). Such nevi have been variously referred to as showing focal dermal hyperplasia, schwannian differentiation, or focal atypical epithelioid components (51). In our experience, this normal variation consists of displacement of larger, more epithelioid and pigmented type A nevus cells among or deep to the smaller, nonpigmented type B nevus cells within the dermal component. The banal cytology, absence of mitoses and necrosis, and nature of the melanization are helpful features in recognizing this common yet frequently problematic variant. Some of these nevi are dysplastic nevi, and deep penetrating nevi may represent a related phenomenon. Pigment in nevi is usually coarse, while conversely, the presence of finely divided "dusty" pigment as well as coarse pigment is suggestive of significant dysplasia or melanoma. Ultrastructurally, the coarse pigment represents compound melanosomes, which are more characteristic of nevi but may be seen in melanomas, while the dusty pigment of melanomas represents a predominant population of individual, poorly melanized premelanosomes (3).

Except in traumatized lesions, where there may be ulceration and neutrophilic inflammation, there is little or no host response in compound nevi, and there is no evidence of spontaneous necrosis except in occasional polypoid nevi with long stalks that may undergo apparent infarction. Most compound nevi contain few lymphocytes, and the finding of numerous lymphocytes should prompt consideration of halo nevus, dysplastic nevus, or melanoma.

The dermal component of ordinary melanocytic nevi is generally free of mitotic activity, although rarely, a mitosis is detected. When such lesions fulfill all other architectural and cytologic criteria for benign melanocytic nevi, we do not attribute biologic significance to this finding, although we generally document it in a note or comment in the pathology report.

If multiple mitoses are detected in the dermal component of otherwise banal common acquired nevi, this is noted in the report as a finding of uncertain biologic significance, and modest complete excision is advised. In some instances, we have found that such lesions have been removed during pregnancy. The ability to easily detect mitoses in the dermal component of a lesion initially resembling a nevus, however, should raise serious consideration of the possibility of nevoid melanoma (see chapter 11).

Selim et al. (52) recently studied 92 cases of traumatized melanocytic nevi, looking for histologic evidence of architectural and cytologic criteria that might be considered atypical. Histologic findings thought to be attributable to trauma included parakeratosis (92 percent of cases), dermal telangiectasias (61 percent), ulceration (51 percent), dermal inflammation (49 percent), melanin within the stratum corneum (24 percent), and dermal fibrosis (25 percent). Pagetoid spread of melanocytes was limited to the site of trauma in 20 percent of cases and was identified away from areas of trauma in 8 percent. Melanocytic atypia was seen in 3 cases. Dermal mitoses were rare. These authors concluded that any traumatized melanocytic lesion that displays cytologic atypia, pagetoid spread outside of the area of the traumatized epidermis, or dermal mitoses should be treated with caution because these findings were rarely seen in their series of traumatized nevi.

The so-called *nevus spilus,* or *speckled lentiginous nevus,* is a variant of a compound nevus that presents clinically as a tan macule within which are more darkly pigmented, flat or slightly raised speckles. Although the clinical appearance is quite striking, the histology is often unimpressive. The flat speckles show lentiginous melanocytic hyperplasia without atypia, the raised spots show banal nevus cells in the superficial dermis, and the tan background shows hyperpigmentation of keratinocytes,

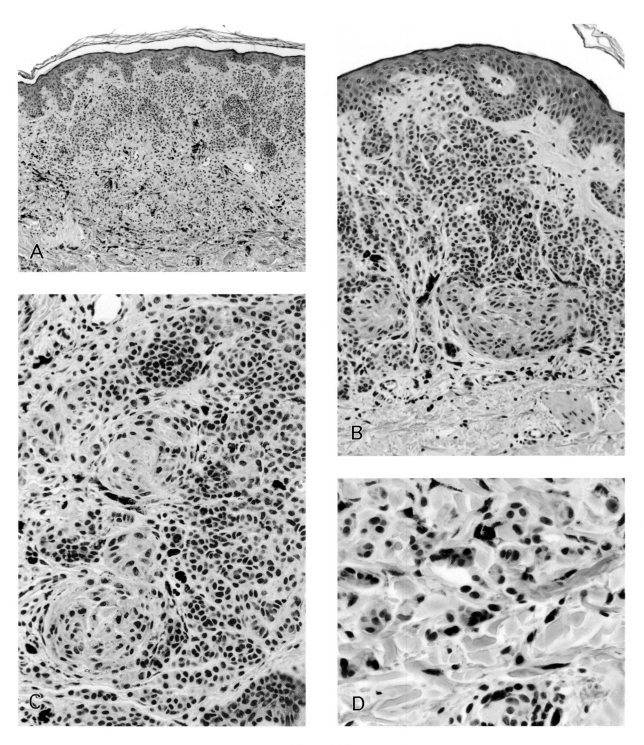

Figure 2-10

COMPOUND NEVUS: INVERTED TYPE A PATTERN (INVERTED TYPE A NEVUS)

In this somewhat unusual nevus, the usual pattern of maturation from superficial to deep is "inverted," with enlarged type A cells at the base of the lesion containing pigment, and smaller type B cells more superficial, lacking cytoplasmic melanin pigment.

Table 2-2

FEATURES HELPFUL IN DIFFERENTIATING PROTOTYPIC COMPOUND NEVUS AND VERTICAL GROWTH MELANOMA

	Compound Nevus	Vertical Growth Melanoma
Architecture		
Single cells above basal layer	Absent or rare	Pagetoid growth frequent[a]
Shoulder within epidermis	Absent	Often present
Symmetry of dermal growth	Present	Incomplete or absent
Expansile nodule formation	Absent	Present
Maturation	Present	Usually absent
Stroma		
Lymphocytic inflammation	Scant or absent	Often prominent, may be absent
Fibrosis	Delicate, scant	May be diffuse, dense, or absent
Reticulin fibers	Surrounds single cells	Surrounds clusters of cells
Cytology		
Nuclear chromatin	Delicate, dispersed	Coarse, clumped
Nuclear membrane	Thin, smooth, uniform	Variably thickened, angular
Nucleoli	Inconspicuous, basophilic	Large, eosinophilic
Atypia	Absent or random/senescent	Present, uniform
Mitoses	Generally absent	Usually present
Necrosis	Absent	Often present
Pigment synthesis	Superficial, uniform[b]	May be deep, nonuniform
Pigment quality	Coarse	Fine (dusty or muddy)
Single cells at base	Present	Absent (cells in nests/nodules)
Type C nevus cells at base	May be present	Absent
HMB45 reactivity[c]	Generally absent in deeper cells	Often present
Ki-67 activity	Very low (<10%)	May be low or very high (>50%)
p16 reactivity	May be high	Often low

[a]By definition, absent in the nodular variant in the adjacent epidermis.
[b]Exception is dermal nevus with focal retention of pigment synthesis (inverted type A pattern).
[c]Must be used in context of histology, since many examples of false positive and negative patterns exist.

sometimes with a slightly increased number of melanocytes. The occasional occurrence of melanoma in a nevus spilus has been reviewed (53). Studies suggest that many such lesions may represent a subtype of congenital melanocytic nevus (54,55).

Table 2-2 summarizes some of the architectural and cytologic features that distinguish compound nevi from vertical growth melanoma (see also chapter 11, Tumorigenic Melanoma). In particular, mitotic activity is rare, although occasionally, otherwise benign nevi, often in children, contain a single mitosis or a few mitoses (fig. 2-11) (56,57). Mitotic activity in benign nevi has also been described in pregnant patients (58). Another curiosity sometimes seen in the cells of benign nevi is balloon cell change (fig. 2-12), which may also be seen in melanomas (see fig. 8-35). Cytologic atypia is usually absent from the dermal component of nevi, although some examples show "random atypia" considered to represent a form of senescence

or "ancient change," and occasionally, benign nevus giant cells are present (fig. 2-13). These changes are seen more commonly in dermal nevi from older subjects (see next section).

Dermal Melanocytic Nevus

Definition. In *dermal melanocytic nevus,* the nevus cells are confined exclusively to the dermis.

Clinical Features. Dermal nevi are circumscribed and symmetric papules, typically pink or flesh colored but occasionally pale tan or light brown. Most range from 2 to 7 mm in size (figs. 2-14, 2-15). The borders of dermal nevi are smooth and regular, and pigment, if present, tends to be uniform in texture and pattern. Most are at least slightly raised to side-lighting, but as evolution into a strictly dermal nevus progresses over many decades and is followed by involution, many of the lesions become flatter and ultimately fade into the surrounding skin (1). In another pathway of involution, some dermal nevi evolve into pedunculated acrochordon-like

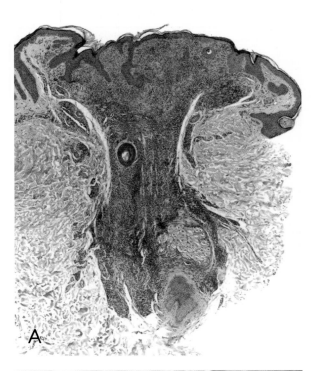

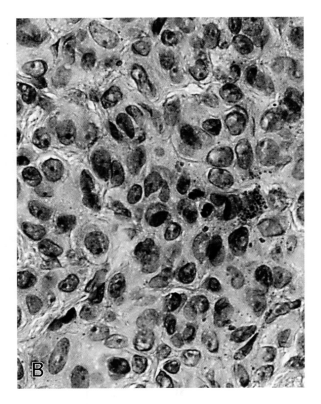

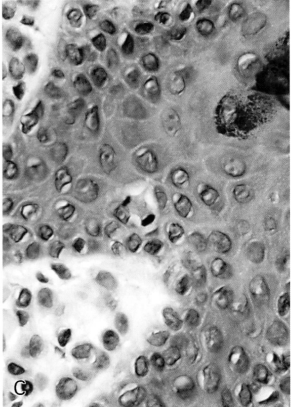

Figure 2-11

NEVUS WITH MITOSIS

A,B: This otherwise banal nevus contains a single dermal mitosis.

C: There is also a mitosis in the epidermis. There is no atypia, no in situ component, and no other evidence of malignancy.

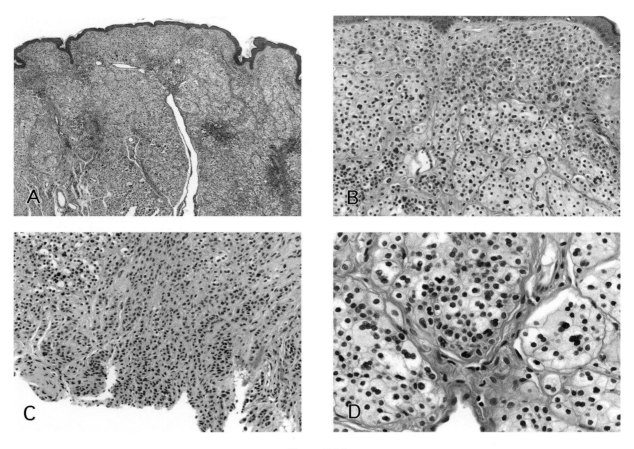

Figure 2-12

COMPOUND NEVUS WITH BALLOON CELL CHANGE (BALLOON CELL NEVUS)

A: This globoid lesion is composed of large cells that are uniform from side to side.
B: The cells have abundant clear "ballooned" cytoplasm.
C: There is evidence of maturation from superficial to deep.
D: There is no cytologic atypia and no mitoses.

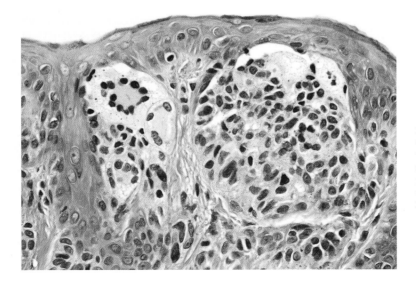

Figure 2-13

COMPOUND NEVUS WITH TOUTON-LIKE BALLOON CELLS

Peculiar enlarged cells may be seen in the dermal component of compound or dermal nevi. This has been likened to the phenomenon of "ancient change" in schwannomas, which is probably a reactive phenomenon. In this example, there are cells with clear or ballooned cytoplasm, reminiscent of Touton giant cells.

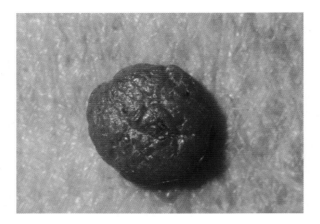

Figure 2-14

DERMAL NEVUS

This dermal nevus is truly papular, without an adjacent macular component. In contrast to a prototypic compound nevus, it has lost pigment and is now flesh colored.

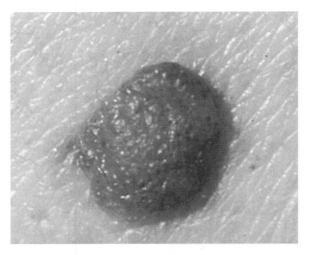

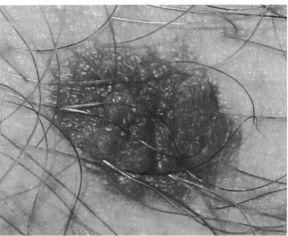

Figure 2-15

DERMAL NEVI

The lesions are flesh colored, with no discernable pigment (top, bottom). The papillomatous or verrucous surface configuration is a common variant of compound or dermal nevi (bottom). (Figs. C and D from Plate I, Fascicle 2, Third Series.)

lesions (fibroepithelial polyps) that ultimately may undergo spontaneous infarction and spontaneous sloughing. Interestingly, solar ultraviolet irradiation, in addition to its role in the genesis of new nevi in children, also has been implicated in the disappearance of nevi in older adult life (59).

Microscopic Findings. At scanning magnification, dermal nevi, like compound nevi, are relatively small, well-circumscribed, symmetric papules. The epidermis is normal or flattened, with effaced rete ridges and without the complex ramifications of elongated rete that characterize many compound nevi. The superficial papillary dermis and basement membrane zone are unremarkable. By definition, there are no nests of melanocytes (nevus cells) in the epidermis and there is no contiguous lentiginous proliferation of nevoid melanocytes. In practice, a few enlarged, arguably nevic melanocytes in the epidermis can reasonably be ignored as there is no clinical importance in distinguishing compound and dermal nevi.

In the dermis, the nevus cells are localized in clusters, either entirely within a widened papillary dermis, in which case the lower border of the cluster is fairly straight, or extending symmetrically from the papillary dermis into the reticular dermis with a more irregular, ill-defined border (fig. 2-16). As is also true in spindle and epithelioid cell (Spitz) nevi, it is characteristic for

the nevus cells to become progressively attenuated as they extend into the reticular dermis, with the deepest cells arranged as single rather than nested or fascicular units, and becoming progressively more difficult to distinguish from neural cells and fibroblasts. Nevus cells that are confined to the papillary dermis, in contrast, often present a more sharply demarcated lower border at the interface with normal tissue. The extension of nevus cells into the lower third of the reticular dermis is suggestive of a congenital

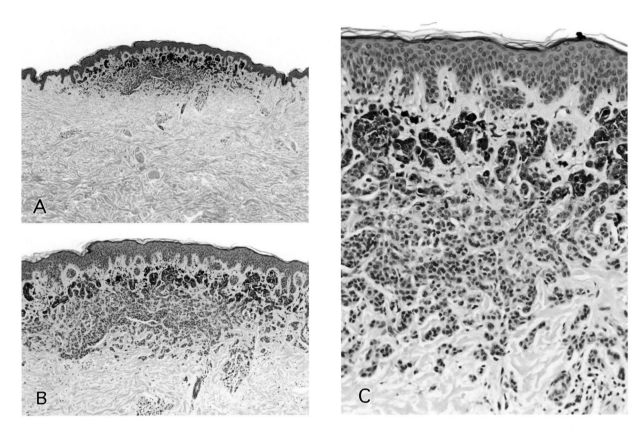

Figure 2-16

DERMAL NEVUS

In this prototypic example of a dermal nevus, the superficial cells are more heavily pigmented (type A cells). The deeper cells have lost their pigment and have become smaller (type B cells).

nevus, especially if the lesion is larger than 1.5 cm in diameter. Lower dermal involvement as an isolated finding is not diagnostic of a congenital nevus (45), however, especially in our experience of lesions of the face and scalp. Although the arrangement of the nevus cells in lesions that involve the reticular dermis may give an impression of infiltrative growth, these are stable lesions clinically, and there is no evidence of the formation of an expansile mass of cells that compresses the stroma or appears to have a selective growth advantage compared to the surrounding nevus cells.

At higher magnification, the dermal nevus cells are usually small and sparsely pigmented round cells (type B), or elongated spindle cells lacking pigment and arranged as "wavy" fibers or as parallel bundles of straight fibers consistent with neural differentiation (type C) (fig. 2-17).

Some lesions also exhibit a population of larger, round pigmented cells (type A) superficially. When spindle and round cell types are both present, there is a superficial to deep progression from the pigmented round cell type, to the non-pigmented smaller cell type, to the spindle cell type at the base of the lesion, with a progressive increase in intercellular basement membrane and reticulin material. The reticulin surrounds individual cells, similar to the pattern described above in compound nevi and different from that in melanomas, where larger clusters of melanoma cells are invested by the fibers.

The pattern of continuous blending of the cell types from superficial to deep within the lesion is most consistent with the hypothesis that the spindle cell neurotized component stems from maturation of cells derived originally from intraepithelial melanocytes. Some

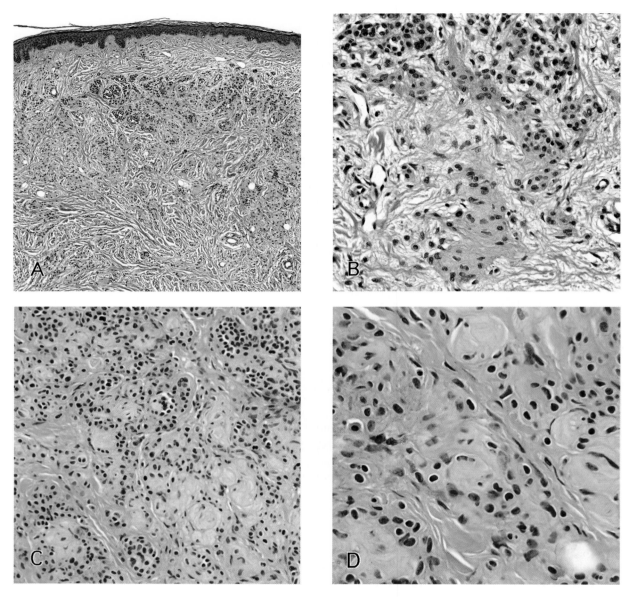

Figure 2-17

DERMAL NEVUS, NEUROTIZED

In this neurotized dermal nevus, the lesional cells enter the reticular dermis in a congenital pattern (A,B). At the base of the lesion, structures reminiscent of Wagner-Meissner corpuscles (sensory end organs) are formed (B–D).

observers, however, have proposed a dual origin of nevi from both epidermal melanocytes and cells associated with nerve fibers or with hair follicles in the dermis (59a).

The spindle cells lack demonstrable tyrosinase, but are positive for cholinesterase; immunohistochemical findings are also consistent with a schwannian or neural phenotype (47). By con-

trast, the type A and B nevus cells are typically tyrosinase positive and cholinesterase negative (nevic or melanocytic phenotype). The type C spindle cells are arranged in bundles of fibers with wavy S-shaped nuclei, and neuroid structures reminiscent of Wagner-Meissner corpuscles are often noted (fig. 2-17). When the process is advanced, there may be little or no residual melanocytic

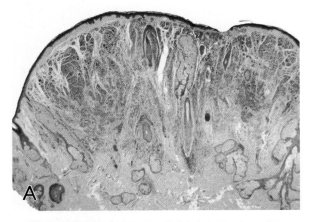

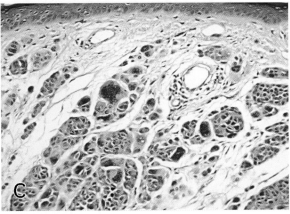

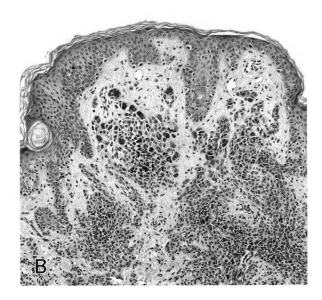

Figure 2-18

DERMAL NEVUS WITH ANCIENT CHANGE

A: Congenital pattern nevus cells enter the reticular dermis, around skin appendages. Maturation is seen from superficial to deep.

B,C: At higher magnification, there are cells with large, hyperchromatic nuclei. This feature, likened to ancient change in schwannomas, is not associated with malignancy. It would be judicious to search carefully for mitoses in such a lesion.

differentiation and the lesion may resemble a neurofibroma. Such lesions were termed "neuronevi" by Masson (60). In most neurotized nevi, both the neural and the melanocytic phenotypes are apparent in the same lesion.

Cytologically, there may be some variation in nuclear size and shape in dermal nevi, especially in the deeper, older cells where there may be startling hyperchromatism and enlargement of individual cells among a population of blander, often neurotized cells (figs. 2-18, 2-19). There are no mitoses and there is no evidence of expansile nodule formation, suggesting that the cells may be senescent rather than proliferative in character. This atypia has been likened to the ancient change that is seen in schwannomas (61) and is of no known clinical significance. In most cells of most dermal nevi, the nuclei are small, with perhaps small blue condensations of chromatin (chromocenters), but with no large eosinophilic nucleoli of the type seen mainly in melanomas. Mitoses are generally absent in

dermal nevi, and spontaneous necrosis is virtually never present.

Typically, there is little or no host inflammatory response and the presence of appreciable lymphocytes, mitotic activity, necrosis, or focal expansile growth should suggest the possibility of melanoma. Clinically, episodes of follicular rupture in nevi may prompt biopsy, but the keratin granulomas so formed are easily recognized histologically.

Balloon cell change is an interesting histologic feature that has no known clinical significance in nevi (37,38,62). Balloon cells may be observed focally in otherwise unremarkable nevi and in melanomas (see fig. 2-13). When they predominate in a lesion, their melanocytic character may be difficult to recognize, and an S-100 protein stain may be helpful. In most instances, however, forms transitional between balloon cells and more characteristic nevus cells can be identified. Ultrastructurally, the clear cytoplasm is due to the presence of

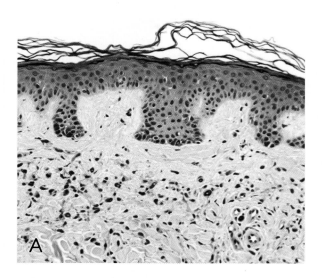

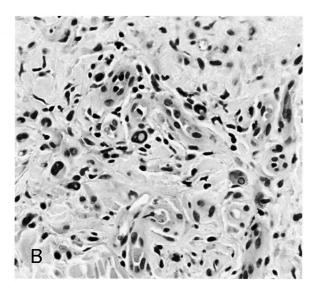

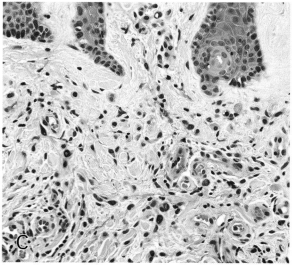

Figure 2-19

DERMAL NEVUS WITH ANCIENT CHANGE

Ancient change in a smaller, less papular lesion than that seen in figure 2-18. Importantly, the atypia is random, that is, confined to a minority of the lesional cells, and not associated with mitoses.

multiple vacuoles that are probably abnormal melanosomes (63). A related phenomenon is the presence of signet ring cells in melanomas, which we have observed in both primary and metastatic lesions (64). Balloon cell nevi and signet ring cell nevi or melanomas are histologic curiosities that do not represent clinicopathologic entities. Rarely, balloon cell change occurs in melanoma, so its presence does not always correlate with benignancy.

The dermal components of nevi are also occasionally associated with marked sclerosis, characterized by deposition of abundant and often hyalinized collagen bundles between nevus cells that otherwise have benign features. We generally designate such lesions in the pathology report as showing a sclerosing dermal component.

Differential Diagnosis. As dermal nevi lose their pigment and involute, they tend to lose attributes of melanocytic differentiation. The differential diagnosis of such amelanotic, involuting dermal nevi includes nodular tumors of round cells and/or spindle cells in the skin. The most important entity in the differential diagnosis, nodular melanoma, is presented in Table 2-2 and is also discussed in chapter 10. Briefly, key features of melanoma are loss of symmetry from side to side and of maturation from superficial to deep, the presence of uniform cytologic atypia, and the presence of mitotic activity in the lesional cells. The presence of an in situ component is very helpful but may be absent in nodular or pure vertical growth phase melanoma, as well as in some nevoid melanomas. Expression of staining for the proliferation marker Ki-67 is increased in most melanomas and low in dermal nevus cells (65–69), and the tumor suppressor p16 is elevated in most nevi and reduced or absent in most vertical growth phase melanomas (17,25,67,70–72). Mitotic figures are rare in benign nevi; however, if there are no other attributes of malignancy, we will sign out such a case as a "nevus with mitotic activity," and recommend complete excision (see fig. 2-11). No single attribute taken alone is diagnostic and in some melanomas, called nevoid or minimal deviation melanomas, a benign nevus may be closely simulated at scanning magnification. This possibility should be seriously considered in any nevoid lesion with mitotic activity.

If a nonmelanocytic round or spindle cell tumor is suggested by routine light microscopy, appropriate immunohistochemical stains should be ordered. HMB45, Mart-1/Melan-A, and tyrosinase antigens with a negative keratin stain aid in confirming melanocytic differentiation (discussed further in the section on metastatic melanoma), although the cells of histiocytosis X, which occasionally simulate nevic cells, are also S-100 protein positive (these are, unlike melanocytic cells, CD1a positive and Melan-A negative) (73,74).

When a lesion is composed of small round uniform cells without pigment or neurotization, a mastocytoma may be simulated. Conversely, an authentic mast cell tumor may be misinterpreted as a dermal nevus. In case of doubt, a Giemsa stain for the metachromatic cytoplasmic granules of mast cells should be performed.

Angioma-like spaces that may be present in dermal as well as compound nevi may suggest the possibility of an angioma, especially if there is associated hemorrhage (38). This diagnosis can usually be ruled out without special stains by recognizing obvious nevus cells elsewhere within the lesion, and by awareness that this pattern is common in nevi (figs. 2-20, 2-21). Moreover, the vascular pattern in "angiomatous" dermal nevi often, at least focally, shows a horizontally stratified "Venetian blind" ar-

chitecture. In situations where doubt persists, a CD31 stain confirms the absence of reactivity in areas of angioma-like change.

Histiocytomas (e.g., xanthogranulomas or reticulohistiocytomas) occasionally resemble dermal nevi, especially when early lesions are sampled or when multinucleated cells are present (see fig. 2-13). In addition to the focal presence of multinucleated cells with foamy or amphophilic ground-glass cytoplasm, early histiocytomas often differ from dermal nevi via a background of mixed inflammatory cells, as well as immunohistochemistry positive for CD68 and negative HMB45 or Melan-A reactivity (74). Epithelioid histiocytoma, which is composed of large epithelioid cells with abundant cytoplasm, but without melanin pigment and devoid of S-100 protein reactivity, is a lesion that is especially likely to be confused with a Spitz tumor or a melanoma and less likely with a banal dermal nevus (74–76).

Cellular neurothekeomas may produce a nested pattern formed by rounded epithelioid cells within the dermis that resembles the architecture of a nevoid melanocytic proliferation. These lesions, however, often show mitotic activity, lack evidence of maturation, and are negative for S-100 protein and positive for the NKI-C3 marker.

Fibrous papules may simulate nevi clinically. Histologically, their prominent vascularity and the presence of plump fusiform and stellate mesenchymal cells suggest the diagnosis at scanning power microscopy. The presence of nevus cells in the dermis readily distinguishes a papillomatous compound or dermal nevus from a verruca (fig. 2-22). Dermatofibromas may simulate nevi, especially if there is prominent reactive epithelial hyperplasia with lentiginous melanocytic proliferation or basal layer hyperpigmentation above the lesion. Recognition of the characteristic underlying spindle cell component that is enriched for factor XIIIa-positive dermal dendrocytes aids in establishing the correct diagnosis in difficult cases. There are occasional neurofibromas that are difficult and even impossible to distinguish from neurotized nevi. If no nevic differentiation is apparent in such a lesion, we usually consider it a neurofibroma. More definitive diagnosis of neurofibroma is often possible by the detection of one or more

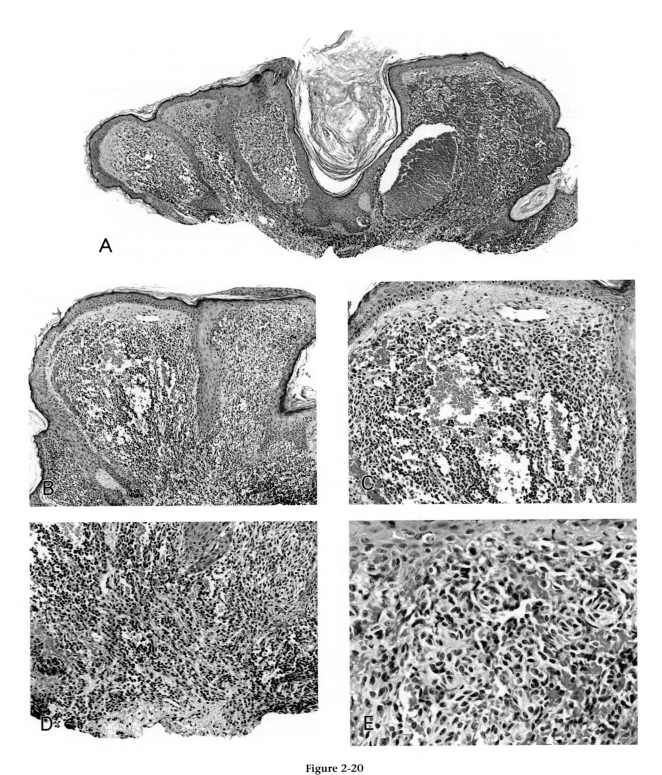

Figure 2-20

COMPOUND NEVUS WITH LYMPHATIC SPACES AND HEMORRHAGE

This nevus contains prominent spaces lined by nevus cells, which resemble lymphatics. Some of the spaces are blood-filled, no doubt the reason for the excision of this benign lesion.

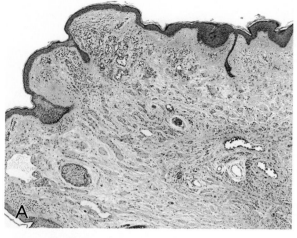

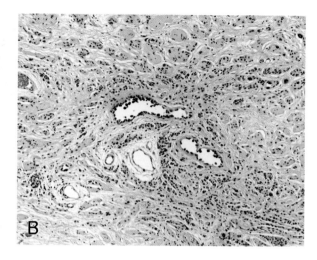

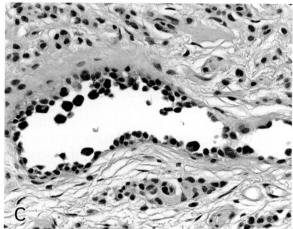

Figure 2-21

DERMAL NEVUS WITH PSEUDOLYMPHATIC SPACES

These spaces are lined by nevus cells and do not represent true lymphatic spaces.

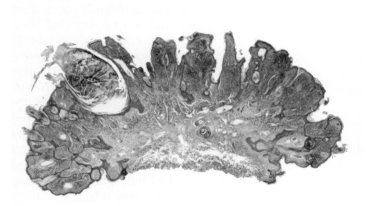

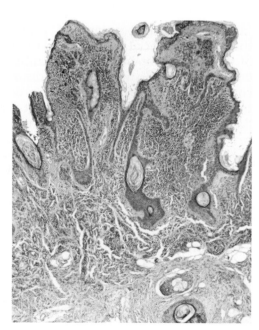

Figure 2-22

DERMAL NEVUS, PAPILLOMATOUS PATTERN

Many compound or dermal nevi exhibit this papillomatous configuration reminiscent, at scanning magnification, of a wart or seborrheic keratosis.

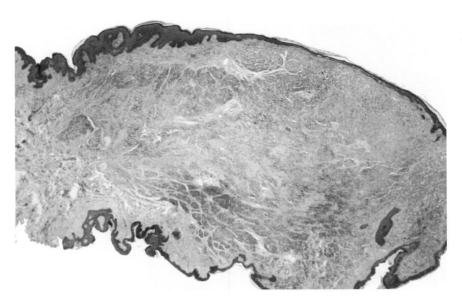

Figure 2-23

DERMAL NEVUS, POLYPOID PATTERN

Many dermal or compound nevi, as in this case, have the configuration of a fibroepithelial polyp.

small axons in cross-section throughout the lesion. Both neurotized nevi and neurofibromas may contain abundant mast cells. Involuting dermal nevi may lose all attributes of nevic differentiation and become replaced by fibrous connective tissue or by mature adipose tissue. Some of these lesions are indistinguishable from or identical to fibroepithelial polyps or acrochordons, a differential diagnosis that is of no clinical significance (fig. 2-23).

VARIANTS OF ACQUIRED MELANOCYTIC NEVI, NONSITE DEPENDENT

There are several variants of acquired nevi that occur in special sites or populations. Some of these represent histologic curiosities, while others, such as halo nevi, represent distinct clinicopathologic entities. The lesions considered in this section, in general, are significant as potential histologic simulants of melanoma.

Halo Nevus

Definition. A *halo nevus* is defined clinically as a small, circumscribed pigmented lesion having the appearance of a common benign compound nevus, surrounded by an area of macular depigmentation, which constitutes the "halo" (77). The lesions are commonly multiple, especially in adolescents (fig. 2-24). The lesions disappear over time, and the area subsequently repigments (fig. 2-25). The nevi are usually completely banal, or occasionally, of the congenital type (fig. 2-26).

The halo is usually symmetric; an asymmetric halo should arouse concern for melanoma, but may be seen in a benign nevus as well (fig. 2-27). The histologic appearance, which is also characteristic and often diagnostic, includes a brisk infiltrative lymphocytic response extending among dermal nevus cells and loss of pigment in the adjacent epidermis. Some lesions exhibiting most of these histologic features do not present with an obvious clinical or histologic depigmented halo. Synonyms for halo nevus include *Sutton nevus* and *leukoderma acquisitum centrifugum* (78).

Clinical Features. Halo nevi are generally small, well-circumscribed, uniformly pigmented tan-brown papules that are surrounded by a symmetric halo of depigmentation (figs. 2-24–2-27). The lesions often present during the summer (perhaps because the halo contrasts better with tanned skin), and they are most common on the trunk. Occasionally, a halo nevus is observed in an individual with generally tanned skin, but with a focal blistering sunburn in the region of the halo. Halo nevi are most often seen in teenagers and young adults, where they are sometimes associated with dysplastic nevi; they are commonly multiple. Less often, a solitary halo lesion develops in an older adult, and in this circumstance a biopsy should be done to rule out the possibility of melanoma, especially if the central pigmented lesion has clinically atypical features or if the halo is eccentric or asymmetric in contour (fig. 2-27).

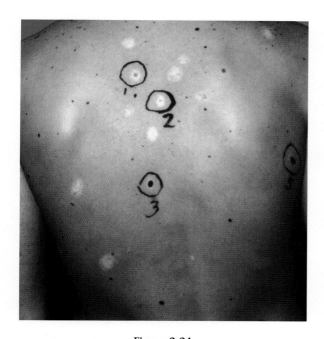

Figure 2-24

MULTIPLE HALO NEVI

Halo nevi commonly present as a zone of depigmentation around a preexisting, clinically benign, symmetric compound nevus, often in a young adult or teenager. Frequently, the lesions are multiple, as in this case. Lesions commonly present in the summer, when tanning of the background skin reveals the halo.

Serial follow-up studies of halo nevi have documented a characteristic time sequence of changes, beginning with the sudden appearance of the halo about a discrete compound nevus (fig. 2-25). Over several months, the nevus gradually fades and ultimately disappears. The halo then gradually repigments, and a year or two later, the lesional site has the appearance of normal skin. During this period, especially in teenagers, other similar halos may appear about preexisting compound nevi, which then undergo a similar involution.

Studies in patients with halo nevi have demonstrated circulating antibodies that are reactive with neoplastic melanocytes including melanoma cells, and the infiltrating cells have been shown to be mainly T lymphocytes (79). Antigen-presenting cells and CD8-positive T cells have been identified in the inflammatory infiltrates of halo nevi, implicating cytotoxic mechanisms in the destruction of nevomelanocytes (80). Moreover, the phenomenon appears to have systemic

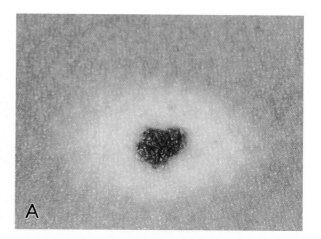

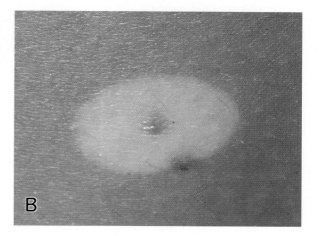

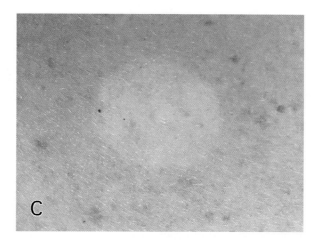

Figure 2-25

HALO NEVI: GOING, GOING, GONE

Three lesions at different stages of regression. Following the disappearance of the central lesion, the halo typically repigments over a period of months or years.

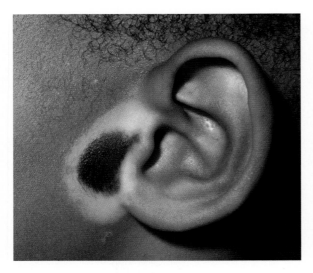

Figure 2-26

**HALO REACTION IN A SMALL TO
INTERMEDIATE CONGENITAL PATTERN NEVUS**

This lesion is larger than most acquired nevi and is surrounded by a symmetric halo.

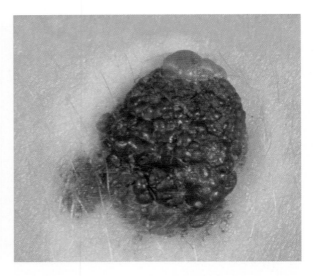

Figure 2-27

**ASYMMETRIC HALO IN A CLINICALLY
ATYPICAL MELANOCYTIC LESION**

This lesion simulates melanoma with a halo reaction, and should be excised for histologic diagnosis.

implications since affected individuals show activated lymphocytes in their peripheral blood (81) as well as T-cell clonal expansion (82) and antinevic IgM antibody production (83). Interestingly, halo nevi appear to be associated with Turner syndrome; in a recent study of 72 patients with this syndrome, the incidence of halo nevi was 18 percent compared to 1 percent in controls, with the halo nevi occurring preferentially in patients with a particular human leukocyte antigen (HLA) subtype (84). These findings are consistent with the idea that halo nevi represent immunologically mediated rejection of a nevus. The halo develops outside the nevus proper, suggesting that there may be a cross-reaction with melanocytes that surround the nevus prior to the onset of the intense inflammation in the dermal component. This does not preclude the idea that some change in these intraepidermal melanocytes is the primary stimulus to a reaction that secondarily involves the dermal component of the nevus, or that an ostensibly normal field of melanocytes may have antigenic overlap with the nevus cells that they surround.

Microscopic Findings. The basic pattern is that of a compound nevus: a small (less than 4 mm as a rule) circumscribed lesion composed of nevus cells that is located in the papillary dermis

and epidermis (figs. 2-28–2-32). As in other benign nevi, the lesion is bilaterally symmetric and composed of uniform cells that tend to mature (become smaller) from top to bottom. The epidermis may be hyperkeratotic with follicular plugging (77). The key feature that distinguishes a halo nevus from a banal nevus is the presence of a striking, dense lymphocytic infiltrate, and this feature may arouse suspicion of melanoma. The lymphocytes extend among the lesional nevus cells, obscuring their underlying nested pattern in some cases (fig. 2-30). By electron microscopy, melanin-laden histiocytes and mast cells, as well as lymphocytes, are seen (79). Occasional halo nevi contain a few giant cells or there may even be a frankly granulomatous response.

With the passage of time (weeks or months), the dermal nevus cells disappear and then the histologic differential diagnosis may include lichenoid inflammatory dermatoses. Histologic examination of the site of a completely resolved halo nevus may disclose essentially normal skin, with no evidence of scarring or residual pigment (77), although fibrovascular proliferation consistent with regression is occasionally seen (fig. 2-31). In most halo nevi, there is little or no readily observable melanocytic abnormality in the epidermis at the "shoulder" of the

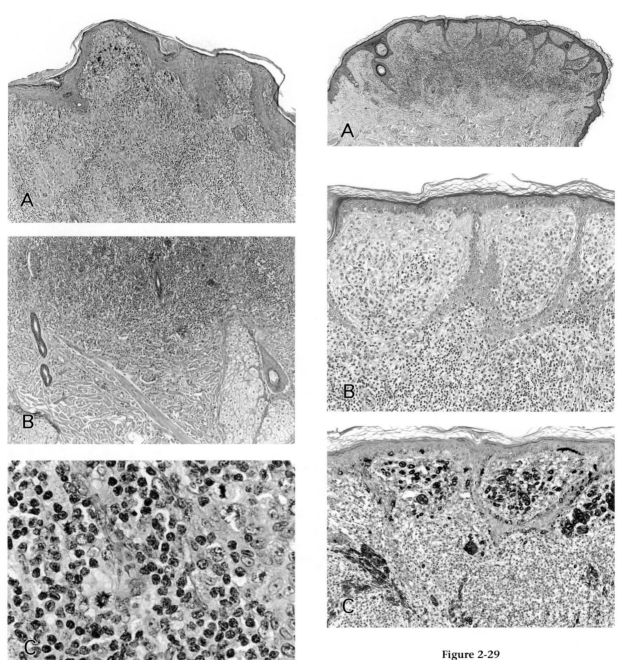

Figure 2-28

HALO NEVUS

This lesion from the temple of a 14-year-old boy shows a prominent lymphocytic infiltrate of the type seen in halo nevi. There is maturation of the lesional cells from superficial to deep (A,B). A single mitosis was found (C); however, the mitosis was in an infiltrating histiocyte rather than in a lesional cell. Mitotic figures in lesional cells of halo nevi are uncommon and should be interpreted with caution.

Figure 2-29

HALO NEVUS WITH MELAN-A STAIN

A: At scanning magnification, the lesion has the characteristics of a dermal nevus.

B: At higher magnification, infiltrating lymphocytes are seen among nevus cells. At the base of the lesion, the nevus cells show evidence of maturation, important in distinguishing this lesion from a nevoid melanoma with brisk tumor infiltrating lymphocytes. Mitoses are rare or absent.

C: The Melan-A stain demonstrates residual nevus cells among the infiltrating lymphocytes. Sometimes, a halo nevus is mistaken for an inflammatory process.

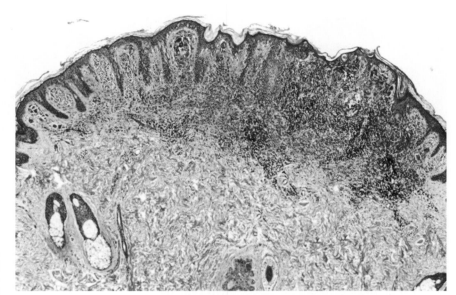

Figure 2-30

HALO NEVUS

Top: At low power, the appearance is that of a compound or dermal nevus, with the impression of increased cellularity resulting from the infiltrating lymphocytes.

Bottom: The lymphocytes permeate among the preexisting lesional nevus cells, tending to obscure them and ultimately resulting in their disappearance.

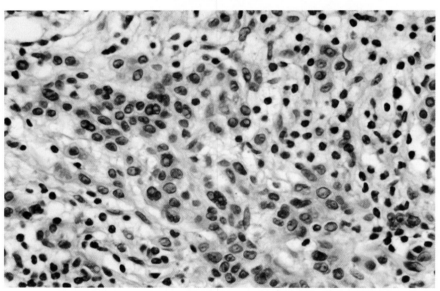

lesion beyond the lateral border of the dermal component, even though it is in this region that the striking clinical halo is located. DOPA stains for tyrosinase and argentaffin stains for melanosomes, however, reveal greatly reduced numbers of melanocytes in the area of the halo compared with the surrounding skin (77).

At higher magnification, the lesional cells in most halo nevi are unremarkable dermal nevus cells of the large pigmented (type A) or small nonpigmented (type B) type. Pigment is located in nevus cells and in melanophages superficially, and is usually coarse in texture. In

some lesions, the dermal cells are larger than is usual in common nevi, and nucleoli are present. These changes may represent a form of inflammatory or reactive atypia, or possibly a Spitz tumor–like cytology (fig. 2-32).

Mitotic figures are absent in most lesions; however, a few lesions judged to be benign halo nevi have shown one or two mitotic figures (85). Such a finding should provoke careful examination of the lesion to rule out melanoma, with deeper sections and embedding of any residual gross tissue. Mitoses and Ki-67 reactivity are also seen in host reactive cells (fig. 2-28). If Ki-67

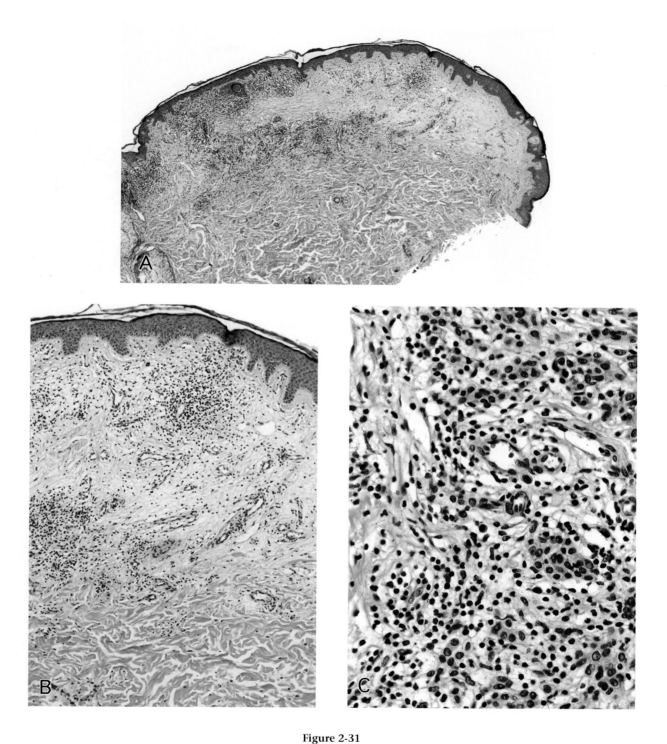

Figure 2-31

HALO NEVUS WITH REGRESSIVE FIBROPLASIA

A: The nevus has been largely replaced by fibrosis or by residual clusters of lymphocytes.

B: At higher magnification, the area of scarring is visible. When this type of histology is observed without residual nevus cells, "regressed pigmented lesion" is often the only diagnosis.

C: In another area, lymphocytes infiltrate among nevus cells.

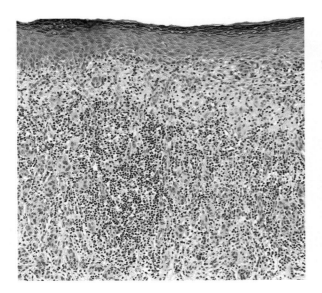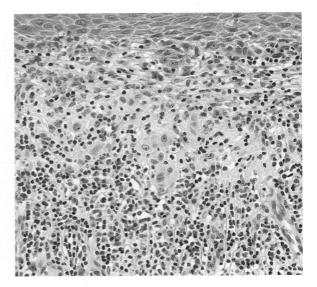

Figure 2-32

HALO NEVUS WITH LARGE EPITHELIOID CELLS (SPITZ NEVUS WITH HALO REACTION)

This lesion, from a young patient, consists of large epithelioid cells with brisk infiltrating lymphocytes. The possibility of a "spitzoid" melanoma with brisk tumor-infiltrating lymphocytes should be seriously considered, and some examples of lesions like this are best interpreted as "melanocytic tumor of uncertain potential," with a differential diagnosis of melanoma versus halo nevus.

immunohistochemistry is employed to further evaluate the potential significance of mitoses in halo nevi, we have found that a combined Mart-1/Ki-67 double staining approach greatly assists in excluding staining within the lymphoid component, which often is itself mitotically active upon immunologic stimulation.

Findings suggestive of melanoma in a lesion simulating a halo nevus include the presence of a separate population of cells with an expansile pattern of growth, severe uniform cytologic atypia, and/or the presence of frequent mitoses, ulceration, or necrosis. It is important to remember that the halo phenomenon occasionally involves other types of nevi, including Spitz nevi (86) and congenital nevi (83), as well as melanomas (79), and therefore careful inspection of the underlying lesional architecture and cytology in multiple sections may be required for definitive classification.

Examination of the halo region at the periphery of the dermal component of the lesion may show a few lymphocytes at the dermal-epidermal interface, and occasionally, a reduction or an absence of identifiable melanocytes. In comparison with adjacent normal epidermis, pigment may be visibly reduced, and this contrast can be enhanced with a melanin stain. In most lesions, there is no intraepidermal melanocytic proliferation adjacent to the dermal component, but in a few lesions a component suggestive of dysplasia is observed (see chapter 6). If a radial growth phase component diagnostic of melanoma is present adjacent to a dermal lesion simulating halo nevus, the entire lesion most likely represents melanoma.

Differential Diagnosis. Since halo nevi are of no significance other than as possible simulants of melanoma, their distinction from common acquired nevi, although usually easy because of the dense lymphocytic infiltrate, is clinically unimportant. Compared to nodular melanoma or the vertical growth phase of superficial spreading melanoma, a halo nevus is usually smaller (the central nevus is usually less than 4 mm in diameter, while most melanomas are larger than 6 mm, although these values are by no means absolute). However, we have observed rare small (less than 5 mm) melanomas with nevoid characteristics but with diffuse cellular atypia sometimes combined with brisk mitotic activity in which diffuse lymphoid infiltration is a dominant pattern. When pigment is present in a halo nevus, it is usually coarse as is the case in most benign nevi, and if there is a junctional component, its character is that of a nevus rather than a melanoma. Thus, there is usually a discontinuous rather than continuous proliferation of predominantly nested rather than predominantly single nevus cells, and there is little or no tendency to single cell, upward (pagetoid) intraepidermal spread of the junctional cells.

Some halo nevi may be difficult to distinguish from dysplastic nevi that have an unusually brisk lymphocytic infiltrate. Not only do halo nevi appear to be common in patients with dysplastic nevi but also a halo response may be seen, clinically and histologically, in the dysplastic nevi themselves. If the characteristic patterns of dysplasia are seen at the shoulder of the compound portion of a lesion whose other features are consistent with a halo nevus, the diagnosis of dysplastic nevus with halo reaction can be made, especially if there is a history of other atypical nevi or a personal or family history of melanoma.

When nevus cells are inconspicuous among a dense lymphocytic infiltrate, inflammatory dermatoses such as lichenoid keratoses may be simulated (87). In these circumstances, an S-100 protein, Melan-A, or HMB45 stain may reveal the hidden nevus cells (care must be taken in interpretation, since histiocytes may weakly express S-100 protein, and activated melanocytes and melanoma cells may express HMB45).

Finally, there are lesions that have an infiltrative lymphocytic response similar to that of a halo nevus but without a clinical halo. These lesions may be signed out descriptively as "compound (or dermal) nevi with halo reaction" (85), or more descriptively as "nevi with a lymphocytic infiltrate of the type seen in halo nevi." Since a description of the presence or absence of a halo is not always available, such a descriptive diagnosis may be the best that can be rendered in many instances.

Deep Penetrating Nevus

Definition. *Deep penetrating nevus*, a recently described lesion, appears to represent a distinctive entity that has some features of combined nevus, cellular variants of blue nevus, and spindle and epithelioid nevus (88). These benign acquired lesions are distinguished by

their characteristic large size, often extending into the deep dermis or fat; by a large nevic cell type with pigment synthesis through the full thickness of the lesion; and by the absence of indicators of malignancy such as frequent mitoses, necrosis, or ulceration.

Clinical Features. In the first report of 70 cases, patients ranged widely in age from 3 to 63 years, with most lesions occurring in the second and third decades (88). The most common sites were the head, neck, and shoulder, and no lesions occurred on the hands or feet. Blue nevus or cellular blue nevus was the most common clinical diagnosis. Malignant melanoma was histologically diagnosed (erroneously) in 9 of 42 cases. In follow-up ranging from 1 to 23 years (mean, 7 years), no lesions recurred or metastasized. The lesions ranged from 2 to 9 mm, and were darkly pigmented papules and nodules. None of the lesions was entirely amelanotic. On cross-section, the lesions extended at least halfway into the dermis, with a smooth, dome-shaped elevation of the epidermis. Similar lesions have also been described as *plexiform spindle cell nevi* (89).

Microscopic Findings. At scanning magnification, the lesions are circumscribed and wedge-shaped, with the broad base abutting the epidermis, and sometimes with extensions pointing toward the fat (fig. 2-33). Nests of nevus cells are found at the dermal-epidermal junction in most cases. The dermal component of the lesion is made up of loosely arranged, coalescent nests or fascicles of large pigmented spindle and epithelioid cells interspersed with melanophages. Many cases show an admixture of smaller, more conventional-appearing nevus cells as well.

The lesional cell nests tend to surround skin appendages and to spread apart at the periphery of the lesion, in an apparently infiltrative and often plexiform pattern. There is only a slight tendency for the cells to become smaller toward the base of the lesion, and this apparent failure of maturation, along with some degree of architectural asymmetry and deep pigment synthesis, may falsely suggest melanoma. Some lesions have a mild lymphocytic infiltrate. Extension into the fat as a pushing, finger-like or expansile protrusion may occur.

At higher magnification, nuclear pleomorphism may be striking in some lesions, with variation in size and shape, hyperchromasia, nuclear

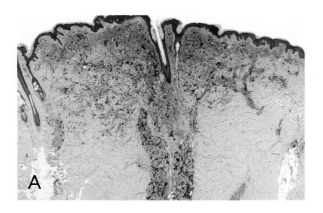

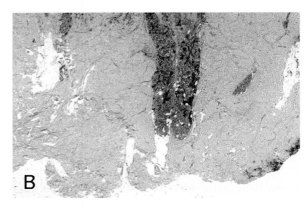

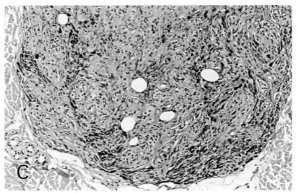

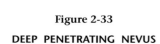

Figure 2-33

DEEP PENETRATING NEVUS

A,B: A pyramidal lesion has its apex in the deep reticular dermis.

C,D: At high magnification, the lesional cells tend to be arranged in clusters, sometimes surrounded by spindle cells reminiscent of sustentacular cells. The cells are heavily pigmented, and there is an admixture of pigmented melanophages.

E: In some areas, the histology overlaps with that of a cellular blue nevus.

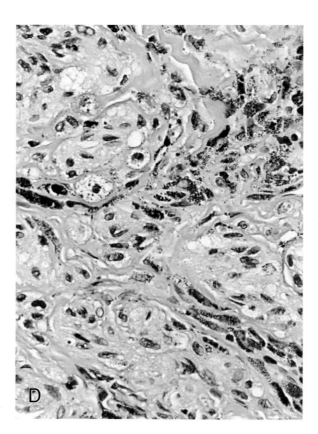

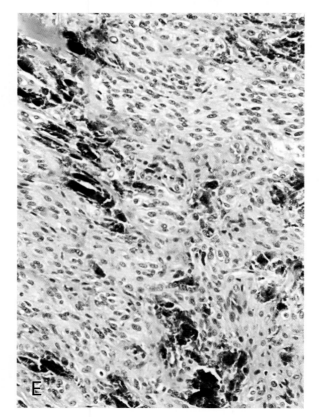

pseudoinclusions, and smudged structureless chromatin. Nucleoli are usually inconspicuous but a few large eosinophilic nucleoli may be observed. Importantly, mitoses are absent or rare, with no more than one or two in multiple sections of a particular lesion. The cytoplasm is abundant, and contains finely-divided brown melanin pigment. The lesional cells react for S-100 protein and HMB45 antigen; stains for keratin are negative. These lesions frequently react with an antibody to a MAGE antigen that had previously been thought to be a useful marker for tumorigenic melanoma (90,91).

While we regard deep penetrating nevi as most likely representing benign nevus variants, their biologic potential has not been studied in enough lesions at this juncture to predict banal clinical behavior in all instances. Accordingly, we recommend that lesions be completely excised and that interval follow-up over time be instituted.

Differential Diagnosis. The most important entity in the differential diagnosis is nodular malignant melanoma. Architectural and cytologic features distinguish the two lesions. Most bulky tumorigenic vertical growth phase melanomas exhibit a more striking pattern of epidermal involvement, with spread of atypical cells into the epidermis and, often, with ulceration. In contrast, the deep penetrating nevus has an inconspicuous epidermal component consisting only of a few basilar nevic cell nests. Melanomas of this bulk usually exhibit a more destructive pattern of infiltration, with displacement and compression of the stroma, and often spontaneous necrosis and ulceration. Such lesions usually exhibit marked nuclear atypia with frequent and often abnormal mitoses, making the distinction easy. A few nodular spindle cell melanomas have lower-grade nuclei, and in these cases, the presence of more than a few mitoses may be decisive. In general, melanomas are likely to be broader than their depth, and to have more poorly circumscribed margins than the deep penetrating nevus, which tends to be vertically oriented like a fully evolved spindle and epithelioid cell nevus.

Benign lesions that can be distinguished from deep penetrating nevi include common and cellular blue nevi and spindle and epithelioid cell nevi. Dendritic melanocytes, a feature of blue nevi and most cellular blue nevi, are not prominent in deep penetrating nevi. The nests of nonpigmented, often clear spindle cells that are characteristic of cellular blue nevi are not a feature of deep penetrating nevi, and blue nevi do not typically exhibit significant nuclear atypia. Rarely, however, we have encountered lesions that seem to possess histopathologic features that fall between those of deep penetrating and cellular blue nevi. Spindle and epithelioid cell nevi (Spitz nevi) tend to involve the dermis and are more superficial than most deep penetrating nevi. The epidermal component of Spitz nevi is usually more cellular, and there is much less pigment in the dermis. The pigmented spindle cell nevus of Reed, which may be quite heavily pigmented, is a strictly superficial lesion confined to the papillary dermis. The lesional cells are usually less plump and more elongated spindle cells. Mitoses are often present in pigmented spindle cell nevi, but not in most deep penetrating nevi, in which a rare mitosis is only seen occasionally (92).

Although the deep penetrating nevus can usually be distinguished from these other benign lesions, the distinction from malignant melanoma is of greatest importance so that unnecessary or disfiguring surgery can be avoided. Problematical examples (for example, those with more than a few mitoses) may be interpreted descriptively as "melanocytic tumor of uncertain potential," and patients may be offered the alternative of minimal treatment for possible melanoma. Neural involvement is not an indicator of malignancy in these lesions. Table 2-3 summarizes the differential diagnostic features that separate deep penetrating nevus from nodular melanoma.

Recurrent Melanocytic Nevus

Definition. *Recurrent melanocytic nevus* presents as a pigmented patch at the site of prior removal of a benign nevus by shave biopsy. Histologically, the lesion may have unusual architectural features that can be misinterpreted as melanoma, and for this reason, some were described by Kornberg and Maize and Ackerman (37,93) under the term "pseudomelanoma." It has also been averred that these lesions are not strictly recurrent but rather "persistent" (94), however, the term "recurrent" seems appropriate due to the appearance of the atypical junctional nevoid

Table 2-3

FEATURES HELPFUL IN DIFFERENTIATING DEEP PENETRATING NEVUS AND NODULAR MELANOMA

	Deep Penetrating Nevus	Nodular Melanoma
Architecture		
Size	Smaller (>1 cm)	Tend to be larger
Epidermal involvement	Occasional junctional nests	May be prominent, pagetoid
Ulceration	Absent	May be present
Symmetry	May be absent	Often absent
Coalescent nests	Present	Present
Involvement of fat	May be present	Present in level V lesions
Maturation	Incomplete or absent	Absent
Destructive expansile growth	Absent	Present
Horizontal:vertical dimension ratio	Often <1	Often >1
Cytology		
Enlarged epithelioid cells	Present	Present
Nuclear atypia	Present	Present
Deep melanin synthesis	Present	Present
Mitoses	Rare	Variable, often numerous
Necrosis	Absent	Often present
Admixed melanophages	Present	Variable

proliferation in the newly formed regenerating epithelium rather than the adjacent undisturbed epithelium and based on the clinical observation of reappearance of pigmentation in a previously unpigmented site. Truly persistent nevus is often present as well, usually at the base.

Clinical Features. Recurrent hyperpigmentation may follow the incomplete removal of any form of benign or malignant melanocytic lesion, but the phenomenon is most commonly seen after shave biopsy of a compound nevus. Recurrence sometimes follows removal of a dermal nevus where there is no epidermal component, and often the initial specimen, on review, does not show nevus cells extending to the margin. This recurrence appears to be different from the simple recurrence of an incompletely excised neoplasm, and may be a proliferation of intraepidermal melanocytes stimulated by growth factors in the healing wound. Accordingly, such lesions are designated as representing the recurrent nevus phenomenon, in contradistinction to residual or persistent nevi, where nevus cells not initially eradicated occur in association with scar tissue. Even so, some authorities prefer the use of the term "persistent nevus," arguing that there must have been a residual nevus as the source of the recurrence (94a). The observation that cells within healing scar tissue are an important source for synthesis of growth factors,

such as c-kit ligand, for which melanocytes and nevus cells express receptors, supports the recurrence associated with scar tissue theory (95).

Repigmentation of a recurrent nevus characteristically occurs rapidly, within 6 weeks or so. This rapid repigmentation helps differentiate recurrent nevus from recurrence of a melanoma which, in our experience, somewhat paradoxically tends to occur over a much slower time course of months or years. By the time a recurrent nevus presents clinically, its growth has usually ceased. Clinically or histologically, the observation of a scar at the site of a pigmented lesion should prompt a careful inquiry as to any history of prior removal at that site, a history that is sometimes not offered spontaneously by patients to clinicians, or by clinicians to pathologists.

The recurrent pigmentation is typically macular, tan to dark brown, with slightly indefinite irregular borders. Importantly, it does not extend beyond the borders of the scar (fig. 2-34), as may happen with the recurrence of incompletely excised radial growth phase melanoma. Most of these lesions do not particularly suggest melanoma clinically, but they are often sampled or excised to rule out melanoma because of the history of recurrence. The observation of pigment activity spreading beyond the original scar suggests recurrent or persistent melanoma, both clinically and histologically.

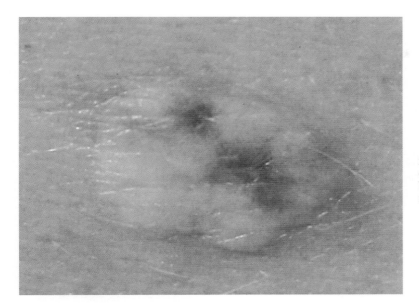

Figure 2-34

RECURRENT ("PERSISTENT") NEVUS

An area of repigmentation has appeared in the scar of a previous shave excision of a nevus. The pigment does not extend beyond the lateral border of the scar. (Fig. B from Plate II, Fascicle 2, Third Series.)

Microscopic Findings. As discussed by Maize and Ackerman (37), a recurrent nevus may have many features in common with melanoma in situ, including breadth greater than 6 mm, variably sized and shaped intraepidermal nests that are sometimes confluent, the presence of single cells and nests above the dermal-epidermal junction (although rarely in the stratum corneum), and marked hyperpigmentation due to melanin synthesis by the recurrent nevus cells (figs. 2-35, 2-36). In recurrent nevus, nests usually predominate over single cells, however, and there is little or no cytologic atypia, although the recurrent junctional cells often are enlarged and epithelioid. Further, mitoses are usually absent (although rare mitoses in the epidermis do not rule out the diagnosis).

The junctional nests of recurrent nevus arise within an atrophic epidermal layer that generally overlies scar tissue. Accordingly, the nests may be dyshesive, irregular in size and shape, and by definition, cannot arise in association with the rete ridges that typify the nonatrophic epidermis. Importantly, the junctional component does not extend beyond the horizontal limits of the underlying scar. Residual nevi tend to consist of banal dermal nevic elements architecturally distorted by associated scar tissue (fig. 2-35). Occasional lesions have junctional changes consistent with the recurrent nevus phenomenon and dermal nevic elements consistent with residual nevus. In these and also in other cases in which there

is no residual nevus, it is judicious to obtain the prior nevus for review (fig. 2-36).

Recurrent Spitz nevus may show features similar to those of more banal nevi, but in addition, shows a greater tendency to proliferation in the dermis (94) (see Spindle and Epithelioid Cell Melanocytic Tumor [Spitz Tumor/Nevus]).

In a study of 173 cases of recurrent/persistent nevi, Park et al. (96) found pagetoid scattering of cells in 3 percent, moderate nuclear atypia in 12 percent, and rare mitoses in 8 percent of cases. None of the original nevi, on review, had these features to a worrisome degree. According to these authors, features suggestive of melanoma in a recurrent melanocytic lesion include an interval of recurrence greater than 6 months, markedly atypical melanocytes, solid infiltrating nests of melanocytes in the dermis (vertical growth phase), and the presence of an atypical intraepidermal melanocytic proliferation away from the scar and beyond the original borders of the nevus.

In a "difficult" lesion of this type, the pathologist's "comfort level" may be improved by noting that even if the intraepidermal component is worrisome, there is certainly no evidence of any tumorigenic malignant proliferation in the dermis. The dermis usually reveals evidence of the previous procedure in the form of fibrosis, with or without residual benign dermal collections of nevus cells. In lesions where the features are at all suggestive of melanoma, we obtain the

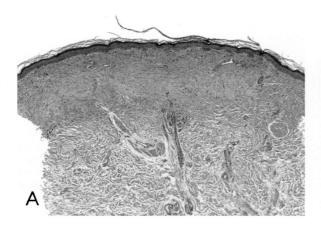

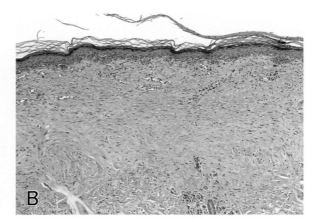

Figure 2-35

RECURRENT NEVUS

A: There is a scar in the dermis.

B: Higher magnification reveals an increased number of nevoid to epithelioid melanocytes at the dermal-epidermal junction. This proliferation is confined to the epidermis above the scar and does not extend into the native epidermis beyond the scar.

C,D: The cells are arranged as single cells and nests that tend to become confluent. There may be pagetoid extension of single cells into the epidermis. In this example, the pigmented keratinocytes add to an impression of pagetoid spread in the epidermis.

E: Intermediate magnification of another field shows extensive continuous proliferation of atypical melanocytes in the epidermis. In the underlying dermis, there is clear evidence of a residual nevus. Although not always seen, this is a valuable clue to the diagnosis of recurrent nevus.

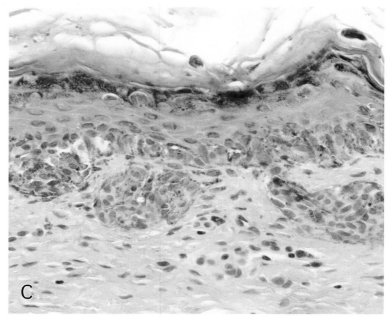

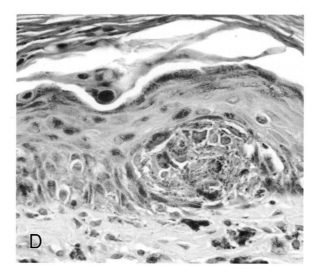

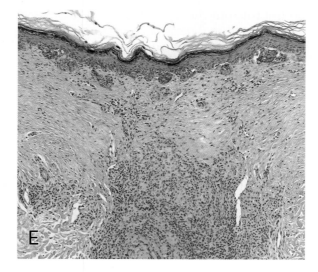

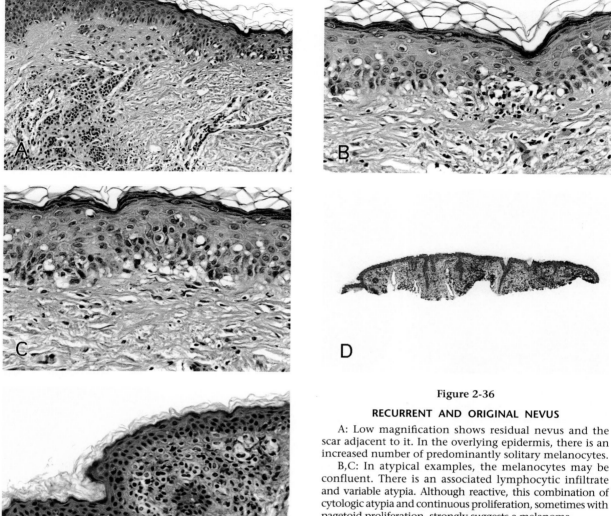

Figure 2-36

RECURRENT AND ORIGINAL NEVUS

A: Low magnification shows residual nevus and the scar adjacent to it. In the overlying epidermis, there is an increased number of predominantly solitary melanocytes.

B,C: In atypical examples, the melanocytes may be confluent. There is an associated lymphocytic infiltrate and variable atypia. Although reactive, this combination of cytologic atypia and continuous proliferation, sometimes with pagetoid proliferation, strongly suggests a melanoma.

D,E: It is always desirable to review the previously excised nevus, which is usually removed by a shave biopsy and not always with positive margins. At high magnification, this nevus is composed of benign nevus cells.

prior biopsy for review (figs. 2-36, 2-37). On review, such lesions have included not only common nevi but also dysplastic nevi, and some of the more florid simulants of melanoma we have seen have in fact been examples of incompletely excised dysplastic nevi. We have observed other cases where the recurrent lesion had diagnostic characteristics of melanoma. In these circumstances, the prior material was malignant on review, even cases in which the malignancy had been missed by the referring pathologists. As long as such a recurrent melanoma is still in the radial growth phase, whether in situ or microinvasive, the patients can be reassured that their prognosis is excellent and has not been altered by the delay. However, we have unfortunately seen some lesions that progressed during the delay from radial to vertical growth phase with potential for metastasis.

Traumatized nevi that have not been previously biopsied also occasionally demonstrate intraepidermal changes in keeping with the recurrent nevus phenomenon. As is the case with recurrent nevi at biopsy sites, the intraepidermal

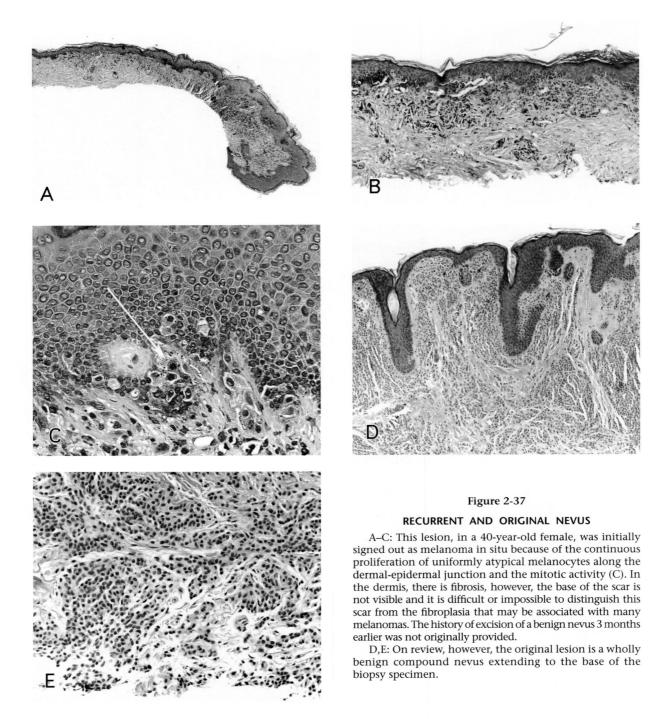

Figure 2-37

RECURRENT AND ORIGINAL NEVUS

A–C: This lesion, in a 40-year-old female, was initially signed out as melanoma in situ because of the continuous proliferation of uniformly atypical melanocytes along the dermal-epidermal junction and the mitotic activity (C). In the dermis, there is fibrosis, however, the base of the scar is not visible and it is difficult or impossible to distinguish this scar from the fibroplasia that may be associated with many melanomas. The history of excision of a benign nevus 3 months earlier was not originally provided.

D,E: On review, however, the original lesion is a wholly benign compound nevus extending to the base of the biopsy specimen.

proliferation subsequent to trauma should be exquisitely localized above a zone of superficial dermal stromal changes consistent with traumatic injury. If there is no clinical history of trauma, however, it is prudent to regard such proliferations as potentially dysplastic, and to recommend complete excision.

Table 2-4 summarizes certain features helpful in separating recurrent melanocytic nevus from recurrent radial growth phase melanoma.

Table 2-4

FEATURES HELPFUL IN DIFFERENTIATING RECURRENT NEVUS PHENOMENON AND RECURRENT RADIAL GROWTH PHASE (RGP) MELANOMA

	Recurrent Nevus	RGP Melanoma
Architecture		
Epidermis	Atrophic, no rete ridges	Variable, rete often present
Dyshesive growth	Often present	Often present
Pagetoid growth	Occasional, low level	Often present, high level
Irregular junctional nests	Often present	Often present
Confluent junctional nests	Often present	Often present
Extension beyond scar	Absent	Present
Breadth >6 mm	Often	Often
Cytology		
Enlarged epithelioid cells	Present	Present
Nuclear atypia	Absent	Present
Melanin synthesis	Present	Often present
Mitoses	Rare to absent	Variable, often present
Necrosis	Absent	Occasionally present

NEVI OF SPECIAL SITES

Nevi on the skin of particular body sites and in physiologic states such as old or young age or pregnancy may show patterns of junctional or dermal proliferation that deviate from ordinary acquired nevi and cause confusion with atypical and dysplastic nevi and melanoma. This relatively common, recently recognized and growing group of nevi has been termed generically, *nevi of special sites*. These lesions may show architectural features that overlap with those of melanoma and may be overdiagnosed as such, or as dysplastic nevi. Many of these lesions appear to be isolated phenomena, not associated with a measurably increased melanoma risk. At the same time, authentic melanomas and dysplastic nevi occur in these same "special sites." Undercalling a melanoma as a nevus of special site could have tragic consequences if the lesion is thereby allowed to persist and progress. Similarly, in our opinion, it is important to recognize truly dysplastic nevi as such, so that patients who are at increased risk for melanoma (which varies from slight to extreme depending on other risk factors) can be identified and offered appropriate follow-up (97). Some special site nevi are difficult to interpret due to atypical or unusual features of the intraepidermal and superficial dermal components, or from frankly tumorigenic proliferation of atypical melanocytes in the dermis.

Nevus of Genital Skin

Definition. *Nevus of genital skin* is a benign melanocytic nevus that has certain histologic features that imperfectly simulate some aspects of dysplastic nevi and melanomas, including the presence of large cells with prominent nucleoli arranged in large dyshesive nests. This nevus is most often seen on the vulva of young (premenopausal) women, but similar lesions also occur, uncommonly, on the male genitalia (37,98–100).

Clinical Features. These are benign nevi that are often removed incidentally during pregnancy, often at the time of delivery. Certain histologic features, however, may arouse suspicion of melanoma on pathologic examination. Clinically, they are typically symmetric and papular, most often smaller than 1 cm in diameter, and usually uniformly pigmented; they have discrete well-circumscribed borders. These atypical changes are rare in vulvar nevi; in a comparative histologic study, all but a few lesions were indistinguishable from control nevi of nonvulvar skin (98). Vulvar nevi are uncommon: in a study of 301 new patients in a gynecology practice, the prevalence of melanocytic nevi on the vulvar skin was only 2.3 percent (101).

Atypical features are a histologic curiosity seen in a minority of vulvar nevi, with no clinical significance except the possibility of diagnostic error. In our consultation practices,

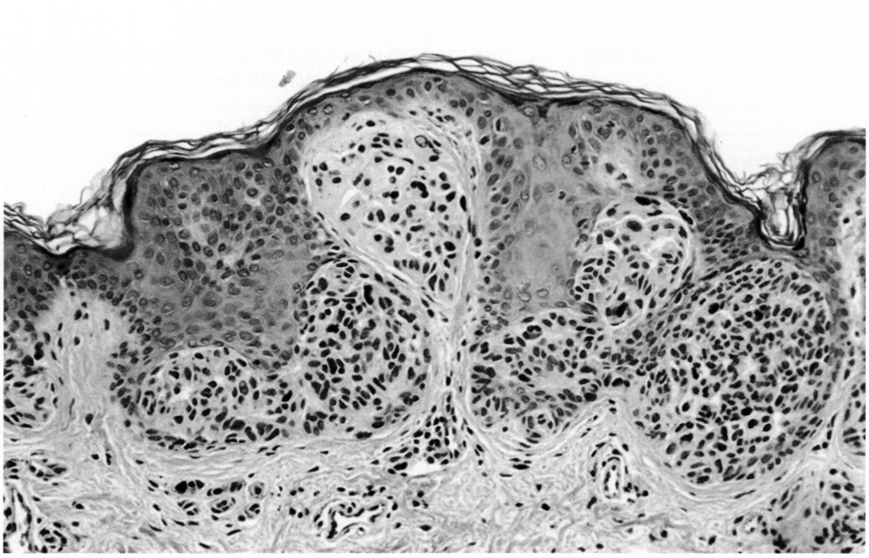

Figure 2-38

GENITAL PATTERN NEVUS

Large cells are present in large nests at the junction.

we have seen tragic examples of diagnostic errors that have been followed by unnecessary ablative surgery in young women. Occasionally, we have observed these lesions in women who have characteristic dysplastic nevi elsewhere on their skin, but we do not regard these genital nevi as indicative, in themselves, of any generalized cutaneous diathesis. If an incompletely excised lesion presents atypical features similar to those described in this section, it is prudent to recommend complete excision so that the whole lesion can be examined and to prevent recurrence; however, wide excision of any kind is not indicated for these benign simulants of dysplastic nevi and malignant melanoma.

Microscopic Findings. The scanning magnification impression is typically that of a small, well-circumscribed papular lesion composed of nevus cells arranged in clusters in the papillary dermis, and arranged mainly in nests in the epidermis where the cells do not extend beyond the shoulder of the dermal component. The epidermal nests may vary considerably in size and shape, tending to become confluent. The position of the nests varies as well, originating from the sides as well as the tips of the rete ridges, and often oriented parallel to the surface (fig. 2-38). Single cells and nests of nevus cells are occasionally seen within the epithelia of skin adnexa (102), a feature shared with congenital nevi. The epidermis may show markedly irregular thickening, resulting in an impression of

asymmetric nevus cell proliferation (fig. 2-39). The keratinocytic proliferation differs from the lentiginous elongation of rete ridges seen in dysplastic nevi because it is less regular.

Cytologically, cells forming nevi of genital skin may be larger than nevus cells occurring elsewhere, particularly within the superficial component, where they also may have eosinophilic nuclei. There is no mitotic activity or individual cell necrosis, however, and generally cells demonstrate maturation with descent into the deeper dermal layers (fig. 2-39).

In a formal study of 56 atypical genital nevi, the median patient age was 26 years (range, 6 to 54 years) (100). The dominant histologic feature was a lentiginous and nested junctional component composed of prominent round or fusiform nests, often with retraction artifact and cellular dyshesion. Cytologic atypia was severe in 20 percent of the cases. Focal pagetoid spread was seen in about 20 percent of the cases, usually not beyond the mid-spinous layer. The lesions had a large common dermal nevus component, often with dermal nuclear atypia. There were occasional dermal mitoses, seen in 7 percent of the cases. Maturation was present in all cases. Only 1 lesion recurred, after incomplete excision, and subsequent follow-up of this and all other lesions was benign. Recognition of this group of melanocytic lesions is important to avoid overdiagnosis and overtreatment (100).

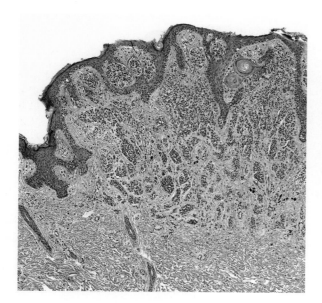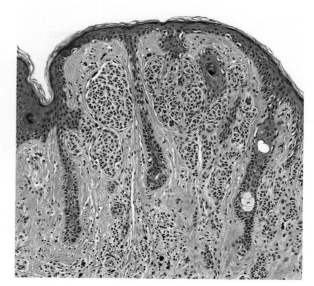

Figure 2-39

GENITAL PATTERN NEVUS

Maturation of lesional cells is seen from superficial to deep (left), with large cells in junctional nests (right).

Differential Diagnosis. Genital lentigines and nevi with concurrent changes of lichen sclerosus may show a lichenoid lymphocytic infiltrate and pigment incontinence, with melanophages in a fibrosed papillary dermis, reminiscent of completely or partially regressed melanoma. Confluent nests varying in size and shape, and pagetoid upward spread of melanocytic nests and single melanocytes, have been described in a few nevi associated with lichen sclerosus (103). Atypical nevi in patients with lichen sclerosus have also been likened to persistent (or recurrent) melanocytic nevi (see Recurrent Melanocytic Nevus) (104).

The suspicion of nodular melanoma that is falsely aroused by the cellular growth patterns and large, dyshesive nests at low magnification may appear to be confirmed by the observation at higher power of large cells in the epidermis and upper dermis. Most genital nevi, however, are small and well circumscribed and show evidence of maturation of the dermal component toward the base of the nevus at the interface of the papillary and reticular dermis. Some of the lesional cells may have eosinophilic nucleoli, but there are usually no mitoses and no necrosis. Occasional lesions with a rare mitosis in our opinion should be interpreted cautiously, and

completely excised (98). Further, there is little or no pagetoid extension of atypical melanocytes into the epidermis, there is no shoulder of intraepidermal proliferation (radial growth phase) at the edge of the dermal component of the lesions, and in the dermis, there is no evidence of an expansile, pushing, or infiltrating destructive mass lesion (vertical growth phase melanoma). When such extension is observed, the possibility that the lesion is a melanoma should be seriously considered. In addition, we have seen an occasional example of melanoma in situ adjacent to a lesion judged to be a vulvar nevus (fig. 2-40). Table 2-5 summarizes the features helpful in differentiating nevi of genital skin from vulvar melanoma.

Distinguishing a nevus of the genital type without high-grade atypia from a banal compound nevus occurring elsewhere is unimportant, because neither lesion has any clinical implication, as long as it is not mistaken for a melanoma. The lentiginous patterns with regular rete ridge elongation that characterize dysplastic nevi are not as a rule seen in genital nevi, and most of these patients do not have dysplastic nevi elsewhere on the skin. We have seen a few unequivocal examples of dysplastic nevi on the skin of the labia, but not on the mucous membrane epithelium.

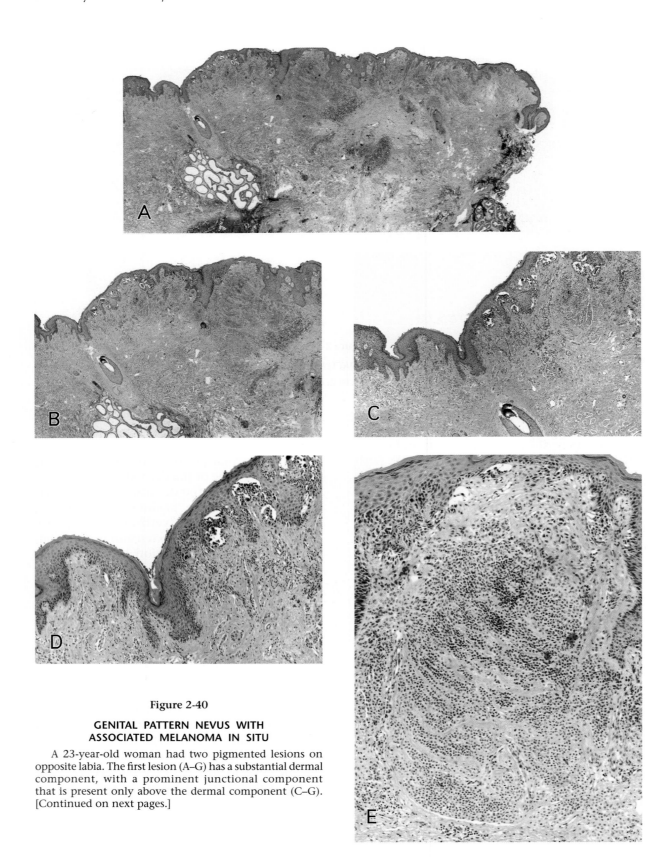

Figure 2-40

**GENITAL PATTERN NEVUS WITH
ASSOCIATED MELANOMA IN SITU**

A 23-year-old woman had two pigmented lesions on opposite labia. The first lesion (A–G) has a substantial dermal component, with a prominent junctional component that is present only above the dermal component (C–G). [Continued on next pages.]

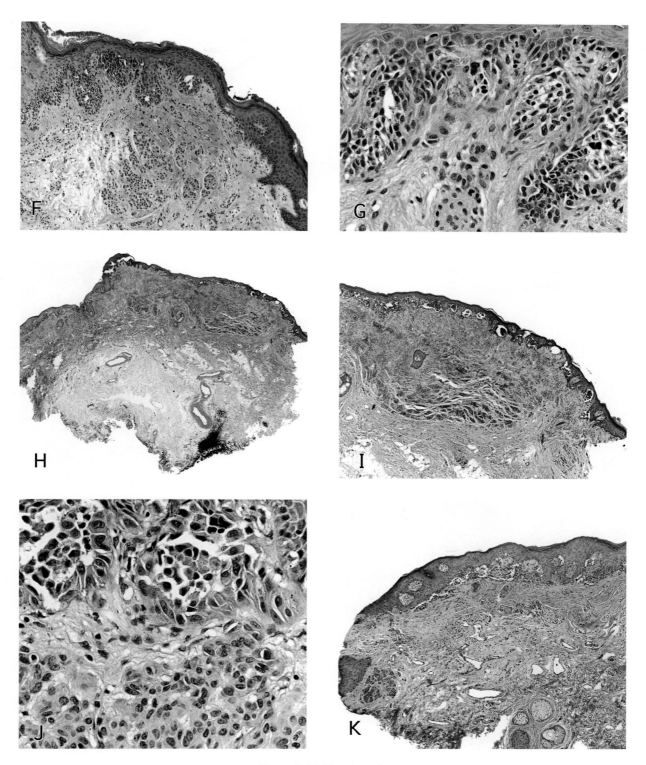

Figure 2-40 (Continued)

At higher magnification, the lesional cells in the epidermis are large and tend to be dyshesive (G), however, there is evidence of maturation from superficial to deep in the dermal component (E,F). In the second lesion (H–K), there is a junctional component that extends beyond the dermal component (J) and close to a margin (K,L).

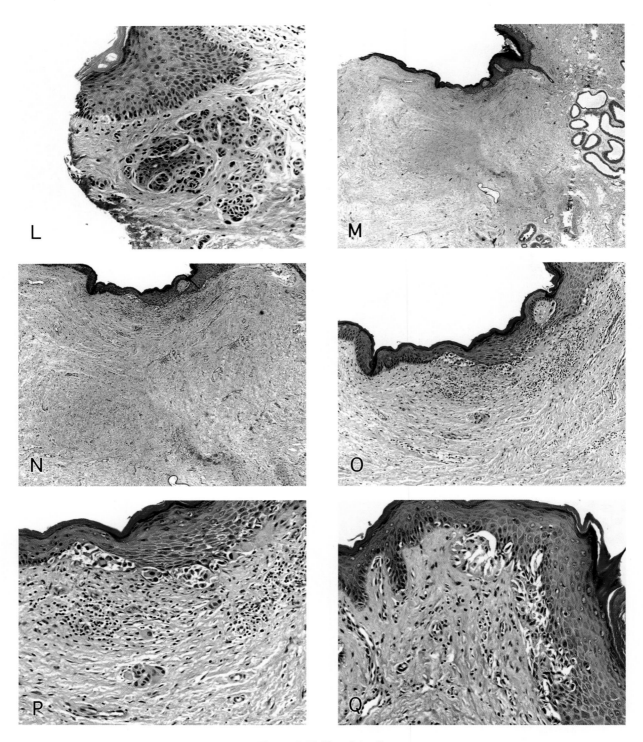

Figure 2-40 (Continued)

This finding was concerning for melanoma in situ arising in association with a nevus of genital skin. In a reexcision specimen (M–Q), there is a scar in the lamina propria (L) within the overlying melanocytic proliferation. This is associated with a lymphocytic infiltrate (M), within which are uniformly atypical cells in the epidermis and a few similar cells in the dermis, consistent with in situ and microinvasive melanoma (N,O). Elsewhere in the epidermis, uniformly atypical melanocytes are in continuity along the basal epidermal layer, consistent with melanoma in situ (P,Q).

Table 2-5

FEATURES HELPFUL IN DIFFERENTIATING COMPOUND NEVUS OF GENITAL SKIN AND VULVAR MELANOMA

	Nevus of Genital Skin	Vulvar Melanoma
Architecture		
Size	Smaller (<1 cm)	Tend to be larger
Shoulder within epidermis	Absent	Often present
Lentiginous epidermal component	Absent	Often present
Pagetoid growth	Absent	Occasionally present
Coalescent junctional nests	Present	Occasionally present
Irregular junctional nests	Present	Occasionally present
Asymmetric keratinocyte proliferation	Present	Variable to absent
Asymmetric junctional component	Absent	Present
Asymmetric dermal component	Absent	Often present
Cytology		
Enlarged cells	Present superficially	Present diffusely
Eosinophilic nucleoli	May be present	Present
Maturation	Present	Generally absent
Mitoses	Absent	Often present
Necrosis	Absent	Often present

Again, nevi of the genital type in young to middle-aged women that show significant cytologic atypia or any mitotic activity are best modestly excised to prevent local persistence or recurrence, and to rule out any additional pathology that might contribute to the diagnosis.

Nevus of the Breast

In a recent study, 101 *nevi from the breast area* were compared with 97 from elsewhere (105). The breast nevi exhibited significantly more atypical features than nevi from other sites. In particular, nevi with intraepidermal melanocytes, melanocytic atypia, and dermal fibroplasia were significantly more numerous in the breast area. Interestingly, there was no gender difference in incidence. Whether this represents a finding related to the site of occurrence of entirely banal nevi (as with genital nevi) or a proclivity for nevi with dysplastic features to favor breast skin has yet to be resolved. At present, we report the atypia and generally recommend conservative complete excision for such lesions. It is important, in our opinion, not to under-report dysplastic nevi in special sites, and it is obviously important as well not to misdiagnose a melanoma as a nevus (figs. 2-41–2-44) (97).

Nevus of Acral Skin

Although some older reports suggested that *acral nevi* should be removed to prevent malig-nant change, these nevi are present in as many as 4 to 9 percent of the population (106), and melanomas are rare in acral sites. Histologically, acral nevi tend to be more cellular than most common nevi, and the nevus cells may be arranged in predominantly lentiginous rather than nested patterns in the epidermis. Occasional low-level pagetoid, single cell migration into the stratum spinosum, and even transepidermal elimination of effete pigmented nevus cells within the normally compacted acral stratum granulosum, may be observed. These features perhaps account for the suspicion traditionally directed toward acral nevi. There is no evidence, however, that these lesions are frequent precursors or risk markers for acral melanoma.

Acral nevi tend to be circumscribed, light brown lesions that are usually impalpable and flat to side-lighting (fig. 2-45). They are generally stable, and are more often junctional than are nevi of the trunk. Like other nevi, they probably involute and disappear over time.

Histologically, lentiginous proliferation of melanocytes is often prominent, with moderate amounts of melanin pigment; there may be variably sized and shaped nests of melanocytes at the interface. Nevus cells in the dermis, unlike melanoma cells, mature to the lesional base (figs. 2-46–2-49). There may be patchy lymphocytes and occasional melanophages in the dermis.

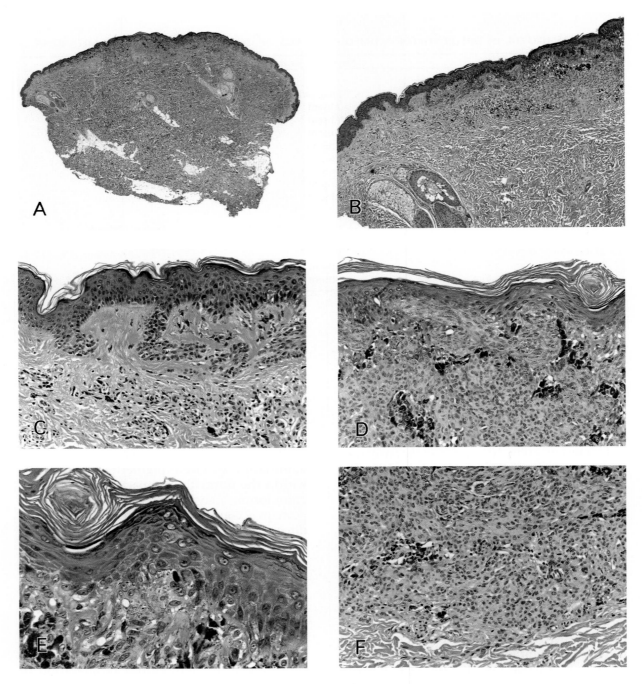

Figure 2-41

NEVUS OF THE BREAST IN A CHILD

A,B: This lesion in an 11-year-old child is broad at scanning magnification.

C: At higher magnification, there are nests bridging adjacent elongated rete ridges, as is seen in melanocytic dysplasia.

D: The cells are uniformly large, with large nuclei and fairly prominent nucleoli.

E,F: The dermal component shows evidence of maturation from superficial to deep. It is not clear whether this lesion should be regarded as a nevus of special sites (breast) or a dysplastic nevus. We favor the latter interpretation, and would recommend evaluation of the patient's other risk factors for melanoma development.

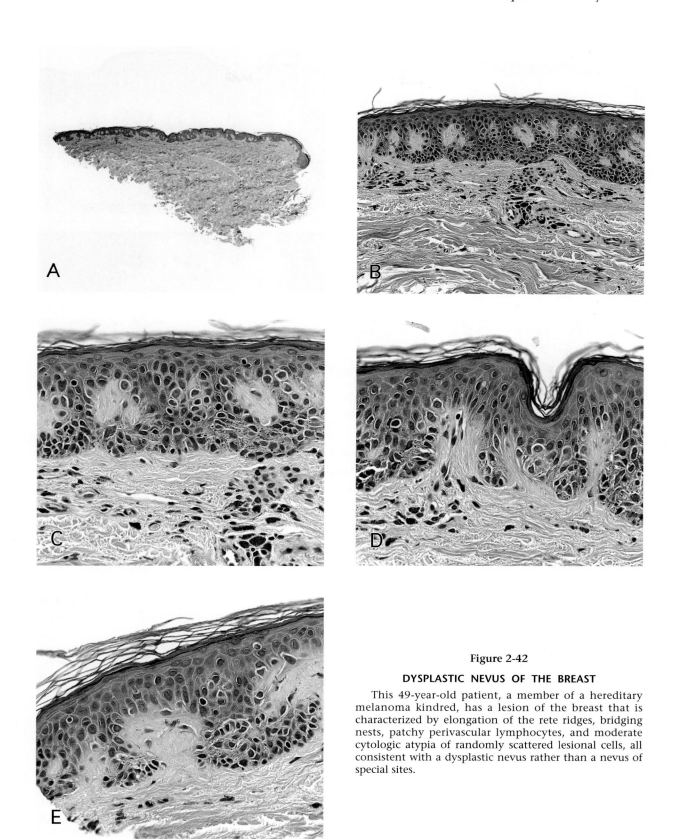

Figure 2-42

DYSPLASTIC NEVUS OF THE BREAST

This 49-year-old patient, a member of a hereditary melanoma kindred, has a lesion of the breast that is characterized by elongation of the rete ridges, bridging nests, patchy perivascular lymphocytes, and moderate cytologic atypia of randomly scattered lesional cells, all consistent with a dysplastic nevus rather than a nevus of special sites.

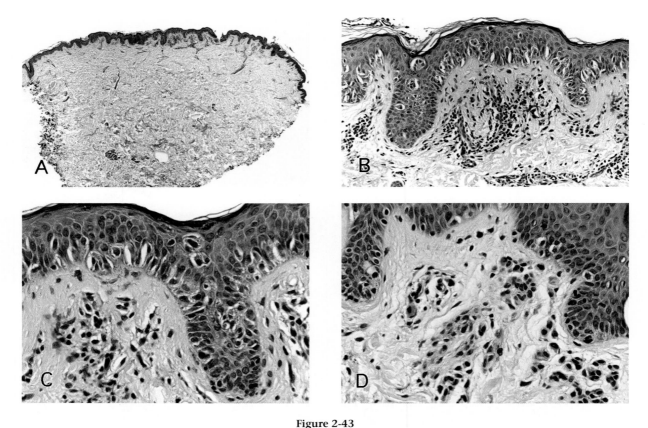

Figure 2-43

MELANOMA IN SITU OF THE BREAST

This lesion in a 42-year-old female is broad and quite cellular, and shows effacement of the rete ridges (A). There is an increased number of uniformly atypical epithelioid melanocytes present in a pagetoid pattern in the epidermis (B,C). Focally, there are mature nevus cells in the dermis (D). These features are consistent with melanoma in situ arising in a nevus. The patient is a member of a hereditary melanoma kindred. Her brother had four melanomas. Such a lesion should not be underdiagnosed as a nevus of special sites.

Some of these features may suggest a dysplastic nevus; however, the rete ridge pattern of keratinocytes does not show the uniform elongation with occasional accentuation of the anastomosing pattern of rete that characterizes dysplastic nevi. If these features are present, and if there is slight to moderate random atypia in a minority of the junctional epithelioid cell population, the diagnosis of dysplastic nevus can reasonably be made in a lesion of acral skin.

Pagetoid proliferation is occasionally striking in an acral nevus. If there is no severe uniform atypia or mitotic activity, and if there is maturation of lesional cells in the dermis, this finding is consistent with a benign nevus. Some other examples may be impossible to distinguish from melanoma in situ and may be reported descriptively as a "superficial atypical melanocytic proliferation of uncertain significance" (SAMPUS), with a recommendation for complete excision (figs. 2-50–2-52). A Spitz tumor may occur on acral skin and should be distinguished from a melanoma (fig. 2-53).

Nevus of Flexural Skin

Like acral regions, other body sites also show lentiginous and nested patterns of junctional proliferation that may deviate from ordinary acquired nevi and cause confusion with atypical and dysplastic nevi. One such recognized site involves *nevi of flexural skin* (107). Such nevi show greater variability in the size of the junctional nests as well as origin of nests at the edges of rete ridges and in inter-rete regions, features that also occur in dysplastic nevi (figs. 2-54–2-57). Cytologic atypia and associated

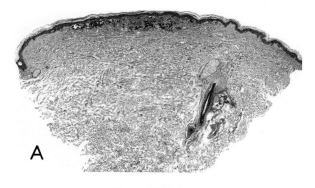

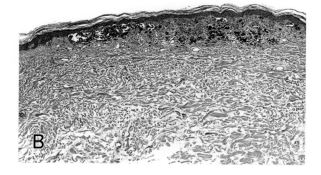

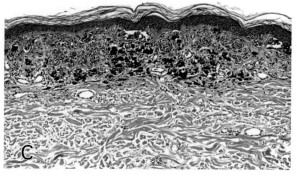

Figure 2-44

NEVUS OF THE BREAST

This lesion, in a 65-year-old woman, shows large nests that become confluent near the dermal-epidermal junction. In the dermis, large cells in nests are uniform in size and shape, and there is some evidence of nevoid maturation. These features are consistent with a nevus of special sites. The possibility of a dysplastic nevus should be considered, in our opinion, and the patient should be offered screening skin examination and possible surveillance, depending on the findings.

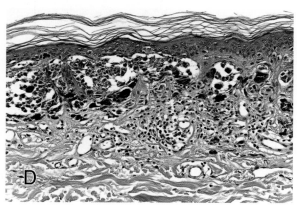

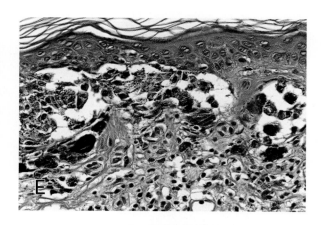

Figure 2-45

ACRAL JUNCTIONAL NEVUS FOLLOWING DERMATOGLYPHS

Although somewhat irregular and asymmetric, this lesion respects the marking patterns of the skin and is uniformly colored, consistent with a benign, predominantly junctional acral nevus.

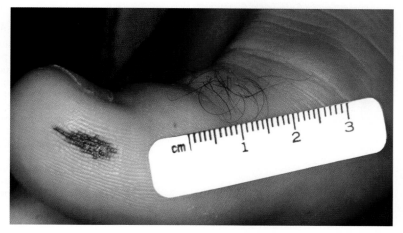

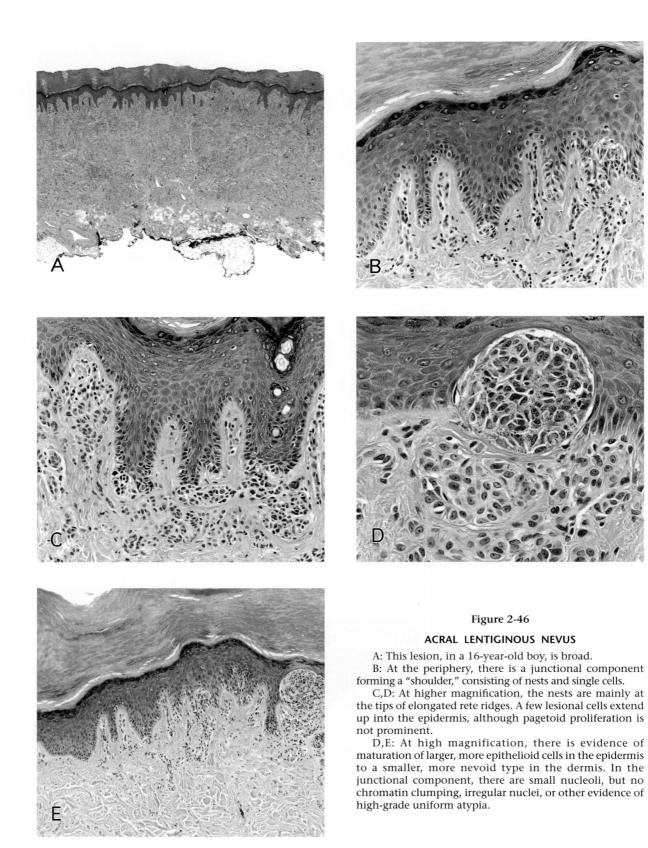

Figure 2-46

ACRAL LENTIGINOUS NEVUS

A: This lesion, in a 16-year-old boy, is broad.

B: At the periphery, there is a junctional component forming a "shoulder," consisting of nests and single cells.

C,D: At higher magnification, the nests are mainly at the tips of elongated rete ridges. A few lesional cells extend up into the epidermis, although pagetoid proliferation is not prominent.

D,E: At high magnification, there is evidence of maturation of larger, more epithelioid cells in the epidermis to a smaller, more nevoid type in the dermis. In the junctional component, there are small nucleoli, but no chromatin clumping, irregular nuclei, or other evidence of high-grade uniform atypia.

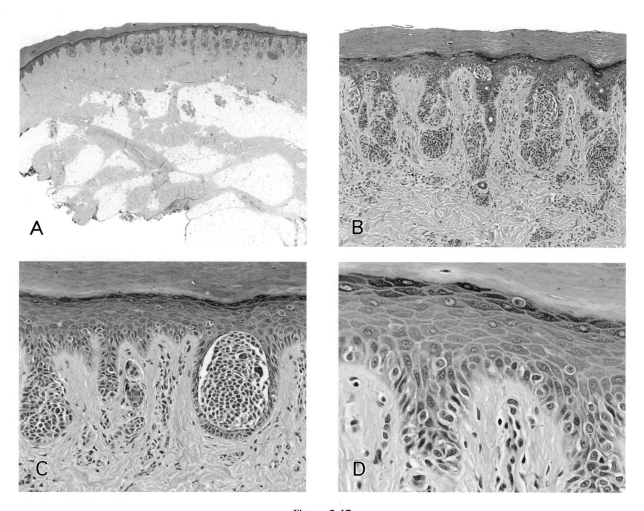

Figure 2-47

ACRAL LENTIGINOUS NEVUS IN A CHILD

A: This lesion, in a 5-year-old boy, is quite broad, with nests in the epidermis, predominantly at the tips of elongated rete ridges.

B,C: Maturation to a smaller, more nevoid cell type is evident in the dermis.

D: Single cells between the nests form a lentiginous pattern, with some pagetoid extension into the epidermis. This latter feature could raise concern for melanoma in situ (especially in an older patient), however, the cytologic atypia is minimal.

stromal alterations typical of dysplastic nevi are, however, lacking in nevi of the flexural type (figs. 2-56, 2-57). The nests of flexural nevi are often separated from adjacent keratinocytes by thin semilunar clefts, a finding that also occurs in Spitz tumors/nevi, but one usually not observed in dysplastic nevi.

Knowledge of the regional anatomy occurrence of a lesion is increasingly important for the accurate interpretation of the biologic significance of variations in growth patterns of acquired melanocytic nevi. At the same time,

care should be taken to recognize dysplastic nevi and melanomas when they occur in these sites (figs. 2-54, 2-55). Melanomas are rare in sun-protected sites, however, dysplastic nevi preferentially occur in such sites. In case of doubt, a lesion can be signed out descriptively, with a note that the differential diagnosis includes a dysplastic nevus. It would then be reasonable for the clinician to reassess the patient's other cutaneous nevi, skin phenotype, and sun-exposure history as well as family history for melanoma risk assessment.

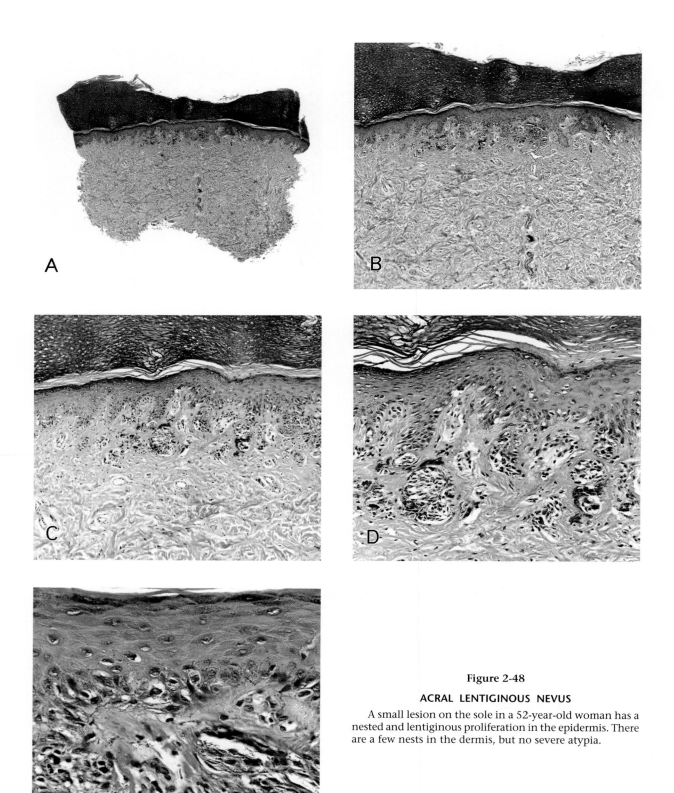

Figure 2-48

ACRAL LENTIGINOUS NEVUS

A small lesion on the sole in a 52-year-old woman has a nested and lentiginous proliferation in the epidermis. There are a few nests in the dermis, but no severe atypia.

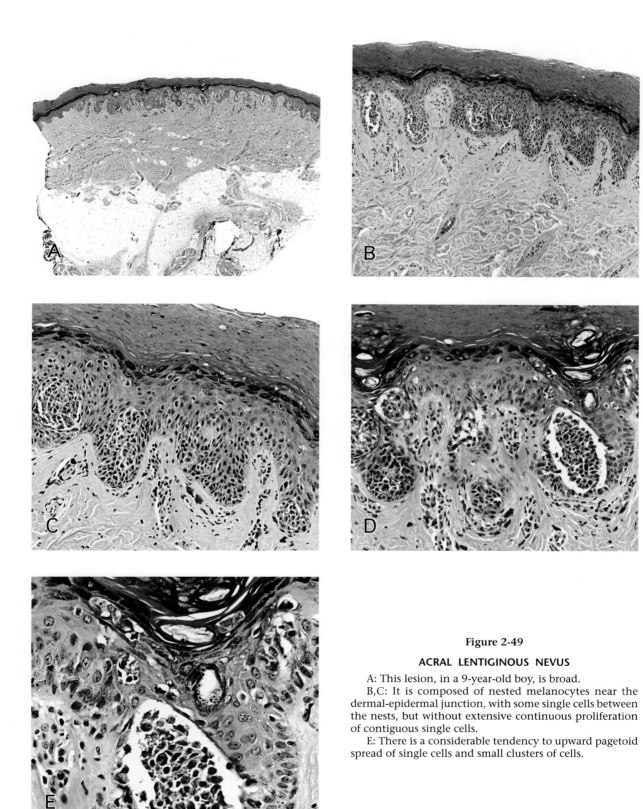

Figure 2-49

ACRAL LENTIGINOUS NEVUS

A: This lesion, in a 9-year-old boy, is broad.

B,C: It is composed of nested melanocytes near the dermal-epidermal junction, with some single cells between the nests, but without extensive continuous proliferation of contiguous single cells.

E: There is a considerable tendency to upward pagetoid spread of single cells and small clusters of cells.

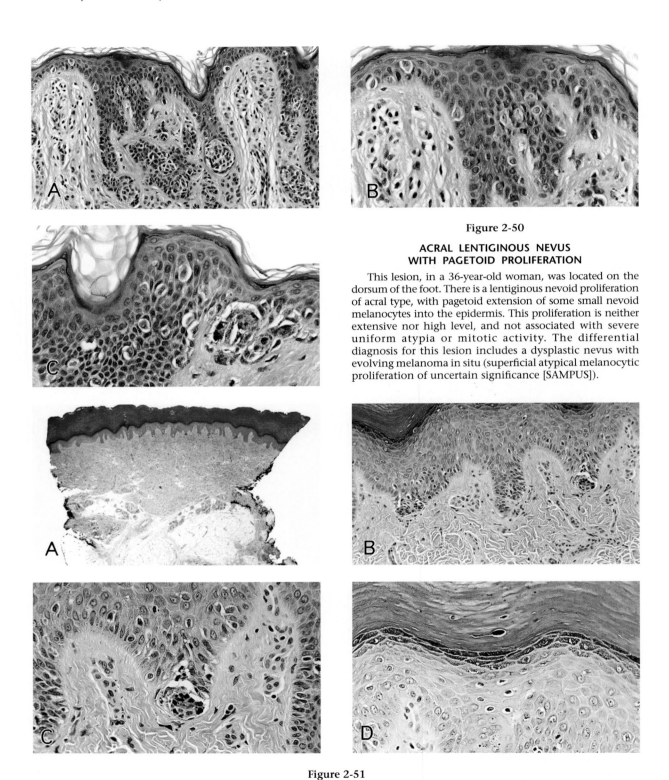

Figure 2-50

**ACRAL LENTIGINOUS NEVUS
WITH PAGETOID PROLIFERATION**

This lesion, in a 36-year-old woman, was located on the dorsum of the foot. There is a lentiginous nevoid proliferation of acral type, with pagetoid extension of some small nevoid melanocytes into the epidermis. This proliferation is neither extensive nor high level, and not associated with severe uniform atypia or mitotic activity. The differential diagnosis for this lesion includes a dysplastic nevus with evolving melanoma in situ (superficial atypical melanocytic proliferation of uncertain significance [SAMPUS]).

Figure 2-51

ACRAL NEVUS WITH PAGETOID PROLIFERATION

A: This is a broad lesion in a 12-year-old.
B,C: The lentiginous proliferation is subtle, with only a few nests.
C,D: A few nevoid melanocytes are seen above the basal layer, some as far as the stratum corneum.

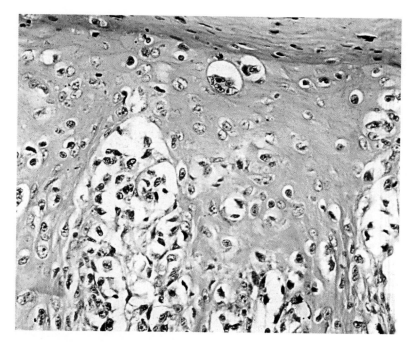

Figure 2-52

ACRAL LENTIGINOUS MELANOMA WITH PAGETOID MELANOCYTIC PROLIFERATION

Included for comparison with nevi with pagetoid proliferation, this lesion shows extensive pagetoid proliferation of uniformly atypical cells into all levels of the epidermis and stratum corneum. In addition, there is continuous basal lentiginous proliferation of uniformly atypical cells.

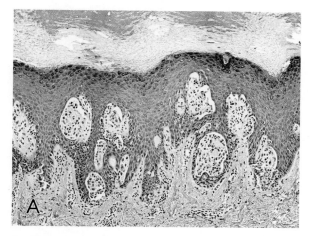

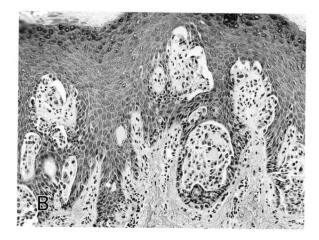

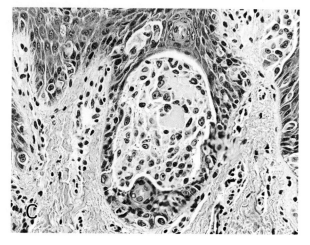

Figure 2-53

ACRAL SPITZ NEVUS

A: Large nests of large spindle and/or epithelioid cells, with clefting artifact at the dermal-epidermal junction.

B,C: Higher magnification shows the presence of globoid eosinophilic Kamino bodies (see chapter 4).

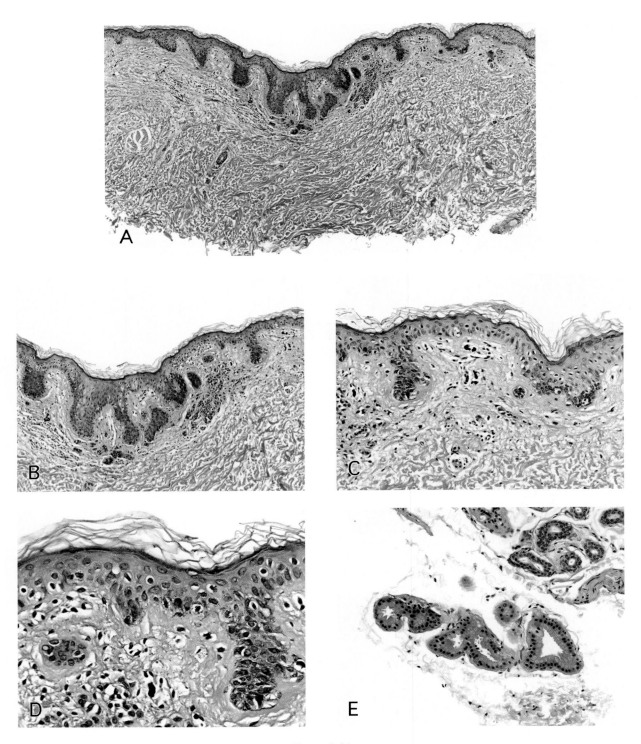

Figure 2-54

COMPOUND NEVUS OF AXILLA WITH MILD ATYPIA

There is elongation of the rete ridges, a few nests near the tips and sides of the rete, few if any bridging nests, no severe cytologic atypia, and patchy lymphocytes in the dermis. The presence of apocrine glands at the base of the biopsy (E) is a clue to its location in the axilla. This lesion should not be overinterpreted as a dysplastic nevus or an evolving melanoma.

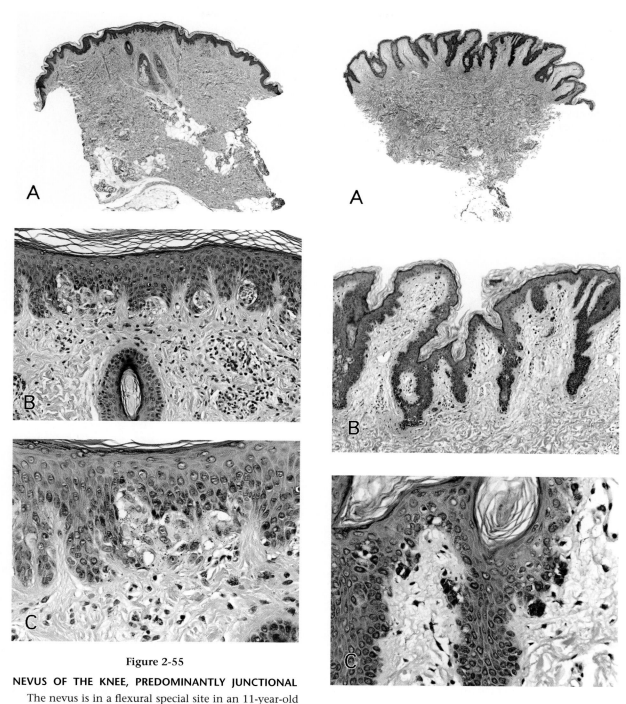

Figure 2-55

NEVUS OF THE KNEE, PREDOMINANTLY JUNCTIONAL

The nevus is in a flexural special site in an 11-year-old girl. Relatively large melanocytes are present in nests that are fairly uniform, mainly near the tips of elongated rete ridges. It is unclear whether this represents a form of melanocytic dysplasia or a nevus of special sites. Such a lesion can be signed out descriptively, with a note that the differential diagnosis includes a dysplastic nevus and that evaluation of other cutaneous nevi, skin phenotype, and family history would be appropriate for melanoma risk assessment.

Figure 2-56

NEVUS OF THE PERINEUM

This nevus shows markedly elongated, almost papillomatous, rete ridges, perhaps a reflection of the site, with nevus cells and small nests at the sides of elongated rete ridges. There is no atypia. This lesion should not be interpreted as a dysplastic nevus or an evolving melanoma.

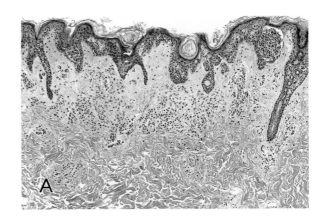

Figure 2-57

FLEXURAL NEVUS

The junctional component of this lesion is composed of large "nested and dyshesive" cells. The dermal component is mature.

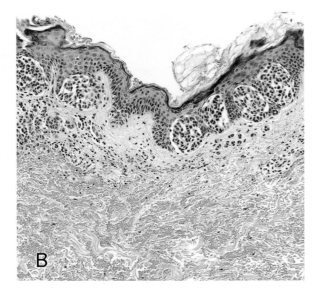

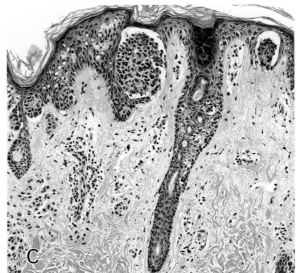

Nevus of the Head and Neck

Clinically, *nevi of the head and neck* tend to be papular lesions that are pigmented compound nevi in childhood and early adult life, and evolve into flesh-colored dermal nevi as the individual becomes older. "Skin tags," which are common on the neck, histologically represent simple fibroepithelial polyps or, occasionally, mature dermal nevi. Such lesions occasionally spontaneously infarct.

In lesions of the face and scalp, it is common to observe nevus cells in the lower third of the reticular dermis, a finding that is rare in nevi from other locations and that is considered suggestive of a small congenital nevus (see figs. 2-9, 2-10). In the absence of more specific findings, such as a lesional size greater than 1.5 cm, the presence of nevus cells within the epithelium of skin appendages, or convincing historical confirmation that the lesion was present at birth (108), we regard these lesions as most likely acquired nevi. Combined nevi, discussed above, are most common on the skin of the face.

Two recent publications (109,110) have described lesions of the ear, judged to be benign, that have shown atypical features, including poor circumscription, asymmetry, lateral extension of the junctional component beyond the dermal component, and elongation of rete ridges with bridging between them. Some cases showed uniformly large melanocytes with large vesicular nuclei and abundant pale, finely granular cytoplasm. Pagetoid spread, moderate to severe cytologic atypia, and nucleoli were also observed. None of the cases showed mitoses or apoptotic melanocytes. These features overlap with those of dysplastic nevi and melanomas, and we would recommend caution in the interpretation of lesions demonstrating combinations of these features to any significant degree. Especially in middle-aged to elderly males, the ear is a very common site for melanoma (111), and such lesions may be associated with considerable risk of local recurrence, progression, and mortality.

A recent study of nevi of the scalp in adolescents described changes characterized by the presence of large, bizarrely shaped nests of nevus cells scattered in a disorderly manner along the junction. The nests of melanocytes had a dyshesive pattern with pagetoid spread of cells above the junction (112). These findings, even when occurring in young patients, are obviously suggestive of melanoma or evolving melanoma or a severely dysplastic nevus, and should not be automatically attributed to special site status. We would agree with the authors' recommendation for complete excision of such lesions, and would add that such findings should also prompt evaluation of the patient's skin and other risk factors for melanoma. Additional evaluation and possible skin surveillance should be considered if there are other clinically atypical nevi or a family or personal history of melanoma (97).

NEVI IN SPECIAL PHYSIOLOGIC STATES

Nevus in Childhood

Nevi in childhood are often considered unusually "active" compared to nevi of adults. There are several reasons why this impression has developed. First, several variants of nevi that are more common in the young are histologically atypical or unusual in some way. Spindle and epithelioid cell nevi and halo nevi, for example, are seen much more often in children and teenagers than in adults. Congenital nevi, of course, occur in childhood, and they may show peculiar patterns of melanocytic proliferation (reviewed below). Dysplastic nevi, the most common atypical nevi in adults, are uncommon before puberty, but are not rare in teenagers. The curious phenomenon of transepidermal elimination of junctional nevus cell nests (see Spitz Nevus) has been said to be more common in juvenile nevi than in adult nevi, and this pattern may simulate the intraepidermal pagetoid spread that is a sign of melanoma (39). This

finding is common in childhood nevi: a study of 200 nevi from a pediatric hospital found 14 lesions that showed prominent upward intraepidermal nevus cell migration (113).

Clinically banal nevi also tend histologically to be more cellular and composed of somewhat larger cells in children than in adults (fig. 2-58). Moreover, superficial nevus cells in lesions from children and young adults occasionally show epithelioid cell differentiation, not dissimilar to the cytologic findings more diffusely expressed in true Spitz nevi. It is possible also that occasional mitoses may be seen in a few childhood nevi that are not melanomas or spindle and epithelioid cell nevi. These differences might be consistent with lesions that are newly evolved and in a stage of transient proliferative activity.

There may be a selection bias in these results since most excisions of nevi in children are probably done for some clinical indication other than cosmetic. In contrast, many nevi in adults are removed for strictly cosmetic reasons. The histologic findings in childhood nevi thus may be representative of abnormal morphology in many of the lesions, or may simply correlate with an evolutionary phase of active growth of the nevi. It must be recognized that melanoma is almost vanishingly rare before puberty, so that criteria must be rigorously applied before a diagnosis of melanoma is made in this age group. Lesions in adolescents are more problematic. Lesions on the scalp that may mimic melanomas in adolescents have been discussed in the section on head and neck nevi (112). Occasional markedly atypical lesions in these as in other "special sites" may show such overlap with melanoma that a descriptive diagnosis with recommendation for complete excision and follow-up is all that can be rendered.

Nevus in Pregnancy

Cutaneous hyperpigmentation is a common occurrence in pregnancy, and some patients also observe darkening or enlargement of their nevi. In our experience, the most common change is a slight uniform darkening of all or the majority of the pigmented nevi, which is usually associated with subtle generalized darkening of the skin and, especially, of the areolae. Most pregnant patients do not notice any changes in their nevi. In one study, about 10 percent of 389

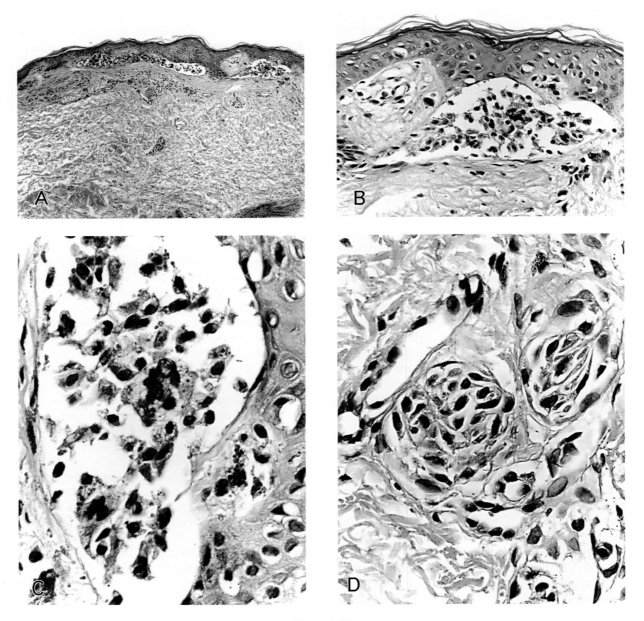

Figure 2-58

COMPOUND NEVUS WITH ATYPICAL FEATURES IN A CHILD

A–C: This lesion, in a 1-year-old child, shows large nests at the dermal-epidermal junction, with dyshesion of the lesional cells.

D: Lesional cells in the dermis mature along nevoid lines. This lesion should not be overinterpreted as a dysplastic nevus or melanoma.

pregnant women reported changes in their nevi (114), but there were no significant histologic changes in the 20 changing nevi that were excised compared to nevi from controls.

There is evidence, however, that such changing nevi do undergo cellular alterations during pregnancy, such as those relating to nevus cell apoptosis (115). Moreover, we have observed occasional nevi with unusually conspicuous epithelioid superficial components in which "blind" predictions that the patient was pregnant were validated. Further evidence that hormonal factors affect nevi may be found in the reported relationship between estrogen and melanocytic nevi with papillomatous epidermal components (116). Since pregnant patients are certainly not immune to melanoma, any changing nevus should be assessed carefully, especially if it is a change occurring in a single lesion that is "out of step" with the patient's other nevi, and especially if any of the features of evolving melanoma (discussed in detail below) are present in the lesion.

Anecdotal cases of changes in nevi induced by birth control pills have not been substantiated in our experience, and again, any changing nevi that are observed in this as in any other context should be carefully evaluated. There is no association between contraceptive use and the total number of nevi (106).

The atypical genital nevi discussed above are often removed in the course of pregnancy. Most of these genital nevi are removed incidentally, with no history of change, and similar lesions are common in patients who are not pregnant. In one study of 128 nevi removed from 86 pregnant patients (58), there were subtle changes compared to nevi from control female patients. These changes were consistent with a mild degree of histopathologic atypia or activation and rare mitoses in 11 nevi from pregnant women but in only 1 nevus from a nonpregnant patient (see also fig. 2-11). The changes were never of sufficient degree to result in diagnostic confusion with melanoma.

We have occasionally encountered nevi from premenopausal women with easily detectable, multiple mitoses within their dermal components, but without other worrisome cytologic or architectural features of melanoma, including the nevoid melanoma variant. A surprising number of these were from women who either were known to be, or proved to be, pregnant. It is cautioned, however, that all mitotically active nevi be carefully evaluated in multiple levels to exclude associated dysplasia or malignancy.

Until the significance of this phenomenon is more fully studied, modest complete excision is recommended.

Nevus in the Elderly

The life history of acquired nevi has already been discussed. As nevi age and mature, they evolve from junctional to compound nevi and then senesce, forming nonpigmented papular dermal nevi which gradually flatten into clinically normal skin. This clinical senescence is accompanied histologically by fatty infiltration or adipocyte metaplasia of the nevus, and often by neurotization, which has been discussed and illustrated earlier (see fig. 2-17).

Kerl et al. (117) have described a subset of nevi generally affecting the face of elderly individuals that contain pleomorphic epithelioid melanocytes admixed with smaller, more uniform nevus cells. These *ancient nevi* have characteristics of Meischer nevi (see above); exhibit other degenerative alterations, including fibrosis, hemorrhage, mucinosis, and vascular thrombosis; and must be recognized as separate from melanoma arising within a dermal nevus (see figs. 2-13, 2-18, 2-19).

The finding of scattered, mitotically inactive cells with enlarged, angulated, hyperchromatic nuclei among otherwise banal dermal nevic elements is another manifestation of such cellular senescence, akin to that described as ancient or degenerative change in schwannomas.

The total number of nevi on the skin declines progressively with age (106), probably mainly due to this process of senescence and disappearance of the lesions. It is also likely that the prevalence of nevi has increased during this century, so that members of older cohorts, known to be at lower risk for melanoma, also have a constitutionally lower prevalence of nevi (118). In addition to these benign phenomena, nevoid lesions that may be in transition to melanoma are commonly biopsied, often from the sun-damaged torso of an elderly patient. These lesions may be difficult to diagnose with complete specificity, and should be treated by complete excision (fig. 2-59).

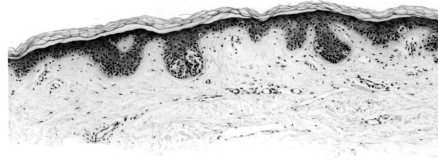

A

Figure 2-59

SUPERFICIAL ATYPICAL MELANOCYTIC PROLIFERATION OF UNCERTAIN SIGNIFICANCE (SAMPUS)

A: This lesion, from the torso of an elderly patient, shows actinic elastosis in the dermis. The epidermis is variably atrophic, with some elongation of rete ridges associated with nests at the tips.

B,C: In another area (B), there is a tendency to confluence of nests, and a tendency to upward pagetoid spread into the epidermis (C). Cytologic atypia is not marked. Such lesions have been described as nevoid lentigo maligna. It is not clear whether they represent unusual nevi, dysplastic nevi, or evolving melanoma in situ of the lentigo maligna type. Complete excision is indicated for these lesions and evaluation of the patient for other melanoma risk factors.

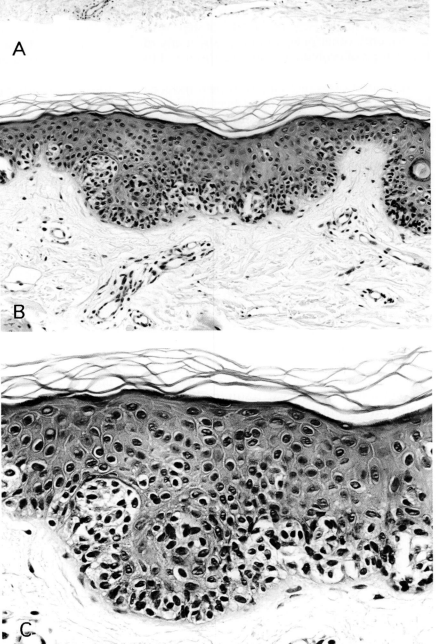

B

C

REFERENCES

1. Elder DE, Greene MH, Bondi EE, Clark WH Jr. Acquired melanocytic nevi and melanoma: the dysplastic nevus syndrome. In: Ackerman AB, ed. Pathology of malignant melanoma. New York: Masson Pub.; 1981:185-216.

2. Whimster IW. Recurrent pigment cell naevi and their significance to the problem of endogenous carcinogenesis. Ann Ital Dermatol Clin Sper 1965;19:168-191.

3. Hu F. Melanocyte cytology in normal skin, melanocytic nevi, and malignant melanomas: a review. In: Ackerman AB, ed. Pathology of malignant melanoma. New York: Masson Pub.; 1981:1-22.

4. Spitz S. Melanomas of childhood, 1948. CA Cancer J Clin 1991;41:40-51.

5. Barnhill RL, Flotte TJ, Fleischli M, Perez-Atayde A. Cutaneous melanoma and atypical Spitz tumors in childhood. Cancer 1995;76:1833-1845.

6. Urso C. A new perspective for Spitz tumors? Am J Dermatopathol 2005;27:364-366.

7. LeBoit P, Burg G, Weedon D, Sarasin A. Melanocytic tumours. In: Le Boit PE, Burg G, Weedon D, Sarasin A, eds. Pathology and genetics of skin tumors. Lyon: IARC Press; 2006:49-120.

8. Nowell PC. The clonal evolution of tumor cell populations. Science 1976;194:23-28.

9. Hui P, Perkins A, Glusac E. Assessment of clonality in melanocytic nevi. J Cutan Pathol 2001;28:140-144.

10. Robinson WA, Lemon M, Elefanty A, Harrison-Smith M, Markham N, Norris D. Human acquired naevi are clonal. Melanoma Res 1998;8:499-503.

11. Harada M, Suzuki M, Ikeda T, Kaneko T, Harada S, Fukayama M. Clonality in nevocellular nevus and melanoma: an expression-based clonality analysis at the X-linked genes by polymerase chain reaction. J Invest Dermatol 1997;109:656-660.

12. Kumar R, Angelini S, Snellman E, Hemminki K. BRAF mutations are common somatic events in melanocytic nevi. J Invest Dermatol 2004;122:342-348.

13. Pollock PM, Harper UL, Hansen KS, et al. High frequency of BRAF mutations in nevi. Nat Genet 2003;33:19-20.

14. Uribe P, Wistuba II, Gonzalez S. BRAF mutation: a frequent event in benign, atypical, and malignant melanocytic lesions of the skin. Am J Dermatopathol 2003;25:365-370.

15. Yazdi AS, Palmedo G, Flaig MJ, et al. Mutations of the BRAF gene in benign and malignant melanocytic lesions. J Invest Dermatol 2003;121:1160-1162

16. Satyamoorthy K, Li G, Gerrero MR, et al. Constitutive mitogen-activated protein kinase activation in melanoma is mediated by both BRAF mutations and autocrine growth factor stimulation. Cancer Res 2003;63:756-759.

17. Mihic-Probst D, Saremaslani P, Komminoth P, Heitz PU. Immunostaining for the tumour suppressor gene p16 product is a useful marker to differentiate melanoma metastasis from lymphnode nevus. Virchows Arch 2003;443:745-751.

18. Wajapeyee N, Serra RW, Zhu X, Mahalingam M, Green MR. Oncogenic BRAF induces senescence and apoptosis through pathways mediated by the secreted protein IGFBP7. Cell 2008;132:363-374.

19. Michaloglou C, Vredeveld LC, Soengas MS, et al. BRAFE600-associated senescence-like cell cycle arrest of human naevi. Nature 2005;436:720-724.

20. Bennett DC. Human melanocyte senescence and melanoma susceptibility genes. Oncogene 2003;22:3063-3069.

21. Sanki A, Li W, Colman M, Karim RZ, Thompson JF, Scolyer RA. Reduced expression of p16 and p27 is correlated with tumour progression in cutaneous melanoma. Pathology 2007;39:551-557.

22. Gallagher RP, McLean DI, Yang CP, et al. Anatomic distribution of acquired melanocytic nevi in white children. A comparison with melanoma: the Vancouver Mole Study. Arch Dermatol 1990;125:466-471.

23. Lund HZ, Kraus JM. Melanotic tumors of the skin. Atlas of Tumor Pathology, 1st Series, Fascicle 3. Washington DC: Armed Forces Institute of Pathology; 1962.

24. Yaar M, Woodley DT, Gilchrest BA. Human nevocellular nevus cells are surrounded by basement membrane components. Immunohistochemical studies of human nevus cells and melanocytes in vivo and in vitro. Lab Invest 1988;58:157-162.

25. Maldonado JL, Timmerman L, Fridlyand J, Bastian BC. Mechanisms of cell-cycle arrest in Spitz nevi with constitutive activation of the MAP-kinase pathway. Am J Pathol 2004;164:1783-1787.

26. Glaessl A, Bosserhoff AK, Buettner R, Hohenleutner U, Landthaler M, Stolz W. Increase in telomerase activity during progression of melanocytic cells from melanocytic naevi to malignant melanomas. Arch Dermatol Res 1999;291:81-87.

27. Gray-Schopfer VC, Cheong SC, Chong H, et al. Cellular senescence in naevi and immortalisation in melanoma: a role for p16? Br J Cancer 2006;95:496-505.

28. Chaudru V, Chompret A, Bressac-de Paillerets B, Spatz A, Avril MF, Demenais F. Influence of genes, nevi, and sun sensitivity on melanoma risk in a family sample unselected by family history and in melanoma-prone families. J Natl Cancer Inst 2004;96:785-795.

29. Rivers JK. Is there more than one road to melanoma? Lancet 2004;363:728-730.

30. Rokuhara S, Saida T, Oguchi M, Matsumoto K, Murase S, Oguchi S. Number of acquired melanocytic nevi in patients with melanoma and control subjects in Japan: nevus count is a significant risk factor for nonacral melanoma but not for acral melanoma. J Am Acad Dermatol 2004;50:695-700.

31. Bauer J, Garbe C. Acquired melanocytic nevi as risk factor for melanoma development. A comprehensive review of epidemiological data. Pigment Cell Res 2003;16:297-306.

32. Wiecker TS, Luther H, Buettner P, Bauer J, Garbe C. Moderate sun exposure and nevus counts in parents are associated with development of melanocytic nevi in childhood: a risk factor study in 1,812 kindergarten children. Cancer 2003;97:628-638.

33. Swerdlow AJ, English J, MacKie RM, et al. Benign melanocytic naevi as a risk factor for malignant melanoma. Br Med J 1986;292:1555-1559.

34. Tucker MA, Halpern A, Holly EA, et al. Clinically recognized dysplastic nevi. A central risk factor for cutaneous melanoma. JAMA 1997;277:1439-1444.

35. Gandini S, Sera F, Cattaruzza MS, et al. Meta-analysis of risk factors for cutaneous melanoma: I. Common and atypical naevi. Eur J Cancer 2005;41:28-44.

36. Holman CD, Armstrong BK. Pigmentary traits, ethnic origin, benign nevi, and family history as risk factors for cutaneous malignant melanoma. J Natl Cancer Inst 1984;72:257-266.

37. Maize JC, Ackerman AB. Pigmented lesions of the skin: clinicopathologic correlations. Philadelphia: Lea & Febiger; 1987.

38. McGovern VJ. Melanoma. Histologic diagnosis and prognosis. New York: Raven Press; 1983:3-24.

39. Kantor G, Wheeland RG. Transepidermal elimination of nevus cells. A possible mechanism of nevus involution. Arch Dermatol 1987;123:1371-1374.

40. Klein LJ, Barr RJ. Histologic atypia in clinically benign nevi. A prospective study. J Am Acad Dermatol 1990;22:275-282

41. Clark WH Jr, Ackerman AB. An exchange of views regarding the dysplastic nevus controversy. Semin Dermatol 1989;8:229-250.

42. Unna PG. Histopathology of diseases of the skin. New York: Macmillan; 1896:1129-1144.

43. Parr MM, Miescher G, von Albertini A. Histologie de 100 cas de naevi pigmentaires d'apres les methodes de Masson. Bull Soc Fr Dermatol Syphiligr 1935;42:1265-1273.

44. Yus ES, del Cerro M, Simon RS, Herrera M, Rueda M. Unna's and Miescher's nevi: two different types of intradermal nevus: hypothesis concerning their histogenesis. Am J Dermatopathol 2007;29:141-151.

45. Clemmensen OJ, Kroon S. The histology of "congenital features" in early acquired melanocytic nevi. J Am Acad Dermatol 1988;19:742-746.

46. Sagebiel RW. Histologic artifacts of benign pigmented nevi. Arch Dermatol 1972;106:691-693.

47. Aso M, Hashimoto K, Eto H, et al. Expression of Schwann cell characteristics in pigmented nevus. Immunohistochemical study using monoclonal antibody to Schwann cell associated antigen. Cancer 1988;62:938-943.

48. Paul E, Wen DR, Cochran AJ. Variations in S-100 protein expression in naevocellular nevi may be related to metabolic activity. Brit J Dermatol 1987;116:371-378.

49. Ahmed I, Piepkorn M, Goldgar DE, et al. HMB-45 staining of dysplastic melanocytic naevi in melanoma risk groups. J Cutan Pathol 1991;18:257-260.

50. Busam KJ, Chen YT, Old LJ, et al. Expression of melan-A (MART1) in benign melanocytic nevi and primary cutaneous malignant melanoma. Am J Surg Pathol 1998;22:976-982.

51. Ball NJ, Golitz LE. Melanocytic nevi with focal atypical epithelioid cell components: a review of seventy-three cases. J Am Acad Dermatol 1994;30:724-729.

52. Selim MA, Vollmer RT, Herman CM, Pham TT, Turner JW. Melanocytic nevi with nonsurgical trauma: a histopathologic study. Am J Dermatopathol 2007;29:134-136.

53. Rhodes AR, Mihm MC Jr. Origin of cutaneous melanoma in a congenital dysplastic nevus spilus. Arch Dermatol 1990;126:500-505.

54. Cohen LM. Nevus spilus: congenital or acquired? Arch Dermatol 2001;137:215-216.

55. Schaffer JV, Orlow SJ, Lazova R, Bolognia JL. Speckled lentiginous nevus: within the spectrum of congenital melanocytic nevi. Arch Dermatol 2001;137:172-178.

56. Eng AM. Solitary small active junctional nevi in juvenile patients. Arch Dermatol 1983;119:35-38.

57. Gottlieb GJ, Ackerman AB. Mitotic figures may be seen in cells of banal melanocytic nevi. Am J Dermatopathol 1985;7(Suppl):87-91.

58. Foucar E, Bentley TJ, Laube DW, Rosai J. A histopathologic evaluation of nevocellular nevi in pregnancy. Arch Dermatol 1985;121:350-354.

59. Gallagher RP, McLean DI. The epidemiology of acquired melanocytic nevi. A brief review. Dermatol Clin 1995;13:595-603.

59a. Cramer SF. Nevus cells of nerve sheath origin? Arch Dermatol 1990;126:1367-1368.

60. Masson P. My conception of cellular nevi. Cancer 1951;4:19-38.

61. Enzinger FM, Weiss SW. Soft tissue tumors. St Louis: CV Mosby; 1983:597.

62. Goette DF, Doty RD. Balloon cell nevus. Summary of the clinical and histological characteristics. Arch Dermatol 1978;114:109-111.

63. Hashimoto K, Bale GF. An electron microscopic study of balloon cell nevus. Cancer 1972;30:530-540.

64. Sheibani K, Battifora H. Signet-ring cell melanoma: a rare morphologic variant of malignant melanoma. Am J Surg Pathol 1988;12:28-34.

65. Lohmann CM, Iversen K, Jungbluth AA, Berwick M, Busam KJ. Expression of melanocyte differentiation antigens and ki-67 in nodal nevi and comparison of ki-67 expression with metastatic melanoma. Am J Surg Pathol 2002;26:1351-1357.

66. Hoang MP, Prieto VG, Burchette JL, Shea CR. Recurrent melanocytic nevus: a histologic and immunohistochemical evaluation. J Cutan Pathol 2001;28:400-406.

67. Talve L, Sauroja I, Collan Y, Punnonen K, Ekfors T. Loss of expression of the $p16^{INK4}/CDKN2$ gene in cutaneous malignant melanoma correlates with tumor cell proliferation and invasive stage. Int J Cancer 1997;74:255-259.

68. Rudolph P, Lappe T, Schubert C, Schmidt D, Parwaresch RM, Christophers E. Diagnostic assessment of two novel proliferation-specific antigens in benign and malignant melanocytic lesions. Am J Pathol 1995;147:1615-1625.

69. Carey WP Jr, Van Belle P, Elder DE. Tumor progression-related reactivity of nevi and melanomas with the MIB-1 (Ki-67) antigen evaluated by streptavidin immunohistochemistry on paraffin sections. Pigment Cell Res 1994;7(Suppl 3):10-31.

70. Ghiorzo P, Villaggio B, Sementa AR, et al. Expression and localization of mutant p16 proteins in melanocytic lesions from familial melanoma patients. Hum Pathol 2004;35:25-33.

71. Radhi JM. Malignant melanoma arising from nevi, p53, p16, and Bcl-2: expression in benign versus malignant components. J Cutan Med Surg 1999;3:293-297.

72. Sparrow LE, Eldon MJ, English DR, Heenan PJ. p16 and p21WAF1 protein expression in melanocytic tumors by immunohistochemistry. Am J Dermatopathol 1998;20:255-261.

73. Furue M, Nindl M, Kawabe K, Nakamura K, Ishibashi Y, Sagawa K. Epitope mapping of CD1a, CD1b, and CD1c antigens in human skin: differential localization on Langerhans cells, keratinocytes, and basement membrane zone. J Invest Dermatol 1992;99:23S-26S.

74. Busam KJ, Granter SR, Iversen K, Jungbluth AA. Immunohistochemical distinction of epithelioid histiocytic proliferations from epithelioid melanocytic nevi. Am J Dermatopathol 2000;22:237-241.

75. Jones EW, Cerio R, Smith NP. Epithelioid cell histiocytoma: a new entity. Br J Dermatol 1989;120:185-195.

76. Glusac EJ, McNiff JM. Epithelioid cell histiocytoma: a simulant of vascular and melanocytic neoplasms. Am J Dermatopathol 1999;21:1-7.

77. Wayte DM, Helwig EB. Halo nevi. Cancer 1968;22:69-90.

78. Sutton RL. An unusual variety of vitiligo (leukoderma acquisitum centrifugum). J Cutan Dis Incl Syph 1916;34:797-800.

79. Schmitt D, Ortonne JP, Haftek M, Thivolet J. Halo nevus and halo melanoma. Immunocytochemical study of the inflammatory cell infiltrate. In: Ackerman AB, ed. Pathology of malignant melanoma. New York: Masson; 1981:333-340.

80. Zeff RA, Freitag A, Grin CM, Grant-Kels JM. The immune response in halo nevi. J Am Acad Dermatol 1997;37:620-624.

81. Baranda L, Torres-Alvarez B, Moncada B, et al. Presence of activated lymphocytes in the peripheral blood of patients with halo nevi. J Am Acad Dermatol 1999;41:567-572.

82. Musette P, Bachelez H, Flageul B, et al. Immune-mediated destruction of melanocytes in halo nevi is associated with the local expansion of a limited number of T cell clones. J Immunol 1999;162:1789-1794.

83. Tokura Y, Yamanaka K, Wakita H, et al. Halo congenital nevus undergoing spontaneous regression. Involvement of T-cell immunity in involution and presence of circulating anti-nevus cell IgM antibodies. Arch Dermatol 1994;130:1036-1041.

84. Steffen C, Thomas D. The man behind the eponyms: Richard L Sutton: periadenitis mucosa necrotica recurrens (Sutton's ulcer) and leukoderma acquisitum centrifugum-Sutton's (halo) nevus. Am J Dermatopathol 2003;25:349-354.

85. Reed RJ, Ichinose H, Clark WH Jr, Mihm MC Jr. Common and uncommon melanocytic nevi and borderline melanomas. Semin Oncol 1975;2:119-147.

86. Harvell JD, Meehan SA, LeBoit PE. Spitz's nevi with halo reaction: a histopathologic study of 17 cases. J Cutan Pathol 1997;24:611-619.

87. Goette DK. Benign lichenoid keratosis. Arch Dermatol 1980;116:780-782.

88. Seab JA Jr, Graham JH, Helwig EB. Deep penetrating nevus. Am J Surg Pathol 1989;13:39-44.

89. Barnhill RL, Mihm MC Jr, Magro CM. Plexiform spindle cell naevus: a distinctive variant of plexiform melanocytic naevus. Histopathology 1991;18:243-247.
90. Kazakov DV, Kutzner H, Rutten A, et al. The anti-MAGE antibody B57 as a diagnostic marker in melanocytic lesions. Am J Dermatopathol 2004;26:102-107.
91. Busam KJ, Iversen K, Berwick M, Spagnoli GC, Old LJ, Jungbluth AA. Immunoreactivity with the anti-MAGE antibody 57B in malignant melanoma: frequency of expression and correlation with prognostic parameters. Mod Pathol 2000;13:459-465.
92. Cooper PH. Deep penetrating (plexiform spindle cell) nevus. A frequent participant in combined nevus. J Cutan Pathol 1992;19:172-180.
93. Kornberg R, Ackerman AB. Pseudomelanoma: recurrent melanocytic nevus following partial surgical removal. Arch Dermatol 1975;111:1588-1590.
94. Harvell JD, Bastian BC, LeBoit PE. Persistent (recurrent) Spitz nevi: a histopathologic, immunohistochemical, and molecular pathologic study of 22 cases. Am J Surg Pathol 2002;26:654-661.
94a. LeBoit PE. Persistent nevus with "no" prior biopsy. Am J Dermatopathol 2004;26:347-348.
95. Ohashi A, Funasaka Y, Ueda M, Ichihashi M. c-KIT receptor expression in cutaneous malignant melanoma and benign melanotic naevi. Melanoma Res 1996;6:25-30.
96. Park HK, Leonard DD, Arrington JH 3rd, Lund HZ. Recurrent melanocytic nevi: clinical and histologic review of 175 cases. J Am Acad Dermatol 1987;17:285-292.
97. Elder DE. Precursors to melanoma and their mimics: nevi of special sites. Mod Pathol 2006;19(Suppl 2):S4-20.
98. Christensen WN, Friedman KJ, Woodruff JD, Hood AF. Histologic characteristics of vulval nevocellular nevi. J Cutan Pathol 1987;14:87-91.
99. Clark WH Jr, Hood AF, Tucker MA, Jampel RM. Atypical melanocytic nevi of the genital type with a discussion of reciprocal parenchymal-stromal interactions in the biology of neoplasia. Hum Pathol 1998;29(Suppl 1):S1-24.
100. Gleason BC, Hirsch MS, Nucci MR, et al. Atypical genital nevi: a clinicopathologic analysis of 56 cases. Am J Surg Pathol 2008;32:51-57.
101. Rock B, Hood AF, Rock JA. Prospective study of vulvar nevi. J Am Acad Dermatol 1990;22:104-106.
102. Friedman RJ, Ackerman AB. Difficulties in the histologic diagnosis of melanocytic nevi on the vulvae of premenopausal women. In: Ackerman AB, ed. Pathology of malignant melanoma. New York: Masson; 1981:119-127.
103. Shabrawi-Caelen L, Soyer HP, Schaeppi H, et al. Genital lentigines and melanocytic nevi with superimposed lichen sclerosus: a diagnostic challenge. J Am Acad Dermatol 2004;50:690-694.
104. Carlson JA, Mu XC, Slominski A, et al. Melanocytic proliferations associated with lichen sclerosus. Arch Dermatol 2002;138:77-87.
105. Rongioletti F, Urso C, Batolo D, et al. Melanocytic nevi of the breast: a histologic case-control study. J Cutan Pathol 2004;31:137-140.
106. MacKie RM, English J, Aitchison TC, Fitzsimmons CP, Wilson P. The number and distribution of benign pigmented moles (melanocytic naevi) in a healthy British population. Br J Dermatol 1985;113:167-174.
107. Rongioletti F, Ball RA, Marcus R, Barnhill RL. Histopathological features of flexural melanocytic nevi: a study of 40 cases. J Cutan Pathol 2000;27:215-217.
108. Rhodes AR. Congenital nevomelanocytic nevi. Histologic patterns in the first year of life and evolution during childhood. Arch Dermatol 1986;122:1257-1262.
109. Lazova R, Lester B, Glusac EJ, Handerson T, McNiff J. The characteristic histopathologic features of nevi on and around the ear. J Cutan Pathol 2005;32:40-44.
110. Saad AG, Patel S, Mutasim DF. Melanocytic nevi of the auricular region: histologic characteristics and diagnostic difficulties. Am J Dermatopathol 2005;27:111-115.
111. Elder DE, Murphy GF. Melanocytic tumors of the skin. AFIP Atlas of Tumor Pathology, 3rd Series, Fascicle 2. Washington, D.C: American Registry of Pathology; 1991:103-206.
112. Fabrizi G, Pagliarello C, Parente P, Massi G. Atypical nevi of the scalp in adolescents. J Cutan Pathol 2007;34:365-369.
113. Cullity G. Intra-epithelial changes in childhood nevi simulating malignant melanoma. Pathology 1984;16:307-311.
114. Sanchez JL, Figueroa LD, Rodriguez E. Behavior of melanocytic nevi during pregnancy. Am J Dermatopathol 1984;6(Suppl):89-91.
115. Lee HJ, Ha SJ, Lee SJ, Kim JW. Melanocytic nevus with pregnancy-related changes in size accompanied by apoptosis of nevus cells: a case report. J Am Acad Dermatol 2000;42:936-938.
116. Morgan MB, Raley BA, Vannarath RL, Lightfoot SL, Everett MA. Papillomatous melanocytic nevi: an estrogen related phenomenon. J Cutan Pathol 1995;22:446-449.
117. Kerl H, Soyer HP, Cerroni L, Wolf IH, Ackerman AB. Ancient melanocytic nevus. Semin Diagn Pathol 1998;15:210-215.
118. Cooke KR, Spears GF, Skegg DC. Frequency of moles in a defined population. J Epidemiol Community Health 1985;39:48-52.

3 SPINDLE AND EPITHELIOID CELL MELANOCYTIC TUMORS/NEVI

Spindle and epithelioid cell melanocytic tumors are neoplastic proliferations of melanocytes that generally behave as benign neoplasms, resembling melanocytic nevi in most respects. They are distinguishable from common melanocytic nevi clinically by their typically rapid onset and history of limited growth, and histologically by their large spindle-shaped and epithelioid or nevoid cell type. The importance of these lesions is that they may simulate melanomas. In addition, there is a small group of related lesions that have the capacity for aggressive behavior, often but not always limited to regional lymph nodes. Because of this group of lesions with malignant potential, the term "tumor" is currently favored over "nevus" because the latter implies an unequivocally benign neoplasm (1–4). Distinction of these lesions from melanomas may be difficult because these large cells may exhibit mitotic activity and prominent nucleoli, as well as an infiltrative pattern of growth. Clinically, however, the lesions usually appear innocuous because of their characteristic symmetry and uniform color.

Two variants of spindle and epithelioid tumor are recognized. The classic *Spitz tumor/nevus*, originally described by Sophie Spitz (5), is a papular or nodular lesion composed of very large and plump spindle and/or epithelioid cells that classically extend into the reticular dermis (deep nevi), with typically scant pigment. These lesions tend to simulate nodular melanomas. The *pigmented spindle cell nevus* (PSCN) described by Richard Reed (6) is usually a superficial plaque-like lesion, confined to the epidermis and papillary dermis, and composed of narrow, elongated spindle cells that are heavily pigmented. These lesions tend to simulate thin, usually nontumorigenic melanomas. Although the existence of overlap lesions suggests that there is a spectrum between the two extremes (7), it is useful, in our opinion, to conceptualize the spindle and epithelioid cell nevi into these two broad classes, if only to facilitate accurate

diagnosis and distinguish between the disparate melanoma patterns that the lesions simulate.

SPINDLE AND EPITHELIOID CELL MELANOCYTIC TUMOR (SPITZ TUMOR/NEVUS)

Definition. *Spindle and epithelioid cell melanocytic tumor*, or *Spitz tumor*, is a benign tumor composed of a single large spindle and/or epithelioid cell type. Clinically, there is a history of rapid but limited growth, frequently in children. The classic term *spindle and epithelioid cell nevus* was introduced by Kernen and Ackerman (8) for a lesion originally described by Spitz in 1948 as *juvenile melanoma* (5), later termed *benign juvenile melanoma* or *Spitz nevus*, and currently more commonly *Spitz tumor*. The term *nevus of large spindle and/or epithelioid cells* (9), although cumbersome, is admirably descriptive of this lesion.

Before Spitz described these tumors, they were regarded as unequivocal malignant melanomas, and Spitz herself regarded them as melanomas with an unusually good prognosis (5). The significance of the vast majority of Spitz tumors today, particularly those occurring in children, is as benign lesions that are of no consequence except as potential melanoma simulants. As noted above, a few lesions, difficult or impossible to distinguish from the wholly benign ones, metastasize, and for this reason the designation of these lesions as "tumors" (or as "tumors/nevi") rather than "nevi" is currently preferred (1–3,10). The lesions are defined histologically, but there are characteristic clinical features that may be of some assistance in reaching a diagnosis.

Clinical Features. Spitz tumors/nevi are uncommon; their incidence in Queensland, Australia was estimated at about 5 percent that of malignant melanoma (11). The lesions are either asymptomatic or cause concern because of a history of growth, which is often rapid (several weeks or even less). They occur anywhere on the skin, but common presentations

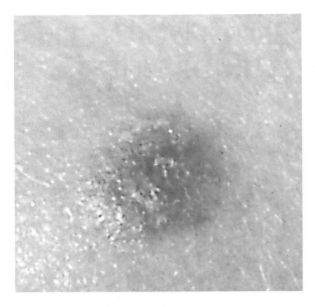

Figure 3-1

SPITZ NEVUS

A pink papule in a child. (Fig. C from Plate II, Fascicle 2, Third Series.)

are a pink papule on the face of a child and a papule, pink or pigmented, on the thigh or leg of a young woman (fig. 3-1). In a recent study, it was found that Spitz tumors were often present on the thighs, especially in persons younger than 40 years of age (12). In contrast, melanomas were more likely to be on the trunk in persons 40 years of age or older. The lesions occur in either sex and at almost any age (although they become progressively more uncommon after the third decade). The diagnosis should be made with particular caution in patients over the age of 40 and certainly with great trepidation in those over 60, although lesions in this age group do occur (13). Most of the lesions occur in Caucasians, but we have seen occasional examples in Blacks, one of which had been interpreted erroneously as a nodular melanoma. Because classic Spitz tumors are often relatively nonpigmented, the clinical diagnosis is often that of a nonmelanocytic lesion, such as a hemangioma, and the diagnosis of melanoma is not often suspected clinically.

Grossly, the lesions are symmetric, small to moderately sized papules (3 to 10 mm or so), with smooth discrete borders and a uniform color, typically pink or flesh-colored. After a pe-

riod of rapid growth, they remain unchanged as stable pigmented or flesh-colored papules. Spitz tumors occasionally present as multiple grouped ("agminated") lesions, a benign phenomenon of cosmetic significance for some patients (14). These multiple lesions often develop in a background tan macule like a café au lait spot or a nevus spilus and may extensively involve large areas of the body (15,16).

In some patients we have observed with multiple Spitz tumors, the lesions gradually acquire clinical characteristics of more banal ordinary acquired nevi over years of follow-up, and have not shown any tendency toward inexorable growth or transformation. Insights as to the developmental biology of Spitz tumors and biologic differences between these melanoma simulants and melanomas as well as common nevi have recently been reported from molecular studies. They are discussed in more detail in the section on differential diagnosis.

There is a developing consensus concerning the management of Spitz tumors. In a survey of American dermatologists and others (17), most recommend biopsies of suspected Spitz tumors, and most completely excise a lesion that is histologically diagnosed as an incompletely removed Spitz tumor. Although most respondents believe Spitz tumors are entirely benign, 7 percent of general dermatologists and 4 percent of pediatric dermatologists have seen metastatic melanomas related to sites of lesions initially diagnosed histologically as Spitz tumors/nevi, and 40 percent of pigmented-lesion clinic directors have seen such lesions. This concern about the possibility of melanoma, or of "malignant Spitz nevus," influences the management of Spitz nevi/tumors and accounts for the usual recommendation that these lesions be completely excised (17,18). In addition, complete excision of these lesions obviates the possibility of their recurrence in scar tissue, an additional complicating factor that could lead to overdiagnosis as overt melanoma.

Microscopic Findings. Although the diagnosis may be suspected clinically, it is confirmed histologically, preferably by complete excisional biopsy. This approach is important to evaluate the base of the lesion in order to accomplish the primary purpose of the biopsy, which is to rule out melanoma or another form of skin cancer. At scanning magnification, the lesions are symmetric papules or nodules that involve the papillary dermis and reticular dermis. They are usually associated with hyperkeratosis and reactive hyperplasia of keratinocytes (figs. 3-2–3-9). Important features visible at scanning power include small lesional size, relative bilateral symmetry (9), uniformity of cell type from side to side, large spindle and/or epithelioid cells (9), lesional cells that become smaller from superficial to deep within the lesion (maturation, or perhaps better termed senescence) (9,11), sharp demarcation of the lateral border of the lesion (9), lack of prominent spread of lesional cells into the epidermis (11), and a characteristic pattern of permeation of the reticular dermis by attenuated fibroblast-like lesional cells, with single cells predominating over nests and fascicles at the base of the nevus (11).

Although there is overlap in size between Spitz tumors and some melanomas, most Spitz tumors are less than 6 mm in diameter, while most melanomas are larger than this. "Symmetry" is present when the two halves of the lesion about a central axis are similar to one another, unlike most melanomas where the two halves are quite disparate in terms of the shape and number of nodules, in situ or microinvasive components, pigment production, and host responses including inflammatory and epithelial reactions. Some nodular melanomas are quite symmetric, however, and then the distinction must be based on evaluation of the cell type and differentiation. The lesion is said to be "well circumscribed" when the most peripheral lesional cells at the lateral borders are arranged in nests rather than as single cells, the latter pattern being more characteristic of melanoma (9). Although the lesional cells of Spitz tumors are large, at scanning power they are uniform from side to side, and become smaller as one looks from superficial to deep within the lesion.

At the base of the lesion, most compound Spitz tumors show some evidence of involvement of the reticular dermis; indeed, this preference for the reticular dermis is for us an important diagnostic attribute of these lesions (6). The reticular dermis at the base is permeated by single cells and single files of cells in a pattern that is different from the pushing or fascicular pattern of invasion seen in most mela-

nomas that involve the reticular dermis, except for desmoplastic melanoma (fig. 3-2).

Also characteristic at scanning magnification is the keratinocytic and stromal host response. There is marked epithelial hyperplasia, which on occasion may be pseudoepitheliomatous, even sometimes simulating a squamous cell neoplasm (19). This hyperplasia is much more prominent than in most other benign melanocytic lesions, including dysplastic nevi. The hyperplasia consists of markedly elongated and often somewhat irregularly thickened rete ridges separated by edematous dermal papillae. Within the papillae are dilated capillaries and patchy aggregates of lymphocytes (fig. 3-2). Frequently, these papillae also contain hyalinized collagen (13).

Near the dermal-epidermal junction, eosinophilic "cytoid," or "Kamino," bodies are commonly, but not always, seen (20). These structures may represent apoptotic degenerate melanocytes or keratinocytes and/or basement membrane material (figs. 3-2, 3-4) (21,22). When present in considerable numbers and especially when arranged in globular clusters, these bodies are much less frequently seen in melanomas than in Spitz tumors, and they serve as a useful criterion in difficult and borderline lesions (22–24).

In a Spitz tumor, the lesional cell population, by definition, includes plump spindle cells; there may or may not be an associated large round or epithelioid cell type. Forms transitional between these cell shapes suggest that the lesion is composed of a single population of cells with a biphasic morphology (fig. 3-4). The lesional cells at the dermal-epidermal junction are arranged in parallel aggregates within large nests, ellipsoid in configuration, with their long axes perpendicular to the epidermis (the "bunches of bananas" or "raining down" pattern) (fig. 3-5). The nests are often separated from the surrounding keratinocytes by a characteristic semilunar clefting artifact (13). Nests and fascicles may merge and coalesce, producing patterns that result in diagnostic confusion with the junctional cells of dysplastic nevi and some melanomas. Pagetoid cells and upward migration of nested lesional cells within the epidermis may be seen in Spitz tumors/nevi, but unlike melanomas, these changes are restricted to the zone of epidermis directly above the dermal component,

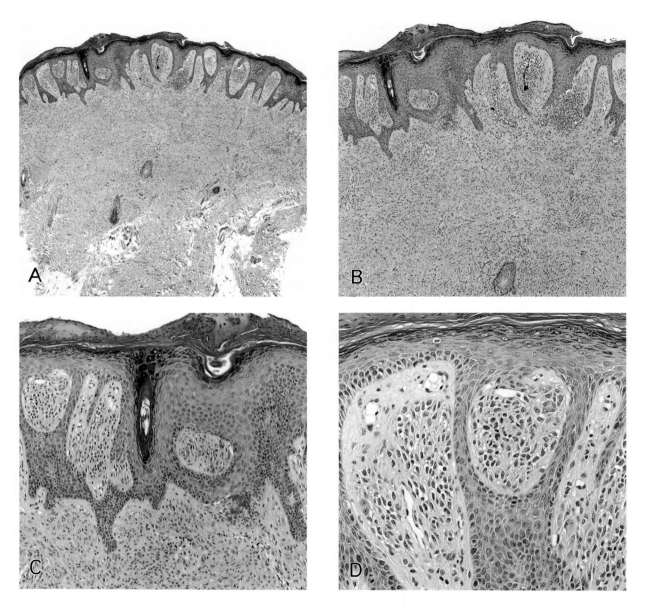

Figure 3-2

SPINDLE AND EPITHELIOID CELL NEVUS (SPITZ NEVUS, CLASSIC TYPE)

A: Scanning magnification of this lesion in a 7-year-old girl shows epithelial hyperplasia with hyperkeratosis and hypergranulosis, and lesional cells extending well into the reticular dermis.

B: Large spindle and epithelioid cells are near the surface.

C: Higher magnification shows nests of spindle and epithelioid cells, tending to be vertically oriented, "raining down" from near the epidermis.

D: The lesional cells superficially are larger and nests near the epidermis tend to be vertically oriented.

and in most lesions, junctional fascicles and nests significantly predominate. The nests and fascicles are best seen in the superficial part of the dermal component, but in thicker lesions, the nested architecture becomes less prominent with descent to the base of the lesion, where the cells may be distributed in a more diffuse pattern. The fascicles are arranged loosely, without compressing, replacing, or obliterating the stroma of the dermis (6).

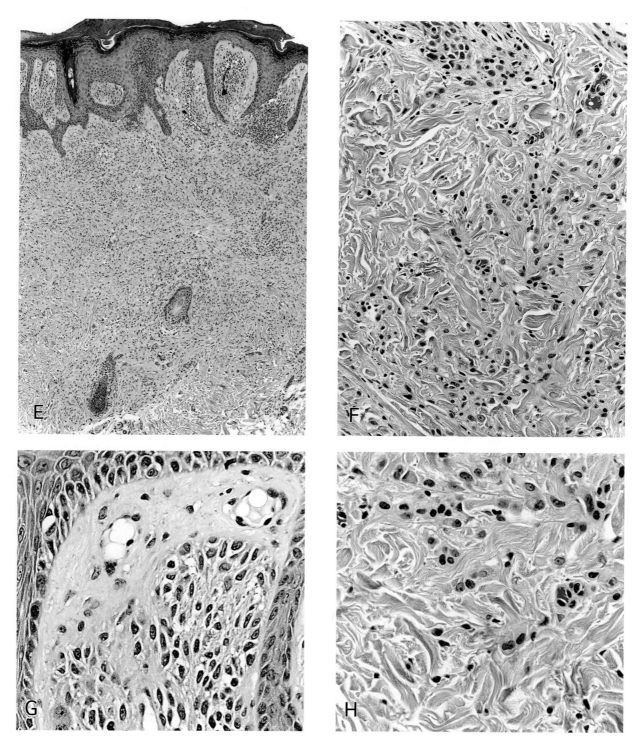

Figure 3-2 (continued)

E: Lesional cells mature to a smaller cell type at the base and are dispersed as single cells into the reticular dermis.
F: Smaller cells at the base are dispersing as single cells into the collagen of the reticular dermis.
G: Basement membrane-like material beneath the epidermis represents a form of ill-defined Kamino body.
H: Single cells disperse into the collagen at the base.

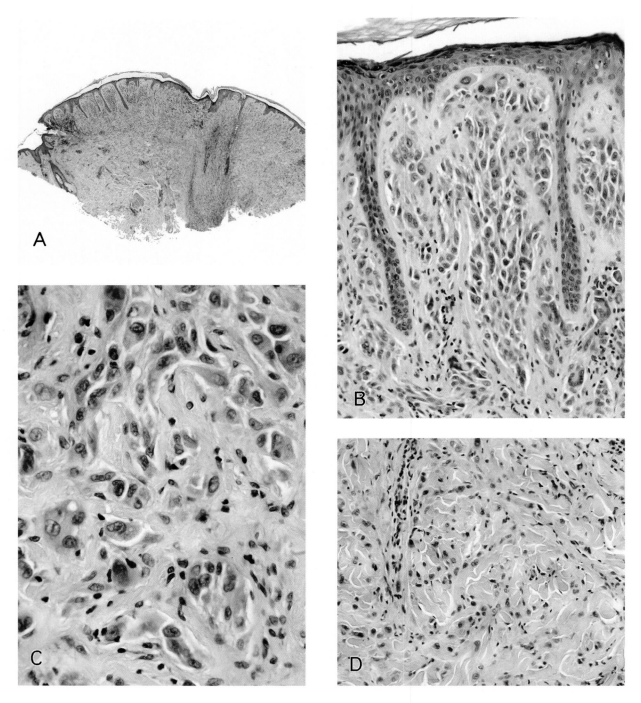

Figure 3-3

SPITZ NEVUS

A: This lesion of the back in a 23-year-old man is larger than most Spitz nevi, almost a centimeter in greatest dimension.

B: Large spindle and epithelioid cells rain down into the dermis from near the epidermis.

C: Larger cells are near the surface.

D: At the base, the lesional cells tend to disperse among reticular dermis collagen fiber bundles as single cells, becoming smaller with descent.

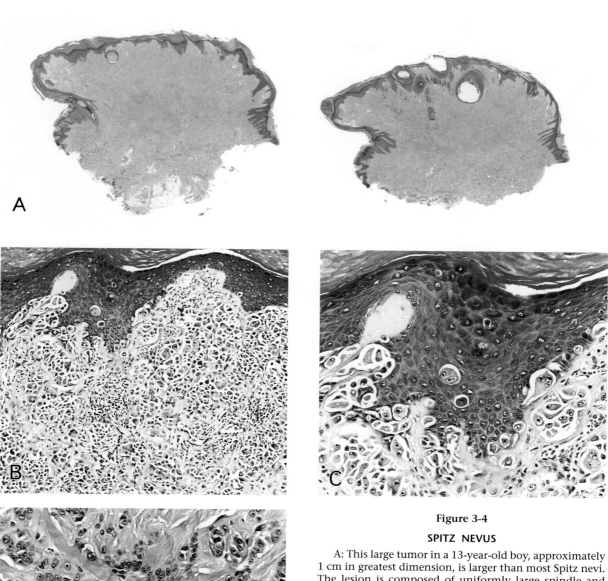

Figure 3-4

SPITZ NEVUS

A: This large tumor in a 13-year-old boy, approximately 1 cm in greatest dimension, is larger than most Spitz nevi. The lesion is composed of uniformly large spindle and epithelioid cells, which are uniform from side to side across the lesion.

B: A globoid eosinophilic Kamino body is seen at top left. The epidermis is irregularly hyperplastic, with hyperkeratosis and a prominent granular layer.

C: Higher magnification shows a Kamino body. These typically represent either apoptotic cells or basement membrane-like material; the latter is likely to be the case in this instance. Lesional cells at the base are smaller than those near the surface.

D: Lesional cells tend to disperse, albeit imperfectly, as single cells among reticular dermis collagen bundles (not seen well in this example). Mitotic figures were absent in this lesion. If a lesion of this type had more than 2 mitoses/mm², we would term it a melanocytic tumor of uncertain malignant potential (MELTUMP), or perhaps a melanoma, depending on the level, distribution, and morphology of the mitotic activity.

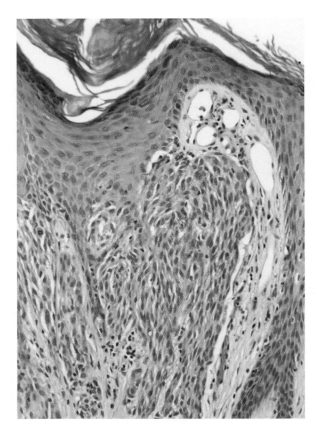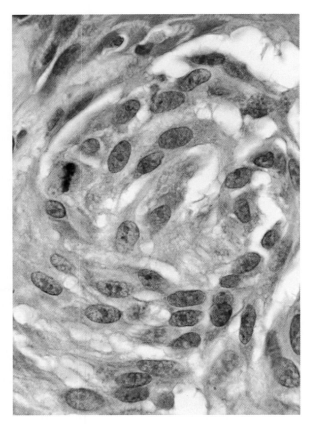

Figure 3-5

MITOSIS IN A SPITZ NEVUS

Mitotic figures occur in Spitz nevi, however, they should not be numerous or abnormal, no more than 2/mm², and not usually two in a single high-power field.

Cytologically, the cells near the surface of the lesion are large, with abundant eosinophilic or amphophilic cytoplasm. At high magnification, the cytoplasm may appear finely vacuolated or net-like, reminiscent of the cytoplasm of ganglion cells. There may be scanty dusty pigment or no pigment in the cytoplasm. The nuclei are large, often with finely particulate and evenly dispersed chromatin, and often with large eosinophilic nucleoli as well as intranuclear cytoplasmic invaginations. Mitotic figures may be present, particularly in the upper third of the tumor, whereas the deepest third is generally devoid of mitotic activity (fig. 3-5). Most Spitz tumors have no mitoses.

With their infiltrative patterns of growth and their large nucleolated and sometimes mitotically active cells, Spitz tumors may simulate vertical growth phase melanoma at both the architectural and cytologic levels, resulting in exceedingly difficult diagnostic dilemmas in some cases. In these problematic cases, evidence of architectural and cytologic symmetry and cytologic maturation should be carefully evaluated. We have found the cytologic features to be especially important in these equivocal lesions. In Spitz tumors, the cells are commonly uniform from side to side (cytologic symmetry). Although the cells may be large and pleomorphic superficially, they become smaller, often losing their macronucleoli, and become less mitotically active, as they descend into the dermis (fig. 3-2). These attributes are considered to represent maturation of the benign nevus cells. In melanomas, such maturation is less likely to occur or is incomplete. In a recent morphometric study, a progressive reduction in nuclear size from the superficial to the deep portions of

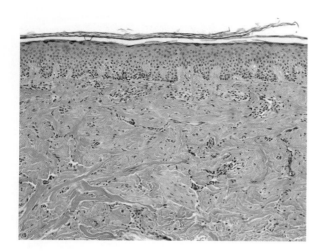 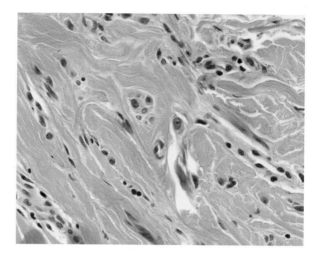

Figure 3-6

SCLEROSING SPITZ NEVUS

Left: The lesion is predominantly dermal and is composed of single cells permeating among abnormal collagen matrix.
Right: At high magnification, the lesional cells have the characteristic large spindle and/or epithelioid cell Spitz phenotype.

Spitz and common nevi was documented, while melanomas as a group showed a tendency to nuclear enlargement with descent (25).

The mature nevoid cells at the base of a characteristic Spitz tumor infiltrate as single cells among reticular dermis collagen fibers, sometimes extending several high-power fields beyond the deepest contiguous lesional cells. In melanomas, fascicles and nests of contiguous tumor cells predominate over single cells at the base, and the cells at the base are usually similar to those at the surface of the tumor. According to the computer simulation model of Smolle et al. (26), the different patterns are likely to depend on the relative degrees of proliferation and motility of the tumor cells. The cells of benign nevi show a low degree of motility, which, however, still exceeds the very low degree of proliferation, so that single cells at the base do not undergo cell division. In contrast, single cells at the base of melanomas tend to divide and form multicellular structures (26). This pattern of maturation and dispersion is of critical importance in establishing the diagnosis, especially in atypical lesions. When the base of the lesion is not available for examination, a descriptive diagnosis must be given so that the lesion can be completely excised for a more definitive interpretation.

Histologic Variants. *Desmoplastic* or *sclerosing Spitz tumor* is a term applied to a lesion composed of spindle cells that are typically somewhat smaller than those of classic Spitz tumors, less likely to have a junctional component, and associated with delicate fibrosis or desmoplasia that tends to separate individual lesional cells (figs. 3-6, 3-7) (27,28). Pigment is typically sparse. Such lesions are categorized in general as desmoplastic nevi, and when the large spindle/epithelioid cell type is prominent, as variants of Spitz tumors (27). In a study of 15 cases by MacKie et al. (28), female patients predominated, ranging in age from 8 to 83 years. The usual site of the lesions was the upper limb. The lesions were characterized by a dense sclerotic or desmoplastic appearance of dermal collagen surrounding a population of predominantly epithelioid nevus cells, some of which had bizarre but nonmalignant cytology. The uncommon and aptly named *angiomatoid Spitz tumor* is considered a variant of desmoplastic Spitz tumor in which there is a prominent vascular as well as fibrogenic stromal response (fig. 3-8) (28a).

Hyalinizing Spitz tumor is an uncommon lesion that is characterized by large and epithelioid-shaped or plump and spindle-shaped cells with prominent eosinophilic nucleoli that are present as isolated individual cells, single cells

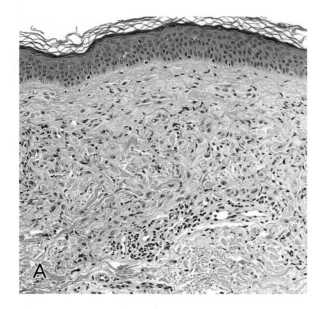

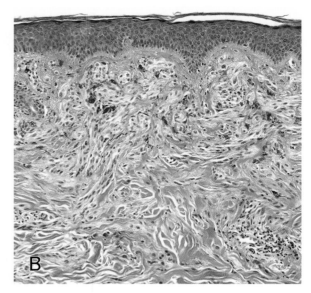

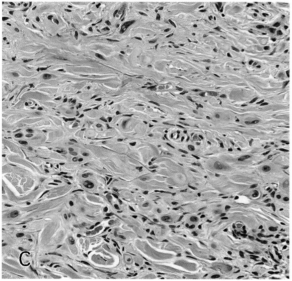

Figure 3-7

DERMAL SPITZ NEVUS WITH SCLEROSIS

A: A uniform population of large spindle cells is arranged in fascicles. The differential diagnosis includes a deep penetrating nevus or possibly a cellular blue nevus. There is evidence of maturation from superficial to deep.

B: At higher magnification, the lesional cells have the characteristic large spindle and/or epithelioid morphology characteristic of a Spitz nevus.

C: There are no mitoses, a very helpful diagnostic feature.

in a linear pattern, small nests, and fascicles in a paucicellular hyalinized stroma. The histologic features can mimic those of dermatofibroma, desmoplastic cellular blue nevus, metastatic carcinoma, or malignant melanoma. Diffuse expression of S-100 protein and absence of staining with antibodies to cytokeratin and HMB45 were observed in one case (29).

Three lesions termed *plexiform Spitz tumors* have been described, and are characterized by a plexiform arrangement of bundles and lobules of enlarged spindle to epithelioid melanocytes throughout the superficial and deep dermis,

with a myxoid stroma, and no junctional component. The lesional cells are similar to those in the classic form of Spitz tumors. Mitoses are rare or absent. Tumor cells were strongly immunoreactive for S-100 protein, but not for HMB45, desmin, and actin (30,31).

Pagetoid Spitz tumors were described by Busam and Barnhill (32) as lesions characterized by a mainly intraepidermal proliferation of large epithelioid melanocytes with a predominantly pagetoid distribution. This melanocytic lesion tends to appear clinically as a small (under 0.4 cm) pigmented macule in young patients (fig.

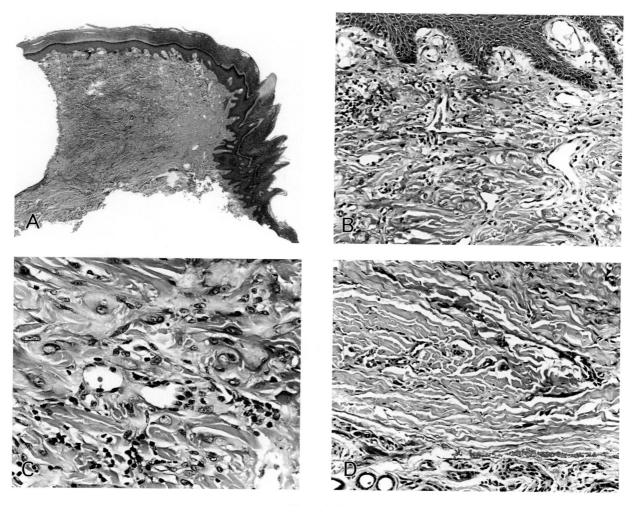

Figure 3-8

ANGIOMATOID SPITZ NEVUS

This lesion could be considered a variant of a desmoplastic or sclerosing Spitz nevus, with not only fibroplasia but also angiogenesis in the stroma.

A: At scanning magnification, the lesion has the appearance of a fibroma or an angioma.

B,C: Higher magnification reveals the presence of large spindle and/or epithelioid cells among the collagen bundles.

D: At the base of the lesion, the cells are smaller than they are superficially. (Courtesy of Dr. Bruce Ragsdale, San Luis Obispo, CA.)

3-9). Histologically, the lesion needs to be distinguished primarily from in situ or microinvasive malignant melanoma with pagetoid spread. Features favoring nevus over melanoma include small size, circumscription, symmetry, even distribution of cells, and lack of marked cytologic atypia (32). However, the natural history of such lesions remains to be fully elucidated, and accordingly, we recommend complete excision. When a pagetoid proliferation is present adjacent to a dermal component of Spitz type,

the diagnosis is especially difficult (fig. 3-10). In such problematic cases, a differential diagnosis can be issued, and the lesion should be managed by minimal criteria for melanoma in situ (complete excision, typically with a 5 mm margin).

Biologic Behavior. Recurrence of Spitz tumors is uncommon but can cause diagnostic difficulty. A series of 22 cases that seemed to have been clinically removed but persisted and recurred at the biopsy site was recently described (33). These authors noted four histopathologic

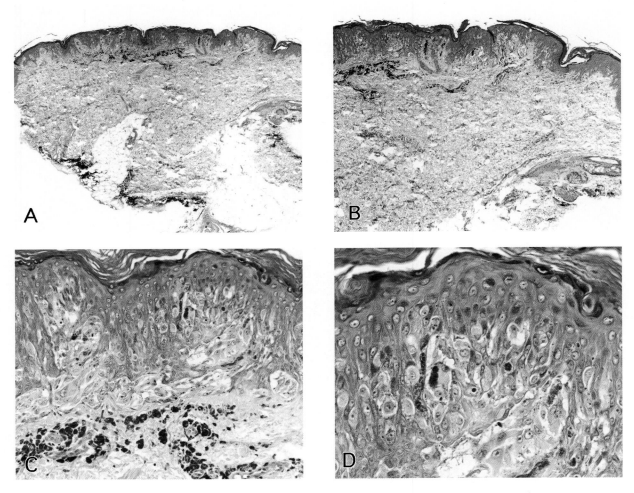

Figure 3-9

PAGETOID SPITZ NEVUS

A,B: This lesion, in a 9-year-old child, is small and well circumscribed, with uniform large spindle and/or epithelioid cells arranged from side to side.

C: There are nests with clefting artifact.

D: The cells have large nuclei, open chromatin, and prominent nucleoli. The differential diagnosis, especially in an older individual, includes severe dysplasia and melanoma in situ (SAMPUS).

patterns in the recurrence: 1) a predominantly intraepidermal pattern resembling pseudomelanoma as seen in recurrent common melanocytic nevi; 2) a compound, mostly nested pattern above or within a scar that was nearly identical to the originally biopsied Spitz tumor; 3) a nodular growth pattern that closely simulated invasive melanoma; and 4) a desmoplastic pattern resembling an intradermal desmoplastic Spitz tumor. Although the majority of recurrent lesions exhibited asymmetry and pagetoid spread, the dermal component usually had a low mitotic rate and retained architectural and cytologic maturation, which allowed distinction from invasive melanoma. The immunostaining pattern with S-100 protein and HMB45 was identical to that previously reported for Spitz tumors, and the Ki-67 index revealed a very low proliferation rate in all cases, including one that eventually behaved as a melanoma. Comparative genomic hybridization (CGH) performed in 10 of the recurrences yielded results consistent

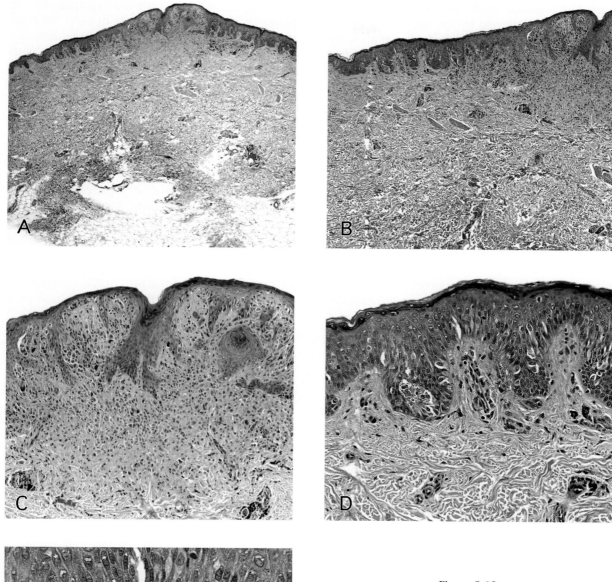

Figure 3-10

MELANOCYTIC TUMOR OF UNCERTAIN MALIGNANT POTENTIAL (MELTUMP)

The tumor favors Spitz nevus with adjacent pagetoid junctional Spitz nevus proliferation.

A,B: The lesion (in a 15-year-old boy) has a central nodule and a peripheral plaque. The nodule consists of uniformly large epithelioid to spindle cells. The nuclei have open chromatin.

D,E: In the adjacent intraepidermal component, there are large spindle and epithelioid cells extending above the basal layer. A lesion such as this should be interpreted with caution. The differential diagnosis includes a level IV melanoma with a thickness of approximately 1.1 mm.

with Spitz tumor in 8. The difficulty of this exercise is exemplified by the fact that 1 of the 22 lesions included in the study was at an early stage but was later recognized as melanoma after metastasis to regional lymph nodes 3 years after the local recurrence. Although the authors concluded that ancillary molecular techniques such as CGH may help in distinguishing recurrence of Spitz tumor from melanoma, this technique is not yet widely available, and its reliability has not been thoroughly evaluated in a sufficiently large number of such difficult cases.

We recommend complete excision of any recurrent Spitz tumor, and if the lesion is tumorigenic, atypical, and difficult to distinguish from melanoma, a sentinel lymph node sampling procedure may be discussed with the patient, at least as an option (34). We would also mention, however, that this procedure has been demonstrated to have staging but not necessarily therapeutic efficacy at this time.

Differential Diagnosis. Since Spitz tumors were first described in children, it is obvious that age plays a role in diagnosis. A "difficult" lesion in a prepubertal child is most likely to be a Spitz tumor, while conversely, this diagnosis should be made with great caution in an adult over the age of 40. Stated differently, the diagnosis of melanoma in a young child, or the diagnosis of Spitz tumor in a middle-aged or older patient, can be made with confidence only when the appearances are absolutely classic. Spitz tumors certainly occur outside the pediatric age group. It has been estimated as a "rule of thumb" that, based on age alone with all else being equal, the odds tend to be more in favor of a benign lesion in patients under the age of approximately 30 (35). Vollmer (36) has recently provided a thoughtful discussion of the influence of patient age in establishing probabilities for the differential diagnosis of melanomas and nevi.

Although the most important entity in the differential diagnosis of the Spitz tumor is malignant melanoma, there are other variants of benign nevi that may be worth distinguishing, if only for nosologic reasons. The pigmented spindle cell nevus described by Reed (6) is probably a variant of a Spitz tumor, but is considered separately in the next section because its characteristic heavy pigmentation is more likely to result in clinical simulation of a melanoma

(37,38). The term spindle and epithelioid cell tumor/nevus can be used, if desired, to refer to either of these lesions. Most spindle and epithelioid cell tumors are compound lesions with a prominent epidermal component. Occasional lesions composed of similar cells in the dermis but lacking an epidermal component may be regarded as dermal Spitz tumors, and a few lesions are entirely intraepidermal (junctional Spitz nevi).

Since most Spitz tumors have no biologic potential for metastasis or progression, and are not associated with melanoma risk, the most important differential diagnostic consideration is malignant melanoma. Architectural and cytologic considerations assist in making this distinction. Although the dermal component is the key to the biologic potential of the lesion, the diagnosis is often accurately made by careful consideration of the junctional component of the lesion. The vertical growth phase of a melanoma of the superficial spreading, lentigo maligna, and acral-lentiginous types can often be distinguished from a Spitz tumor by the presence of an adjacent junctional proliferation that represents the radial growth phase of one of these forms of melanoma. Stated differently, the presence of an indubitable radial growth phase adjacent to a somewhat "spitzoid" tumor essentially rules out the diagnosis of Spitz tumor.

Although a tendency of single cells and nests of cells to spread into the epidermis directly above the dermal component of a Spitz tumor is not necessarily indicative of malignancy (11), such pagetoid changes adjacent to a spindle and/or epithelioid cell dermal tumor suggest that the lesion is melanoma (39). Single cell pagetoid epidermal involvement may be prominent in pagetoid Spitz tumors, which are typically small superficial lesions in children (32). Transepidermal elimination of junctional nevus cell nests is common in Spitz tumors, and should not be confused with pagetoid spread of individual melanoma cells (40). The junctional component of those Spitz tumors that are composed mainly of spindle cells is usually discontinuous (there are zones of sparing of the epidermis within the borders of the dermal tumor), and is often minimal and sometimes absent. Conversely, a spindle cell melanocytic neoplasm that has an extensive and continuous junctional component is suspicious for melanoma (39). Spitz tumors that are composed predominantly of epithelioid cells, however, often have a fairly prominent junctional component. Even so, continuous basal proliferation of lesional cells or extensive confluence of lesional cell nests is a feature of concern in a putative Spitz tumor.

Features in the dermal component that may simulate nodular malignant melanoma histologically include the large cell type, the presence of large eosinophilic nucleoli, the mitotic activity observed in some lesions, ulceration or necrosis, areas of high cellularity with sheet-like growth, and the pattern of permeation of the reticular dermis by the lesional cells which may be interpreted as invasion but is not indicative of malignancy. Multinucleate giant cells are commonly present in Spitz tumors, usually in the papillary dermis (5,13). Their nuclei are uniform, similar to those of the single cells of the lesion. Multinucleated melanoma cells, in contrast, usually have variably sized and shaped nuclei, often with high-grade atypia (39), but some melanomas may have giant cells indistinguishable from those of Spitz tumors (13). Most Spitz tumors do not show bizarre nuclear hyperchromatism and pleomorphism as may be seen in many (but by no means all) nodular melanomas. Perineural and arrector pili muscle involvement, as well as lesional cells in endothelial-lined channels (pseudovascular invasion), have been reported in benign Spitz tumors (6,11,13). The latter features, in particular, are concerning for us and would usually lead to a diagnosis of "atypical Spitz tumor," "melanocytic tumor of uncertain malignant potential" (MELTUMP), or melanoma. All of these features, except involvement of the reticular dermis, are rare in common acquired nevi.

Desmoplastic or sclerosing Spitz tumor must be distinguished from desmoplastic malignant melanoma (27,28,41). Generally, desmoplastic nevi are less cellular than most desmoplastic melanomas, with few if any mitoses. In a recent study by Harris et al. (41), the similarities between desmoplastic nevi and desmoplastic melanomas included the presence of atypical cells and possible HMB45 expression in the superficial portion of both lesions. In addition, desmoplastic melanomas, like desmoplastic nevi, may lack severe cellular atypia and usually do not show prominent macronucleoli. The infrequent location on the head or neck, the absence of mitotic figures, and a significantly lower

number of Ki-67–reactive cells help to distinguish desmoplastic nevi from desmoplastic melanoma (27). The nodular peripheral clusters of lymphocytes so characteristic of desmoplastic melanoma are not seen in the dermal component of desmoplastic nevi, and there is usually a tendency to maturation toward the base of the lesion in the upper reticular dermis. Extension into the fat is common in desmoplastic melanoma but rare in nevi including desmoplastic nevi. Finally, desmoplastic melanomas are usually associated with an adjacent or superficial component of characteristic microinvasive or in situ radial growth phase in the epidermis and papillary dermis (41), and the presence of such an adjacent radial growth phase effectively rules out the diagnosis of Spitz tumor.

Desmoplastic nevi may also resemble dermatofibroma. In the study by Harris et al. (41), the similarities between desmoplastic nevi and dermatofibromas included epidermal hyperplasia, presence of keloidal collagen, hypercellularity, and increased numbers of factor XIIIa-positive dendritic cells. The absence of adnexal induction within the overlying epidermis, the rarity of lesions with multinucleated cells or epidermal hyperpigmentation, and the presence of S-100 protein immunoreactivity and melanocytic proliferation helped differentiate desmoplastic nevi from dermatofibromas (39). HMB45 and Melan-A immunoreactivities are absent in dermatofibromas. Since both lesions are benign, differentiation may not be significant.

Although it is well known that mitoses may be seen in Spitz tumors, the mitotic rate is generally very low (fig. 3-11); commonly, there are no mitoses in a Spitz tumor. Failure to find mitoses after a careful search is a very reassuring negative finding in a lesion that gave rise to concern for some other reason, such as the presence of a few cells in the epidermis, or its size and depth. When mitoses are present in Spitz tumors, they are most common in the epidermis and in the upper third of the dermis; mitoses in the lower third of the lesion are uncommon except in young children (13). Abnormal mitoses are rare in Spitz tumors (24), although it is said that they occur (13). Certainly, a clearly abnormal mitotic figure should prompt careful consideration of other aspects of the lesion before an unqualified benign diagnosis is issued. Few if any benign Spitz tumors

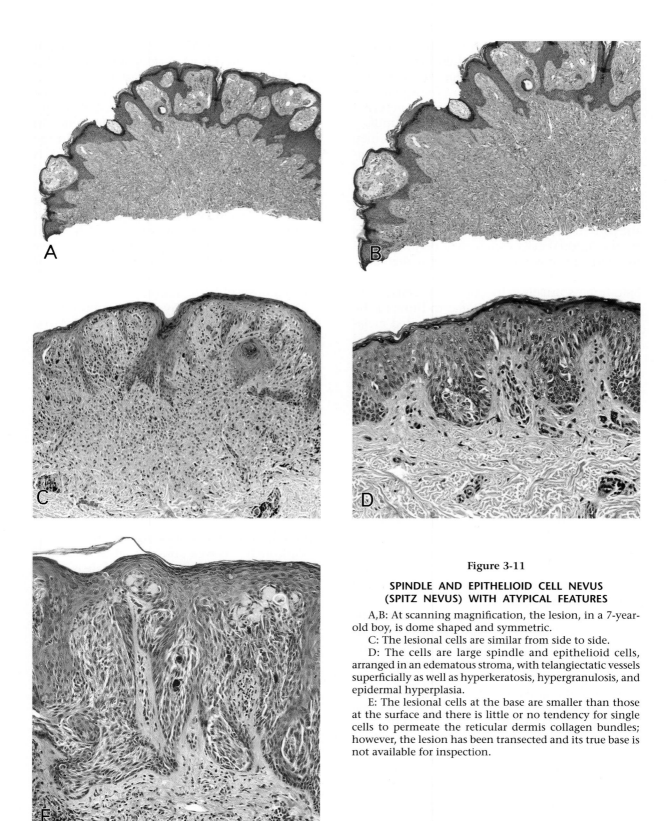

Figure 3-11

SPINDLE AND EPITHELIOID CELL NEVUS (SPITZ NEVUS) WITH ATYPICAL FEATURES

A,B: At scanning magnification, the lesion, in a 7-year-old boy, is dome shaped and symmetric.

C: The lesional cells are similar from side to side.

D: The cells are large spindle and epithelioid cells, arranged in an edematous stroma, with telangiectatic vessels superficially as well as hyperkeratosis, hypergranulosis, and epidermal hyperplasia.

E: The lesional cells at the base are smaller than those at the surface and there is little or no tendency for single cells to permeate the reticular dermis collagen bundles; however, the lesion has been transected and its true base is not available for inspection.

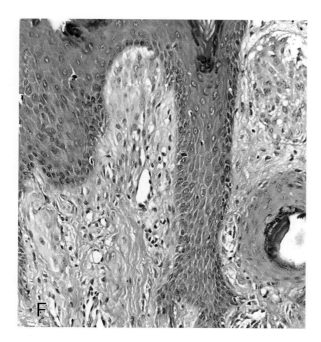
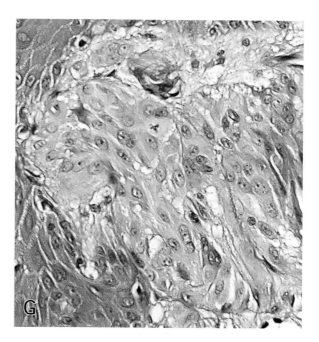

Figure 3-11 (continued)

E,F: The characteristic large epithelioid and spindle cells, vertically oriented, rain down from the dermal-epidermal junction. Mitotic figures were rare in this lesion and confined to its upper third, without abnormal mitoses.

G: The nuclei have open chromatin with small nucleoli and regular nuclear membranes. This lesion was judged to be benign because of its low mitotic rate and the patient's age, as well as the uniformity of the cells from side to side and other characteristic architectural features.

exhibit a high mitotic rate (more than 6 mitoses/mm²). In the study of Crotty et al. (42), the presence of abnormal mitoses, a dermal mitotic rate of more than 2/mm², and mitotic figures within 0.25 mm of the deep border of the lesion were features that favored melanoma. In Spitz tumors, mitotic figures may be seen in hyperplastic keratinocytes, a finding rare in common nevi, but not unusual in melanomas.

Spontaneous ulceration or necrosis is uncommon (24), but we have seen a few ulcerated Spitz tumors that presented with a history of trauma, especially in children who pick at these occasionally itchy lesions. A study of 33 Spitz tumors and 19 malignant melanomas in patients aged 20 years or less identified prominent pagetoid spread, cellular pleomorphism, nuclear hyperchromasia, and mitotic activity as the most striking differences between Spitz tumors and melanomas (24). These authors stressed the importance of cytologic as well as architectural features in distinguishing between the lesions, and emphasized that there is overlap in the histologic features.

Immunohistochemistry and other marker studies have been of limited value in differentiating Spitz tumor and melanoma, since both may express melanoma-associated activation and lineage-related antigens such as HMB45 and Melan-A, respectively, which may be expressed as well in normal melanocytes and ordinary nevus cells (43,44). The zonation of expression may differ between Spitz tumors and melanomas: Spitz tumors tend to show a "top heavy" gradation from superficial to deep, while melanomas tend to be more diffusely reactive or even "bottom heavy." In a recent study, the positivity and pattern of immunoreactivity of S-100A6 protein was found to vary among Spitz tumors, melanomas, and common nevi (45). All of 42 Spitz tumors showed strong and diffuse S-100A6 protein expression, both in junctional and dermal components of the nevi. Only 33 percent of melanomas (35/105) expressed S-100A6 protein; the expression was mainly weak (30/35) and patchy in the dermal component and negative or minimal in the junctional component ($p < 0.001$).

Recent interest in utilizing antibodies to antigens that gauge cell proliferative activity, such as Ki-67 (MIB-1), holds considerable promise for their use as adjuncts for differentiating Spitz tumors and tumorigenic melanomas (46–48). Li and colleagues (49–52) have recently presented an elegant series of studies in which cytometric features were investigated, including nuclear DNA content and chromatin compactness, measured by video-imaged DNA microdensitometry; nuclear morphology, measured by nuclear morphometry (karyometry); transcriptional activity of nucleolar organizer regions, measured as the number and size of argyrophilic staining of nucleolar organizer regions (AgNORs); and cellular proliferative activity, detected by quantifying the immunoreactivity of the Ki-67 antigen. These variables were evaluated in the superficial, middle, and deep zones of each lesion. Using multivariate discriminant analysis, a diagnostic effectiveness of 100 percent could be achieved in a test set of 27 benign compound nevi, 20 dysplastic nevi, 10 Spitz tumors, and 24 melanomas.

A recent elaborate study assessed cell cycle and apoptosis regulators in Spitz nevi in order to appraise the value of these markers as a diagnostic adjunct in differential diagnosis. It was found that the expression of bax, Ki-67, Rb, p16, cyclin A, and cyclin B1 was significantly higher in melanomas than Spitz nevi, whereas p27 expression was significantly higher in Spitz nevi. It was concluded that Spitz nevi differ from melanomas in their immunohistochemical pattern of expression of cell cycle and apoptosis regulators and more closely resemble common benign nevi (53). While these types of studies are promising, it is likely that these methods will be difficult to generalize into practice.

Molecular testing may offer a more specific distinction between atypical Spitz tumors and melanomas in the near future. Spitz tumors appear to differ from most common nevi and from melanomas in that the oncogenes *BRAF* and *NRAS* are not mutated in Spitz tumors (10,54–59), except in a small subset of Spitz-like lesions, some of which may have atypical features (60). In contrast, *BRAF* or *NRAS* mutations have been identified in a high proportion of melanomas and in common nevi (61–63). These mutations typically result in an activated BRAF oncogene protein that activates the mitogen-

activated protein (MAP) kinase pathway, which is constitutively activated in most melanomas, and can, in the absence of inhibitory factors, lead to cell proliferation (64). Interestingly, the MAP kinase pathway is activated in Spitz tumors (63,65) but not in most common acquired nevi (64). MAP kinase pathway activation in Spitz tumors appears to occur through mutation or activation of an oncogene different from *BRAF* (66). In some Spitz tumors, a mutation has been identified in the *HRAS* oncogene, which is found in a subset of cases and is frequently accompanied by the finding of increased copies of the 11p locus of this gene by comparative genomic hybridization (CGH) (10,65). In a subset of Spitz tumors (many of them atypical), this 11p copy increase is the only genetic aberration found by CGH, in contrast to most nevi (including most Spitz tumors) in which there are no consistent aberrations and also in contrast to melanomas in which there are numerous aberrations (67). In another study, activated *Akt* oncogene expression was found to be increased in Spitz nevi and melanomas as compared with benign intradermal nevi, but was considered unlikely to prove diagnostically useful (68). Levels of the cell cycle inhibitor p16 are high in both Spitz (66) and in common nevi (69,70) and it is likely that this and other suppressors such as p21, p27, p14^{ARF}, p53, and IGFBP7 may hold proliferation in check in these lesions as in ordinary nevi (71–73). These CGH and oncogene mutational differences may form the basis for genetic diagnostic testing to distinguish Spitz tumors and melanomas in the future (33,58,67,74–76), however, the sensitivity, specificity, and predictive value of these tests remain to be determined, especially for the difficult cases in which they are likely to be applied.

Atypical and Malignant Spitz Tumors

Spitz tumors that show several of the atypical features discussed above may be very difficult to distinguish from melanoma, and indeed, sometimes a descriptive diagnosis is all that can be rendered in a difficult case (fig. 3-10). In a study in which nine cases selected for their diagnostic difficulty were circulated among "expert" pathologists, the reproducibility of the diagnosis of Spitz tumor was very poor (77). In another study of diagnostic reproducibility for selected difficult and metastasizing lesions,

Table 3-1

FEATURES HELPFUL IN DIFFERENTIATING SPITZ TUMOR AND NODULAR MELANOMA[a]

	Spitz Tumor	Nodular Melanoma
Architecture		
*Diameter[b]	Usually <10 mm	Usually >10 mm
*Symmetry	Usually present	Often absent
*Lateral borders	Sharply demarcated	Often poorly demarcated
*Irregular nesting	Uncommon	Common
*Ulceration	Absent	Often present
*Deep extension (into fat)	Uncommon	Common in thick tumors
*Expansile nodule	Uncommon	Common
*Cellularity	Variable, nested	Dense, sheet-like, cohesive
Epidermal hyperplasia	Present	Minimal or absent
Junctional proliferation	Discontinuous	Often continuous
Junctional nest orientation	Perpendicular to epidermis	Random
Pagetoid spread	Inconspicuous or absent	Often apparent
Pigment distribution	Little or no pigment	Patchy, asymmetric
Nesting pattern at base	Small, uniform	Larger, variable
Nuclear pleomorphism	Mild or moderate	May be severe
Cytology		
*Mitoses in lower third	Absent	Often present
*Maturation/zonation	Present	Generally absent
*Deep border	Infiltrating	Rounded, pushing, fascicular
Kamino bodies	Single and confluent	Inconspicuous or absent
Chromatin pattern	Delicate, evenly dispersed	Coarse, clumped
Necrosis	Absent	Often present

[a]Nodular melanomas lack radial growth phase at the periphery, which if diagnostic of melanoma, rules out Spitz tumor.
[b]Items marked with an * are elements of the Barnhill et al. (3,79) and Spatz et al. (80) grading systems for atypical Spitz tumors.

each of which exhibited some criteria of Spitz tumor, 17 spitzoid lesions, some of which had metastasized, yielded no clear consensus as to diagnosis; in only one case did six or more pathologists agree on a single category, regardless of clinical outcome (3). Notably, some lesions that proved fatal were categorized by most observers as either Spitz nevi or atypical Spitz tumors. Yet another study of diagnostic reproducibility found disagreement to be concentrated in the category of Spitz tumors and "spitzoid" melanomas, for which there was a 35 to 40 percent overall disagreement rate among six reference pathologists who reviewed 72 cases chosen for their potential diagnostic difficulty; in contrast, the percent of agreement was high for most other categories of lesions (78).

Criteria for Spitz tumor are summarized in Table 3-1, along with other criteria that we believe are useful in distinguishing this lesion from invasive melanoma. Hybrid lesions, however, have characteristics that fall between those of classic Spitz tumor and vertical growth phase melanoma. These diagnostically challenging le-

sions have been termed *atypical Spitz tumors*, as has been proposed by Barnhill et al. and Spatz et al. (3,79,80). For such lesions, it has been proposed that points be assigned if certain features are present (designated by asterisks in Table 3-1). A patient over 10 years of age or a tumor diameter over 10 mm is assigned 1 point; fat involvement, ulceration, or a mitotic rate of 6 to 8 mitoses/mm^2 is assigned 2 points; and a mitotic rate of over 8 is assigned 5 points. On this scale, 0-2 points indicates low risk, 3-4 indicates intermediate risk, and 5-11 indicates high risk. This system worked well in 30 children with Spitz tumors, 11 of whom had a history of metastasis and 19 of whom had long disease-free follow-up. Validation in an external system is required, however, and therapeutic guidelines do not readily flow from this classification. Although as a gross generalization it is true that "difficult" lesions are usually benign in terms of long-term follow-up (39), this is not invariably so. In our opinion, equivocal lesions exhibiting the features listed in Table 3-1, if considered to fall short of an unequivocal diagnosis of melanoma, should be

Figure 3-12

MELANOCYTIC TUMOR OF UNCERTAIN MALIGNANT POTENTIAL THAT FAVORS "SPITZOID" MELANOMA

A: This lesion, in a 24-year-old man, is comprised predominantly of epithelioid cells.

B: The cells are arranged in nests that vary in size and shape.

C: There is an abnormal mitosis. The differential diagnosis could include malignant melanoma, nodular type, Clark level III, Breslow thickness 1.1 mm. There is no ulcer, and the dermal mitotic rate is low. We would recommend management with this differential diagnosis taken into consideration.

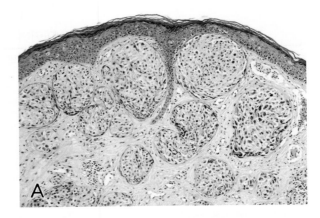

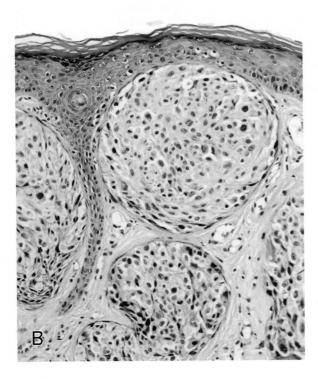

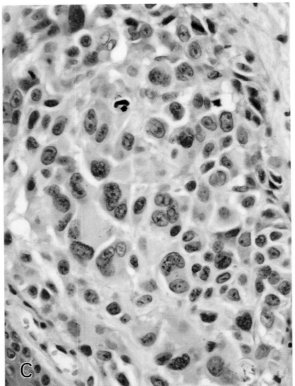

classified as a MELTUMP and the differential diagnosis of melanoma should be presented, with a discussion of staging attributes (fig. 3-12). More aggressive management of these atypical Spitz lesions may be warranted (17), and in our opinion should be tailored to the individual case, including analysis of prognostic attributes that might apply if the lesion is interpreted as a melanoma.

As discussed above, metastasis of spitzoid lesions, although uncommon, is a possibility in an atypical Spitzoid lesion. In a literature review, Urso (81) found about 100 cases of metastasizing Spitz tumors. Although histologic data were not uniformly recorded, this review indicated that any number of the following histologic features could be found in a metastasizing lesion: 1) nodular growth in the dermis and/or large confluent, solid, cellular sheets with no collagen fibers interposed between cells; 2) extension of the neoplastic proliferation to the mid-deep dermis or to subcutaneous fat, especially if associated with absent or impaired maturation; 3) dermal mitoses, especially in the deeper part of the tumor; 4) marked nucleolar and/or nuclear pleomorphism; 5) heavy melanization in the deeper part of the tumor; 6) asymmetry; 7) necrosis; 8) epithelioid epidermal melanocytes below parakeratosis and/or epidermal ulceration; and 9) neoplastic cells in lymphatic vessels.

Management of problematical spitzoid lesions should usually include a re-excision procedure and follow-up of the patient. A sentinel lymph node sampling procedure may also be considered, and in several reported studies was occasionally positive (43,81–84). Interestingly, among 25 reported patients with atypical spitzoid lesions and positive sentinel nodes, not a single death occurred, although follow-up intervals have generally been short. Nevertheless, it seems likely that atypical spitzoid lesions may be associated with excellent survival rates after positive sentinel node metastasis, especially in children.

Many of these tumors, in our opinion, are best regarded as MELTUMPs. Recently, a group of cases assembled by Lorenzo Cerroni, MD, was studied by experts and discussed at the annual meeting of the International Society of Dermatopathology in Graz, Austria (85). These cases were selected as bulky tumors composed of a uniform population of epithelioid or spindled cells. Not all were especially "spitzoid"; some had features of deep penetrating nevi, pigmented epithelioid melanocytomas, or cellular blue nevi. Despite the size of the lesions, only a few small ulcers were observed and there was no in situ melanoma component. The lesional cells had abundant cytoplasm and large round or ovoid nuclei with regular nuclear membranes, pale chromatin, and a single prominent nucleolus. Mitoses were absent in many of the lesions and if present the rate was low. About one third of these lesions had metastases, most often to regional nodes, and about 20 percent were fatal, often after a protracted, at least initially, indolent course. There were several instances of long-term survival after regional metastases, suggesting that some of these metastases, like the primary lesions, were of uncertain malignant potential. It was considered that these lesions represented a form of relatively low-grade malignancy compared to ordinary melanomas of similar depth, and the use of the term "melanocytoma" was

suggested as an expression of their characteristics intermediate between benign nevi and malignant melanomas. In addition to being noncommittal about prognosis, this term could encompass the range of morphologies observed in these lesions. Risk factors for aggressive behavior in these "melanocytomas" included the presence of mitoses, mitoses in the lower third of the lesion, and the presence of inflammation. It was proposed to tentatively classify these lesions into three risk groups: low risk—no inflammation, no mitoses; medium risk—presence of inflammation and/or mitoses not located at the base of the lesion; and high risk—presence of inflammation and/or mitoses near the base.

PIGMENTED SPINDLE CELL NEVUS OF REED

Definition. *Pigmented spindle cell nevus* (PSCN) *of Reed* is a relatively small, well-circumscribed and uniformly darkly pigmented lesion composed histologically of elongated spindle-shaped and nevoid cells that are confined to the epidermis and papillary dermis (6,37,38). The lesions may simulate melanoma histologically and clinically, but the biologic behavior is benign. PSCN is defined histologically but may be suspected clinically, and is probably best regarded as a pigmented variant of a Spitz tumor. It is also known as *spindle cell non-Spitz nevus* (39), and commonly referred to in practice as *pigmented Spitz nevus*. Being superficial and usually nontumorigenic, PSCNs are almost invariably benign and are appropriately termed nevi. A few possibly related lesions with expansile proliferation of spindle cells in the papillary dermis or infiltration of the reticular dermis may be problematic and best interpreted as melanocytic tumors of uncertain malignant potential.

Clinical Features. Patients are usually asymptomatic, or present with a history of recent onset and initial rapid growth followed by stability. Unlike the classic Spitz tumor, however, the dark color of the lesion is often alarming to the patient or suggestive of melanoma to the physician. Although PSCNs occur anywhere on the skin and in either sex, the classic presentation is that of a black papular or plaque-like lesion on the thigh or leg of a young adult woman. A characteristic PSCN is a solitary, symmetric, small to moderately sized papule or plaque, 3 to 10 mm or so in diameter, with a smooth

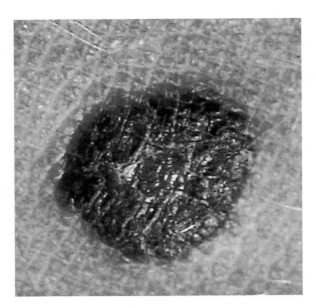

Figure 3-13

PIGMENTED SPINDLE CELL NEVUS

The lesion is relatively small, symmetric, well circumscribed, and homogeneously blue-black. (Fig. D from Plate II, Fascicle 2, Third Series.)

discrete border and a uniform black or blue-black color (fig. 3-13). The dark color often leads to consideration of melanoma, but the lesion is symmetric and uniformly colored.

Microscopic Findings. As with a Spitz tumor, the diagnosis may be suspected clinically but must be confirmed histologically by excision biopsy. At scanning power, the lesion is bilaterally symmetric (figs. 3-14–3-18). The elongated spindle cells in the basal epidermis are arranged in nests with borders that often seem to "blend" with surrounding keratinocytes (fig. 3-15). In most Spitz tumors, by contrast, there may be a sharp separation with clefts between the two cell types (see fig. 3-11). Nests and fascicles may coalesce, leading to confusion with a similar feature in dysplastic nevi, which characteristically bridge across adjacent rete ridges. Pagetoid spread into the epidermis may be prominent, although in such cases the possibility of melanoma should always be given serious consideration. The peripheral border is well circumscribed (there are few or no single cells beyond the last nest).

Important histologic features in common with Spitz tumors include a relatively small size compared to most melanomas, lesional symme-try, uniformity of cell type, good circumscription, and maturation of cells from superficial to deep within the papillary dermis. In contrast to classic Spitz nevi, the lesions are typically heavily pigmented, with abundant coarse melanin granules in lesional cells and in keratinocytes, and in melanophages within the subjacent papillary dermis. The lesions are almost always confined to an expanded and often fibrotic papillary dermis, with compression but not infiltration of the reticular dermis (fig. 3-14) (6). Involvement of the reticular dermis, a diagnostic hallmark of classic Spitz tumors, is a finding that may be suggestive of melanoma in a PSCN. In such cases, it is important to recall that spindle melanoma cells invade the reticular dermis as pushing fascicles, and do not show the attenuated single cell infiltrative pattern that characterizes Spitz tumors and their variants. As in Spitz tumors, PSCNs show an associated, although generally less prominent, keratinocytic reaction, often presenting a uniform pattern of elongated rete ridges across the lesion. There is typically a patchy lymphocytic response in the dermis.

At higher magnification, the lesional cells are more elongated and less plump than those of Spitz tumors, with scanty cytoplasm that contains abundant coarse pigment and may show a degree of cytoplasmic retraction artifact similar to that of normal melanocytes. In contrast to classic Spitz tumors, nucleoli are generally not prominent, or small blue nucleoli may be present. Mitoses may be quite numerous in the epidermis (2 to 3 figures/section). A high mitotic rate in the dermis is suggestive of melanoma, especially if abnormal mitoses are observed or if the lesion prominently involves the reticular dermis and is mitotically active in that location. Spontaneous ulceration or necrosis is unusual. There is usually no associated large "epithelioid" cell type, but the lesional cells often mature to a small round nevoid cell type at the base of the lesion, which often impinges upon and compresses the reticular dermis.

Differential Diagnosis. The major differential diagnostic considerations are the radial growth phase of superficial spreading melanoma (Table 3-2) and dysplastic nevus. PSCN also needs to be separated from other superficial nevi with marked pigment synthesis. Cohen et. al. (86) described 316 patients with nevi forming dark

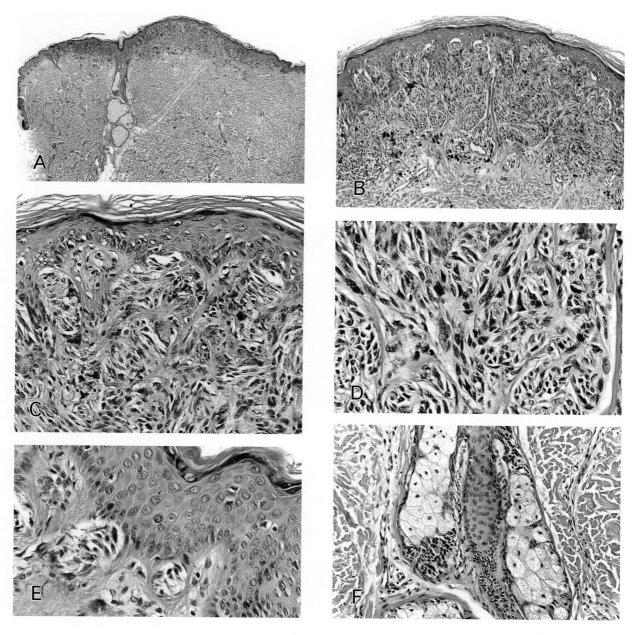

Figure 3-14

PIGMENTED SPINDLE CELL NEVUS

A: The symmetry of this lesion is somewhat altered by the presence of a hair follicle.

B: The lesion is composed of narrow, elongated spindle cells arranged in nests that tend to be vertically oriented. There is some clefting artifact, however, and some of the nests appear to "blend" with adjacent keratinocytes, a feature differentiating these lesions from classic Spitz nevi.

C: There is a tendency to maturation from larger cells superficially to smaller, more nevoid cells at the base, while the cells remain similar from side to side at any level of the lesion.

D: Although there is some variation in size and shape, the nuclei tend to have clear chromatin, small to medium nucleoli, and smooth nuclear membranes.

E: At the periphery, the lesion is well circumscribed; the last lesional cells form nests rather than single cells.

F: An unusual feature in this lesion is the presence of nevoid cells in relation to the sebaceous gland beneath the lesion, as is also seen in congenital pattern nevi.

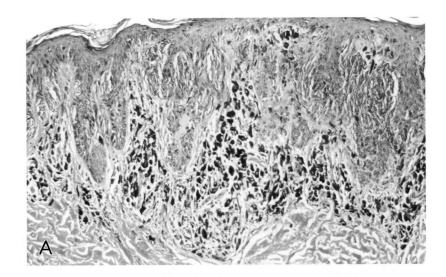

Figure 3-15

PIGMENTED SPINDLE CELL NEVUS

These lesions are small, typically less than 4 mm in diameter, and well circumscribed, with irregularly elongated rete ridges and vertically oriented nests of elongated spindle cells. The lesions may be junctional, or there may be a few nevus cells in the dermis showing evidence of maturation compared to the junctional component (A). The typical narrow elongated spindle cells are arranged in nests that tend to blend with adjacent keratinocytes rather than showing the clefting artifact characteristic of Spitz nevi (B). Cells contain abundant melanin pigment arranged in coarsely divided pigment granules. Like Spitz nevus cells, the nuclei are large, with regular nuclear membranes and fairly prominent nucleoli. Melanophages may be prominent in the stroma, as here (C).

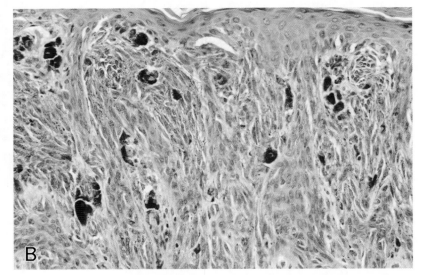

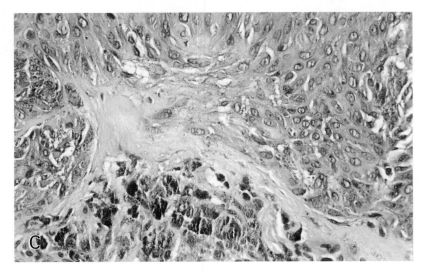

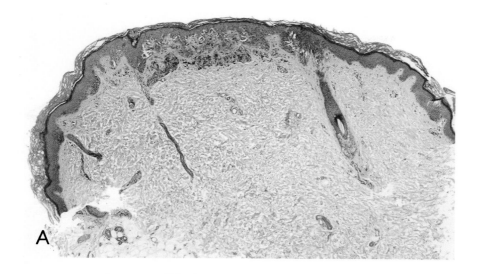

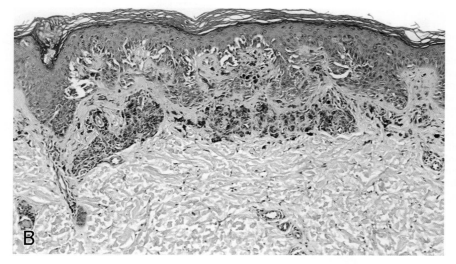

Figure 3-16

**PIGMENTED SPINDLE
CELL NEVUS**

A: This lesion is small and well circumscribed. Symmetry is often not perfect in these lesions.

B: The nests of lesional cells are somewhat haphazardly arranged rather than showing the more characteristic vertical orientation.

C: The lesion is composed of large spindle and/or epithelioid cells, with large nuclei with nucleoli, cleared chromatin, and smooth nuclear membranes. The differential diagnosis includes a dysplastic nevus or a pigmented Spitz nevus.

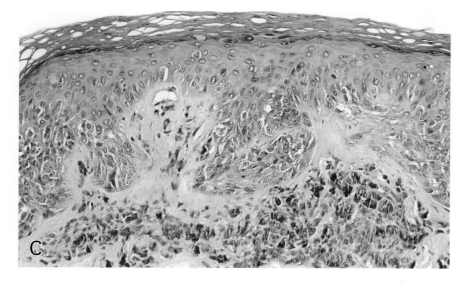

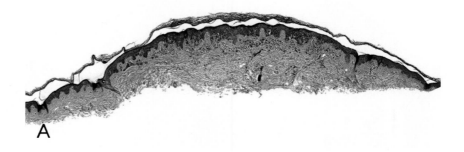

A

Figure 3-17

PIGMENTED SPINDLE CELL NEVUS WITH PAGETOID MELANOCYTIC PROLIFERATION

This lesion, in a 9-year-old child, is small, well circumscribed, and symmetric.

B: At high magnification, spindle to epithelioid cells are arranged in nests that blend with adjacent keratinocytes. A few single cells and small nests of cells are present in the upper layer of the epidermis.

C: Higher magnification shows the focal pagetoid proliferation, which is common in pigmented spindle cell nevi of children especially. This lesion could be considered a pagetoid Spitz nevus.

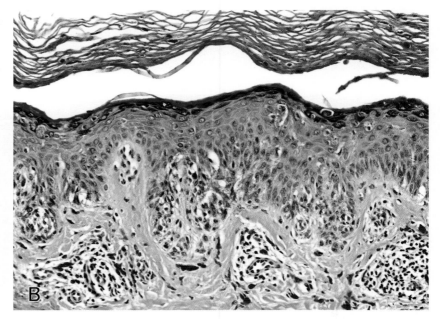

B

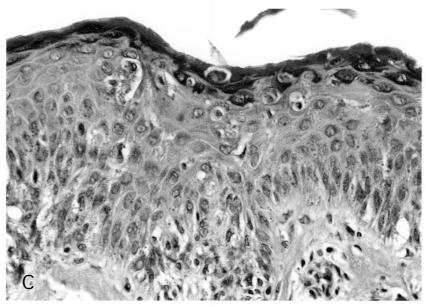

C

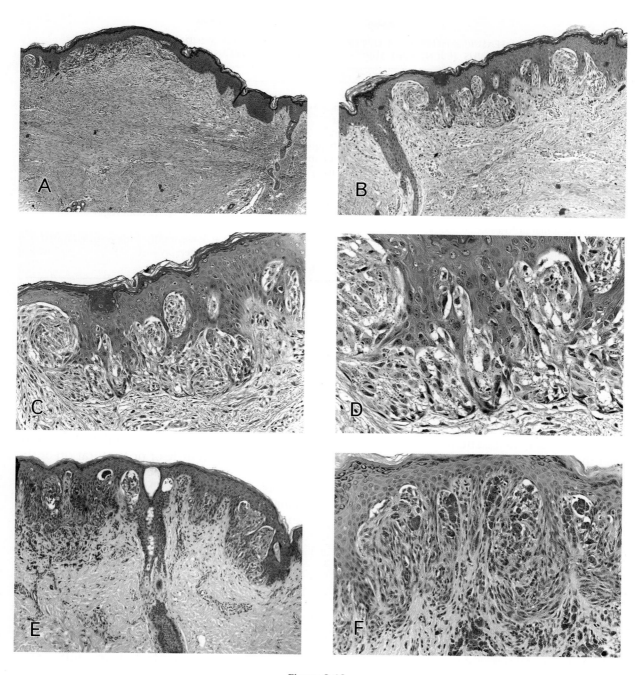

Figure 3-18

RECURRENT PIGMENTED SPINDLE CELL NEVUS

A: This lesion, in a 2-year-old, shows a cellular proliferation of large spindle-shaped melanocytes above the scar of a prior procedure.

B: At high magnification, the cells have the characteristics of a pigmented spindle cell nevus. There is abundant cytoplasmic pigment. The nests show clefting artifact.

C,D: The cells have regular nuclear membranes and small nucleoli.

E: The lesion shown in this figure had been removed from the site 3 months before. It shows narrow, elongated, heavily pigmented spindle cells arranged in vertically oriented nests.

F: Higher magnification shows the characteristic cytology of a pigmented spindle cell nevus.

Table 3-2

FEATURES HELPFUL IN DIFFERENTIATING PIGMENTED SPINDLE CELL NEVUS (PSCN) AND SUPERFICIAL SPREADING MELANOMA (SSM)

	PSCN	SSM
Architecture		
Diameter	Usually <6 mm	Usually >6 mm
Symmetry	Usually present	Usually absent
Junctional nest shape	Ovoid, uniform	Variable in size and shape
Junctional nest orientation	Perpendicular to epidermis	Random
Pagetoid spread	Inconspicuous or absent	Conspicuous
Pigment	Abundant, coarse	Less conspicuous, "dusty"
Cytology		
Cell size	Dermal cells < junctional cells	Dermal cells = junctional cells
Cell shape	Elongated spindle cells	Large epithelioid cells
Intraepidermal mitoses	Common	Common
Intradermal mitoses	Absent	Present only with vertical growth
Necrosis	Absent	Often present
Maturation	Present	Absent

brown-black macules and papules on the back. There was a slight female predominance and a median age of 40 years. These hypermelanotic nevi were characterized by junctional and papillary dermal nevus nests without atypia and heavy melanin content within keratinocytes, stratum corneum, and dermal melanophages. Although such lesions superficially resemble PSCN, they lack the essential cytologic features that make the latter a variant of a Spitz tumor.

Major differences from radial growth phase melanomas include the symmetry of PSCN at scanning magnification, the uniformity of the spindle cell type, the predominance of elongated spindle cells rather than epithelioid cells, the tendency to coarse rather than finely particulate "dusty" cytoplasmic melanin pigment, and the marked tendency to differentiation along nevoid lines as the lesional cells descend into the papillary dermis (Table 3-2). PSCNs usually do not exhibit the characteristic delicate elongation of the rete ridges that characterizes dysplastic nevi. Spindle cell nevi are usually more cellular than dysplastic nevi and, while dysplastic nevi may have some spindle-shaped melanocytes, these are not a uniform predominant popula-

tion. The spindle cells in dysplastic nevi tend to be oriented horizontally, while those in PSCN tend to "rain down" vertically.

Cellular and thicker examples of PSCN must be distinguished from spindle cell nodular melanoma. Spindle cell melanoma usually occurs in an older population, and in obviously sun-damaged skin. Histologically, the reticular dermis of melanomas show a pushing or fascicular pattern of invasion, with little or no maturation of the cells to the base of the lesion. In contrast, the cells of a characteristic PSCN mature to a small banal nevoid cell at the interface of the papillary and reticular dermis; invasion of the reticular dermis by a spindle cell lesion of this type (not a blue nevus) is a feature that suggests the possibility of malignancy.

PSCNs are probably closely related to Spitz tumors and banal acquired nevi. The differential diagnostic considerations that separate PSCN from ordinary acquired nevi are unimportant, since both are benign lesions. Differentiation of PSCN from Spitz tumors, particularly in adults, is potentially important for the reasons discussed in detail above dealing with the latter entity.

REFERENCES

1. Urso C. A new perspective for Spitz tumors? Am J Dermatopathol 2005;27:364-366.

2. Cerroni L. A new perspective for Spitz tumors? Am J Dermatopathol 2005;27:366-367.

3. Barnhill RL, Argenyi ZB, From L, et al. Atypical Spitz nevi/tumors: lack of consensus for diagnosis, discrimination from melanoma, and prediction of outcome. Hum Pathol 1999;30:513-520.

4. Spatz A, Barnhill RL. The Spitz tumor 50 years later: revisiting a landmark contribution and unresolved controversy. J Am Acad Dermatol 1999;40:223-228.

5. Spitz S. Melanomas of childhood. Am J Pathol 1948;24:591-609.

6. Reed RJ, Ichinose H, Clark WH Jr, Mihm MC Jr. Common and uncommon melanocytic nevi and borderline melanomas. Semin Oncol 1975;2:119-147.

7. Ferrara G, Argenziano G, Soyer HP, et al. The spectrum of Spitz nevi: a clinicopathologic study of 83 cases. Arch Dermatol 2005;141:1381-1387.

8. Kernen JA, Ackerman LV. Spindle cell nevi and epithelioid cell nevi (so-called juvenile melanomas) in children and adults. A clinicopathologic study of 27 cases. Cancer 1960;13:612-625.

9. Paniago-Periera C, Maize JC, Ackerman AB. Nevus of large spindle and/or epithelioid cells (Spitz's nevus). Arch Dermatol 1978;114:1811-1823.

10. Bastian BC, LeBoit PE, Pinkel D. Mutations and copy number increase of HRAS in Spitz nevi with distinctive histopathological features. Am J Pathol 2000;157:967-972.

11. Weedon D, Little JH. Spindle and epithelioid cell nevi in children and adults. A review of 211 cases of the Spitz nevus. Cancer 1977;40:217-225.

12. Schmoeckel C, Wildi G, Schafer T. Spitz nevus versus malignant melanoma: Spitz nevi predominate on the thighs in patients younger than 40 years of age, melanomas on the trunk in patients 40 years of age or older. J Am Acad Dermatol 2007;56:753-758.

13. Echevarria R, Ackerman LV. Spindle and epithelioid cell nevi in the adult. Clinicopathologic report of 26 cases. Cancer 1967;20:175-189.

14. Bullen R, Snow SN, Larson PO, Kircik LH, Nychay S, Briggs P. Multiple agminated Spitz nevi: report of two cases and review of the literature. Pediatr Dermatol 1995;12:156-158.

15. Prose NS, Heilman E, Felman YM, Tanzer F, Silber J. Multiple benign juvenile melanoma. J Am Acad Dermatol 1983;9:236-242.

16. Aloi F, Tomasini C, Pippione M. Agminated Spitz nevi occurring within a congenital speck-led lentiginous nevus. Am J Dermatopathol 1995;17:594-598.

17. Gelbard SN, Tripp JM, Marghoob AA, et al. Management of Spitz nevi: a survey of dermatologists in the United States. J Am Acad Dermatol 2002;47:224-230.

18. Murphy ME, Boyer JD, Stashower ME, Zitelli JA. The surgical management of Spitz nevi. Dermatol Surg 2002;28:1065-1069.

19. Scott G, Chen KT, Rosai J. Pseudoepitheliomatous hyperplasia in Spitz nevi: a possible source of confusion with squamous cell carcinoma. Arch Pathol Lab Med 1989;113:61-63.

20. Kamino H, Flotte TJ, Misheloff E, Greco MA, Ackerman AB. Eosinophilic globules in Spitz's nevi. New findings and a diagnostic sign. Am J Dermatopathol 1979;1:319-324.

21. Wesselmann U, Becker LR, Brocker EB, LeBoit PE, Bastian BC. Eosinophilic globules in Spitz nevi: no evidence for apoptosis. Am J Dermatopathol 1998;20:551-554.

22. Arbuckle S, Weedon D. Eosinophilic globules in the Spitz nevus. J Am Acad Dermatol 1982;7:324-327.

23. Maize JC, Ackerman AB. Pigmented lesions of the skin. Clinicopathologic correlations. Philadelphia: Lea & Febiger; 1987.

24. Peters MS, Goellner JR. Spitz naevi and malignant melanomas of childhood and adolescence. Histopathology 1986;10:1289-1302.

25. Smolle J, Soyer HP, Juettner FM, Hoedl S, Kerl H. Nuclear parameters in the superficial and deep portion of melanocytic lesions—a morphometrical investigation. Pathol Res Pract 1988;183:266-270.

26. Smolle J, Smolle-Juettner FM, Stettner H, Kerl H. Relationship of tumor cell motility and morphologic patterns. Part 1. Melanocytic skin tumors. Am J Dermatopathol 1992;14:231-237.

27. Barr RJ, Morales RV, Graham JH. Desmoplastic nevus: a distinct histologic variant of mixed spindle cell and epithelioid cell nevus. Cancer 1980;46:557-564.

28. MacKie RM, Doherty VR. The desmoplastic melanocytic naevus: a distinct histological entity. Histopathology 1992;20:207-211.

28a. Tetzlaff M, Xu X, Elder DE, Elenitsas R. Angiomatoid Spitz nevus: a clinicopathologic study of six cases and a review of the literature. J Cutan Pathol 2009;36:471-476.

29. Liu J, Cohen PR, Farhood A. Hyalinizing Spitz nevus: spindle and epithelioid cell nevus with paucicellular collagenous stroma. South Med J 2004;97:102-106.

30. Clarke B, Essa A, Chetty R. Plexiform Spitz nevus. Int J Surg Pathol 2002;10:69-73.

31. Spatz A, Peterse S, Fletcher CD, Barnhill RL. Plexiform Spitz nevus: an intradermal Spitz nevus with plexiform growth pattern. Am J Dermatopathol 1999;21:542-546.

32. Busam KJ, Barnhill RL. Pagetoid Spitz nevus. Intraepidermal Spitz tumor with prominent pagetoid spread. Am J Surg Pathol 1995;19:1061-1067.

33. Harvell JD, Bastian BC, LeBoit PE. Persistent (recurrent) Spitz nevi: a histopathologic, immunohistochemical, and molecular pathologic study of 22 cases. Am J Surg Pathol 2002;26:654-661.

34. Su LD, Fullen DR, Sondak VK, Johnson TM, Lowe L. Sentinel lymph node biopsy for patients with problematic spitzoid melanocytic lesions: a report on 18 patients. Cancer 2003;97:499-507.

35. Shapiro PE. Spitz nevi. J Am Acad Dermatol 1993;29:667-668.

36. Vollmer RT. Patient age in Spitz nevus and malignant melanoma: implication of Bayes rule for differential diagnosis. Am J Clin Pathol 2004;121:872-877.

37. Sagebiel RW, Chinn EK, Egbert BM. Pigmented spindle cell nevus. Clinical and histologic review of 90 cases. Am J Surg Pathol 1984;8:645-653.

38. Smith NP. The pigmented spindle cell tumor of Reed: an underdiagnosed lesion. Semin Diagn Pathol 1987;4:75-87.

39. McGovern VJ. Melanoma. Histologic diagnosis and prognosis. New York: Raven Press; 1983:3-24.

40. Kantor G, Wheeland RG. Transepidermal elimination of nevus cells. A possible mechanism of nevus involution. Arch Dermatol 1987;123:1371-1374.

41. Harris GR, Shea CR, Horenstein MG, Reed JA, Burchette JL Jr, Prieto VG. Desmoplastic (sclerotic) nevus: an underrecognized entity that resembles dermatofibroma and desmoplastic melanoma. Am J Surg Pathol 1999;23:786-794.

42. Crotty KA, Scolyer RA, Li L, Palmer AA, Wang L, McCarthy SW. Spitz naevus versus Spitzoid melanoma: when and how can they be distinguished? Pathology 2002;34:6-12.

43. Lazzaro B, Rebers A, Herlyn M, Menrad A, Johnson B, Elder DE. Immunophenotyping of compound and Spitz nevi and vertical growth phase melanomas using a panel of monoclonal antibodies reactive in paraffin sections. J Invest Dermatol 1993;100:313S-317S.

44. Evans MJ, Sanders DS, Grant JH, Blessing K. Expression of Melan-A in Spitz, pigmented spindle cell nevi, and congenital nevi: comparative immunohistochemical study. Pediatr Dev Pathol 2000;3:36-39.

45. Ribe A, McNutt NS. S100A6 protein expression is different in Spitz nevi and melanomas. Mod Pathol 2003;16:505-511.

46. Bergman R, Malkin L, Sabo E, Kerner H. MIB-1 monoclonal antibody to determine proliferative activity of Ki-67 antigen as an adjunct to the histopathologic differential diagnosis of Spitz nevi. J Am Acad Dermatol 2001;44:500-504.

47. Kaleem Z, Lind AC, Humphrey PA, et al. Concurrent Ki-67 and p53 immunolabeling in cutaneous melanocytic neoplasms: an adjunct for recognition of the vertical growth phase in malignant melanomas? Mod Pathol 2000;13:217-222.

48. Rudolph P, Schubert C, Schubert B, Parwaresch R. Proliferation marker Ki-S5 as a diagnostic tool in melanocytic lesions. J Am Acad Dermatol 1997;37:169-178.

49. Li LX, Crotty KA, McCarthy SW, Palmer AA, Kril JJ. A zonal comparison of MIB1-Ki67 immunoreactivity in benign and malignant melanocytic lesions. Am J Dermatopathol 2000;22:489-495

50. Li LX, Crotty KA, Palmer AA, et al. Differentiating benign nevi from malignant melanoma using DNA microdensitometry and karyometry and maturation: a zonal comparison, correlation and multivariate analysis. Anal Quant Cytol Histol 2002;24:234-243.

51. Li LX, Crotty KA, Scolyer RA, et al. Use of multiple cytometric markers improves discrimination between benign and malignant melanocytic lesions: a study of DNA microdensitometry, karyometry, argyrophilic staining of nucleolar organizer regions and MIB1-Ki67 immunoreactivity. Melanoma Res 2003;13:581-586.

52. Li LX, Crotty KA, Palmer AA, et al. Argyrophilic staining of nucleolar organizer region count and morphometry in benign and malignant melanocytic lesions. Am J Dermatopathol 2003;25:190-197.

53. Stefanaki C, Stefanaki K, Antoniou C, et al. Cell cycle and apoptosis regulators in Spitz nevi: comparison with melanomas and common nevi. J Am Acad Dermatol 2007;56:815-824.

54. Yazdi AS, Palmedo G, Flaig MJ, et al. Mutations of the BRAF gene in benign and malignant melanocytic lesions. J Invest Dermatol 2003;121:1160-1162.

55. Gill M, Renwick N, Silvers DN, Celebi JT. Lack of BRAF mutations in Spitz nevi. J Invest Dermatol 2004;122:1325-1326.

56. Mihic-Probst D, Perren A, Schmid S, Saremaslani P, Komminoth P, Heitz PU. Absence of BRAF gene mutations differentiates spitz nevi from malignant melanoma. Anticancer Res 2004;24:2415-2418.

57. Palmedo G, Hantschke M, Rutten A, et al. The T1796A mutation of the BRAF gene is absent in Spitz nevi. J Cutan Pathol 2004;31:266-270.

58. Yazdi AS, Palmedo G, Flaig MJ, Kutzner H, Sander CA. Different frequencies of a BRAF point mutation in melanocytic skin lesions. Pigment Cell Res 2003;16:580.

59. Indsto JO, Kumar S, Wang L, Crotty KA, Arbuckle SM, Mann GJ. Low prevalence of RAS-RAF-activating mutations in Spitz melanocytic nevi compared with other melanocytic lesions. J Cutan Pathol 2007;34:448-455.

60. Fullen DR, Poynter JN, Lowe L, et al. BRAF and NRAS mutations in spitzoid melanocytic lesions. Mod Pathol 2006;16:1324-1332.

61. Pollock PM, Harper UL, Hansen KS, et al. High frequency of BRAF mutations in nevi. Nat Genet 2003;33:19-20.

62. Davies H, Bignell GR, Cox C, et al. Mutations of the BRAF gene in human cancer. Nature 2002;417:949-954.

63. Saldanha G, Purnell D, Fletcher A, Potter L, Gillies A, Pringle JH. High BRAF mutation frequency does not characterize all melanocytic tumor types. Int J Cancer 2004;111:705-710.

64. Satyamoorthy K, Li G, Gerrero MR, et al. Constitutive mitogen-activated protein kinase activation in melanoma is mediated by both BRAF mutations and autocrine growth factor stimulation. Cancer Res 2003;63:756-759.

65. Maldonado JL, Timmerman L, Fridlyand J, Bastian BC. Mechanisms of cell-cycle arrest in Spitz nevi with constitutive activation of the MAP-kinase pathway. Am J Pathol 2004;164:1783-1787.

66. Kumar R, Angelini S, Snellman E, Hemminki K. BRAF mutations are common somatic events in melanocytic nevi. J Invest Dermatol 2004;122:342-348.

67. Bastian BC, Wesselmann U, Pinkel D, LeBoit PE. Molecular cytogenetic analysis of Spitz nevi shows clear differences to melanoma. J Invest Dermatol 1999;113:1065-1069.

68. Kantrow SM, Boyd AS, Ellis DL, et al. Expression of activated Akt in benign nevi, Spitz nevi and melanomas. J Cutan Pathol 2007;34:593-596.

69. Talve L, Sauroja I, Collan Y, Punnonen K, Ekfors T. Loss of expression of the p16^{INK4}/CDKN2 gene in cutaneous malignant melanoma correlates with tumor cell proliferation and invasive stage. Int J Cancer 1997;74:255-259.

70. Sparrow LE, Eldon MJ, English DR, Heenan PJ. p16 and p21WAF1 protein expression in melanocytic tumors by immunohistochemistry. Am J Dermatopathol 1998;20:255-261.

71. Wajapeyee N, Serra RW, Zhu X, Mahalingam M, Green MR. Oncogenic BRAF induces senescence and apoptosis through pathways mediated by the secreted protein IGFBP7. Cell 2008;132:363-374.

72. Gray-Schopfer VC, Cheong SC, Chong H, et al. Cellular senescence in naevi and immortalisation in melanoma: a role for p16? Br J Cancer 2006;95:496-505.

73. Ha L, Ichikawa T, Anver M, et al. ARF functions as a melanoma tumor suppressor by inducing p53-independent senescence. Proc Natl Acad Sci U S A 2007;104:10968-10973.

74. Harvell JD, Kohler S, Zhu S, Hernandez-Boussard T, Pollack JR, van de Rijn M. High-resolution array-based comparative genomic hybridization for distinguishing paraffin-embedded Spitz nevi and melanomas. Diagn Mol Pathol 2004;13:22-25.

75. Takata M, Maruo K, Kageshita T, et al. Two cases of unusual acral melanocytic tumors: illustration of molecular cytogenetics as a diagnostic tool. Hum Pathol 2003;34:89-92.

76. Bastian BC. Molecular cytogenetics as a diagnostic tool for typing melanocytic tumors. Recent Results Cancer Res 2002;160:92-99.

77. Schmoeckel C. How consistent are dermatopathologists in reading early malignant melanomas and lesions "precursor" to them? An international survey. Am J Dermatopathol 1984;6(Suppl):13-24.

78. Cerroni L, Kerl H. Tutorial on melanocytic lesions. Am J Dermatopathol 2001;23:237-241.

79. Barnhill RL, Flotte TJ, Fleischli M, Perez-Atayde A. Cutaneous melanoma and atypical Spitz tumors in childhood. Cancer 1995;76:1833-1845.

80. Spatz A, Calonje E, Handfield-Jones S, Barnhill RL. Spitz tumors in children: a grading system for risk stratification. Arch Dermatol 1999;135:282-285.

81. Urso C. A new perspective for spitz tumors? Am J Dermatopathol 2005;27:364-366.

82. Urso C, Borgognoni L, Saieva C, et al. Sentinel lymph node biopsy in patients with "atypical Spitz tumors." A report on 12 cases. Hum Pathol 2006;37:816-823.

83. Roaten JB, Partrick DA, Pearlman N, Gonzalez RJ, Gonzalez R, McCarter MD. Sentinel lymph node biopsy for melanoma and other melanocytic tumors in adolescents. J Pediatr Surg 2005;40:232-235.

84. Lohmann CM, Coit DG, Brady MS, Berwick M, Busam KJ. Sentinel lymph node biopsy in patients with diagnostically controversial spitzoid melanocytic tumors. Am J Surg Pathol 2002;26:47-55.

85. Cerroni L, et al. . . . . Am J Surg Pathol 2010. (in press.) [Author needs to provide more info.]

86. Cohen LM, Bennion SD, Johnson TW, Golitz LE. Hypermelanotic nevus: clinical, histopathologic, and ultrastructural features in 316 cases. Am J Dermatopathol 1997;19:23-30.

4 BLUE NEVI AND RELATED LESIONS

Blue nevi are benign dermal melanocytic tumors defined originally in terms of their clinically characteristic blue-black color. The color is not pathognomonic, however, since other lesions may be blue, especially primary and metastatic melanomas. Histologically, blue nevi are characterized by the presence of slender spindle-shaped to dendritic melanocytes, often exclusively located in the reticular dermis. These cells have sometimes been assumed to be derived from Schwann cells, but the occasional finding of subtly increased numbers of melanocytes in the overlying epidermis and the location of some lesions close to the epidermis suggest the alternative possibility of an epidermal origin (1).

The characteristic blue hue has been explained in terms of the "Tyndall effect," which results in blue coloration of any deep-seated pigment because of the scattering of light by dermal collagen, with preferential transmission of the blue wavelengths. Thus, blood in veins, old tattoos where the pigment has migrated deeply, and metastatic melanomas where brown pigment is synthesized in the dermis or subcutis all appear predominantly dark blue to the clinical observer. Common acquired nevi, in contrast to blue nevi, are composed of round cells that tend to produce pigment only within the cells that are superficially located in the papillary dermis (with the possible exception of the rare inverted type A and deep penetrating variants). Melanin pigment that is located near the dermoepidermal junction, as in normal pigmented skin, tends to appear as various shades of brown to external observation.

Blue nevi can be placed along a spectrum of cellularity and atypia from the common small and sparsely cellular type, to cellular and/or atypical blue nevi, to rare malignant blue nevi. The latter are discussed with malignant melanocytic tumors.

COMMON BLUE NEVUS

Definition. The *common blue nevus* is a benign melanocytic tumor composed of heavily pigmented, spindle-shaped and/or dendritic melanocytes that are located mainly in the reticular dermis (1).

Clinical Features. Typical lesions range from a few millimeters to a centimeter or so in diameter (fig. 4-1). Cellular blue nevi may be considerably larger, up to several centimeters. Common blue nevi occur anywhere on the skin, while cellular blue nevi tend to occur frequently in the sacral and buttock regions and around the ankles. Rare subungual blue nevi have been described (2). Occasionally, multiple lesions occur in a single patient, and rare familial lesions have been described (3).

A characteristic blue nevus is a dark blue-black, small (4 to 10 mm), slightly raised papule with a regular but somewhat ill-defined border. Combined (blue admixed with common acquired) nevi are more likely to resemble

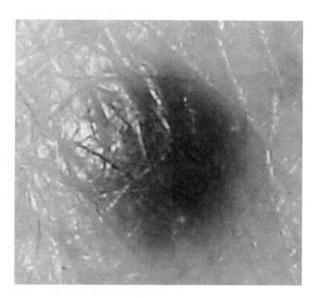

Figure 4-1

BLUE NEVUS

A circumscribed, symmetric, round, blue-black papule. (Fig. F from Plate II, Fascicle 2, Third Series.)

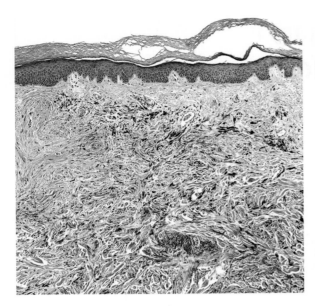
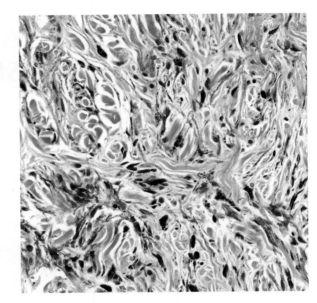

Figure 4-2

BLUE NEVUS

Left: Heavily and uniformly pigmented spindle to dendritic cells are placed among reticular dermis collagen fiber bundles. There is no junctional or in situ component in the overlying epidermis.

Right: At high magnification, the cells are stuffed with coarsely divided melanin pigment granules, which often obscure the nucleus. The nuclei have clear chromatin and smooth nuclear membranes.

common nevi, having a circumscribed border and brown or tan coloration, although some lesions are bicolored. Cellular blue nevi are large nodules, about as tall as they are broad.

All benign blue nevi are typically stable lesions, with no history of change or growth. There is no evidence of any significant propensity for malignant change. The patients are typically asymptomatic, and ulceration, even after trauma, is uncommon. Excision or biopsy may be performed because of the dark color of the lesion to rule out melanoma or for cosmetic indications. If a blue nevus is recognized as such clinically, however, there is no reason to remove it.

Unlike most common nevi, blue nevi do not contain mutations of the oncogene *BRAF* (4,5). As is also the case in common nevi, blue nevi may persist after incomplete excision and present as apparent clinical recurrence (6).

Microscopic Findings. The presence of dendritic and/or spindle cells in the dermis that contain abundant coarse melanin pigment is the hallmark of blue nevi and their variants (figs. 4-2–4-9). The cells are "placed" between dermal collagen bundles, separating

them without tissue destruction, and forming a well-defined but irregular collection of dark-pigmented cells in the reticular dermis. There may be an associated subtle proliferation of nonpigmented fibroblast-like cells and the dermal collagen bundles may appear slightly thickened. The pattern of placement of the cells in the dermis results in separation of most of them from their neighbors, leading to an appearance of low cellularity, with no evidence of expansile contiguous tumorigenic growth of the type seen in a nodule of metastatic melanoma in the dermis. Indeed, pigmented dendritic cells may be so sparsely situated in some lesions that they may be entirely overlooked on low-power inspection, or dismissed as areas of nonspecific dermal hypercellularity (e.g., mild fibrosis). There is a considerable range of cellularity, however, and in some lesions, the architecture of the dermis is largely replaced by the spindle cell proliferation. In other lesions, there is a brisk fibrogenic reaction, with broad collagen bundles that suggest a fibrohistiocytic lesion.

At higher magnification, the lesional cells are elongated, narrow spindle or dendritic

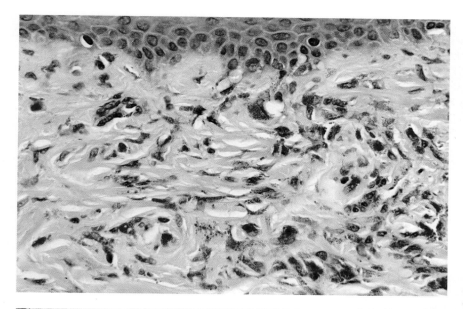

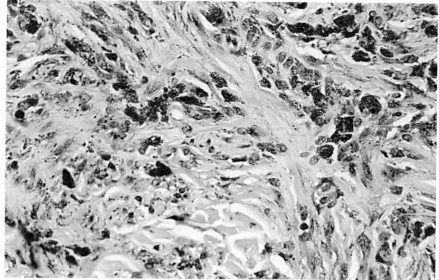

Figure 4-3

BLUE NEVUS

Top: The spindle to dendritic cells placed among reticular dermis collagen fibers have coarse melanin pigment granules.

Bottom: There may be a subtle admixture of more nevoid melanocytes, as here in the top right quadrant.

cells, containing variable but usually quite prominent coarse melanin pigment granules. Unlike melanophages, which also may contain abundant melanin pigment within the perinuclear cytoplasm, blue nevus cells characteristically have pigmented dendrites, visible as thin melanin-laden cytoplasmic extensions upon careful inspection. The more central pigment may obscure the nucleus, but if the nuclei are visualized they are small, with occasional small blue "chromocenters" but no large eosinophilic nucleoli and no mitoses. There is no ulceration or spontaneous necrosis. Nevus cells may be seen in and around nerves and in the walls of blood vessels, and these findings should not be regarded with any concern in an otherwise characteristic lesion.

Although, in general, blue nevi are not associated with a junctional component, five cases of *compound blue nevus* have been described (7). They are characterized by single dendritic melanocytes at the dermoepidermal junction with striking intraepidermal prolongations. These lesions may mimic cutaneous melanoma both upon gross clinical examination and dermoscopically.

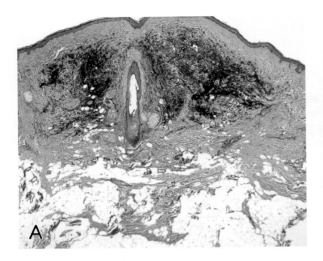

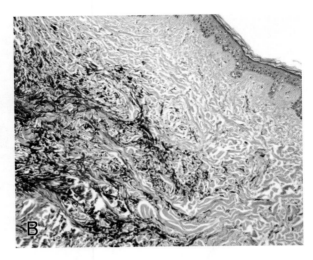

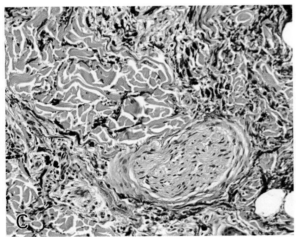

Figure 4-4

BLUE NEVUS

A: In this heavily pigmented example, there appears to be an associated abnormality of cutaneous nerves, which are unusually prominent compared to the surrounding skin.

B: The heavily pigmented spindle cells are placed among reticular dermis collagen fiber bundles.

C: Lesional cells extend around nerves and may be present within the perineurium in blue nevi, without signifying malignancy.

Differential Diagnosis. The most important entity in the differential diagnosis is malignant melanoma. Although some blue nevi simulate a desmoplastic melanoma, the lack of an in situ component, cellular atypia, and nodular peripheral clusters of lymphocytes that are characteristic of desmoplastic melanoma, usually facilitates this distinction. In addition, immunohistochemical studies may be helpful: blue nevi are usually diffusely positive for Melan-A/MART-1 and HMB45, while desmoplastic melanoma is usually negative for these antigens, at least in the dermal spindle cell population. Conversely, metastatic malignant melanoma may simulate a blue nevus. In a study of 10 lesions from three patients, pigmented melanocytes and melanophages were arranged in the dermis in a blue nevus-like growth pattern. Histologic clues to the diagnosis of metastatic melanoma

included the presence of atypical epithelioid melanocytes, mitotic figures, and an associated inflammatory cell infiltrate at the periphery of the lesion (8).

Cellular blue nevus is a related lesion that includes focal areas of increased cellularity without necrosis or mitotic activity (see below). Combined nevi most typically combine the morphology of a common acquired nevus with that of a blue nevus. Most such lesions either show a more superficial common acquired nevus with an underlying blue nevus component, or less commonly, an intimate admixture of common acquired nevus cells with dendritic pigmented blue nevus cells.

Some blue nevi are quite cellular, with storiform-like whorls that may simulate dermatofibromas, especially those variants with abundant hemosiderin pigment that are also known as

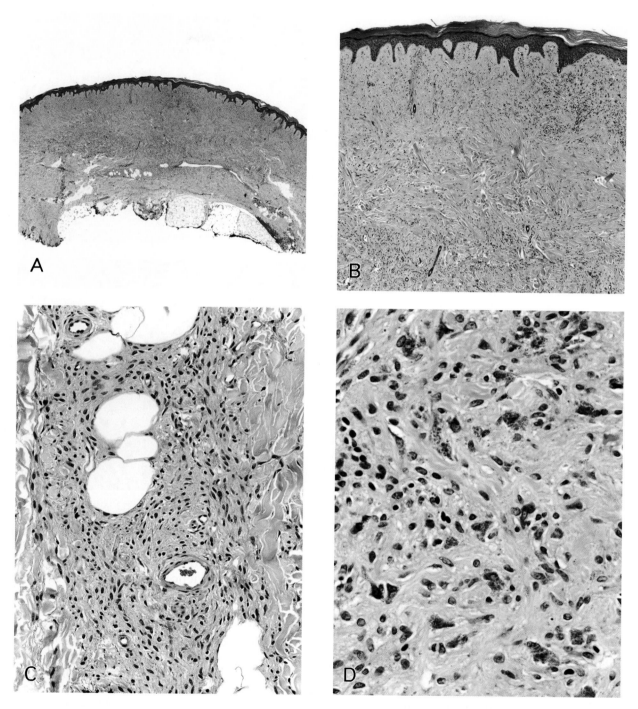

Figure 4-5

BLUE NEVUS, DESMOPLASTIC AND OLIGOMELANOTIC

A: There is extensive alteration of the dermal collagen in this large lesion compared to the surrounding dermis.

B: At higher magnification, lesional cells are present within sclerotic collagen fiber bundles. In this area, the lesional cells are in contiguity with one another, a feature of a cellular blue nevus.

C: Cytoplasmic melanin pigment is sparse in this lesion (oligomelanotic blue nevus).

D: In this field, pigment is present mainly in melanophages.

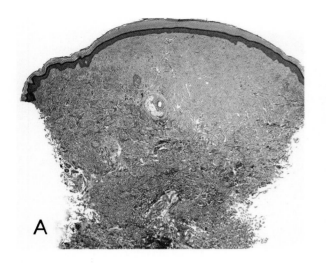

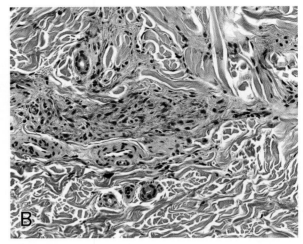

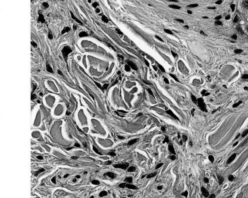

Figure 4-6

BLUE NEVUS, DESMOPLASTIC AND OLIGOMELANOTIC

A: Scanning magnification clearly shows the alteration of collagen in the lesion.

B: High magnification shows heavily pigmented spindle cells, present here around blood vessels and nerves.

C: Pigmented spindle cells are placed among reticular dermis collagen bundles and embedded in a delicate desmoplastic stroma.

sclerosing hemangiomas or aneurysmal variants of blue nevi. Occasional blue nevi are hypopigmented (oligomelanotic) (figs. 4-5–4-7) or frankly amelanotic (9,10), and immunohistochemistry may be required to definitively differentiate them from benign fibrohistiocytic proliferations.

Occasionally a tattoo (post-traumatic or "decorative") may cause difficulty because of pigment in histiocytes that may appear somewhat dendritic. In case of doubt, the pigment can be confirmed as melanin with a silver stain and permanganate bleach (see chapter 11).

Postinflammatory hyperpigmentation and other forms of pigmentary incontinence can usually be distinguished from blue nevi because the architectural patterns differ. The former lesions are usually plaques with pigment disposed in round cells (melanophages) in the papillary

dermis, while blue nevi are composed of clusters or ill-defined nodules of pigmented dendritic cells in the reticular dermis. In certain cases, pigment incontinence primarily involves more stellate dermal dendrocytes, as may be the case with minocycline-induced hyperpigmentation. These lesions form patches that differ clinically from blue nevi, the pigment tends to be positive for iron as well as melanin stains, and the dendritic cells in question express coagulation factor XIIIa by immunohistochemistry.

Oculodermal melanoses, such as nevus of Ota or nevus of Ito, as well as Mongolian spots, may also present with pigmented melanin-containing cells in the reticular dermis. These lesions are much broader than most blue nevi, generally less cellular, and have typical clinical presentations.

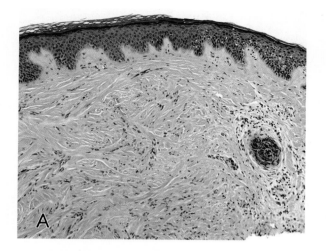

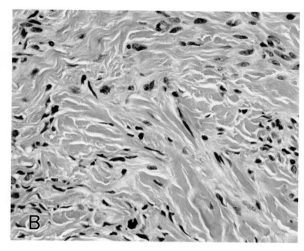

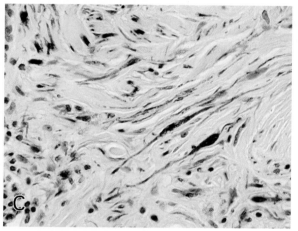

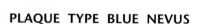

Figure 4-7

BLUE NEVUS, DESMOPLASTIC AND AMELANOTIC

A: Scanning magnification shows altered collagen with spindle cells placed among the fiber bundles.

B: Higher magnification shows elongated spindle cells without melanin pigment embedded in delicate reticulin fibers in a coarser collagenous matrix.

C: S-100 protein stain is strongly and diffusely positive in the lesional cells.

PLAQUE TYPE BLUE NEVUS

Lesions termed *plaque type blue nevi* have been described in a number of case reports. These are large lesions (15 cm or more), distributed anywhere on the skin. They are typically congenital or evolve in childhood (11,12). In a report of two cases in adults, there was a history of slow enlargement during adolescence and subsequent nodule formation (12). The lesions are characterized by a multifocal dermal and subcutaneous proliferation of spindle-shaped and dendritic pigmented melanocytes, with individual foci that range from dermal melanocytosis to common blue nevus and cellular blue nevus (fig. 4-10). In the two reported cases, cellular foci were present in the subcutis and in one patient the stroma of the breast was involved. The cells were immunoreactive for S-100 protein, gp100 (HMB45), and Melan-A (A103).

Ultrastructural analysis revealed melanocytes typical of blue nevus. The lesions were termed "large plaque type blue nevus with subcutaneous cellular nodules."

Plaque type blue nevi are typically benign and may be misdiagnosed as melanomas (11,12). Rare examples of clinically similar lesions with histologically malignant phenotypes have been reported (11,13,14).

NEUROCRISTIC HAMARTOMA

Neurocristic hamartoma may be closely related to plaque type blue nevus. The lesion tends to involve hair follicles preferentially (*pilar neurocristic hamartoma*) (15), or may be more diffuse like a plaque type blue nevus (16). There is usually a more complex mixture of cell types including subpopulations exhibiting schwannian differentiation. Malignant change has been reported in these lesions (13,17).

121

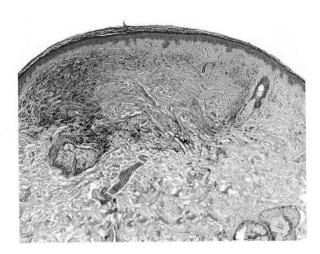
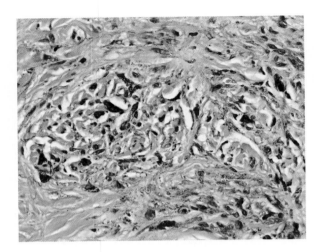

Figure 4-8

BLUE NEVUS, SCLEROTIC

Left: At scanning magnification, the lesion resembles a dermatofibroma.
Right: Higher magnification shows the typical heavily pigmented cells placed among thickened collagen bundles.

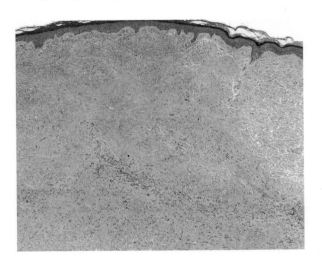
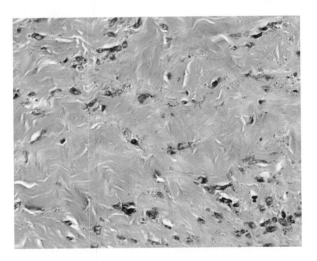

Figure 4-9

BLUE NEVUS, SCLEROTIC

Left: A large lesion has altered collagen, with lesional cells placed among the fiber bundles.
Right: The thickened collagen bundles have scattered lesional cells, most of which are pigmented.

EPITHELIOID BLUE NEVUS

Definition. *Epithelioid blue nevus* is a rare variant of blue nevus that is composed predominantly of plump, heavily pigmented epithelioid to spindle cells. This lesion was first described in association with the Carney complex, a familial multitumoral syndrome consisting of myxomas of the heart, skin, and breast; endocrine tumors of the adrenal cortex, pituitary gland, testis, and thyroid gland; schwannomas; and spotty skin pigmentation. The pigmented skin lesions include lentigines, blue nevi, epithelioid blue nevi, and psammomatous melanotic schwannomas. Psammomatous melanotic schwannoma is a low-grade malignancy and is described in a later section, Malignant Melanocytic Schwannoma. Since the original description by Carney (18), similar epithelioid blue nevi have

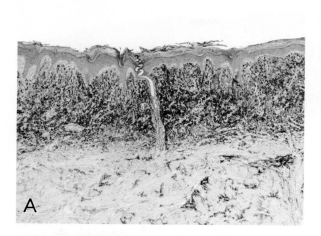

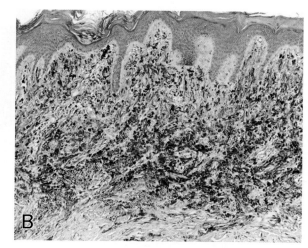

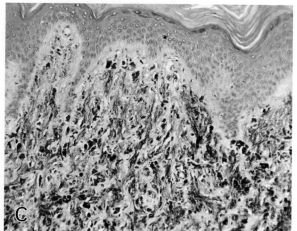

Figure 4-10

PLAQUE TYPE BLUE NEVUS

A: The lesion is broad and heavily pigmented.

B,C: The cells are heavily pigmented spindle cells. This histology may overlap with that of cellular blue nevus and pigmented epithelioid melanocytoma. (Courtesy of Dr. Alain Spatz, Ottawa, Canada.)

been described as sporadic lesions in the absence of the Carney complex (19,20).

Clinical Features. The epithelioid blue nevi in the Carney complex are multiple and widely distributed on the skin, with a predilection for the extremities and trunk. Clinically, these lesions are small (less than 1 cm) and pigmented, and exhibit a dome-shaped architecture. None of the originally described lesions recurred or metastasized (18). In a subsequent study of 33 lesions without evidence of the Carney complex, again there were no metastases (21). More recently, however, a group of lesions categorized as "pigmented epithelioid melanocytoma," including some lesions previously labeled as "animal type" and "melanophagic" melanomas, has been described as being indistinguishable from epithelioid blue nevi, and a few of these have recurred or metastasized, indicating that

at least some of these lesions must be regarded as potential low-grade malignancies whose biologic significance is uncertain (22). These lesions are discussed further with pigmented epithelioid melanocytic tumors (see Pigmented Epithelioid Melanocytoma).

Microscopic Findings. The lesions are intradermal melanocytic nevi composed of polygonal epithelioid cells laden with melanin. The nuclei are vesicular and have pale chromatin and a single prominent nucleolus. The cells show no maturation at the base of the lesion and, in contrast with the usual stromal changes in blue nevi, no fibrosis of the dermis (19). Moderate pleomorphism and rare mitotic figures were described in one series, with no metastatic events in a relatively short follow-up period (average, 31 months; range, 6 to 162 months) (21). In this series, the neoplasms showed a morphologic

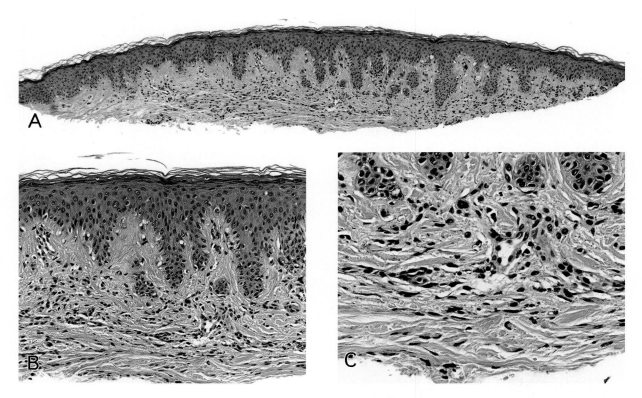

Figure 4-11

EPITHELIOID BLUE NEVUS

This lesion is composed of epithelioid and/or spindle cells that seem to mature from superficial to deep. There is no in situ component of a melanoma in the overlying epidermis (B). Lesions like this should be interpreted with caution, especially in adults and especially if there is cytologic atypia or any mitotic activity.

spectrum that encompassed a group of combined blue nevi with epithelioid melanocytes and other characteristics of Spitz tumors, and there was another group that overlapped with deep penetrating nevi. Epithelioid combined nevus was thought to be a fitting nosologic designation for all of these lesions (figs. 4-11, 4-12).

CELLULAR BLUE NEVUS

Definition. *Cellular blue nevus* is a large, benign, acquired melanocytic tumor composed of pigmented spindle cells that form a bulky cellular nodule. The nodule typically spans the reticular dermis, extending from the papillary dermis to the panniculus. These lesions were first distinguished from malignant melanoma by Allen in 1949 (23).

Clinical Features. The tumor is large (one to several centimeters), blue-black, and nodular. It is usually symmetric and well circumscribed, often located in the lower lumbosacral region, and typically acquired in young adulthood (24). There is a history of slowly progressive or limited growth followed by stability. Other common sites include distal extremities, especially involving the ankle. The sex ratio is about equal, and in one study, two thirds of the patients were under 40 years of age (25). The overlying epidermis is smooth and ulceration is uncommon.

Gross Findings. The cut surface is usually a homogeneous dark brown-blue-black, although some sparsely pigmented lesions are pink or gray. Uncommonly, areas of cystic degeneration or hemorrhage have been described (26). On rare occasions, deep extension may result in compression and destruction of adjacent tissues, as has been reported in certain lesions that have caused osteolysis of underlying bone (27).

Microscopic Features. Cellular blue nevi typically involve the full thickness of the reticular

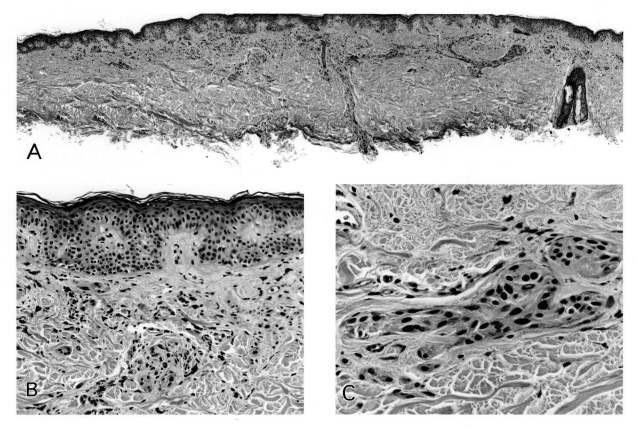

Figure 4-12

EPITHELIOID BLUE NEVUS

This lesion has plumper, more epithelioid cells than the cells in the previous example. At high magnification there is hyperchromatism and nuclear irregularity (C). A careful study should be made for any evidence of an in situ component in the overlying epidermis or for dermal mitoses. There is overlap between lesions of this type and pigmented epithelioid melanocytoma, as well as Spitz nevus, cellular blue nevus, and deep penetrating nevus. We recommend complete excision of this lesion if it is present at the margins.

dermis. They often have a highly characteristic "dumbbell" configuration, with a nodule in the upper reticular dermis connected to a similar nodule in the fat by a narrower isthmic zone (figs. 4-13–4-16). In this manner, a deep expansile nodule may be formed, giving rise to an alarming appearance on gross section and on low-power microscopic examination. This pattern is characteristic of cellular blue nevus and may be essentially diagnostic at scanning magnification.

The lesions are composed mainly of spindle cells, and at the periphery there may be a less cellular component that is indistinguishable from a common blue nevus. Toward the center of the lesion is a much more cellular component, with heavily pigmented spindle cells lying in contiguity. Cytologically, the most characteristic

feature of cellular blue nevi is the biphasic pattern of clear (relatively unmelanized) plumper cells alternating with heavily pigmented spindle cells (figs. 4-13, 4-14, 4-16) (28).

There are several cytoarchitectural variants, although some overlap (24,29). The most common is the *mixed-biphasic*, or *"patternless," variant*, composed of an intermingling of oval to plump spindle and/or epithelioid cells with elongated dendritic melanocytes containing fine melanin granules. The *alveolar variant* is the most distinctive and is characterized by rounded nests of clear spindle cells embedded in a matrix of dendritic and spindle-shaped, more heavily pigmented melanocytes, similar to those of the mixed-biphasic pattern. In the less frequent *fascicular*, or *neuronevoid, pattern*, the background spindle

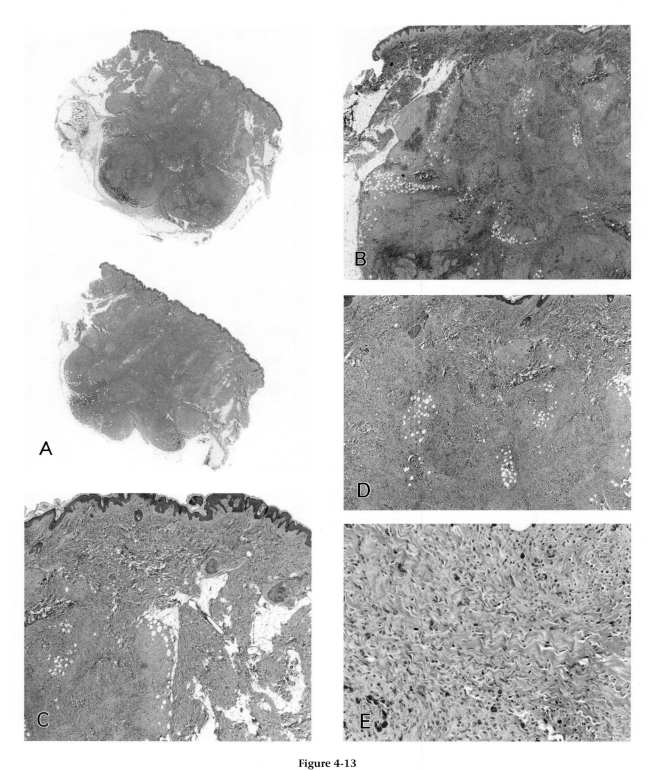

Figure 4-13

CELLULAR BLUE NEVUS

A–C: A bulky tumor in a 7-year-old child spans the full thickness of the reticular dermis.
D,E: Spindle cell areas are reminiscent of banal blue nevus.

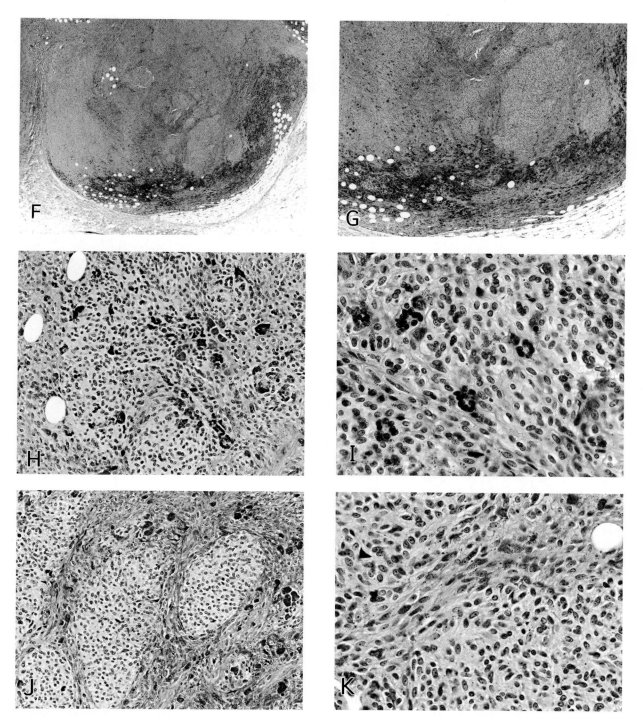

Figure 4-13 (Continued)

F,G: The bulbous extensions at the base are a characteristic feature.

H,I: Focally, peculiar nevus giant cells are present.

J,K: Typical mixed-biphasic pattern of a cellular blue nevus is seen focally. Spindle to cuboidal cells with clear cytoplasm are arranged in clusters, and separated by infiltrating heavily pigmented spindle cells placed among reticular dermis collagen fibers. The lesional cells have bland nuclei, with uniform chromatin and regular nuclear membranes. Mitotic figures are typically rare or absent.

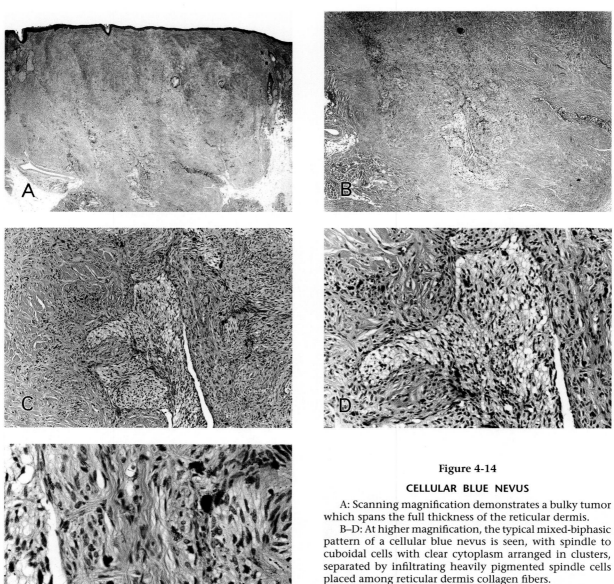

Figure 4-14

CELLULAR BLUE NEVUS

A: Scanning magnification demonstrates a bulky tumor which spans the full thickness of the reticular dermis.

B–D: At higher magnification, the typical mixed-biphasic pattern of a cellular blue nevus is seen, with spindle to cuboidal cells with clear cytoplasm arranged in clusters, separated by infiltrating heavily pigmented spindle cells placed among reticular dermis collagen fibers.

E: The lesional cells have bland nuclei, with uniform chromatin and regular nuclear membranes. Mitotic figures are typically rare or absent.

cells exhibit schwannian differentiation, with fascicles composed of wavy fibers resembling peripheral nerves. This designation from the older literature may overlap with the more recent designation of similar lesions as deep penetrating nevi or as pigmented epithelioid melanocytomas. In cellular blue nevi, lesional cells may be observed in the perineurium of authentic cutaneous nerves, an appearance that

should not suggest malignancy in a blue nevus. Although these patterns are useful in diagnosis and descriptive nosology, they have no known prognostic significance. A fourth pattern, *atypical cellular blue nevus*, may have some prognostic significance, but this is yet unclear as most of the described cases have followed a benign course after excision (see below). Many of the diagnostic features of atypical cellular blue nevi

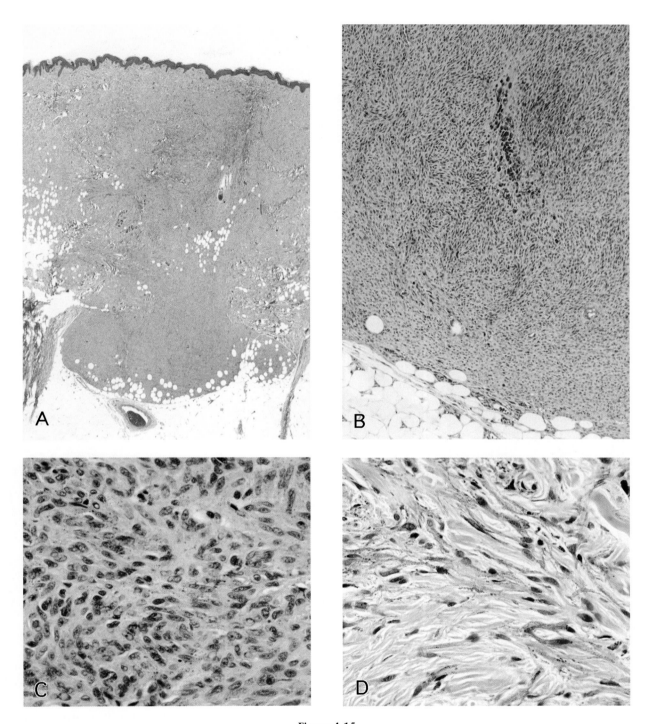

Figure 4-15

CELLULAR BLUE NEVUS

A: A bulky tumor spans the reticular dermis, with bulbous expansion at the base, resembling a "dumbbell." Sheets of spindle cells are arranged in an ill-defined nested pattern, with variable pigmentation.

B: The lesion appears to infiltrate the fat.

C: Higher magnification shows pigment and coarsely divided melanin granules, which are relatively sparse in this case.

D: In another area, the histology is that of a common blue nevus.

Figure 4-16

CELLULAR BLUE NEVUS

A: A bulky tumor spans the reticular dermis and extends into the panniculus at the base of the image.

B: Spindle cells are in a vaguely nested pattern, extending into the panniculus.

C: This field shows the characteristic mixed-biphasic pattern of a cellular blue nevus, with clear cells in the nests, separated by spindle cells which tend to be more heavily pigmented.

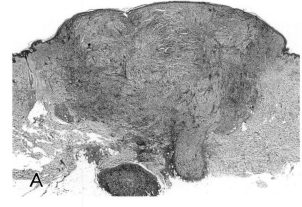

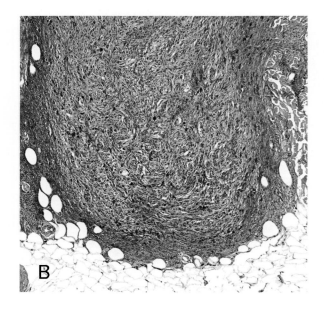

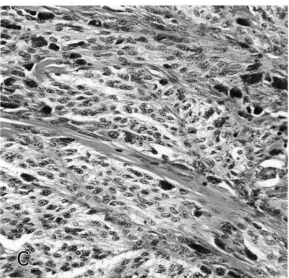

overlap with those of malignant blue nevi, however, so that a cautious approach to diagnosis and management is appropriate (29).

At higher magnification, the predominant lesional cells are long and plump, with abundant cytoplasm that contains, in the pigmented cells, abundant conspicuous, predominantly coarse melanin pigment. The nuclei are usually not completely obscured by the pigment, and they are typically quite regular, without prominent nucleoli and with few if any mitoses. These lesions should be carefully examined at both scanning and high magnification for indicators of possible malignancy (see Malignant Blue Nevus), particularly in the setting of changing lesions or those of large clinical size with evidence of expansile destructive growth, frequent

mitoses, severe cellular atypia, and spontaneous necrosis. Mitotic figures are rare or absent in most cellular blue nevi.

Most cellular blue nevi are heavily pigmented lesions. An unusual *amelanotic variant* of cellular blue nevus was recently reported, however (30). The clinical demographics were similar to those of pigmented cellular blue nevi. The lack of pigmentation resulted in an atypical clinical appearance, so that a diagnosis of blue nevus was not considered by the attending physician in any of the cases. All of the tumors extended deep into the reticular dermis or subcutaneous fat to a mean thickness of 5.5 mm (range, 1.7 to 11 mm). Ulceration was present in two lesions, however, tumor necrosis was not observed. Mild cytologic atypia and pleomorphism were present in five cases. Mitotic activity (up to 3 mitoses/mm^2) was observed in 11 lesions. A brisk lymphocytic host response was present in only one lesion. In contrast to desmoplastic melanomas, which could enter the differential diagnosis, most, but not all, tumors were reactive not only for S-100 protein but also for HMB45. Clinical follow-up for a mean of 32 months was consistent with a benign course in that local recurrence was not observed after complete excision, and none of the cases was associated with clinical evidence of lymph node or distant metastases. These lesions must be distinguished from malignant cellular blue nevus and other variants of melanoma (30).

Harvell and White (31) demonstrated that blue nevi of all histologic subtypes and combinations are capable of persistence and clinical recurrence. In their study, the persistence usually was histologically similar to the original, but in some cases was more "cellular" because, for the most part, excision of the persistent lesion revealed a deeper spindle-fascicular (cellular) component not evident in the original superficial biopsy. In two cases, the original blue nevus appeared completely banal, but the persistent/recurrent lesions were histologically distinct and demonstrated atypical histologic features. Yet follow-up (average, 3.7 years) supported benign biology. Atypical changes in some lesions were worrisome for malignancy, including increased cellularity, cellular pleomorphism, mitotic figures, and a lymphocytic infiltrate. The interval from initial biopsy to biopsy of the recurrent lesion was often longer (mean, 2.7 years) for recurrent blue nevi than for recurrent common compound or intradermal melanocytic nevi. In contrast to recurrent common melanocytic nevi, the recurrence, in at least one case, extended beyond the scar of the original excision. The authors consider that the described atypical morphologic parameters in previously biopsied small blue nevi are probably reactive and "pseudomalignant." Necrosis en mass, marked cytologic atypia, and frequent mitotic figures are, as always, features that should suggest a malignant diagnosis (24,32).

Several cases have recently been described as *ancient blue nevi* or *cellular blue nevi with degenerative stromal changes*. These have had cystic degeneration or hyalinization of stroma, coupled with cytologic atypia but without mitoses (33).

Although mitotic figures are observed in apparently characteristic cellular blue nevi, and some patients have been disease-free for long periods, we are suspicious of lesions with more than an occasional mitosis. A rate greater than 1 mitosis/mm^2 (9 to 10 high-power fields) in our opinion should lead to a qualification of the lesion as an "atypical" cellular blue nevus (22), and a recommendation for complete excision. Similarly, the presence of any necrosis or high-grade nuclear atypia should lead to a careful evaluation of the lesion, a heightened search for other atypical features, and a recommendation for complete excision. In our own practices, we descriptively report some lesions with features of cellular blue nevus, but with occasional mitoses and a history of slow growth, as "melanocytic tumors of uncertain malignant potential" (MELT-UMP). Some perhaps related lesions may also be called "pigmented epithelioid melanocytoma," a term that connotes a low-grade malignancy of uncertain potential (22). Metastasis from such lesions is rare but does occur.

The interobserver agreement for the diagnosis of cellular and atypical cellular blue nevi and their distinction from melanoma has been recently studied by a group of 14 dermatopathologists from the North American Melanoma Study Group. It was concluded that there was substantial disagreement and confusion among these expert pathologists regarding the definitions and biologic potential of cellular blue lesions, especially those thought to have atypical features (34).

A curious phenomenon of "metastasis" to regional lymph nodes has been described in association with benign cellular blue nevi. In reviewing 14 early cases, Rodriguez and Ackerman (25) noted that the patients were younger than average (7 to 26 years), that the sites of the nevi were sacrococcygeal or in the distal limbs, and that the nodes involved were inguinal or axillary. Importantly, the metastases were usually noted at excision of the cutaneous primary and presumably were clinically impalpable. In some cases the metastases consisted of small well-differentiated groups of nevus cells in the marginal sinuses (25). Nodal cells in association with blue nevi have been reported in lymph node sinuses and parenchyma and occasionally have presented as a histologically or clinically expansile and destructive mass. In the latter case, it may perhaps be a true metastasis rather than a developmental abnormality. The limited evidence suggests that survival of patients with cellular blue nevi that give rise to "metastases" in follow-up may be better than expected. Nevertheless, such a finding should prompt careful

evaluation of the primary lesion. The patient should be followed with an attitude of optimism for cure. Adjuvant therapy and additional surgery, including completion lymphadenectomy, may be discussed. The well-recognized phenomenon of capsular nevi in regional lymph nodes should be clearly distinguished from these regional "metastatic tumors of uncertain potential."

REFERENCES

1. Leopold JG, Richards DB. The interrelationship of blue and common naevi. J Pathol Bacteriol 1968;95:37-46.
2. Causeret AS, Skowron F, Viallard AM, Balme B, Thomas L. Subungual blue nevus. J Am Acad Dermatol 2003;49:310-312.
3. Knoell KA, Nelson KC, Patterson JW. Familial multiple blue nevi. J Am Acad Dermatol 1998;39:322-325.
4. Yazdi AS, Palmedo G, Flaig MJ, et al. Mutations of the BRAF gene in benign and malignant melanocytic lesions. J Invest Dermatol 2003;121:1160-1162.
5. Saldanha G, Purnell D, Fletcher A, Potter L, Gillies A, Pringle JH. High BRAF mutation frequency does not characterize all melanocytic tumor types. Int J Cancer 2004;111:705-710.
6. Munoz C, Quintero A, Sanchez JL, Ruiz-Santiago H. Persistent blue nevus simulating melanoma. J Am Acad Dermatol 2004;50(Suppl):S118-S120.
7. Ferrara G, Argenziano G, Zgavec B, et al. "Compound blue nevus": a reappraisal of "superficial blue nevus with prominent intraepidermal dendritic melanocytes" with emphasis on dermoscopic and histopathologic features. J Am Acad Dermatol 2002;46:85-89.
8. Busam KJ. Metastatic melanoma to the skin simulating blue nevus. Am J Surg Pathol 1999;23:276-282.
9. Bhawan J, Cao SL. Amelanotic blue nevus: a variant of blue nevus. Am J Dermatopathol 1999;21:225-228.
10. Bolognia JL, Glusac EJ. Hypopigmented common blue nevi. Arch Dermatol 1998;134:754-756.
11. Pittman JL, Fisher BK. Plaque-type blue nevus. Arch Dermatol 1976;112:1127-1128.
12. Busam KJ, Woodruff JM, Erlandson RA, Brady MS. Large plaque-type blue nevus with subcutaneous cellular nodules. Am J Surg Pathol 2000;24:92-99.
13. Pathy AL, Helm TN, Elston D, Bergfeld WF, Tuthill RJ. Malignant melanoma arising in a blue nevus with features of pilar neurocristic hamartoma. J Cutan Pathol 1993;20:459-464.
14. Wlotzke U, Hohenleutner U, Hein R, Szeimies RM, Landthaler M. [Malignant infiltrating blue nevus of the plaque type. Case report and literature review]. Hautarzt 1995;46:860-864. [German]
15. Tuthill RJ, Clark WH Jr, Levene A. Pilar neurocristic hamartoma: its relationship to blue nevus and equine melanotic disease. Arch Dermatol 1982;118:592-596
16. Bevona C, Tannous Z, Tsao H. Dermal melanocytic proliferation with features of a plaque-type blue nevus and neurocristic hamartoma. J Am Acad Dermatol 2003;49:924-929.
17. Pearson JP, Weiss SW, Headington JT. Cutaneous malignant melanotic neurocristic tumors arising in neurocristic hamartomas. A melanocytic tumor morphologically and biologically distinct from common melanoma. Am J Surg Pathol 1996;20:665-677.
18. Carney JA, Ferreiro JA. The epithelioid blue nevus. A multicentric familial tumor with important associations, including cardiac myxoma and psammomatous melanotic schwannoma. Am J Surg Pathol 1996;20:259-272.
19. Moreno C, Requena L, Kutzner H, de la Cruz A, Jaqueti G, Yus ES. Epithelioid blue nevus: a rare variant of blue nevus not always associated with the Carney complex. J Cutan Pathol 2000;27:218-223.

20. O'Grady TC, Barr RJ, Billman G, Cunningham BB. Epithelioid blue nevus occurring in children with no evidence of Carney complex. Am J Dermatopathol 1999;21:483-486.
21. Groben PA, Harvell JD, White WL. Epithelioid blue nevus: neoplasm Sui generis or variation on a theme? Am J Dermatopathol 2000;22:473-488.
22. Zembowicz A, Carney JA, Mihm MC. Pigmented epithelioid melanocytoma: a low-grade melanocytic tumor with metastatic potential indistinguishable from animal-type melanoma and epithelioid blue nevus. Am J Surg Pathol 2004;28:31-40.
23. Allen AC. A reorientation on the histogenesis and clinical significance of cutaneous nevi and melanomas. Cancer 1949;2:28-56.
24. Temple-Camp CR, Saxe N, King H. Benign and malignant cellular blue nevus. A clinicopathological study of 30 cases. Am J Dermatopathol 1988;10:289-296.
25. Rodriguez HA, Ackerman LV. Cellular blue nevus. Clinicopathologic study of forty-five cases. Cancer 1968;21:393-405.
26. Micali G, Innocenzi D, Nasca MR. Cellular blue nevus of the scalp infiltrating the underlying bone: case report and review. Pediatr Dermatol 1997;14:199-203.
27. Maize JC, Ackerman AB. Pigmented lesions of the skin. Clinicopathologic correlations. Philadelphia: Lea & Febiger; 1987.
28. McGovern VJ. Melanoma. Histologic diagnosis and prognosis. New York: Raven Press; 1983:3-24.
29. Tran TA, Carlson JA, Basaca PC, Mihm MC. Cellular blue nevus with atypia (atypical cellular blue nevus): a clinicopathologic study of nine cases. J Cutan Pathol 1998;25:252-258.
30. Zembowicz A, Granter SR, McKee PH, Mihm MC. Amelanotic cellular blue nevus: a hypopigmented variant of the cellular blue nevus: clinicopathologic analysis of 20 cases. Am J Surg Pathol 2002;26:1493-1500.
31. Harvell JD, White WL. Persistent and recurrent blue nevi. Am J Dermatopathol 1999;21:506-517.
32. Avidor I, Kessler E. 'Atypical' blue nevus—a benign variant of cellular blue nevus. Presentation of three cases. Dermatologica 1977;154:39-44.
33. Cerroni L, Borroni RG, Massone C, Kerl H. "Ancient" blue nevi (cellular blue nevi with degenerative stromal changes). Am J Dermatopathol 2008;30:1-5.
34. Barnhill RL, Argenyi Z, Berwick M, et al. Atypical cellular blue nevi (cellular blue nevi with atypical features): lack of consensus for diagnosis and distinction from cellular blue nevi and malignant melanoma ("malignant blue nevus"). Am J Surg Pathol 2008;32:36-44.

5 CONGENITAL MELANOCYTIC NEVI

Congenital melanocytic nevi are circumscribed benign lesions of nevoid melanocytes that are present at birth. This seemingly simple definition conceals certain difficulties and ambiguities. For example, documentation of congenital origin may be difficult when a parental history is not available, especially for relatively small lesions that a patient may not have discussed with his or her parents as a "birthmark" in childhood. Since most nevi are acquired in childhood and young adulthood, a history that a nevus was "present all my life" cannot be regarded as evidence that it was congenital. Also, some lesions that appear to have developed during early infancy and to have been absent at birth may exhibit clinical or histologic features usually associated with congenital nevi. Some of these may indeed have been present at birth but not pigmented at that time. It is not known whether these nevi with "congenital features" ("congenital pattern nevi") have the same significance as true congenital lesions. Interestingly, studies of genetic mutations in congenital nevi have found activating mutations of the oncogene *NRAS* in 60 to 80 percent, a much higher frequency than in noncongenital nevi (in which *BRAF* mutations predominate), perhaps reflecting a different pathogenesis (1).

Congenital nevi are divided into three arbitrary size categories, which are based for practical purposes on the complexity of surgical removal. Small congenital nevi (up to 1.5 cm) are removed at simple outpatient surgery, intermediate congenital nevi often require a skin graft for closure, and giant congenital nevi (20 cm or larger), which cover large geographic areas of the body, may not be removable at all. Congenital nevi are significant for two reasons: they are potential precursors of melanoma and they may be cosmetically deforming. For those with giant congenital nevi, the lifetime risk of acquiring melanoma is as high as 5 to 10 percent, and these highly disfiguring lesions are often the cause of major psychological problems in affect-ed patients. Fortunately, giant and intermediate congenital nevi are rare (about 1/20,000 births [2,3]). Small congenital nevi, in contrast, occur in 1 to 6 percent of newborns, so that they are common in the general population (4,5).

Other lesions that may present as congenital nevi have a distinctive histology and are discussed elsewhere in this Fascicle. These include congenital Spitz nevi (6–8), cellular blue nevi (9–16), epithelioid cell nevi (12), congenital blue nevi (15,16), and congenital neurocristic hamartoma (17).

SMALL CONGENITAL NEVI

Definition. A *small congenital nevus* is a melanocytic nevus that is present at birth and measures less than 1.5 cm in diameter.

Clinical Features. Examination of newborns suggests that congenital nevi occur in any size, from a few millimeters to many centimeters (2). The etiology of congenital nevi is unknown. They appear to aggregate in families, but a clear genetic transmission pattern has not been defined (18). The smallest lesions, unnoticed by parents or growing children and overlapping morphologically with common nevi, are not likely to be recognizable as congenital after the neonatal period. Larger congenital nevus-like lesions may be acquired; in an interesting epidemiologic study, these nevi were strongly influenced by geographic location and, by implication, degree of solar radiation, suggesting that many so-called congenital nevi are in fact acquired early in life (19). Lesions closer to the arbitrary size limit of 1.5 cm are larger than most common acquired nevi, and may come to clinical attention because of their size alone. These larger lesions are also more likely to be remembered as true "birthmarks."

Smaller congenital nevi are circumscribed and symmetric, tan or brown pigmented lesions that occur anywhere on the skin. The larger lesions in this size range or above may have an irregular border, but one that is usually well-defined

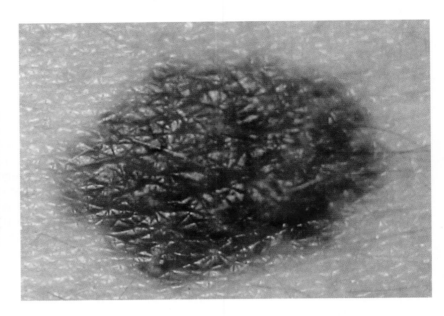

Figure 5-1

**SMALL CONGENITAL
MELANOCYTIC NEVUS**

By definition, a small congenital nevus measures less than 1.5 cm. Nevertheless, these lesions are larger than most banal nevi. They tend to have well-defined, slightly raised edges and lack the "fuzzy" indefinite border of a dysplastic nevus. Intermediate congenital nevi are larger than 1.5 cm, and generally amenable to conservative local excision. (Fig. A from Plate III, Fascicle 2, Third Series.)

in contrast to the "fuzzy" border of dysplastic nevus, which constitutes the major clinical and gross differential diagnostic consideration (fig. 5-1). Most congenital nevi are at least slightly raised to side lighting. The prototypic lesion is considerably broader than it is tall, with a smooth, regular border and uniform pigment distribution. Lesions with marked pigmentary variegation or with prominent black coloration have been termed *atypical congenital nevi*, and if these changes are prominent, the lesions should be biopsied to rule out melanoma (20) .

As noted above, there appears to be a fundamental difference between congenital and acquired nevi in that the former tend to be associated with activating mutations of *NRAS* instead of the *BRAF* mutations that characterize most acquired nevi. Interestingly, "congenital pattern nevi," which resemble small congenital nevi clinically and histologically but are not present at birth, tend to share the *BRAF*-predominant mutation pattern of acquired nevi, rather than the *NRAS*-predominant pattern of congenital nevi, indicating that they are genetically distinct lesions (1).

Congenital nevi are characteristically stable or show a tendency to slight fading over the years, and any lesion that shows progressive changes in size, shape, or color should be biopsied to rule out melanoma. At least some, if not most, examples of so-called *speckled lentiginous nevus* (*nevus spilus*) are small congenital nevi, although others are

certainly acquired. The speckles of such lesions are similar histologically to simple lentigines, and the tan background lesion within which the speckles occur may be similar to a café au lait spot. These lesions do not typically involve the deep dermis (21).

Small congenital nevi are rarely disfiguring. The risk for malignant change is unknown, but much less than that of giant nevi. Nevertheless, melanomas do occur in association with small "congenital pattern" nevi. In a recent study of 667 consecutive cases of primary cutaneous melanoma, 22.1 percent had an associated nevus; 55 percent of these were dysplastic nevi, 40 percent were congenital pattern nevi, and only 5 percent were considered to be ordinary acquired nevi (22). This finding may indicate a more important role for superficial congenital nevus as a precursor lesion of melanoma than previously recognized (22). Removal of small congenital nevi is a simple matter, and is often recommended as an alternative to follow-up, but the risk posed by these lesions appears to be insufficient to justify major efforts at case-finding for prophylactic excision in the community at large (20).

Microscopic Findings. Similar to acquired nevi, at scanning magnification, congenital nevi of any size are composed of nevus cells located in the epidermis and/or dermis, with a variable degree of pigment, mostly in the epidermal and superficial dermal lesional cells (figs. 5-2–5-5). In contrast to most acquired nevi, the nevus cells

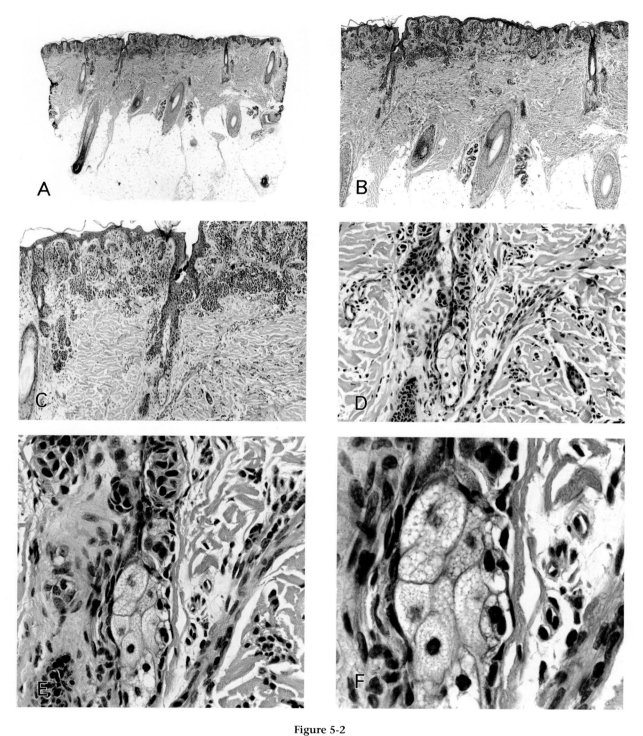

Figure 5-2

SMALL CONGENITAL MELANOCYTIC NEVUS

A–C: This broad and deep lesion from the scalp of a 2-year-old is composed of orderly nevus cells which extend down into the reticular dermis and around the skin appendages.

D–F: Nevus cells are present not only "around" but also "within" the epithelium of skin appendages, including a sebaceous unit. This finding is considered to be quite specific for true congenital onset of a nevus.

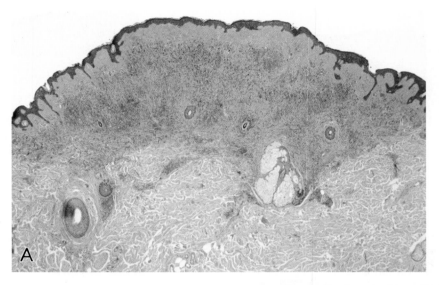

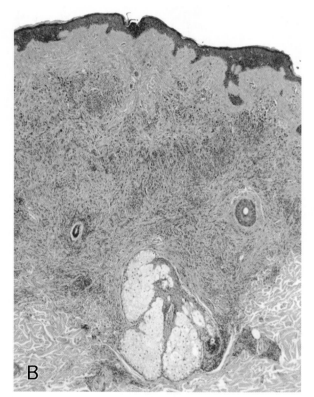
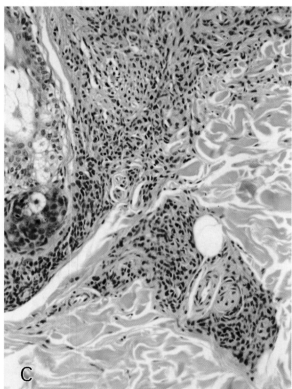

Figure 5-3

SMALL CONGENITAL MELANOCYTIC NEVUS

A: This broad and deep lesion consists of orderly nevus cells which extend down into the reticular dermis and around skin appendages. Although this lesion is large by comparison with most acquired nevi, small congenital nevi, by definition, measure less than 1.5 cm in greatest dimension.

B,C: The presence of nevus cells around skin appendages is a characteristic feature of many, but not all, truly congenital nevi but is not diagnostic of a congenital origin as some acquired nevi show this feature. We refer to these lesions as congenital pattern nevi.

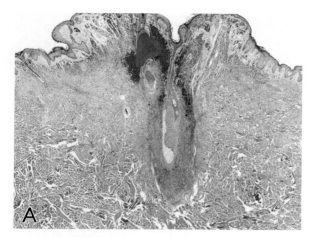

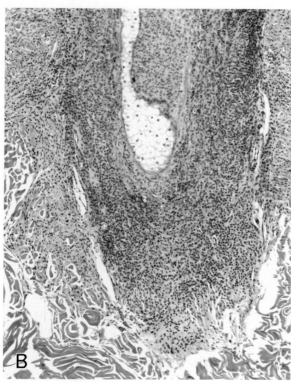

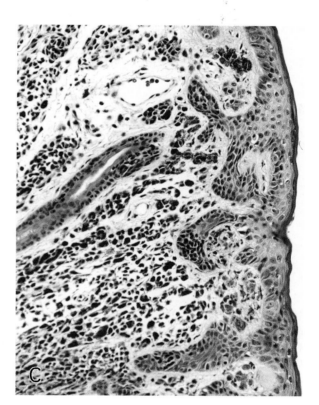

Figure 5-4

SMALL CONGENITAL MELANOCYTIC NEVUS, WITH HEMORRHAGE

A: The nevus cells in an African-American patient extend into the upper reticular dermis and down around a hair follicle.

B: High magnification shows lesional cells around the follicle.

C: Superficially, the lesional cells contain abundant pigment (epidermal surface oriented to the right).

of congenital nevi often extend into the lower third of the reticular dermis, and solitary or nested cells involve the skin appendage epithelium. Features specific to the histologic recognition of the congenital nature of a benign nevus include a size greater than 1.5 cm (a feature not applicable to the small lesions under consideration here) and the presence of nevus cells, singly or in nests, "within" follicular epithelium, eccrine ducts, sweat glands, arrector pili muscles, nerves, and blood vessels in the mid-

reticular dermis or deeper (fig. 5-2) (23). The finding of nevus cells in the adventitial dermis "around" but not within skin appendages (as in fig. 5-2) is a more common, but less specific, feature (23,24). A pattern of "splaying" of cells between collagen bundles of the lower third of the reticular dermis is another characteristic but not specific finding (21). Some (perhaps many) truly congenital nevi fail to show any of these features, and thus are indistinguishable from acquired nevi except by history (25). In a study

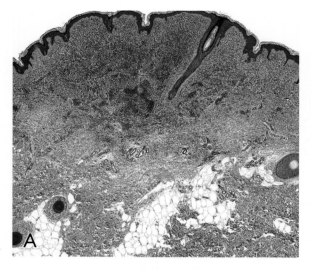

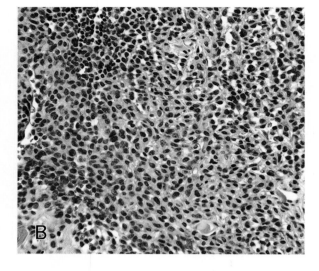

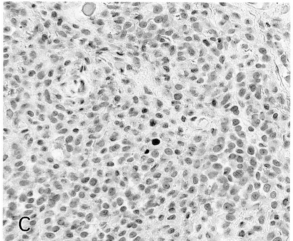

Figure 5-5

SMALL CONGENITAL MELANOCYTIC NEVUS

A: Scanning magnification shows a broad and deep lesion.

B: Higher magnification shows nevoid melanocytes with slight nuclear enlargement and irregularity.

C: Because of a suggestion of cytologic atypia, a Ki-67 stain was done, which shows only a few reactive cells, consistent with a benign nevus.

of 85 nevi biopsied in the first 12 months of life, the depth and pattern of the nevus cells was directly related to the size of the lesion (26). Although the microscopic outlines of the lesions in the dermis are characteristically irregular, with nevus cells that may appear to infiltrate as single cells among reticular dermis collagen fibers, the lesions are typically completely stable clinically, and there is no suggestion of focal expansile growth of cells that compress or destroy adjacent structures.

At higher magnification, congenital nevus cells are generally indistinguishable from those of common acquired nevi. Mitoses and severe cellular atypia are usually absent, especially in the dermis. The possibility of melanoma should be seriously considered if there is any sugges-

tion of a discrete, well-demarcated expansile nodule of cells that appears to have a selective growth advantage compared to the background nevus cells (27), especially if more than a few mitoses are present or if the cells show severe cytologic atypia with large eosinophilic nucleoli or abundant amphophilic cytoplasm with dusty melanin pigment. Atypia is usually absent in congenital nevi, but sometimes degenerative nuclear changes in the dermis, analogous to those seen in ancient schwannomas and in some acquired dermal nevi, arouse concern. Such cellular atypia appears to be of no clinical significance unless seen as part of an expansile nodule, in association with mitotic activity and apoptosis, or in the epidermis as part of an in situ or microinvasive radial growth phase melanoma. One interesting study, however, correlated DNA aneuploidy as determined by flow cytometry with histologic nuclear pleomorphism in 4 of 39 congenital melanocytic nevi, and the authors speculated that the findings might represent premalignant changes (28).

The junctional component of congenital melanocytic nevi often involves lentiginous melanocytic proliferation in addition to junctional nest formation; the former is associated with some degree of thinning and elongation of the rete ridges. This, along with some degree of papillary dermal fibrosis, may initially give the impression of a dysplastic nevus. However, such a junctional component does not generally extend beyond the dermal component as a "shoulder," and cytologic atypia should not be present. This common junctional pattern should not be confused with the less common occurrence of a true dysplastic nevus developing in association with a dermal component with congenital features. The dermal stroma associated with cells of congenital pattern nevi, in addition to variable degrees of fibrosis, may also show zones of neurovascular proliferation, and these mesenchymal features, along with occasional zones of papillomatous proliferation of the associated epidermis and foci of aberrant adnexal differentiation, suggest that in some lesions a more diffuse hamartomatous process is involved.

The specificity, sensitivity, and significance of the histologic findings discussed above for diagnosing a nevus as congenital have been the subject of considerable discussion. Everett (29) studied 39 lesions with a convincing history of presence at birth, classifying them into three patterns: "superficial" congenital nevi had nevus cells in the papillary and upper reticular dermis only; "intermediate" nevi had reticular dermal involvement but no extension into the fat or prominent involvement of adnexal structures; and "deep" congenital nevi exhibited most of the classic architectural features discussed above (reticular dermal and skin appendage involvement, for example). Nine lesions were less than 1.5 cm in diameter, and thus not specifically recognizable as a congenital nevus by histology. Of the 30 lesions larger than 1.5 cm, 12 were deep and 10 were superficial. In another study, the depth and pattern of the nevus cells were directly related to the size of congenital nevi

in infants (26). For larger nevi, however, the lesional diameter alone is virtually diagnostic of a congenital nevus, and historical confirmation is usually more readily available.

The specificity of the histologic diagnosis was called into question by another study in which 15 of 50 nevi documented to have been acquired after birth in a population of 313 consecutive newborns were biopsied (25). Seven lesions (all less than 1.5 cm in diameter but in general larger and more variegated than the other acquired nevi in the study) had one or more of the histologic features of a small congenital melanocytic nevus. In another study, the prevalence of these acquired nevi with "congenital features" was higher than that of true congenital nevi (30). In an extensive study of 1,349 nevi from children in whom a clear parental or clinical history of onset was available, 32 nevi with the histologic criteria of congenital nevi were actually acquired, and 179 nevi present at birth did not fulfill these criteria. This study suggests, like those reviewed above, that it is not possible to predict, by histologic analysis alone, whether a nevus is present at birth, except perhaps for very deep or large nevi. Studies dealing with congenital nevus-associated melanoma should take into account the lack of sensitivity of these criteria (4,5,31). As already mentioned, congenital pattern nevi tend to share the *BRAF*-predominant mutation pattern of acquired nevi, rather than the *NRAS*-predominant pattern of congenital nevi, indicating that they are genetically distinct lesions (1).

This issue is important because in 5 to 10 percent of patients with melanoma, nevi with congenital features (especially involvement of the reticular dermis and the adventitia of skin appendages) have been found in contiguity (32–36). Although this finding demonstrates that some small nevi with congenital features may be potential precursors of melanoma, the individual risk of progression is likely to be quite low since their number in the population, although not known with certainty, is certainly large relative to the rate of occurrence of melanomas. It will be interesting to discover in future studies whether these melanoma-associated congenital nevi (and their associated melanomas) tend to be of the *BRAF* or of the *NRAS* mutational genotype.

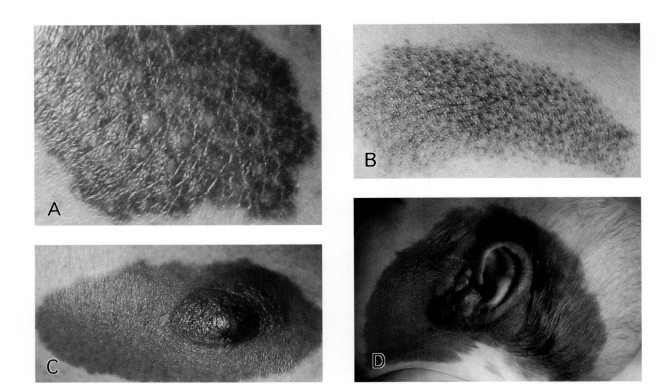

Figure 5-6

INTERMEDIATE TO GIANT CONGENITAL MELANOCYTIC NEVUS

A,B: These lesions are of little consequence as they can easily be excised if indicated.

C: Tumefactions should be evaluated carefully, usually with biopsy.

D: Although not one of the largest, or "garment," nevus this intermediate-sized lesion has considerable cosmetic significance because of its location. (Figs. A–C are figs. B–D from Plate III, Fascicle 2, Third Series.)

INTERMEDIATE AND GIANT CONGENITAL NEVI

Definition. *Intermediate* and *giant congenital nevi* are melanocytic nevi that are present at birth and are greater than 1.5 cm in diameter. The distinction between intermediate and giant nevi is arbitrary, but in general terms, giant nevi are lesions for which complete excision may be impracticable or at least may involve a major, often multistage, surgical exercise. Giant congenital nevi are important as potentially premalignant lesions, and are also of major cosmetic concern to patients and their families.

Clinical Features. Giant nevi typically cover large areas of the body ("garment nevi," "bathing trunk nevi"). They range in color from pale tan to jet black, but most are dark brown. The pigment may be completely uniform, but is usually somewhat variegated. Sometimes darker focal pigmented areas of up to a centimeter or so in diameter are scattered within the larger background lesion. These focal pigmented areas may be elevated or otherwise altered in texture, so that the surface of the entire lesion appears mottled and lumpy (figs. 5-6, 5-7). The growth of the nevus is commensurate with that of the child. The pigment tends to fade somewhat, the colors become more homogeneous, and lumpy areas become smoother. In addition, most giant congenital nevi, like some smaller congenital and acquired nevi, contain abnormally large, coarse terminal hairs. In some lesions, this hypertrichosis is massive, giving rise to a lesion that has the appearance of an animal pelt. Indeed, it has been suggested that the tradition of the werewolf arose from observations of reclusive sufferers of giant hairy nevi in medieval times (fig. 5-7) (some also believe that others so designated suffered from porphyria cutanea

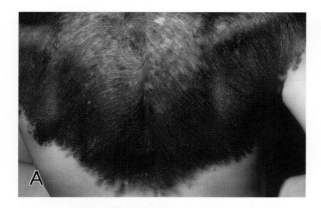

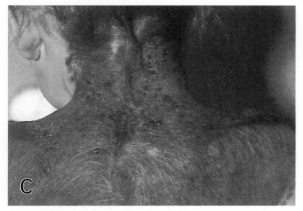

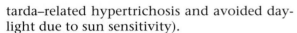

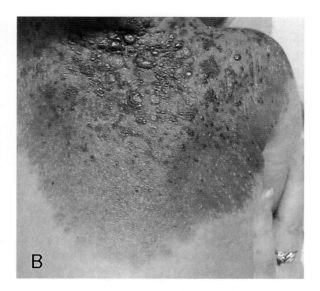

Figure 5-7

CONGENITAL MELANOCYTIC NEVUS, GARMENT TYPE

Hyperpigmentation and hypertrichosis are characteristic of these lesions. Variability in pigmentation may create concern in follow-up. Photographic follow-up, with careful palpation for the development of nodules, is important. The nodularity in lesion B from a neonate diminished progressively over the next 2 years. (B and C are figs. E and F from Plate III, Fascicle 2, Third Series.)

tarda–related hypertrichosis and avoided daylight due to sun sensitivity).

In patients with giant congenital nevi, "satellite" nevi are often present elsewhere on the skin. These are benign nevi that have clinical and histologic features of small or intermediate congenital nevi. The number of satellite nevi in patients with giant congenital nevi correlates with the risk that central nervous system (CNS) involvement (*neurocutaneous melanocytosis*) is present (37).

In addition to their tremendous cosmetic and psychosocial significance for affected individuals, intermediate and giant congenital nevi are potentially premalignant lesions. There are no reliable estimates of the lifetime melanoma risk for patients with intermediate lesions. Illig et al. (38) presented a study of 52 cases of melanoma that occurred in precursor congenital nevi less than 10 cm in size, thus including small as well as intermediate-sized congenital nevi. Of 570 consecutive cases at one of the clinics contributing to this study, the incidence of congenital nevus-associated melanoma was 2.8 percent.

The age of onset ranged from 19 to 79 years, so that no cases occurred in the prepubertal period. Most of the melanomas were of the superficial spreading type, with evidence of origin in the epidermal component of the nevi. This is in contradistinction to previous dogma that suggested that significant numbers of melanomas that arise in congenital nevi develop within their deeper dermal components. The survival experience of the patients was not reported. In contrast, Sahin et al. (39) examined 230 intermediate-sized congenital nevi ranging in diameter from 1.5 to 19.9 cm in 127 patients over a relatively short-term average follow-up period of 6.7 years, and observed no melanomas. They concluded that the results of this short-term follow-up study do not support the view that there is a clinically significantly increased risk for melanoma arising in banal-appearing medium-sized congenital nevi or that prophylactic excision of all such lesions is mandatory. Lifelong medical observation, or excision if this is a simpler option, appears to be a reasonable alternative for many medium-sized congenital nevi.

The incidence of melanoma in giant congenital nevi is also controversial, but numerous case reports and small series attest to its occasional occurrence. The subject has been extensively reviewed (4,40–45). In a recent review of data from eight studies containing a total of 432 large congenital melanocytic nevi, 12 patients (2.8 percent) developed cutaneous malignant melanoma during the reported follow-up periods (40). Two population-based follow-up studies are available. In the one from the Danish health system, the incidence of malignant transformation in 151 patients with congenital giant nevi registered over a 60-year period was 4.6 percent (46). In contrast, a similar Swedish study of 3,922 congenital melanocytic nevi, including 146 large nevi followed for a much shorter period of up to 15 years, found no melanomas (47). In a study of 92 patients followed in a specialty clinic, the 5-year cumulative risk of melanoma was calculated at 4.5 percent (43), and in another such study, the cumulative 5-year risk was 5.7 percent while the observed-to-expected melanoma incidence increased 148-fold, indicating a substantially increased risk of melanoma in patients with large congenital nevi (41). Other estimates of the lifetime risk have ranged up to 10 percent, with a few higher "outlier" estimates that probably reflect ascertainment bias (42). Melanomas (including fatal metastasizing lesions) may occur in giant congenital nevi during childhood as well as in adult life, while childhood onset of melanoma appears to be distinctly unusual in smaller congenital nevi (38). Studies have provided suggestive evidence that when melanoma does arise within large congenital nevi, axial lesions are more often involved than extremity lesions (41). Extracutaneous melanomas also occur: in one recent study of patients with large congenital nevi, two melanomas occurred in the CNS, and one was retroperitoneal (4). Melanomas appear to develop rarely or not at all in satellite lesions (42).

Specimens from giant congenital nevi are received in a pathology laboratory as a major resection or as a biopsy of a focal clinically suspicious area from a larger lesion. Large resections are generally done for prophylaxis, and there may be little or no clinical or gross suspicion of malignancy. The lesion should be bread-loafed to look for nodules or hyperpigmented areas on the surface or in the dermal component. Any such grossly atypical areas should be sampled liberally, but if the lesion is uniform in color and texture, a few survey sections usually suffice. If evaluation of the margins is considered necessary, these should preferably be inked prior to step-sectioning the lesion, and perpendicular sections should be taken at intervals around the border. Biopsies performed in response to clinical atypia (focal hyperpigmentations or nodules) are usually comparatively small and should, in general, be submitted in their entirety with inked margins.

Microscopic Findings. At scanning magnification, the great breadth of the lesion is readily apparent, with constituent nevus cells typically extending to the borders and the base of the tissue section (figs. 5-8–5-12). Essentially all giant nevi show conspicuous nevic cell permeation not only of the reticular dermis, but typically also of the subcutis and even the fascia. The pattern of involvement of the reticular dermis has been described as a form of splaying of cells between the collagen bundles (21). At the base of the lesion in the panniculus, the nevic cells are typically small and "mature," resembling fibroblasts. Indeed, it is sometimes possible to overlook nevus cells in the panniculus, thus missing a valuable clue to the diagnosis (involvement of subcutis, even including fascia, is common in giant congenital nevi, but hardly if ever seen in acquired lesions). Staining for S-100 protein may reveal lesional cells that can be overlooked in routine sections, and is sometimes useful when there is doubt as to whether or not a margin is involved.

In many giant congenital nevi, there are spindle cell areas with bundles of wavy fibers and cells reminiscent of neural structures, as is also seen in neurotized nevi (fig. 5-10). In the superficial part of the lesions, the nevus cells and their patterns of growth are usually similar to those in small congenital nevi and in acquired nevi. In contrast to these smaller lesions, however, many giant congenital nevi exhibit complex and fascinating abnormalities of neural crest-derived tissues, including neurofibroma-like areas of schwannian differentiation, areas of mature cartilage, and pseudo-Meissnerian corpuscles, as well as areas resembling blue nevi

Figure 5-8

GIANT CONGENITAL MELANOCYTIC NEVUS

A: This lesion, in a 1-year-old child, involves the full thickness of the reticular dermis and extends into the subcutis.

B: Nevus cells extend down and not only around but also within skin appendages.

C,D: Nevus cells within a sebaceous gland, as here, are considered to be highly specific for a truly congenital nevus, as is a size greater than 1.5 cm.

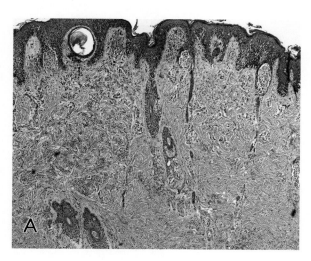

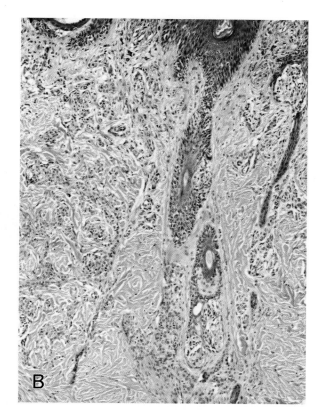

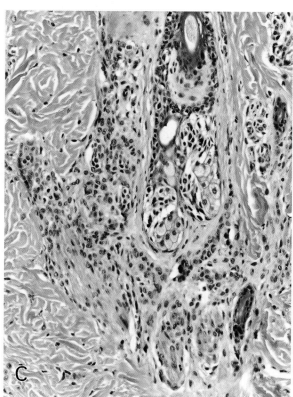

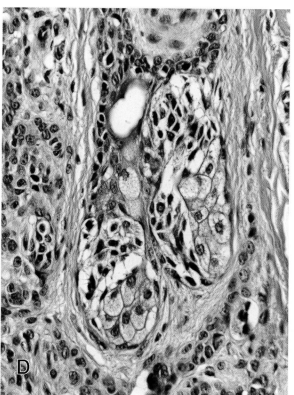

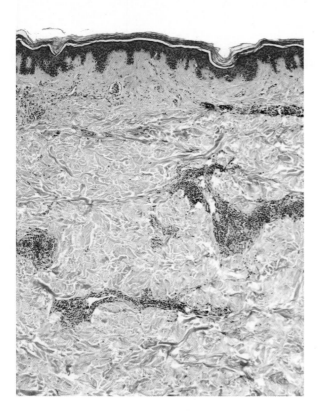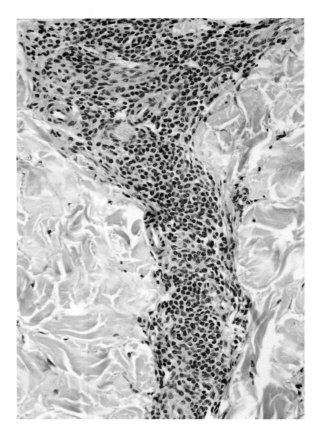

Figure 5-9

GIANT CONGENITAL MELANOCYTIC NEVUS, PSEUDOINFLAMMATORY PATTERN

Left: The nevus cells are arranged around blood vessels, resembling a lymphocytic infiltrate of the skin.
Right: Higher magnification demonstrates the nevoid character of the cells.

and cellular blue nevi (48,49). These changes suggest that giant congenital melanocytic nevi should be regarded as complex hamartomas of neural crest origin, and perhaps this concept explains in part the complexity of the proliferative nodules and malignant tumors that occasionally arise in these lesions (48,49). Involvement of the walls of blood vessels and nerves seen in benign congenital nevi (and also in blue nevi and Spitz nevi) is consistent with a hamartomatous process (figs. 5-11, 5-12). Gene expression profiles of giant congenital nevi have shown potentially informative alterations in the expression of many genes (50).

Melanomas and other malignant neoplasms that may occur in congenital nevi are discussed later in the chapter. Here, certain benign proliferations that may occur in these lesions, and may simulate melanomas, are described.

ATYPICAL PROLIFERATIONS IN CONGENITAL NEVI

Atypical proliferations in congenital nevi may occur in the dermis and simulate nodular melanoma, or may occur in the epidermis and simulate a superficial spreading melanoma.

Cellular and Proliferative Dermal Nodules in Congenital Nevi

Definition. *Cellular* and *proliferative dermal nodules* are clusters or nodules of increased cellularity within otherwise unremarkable congenital pattern nevi. We term these lesions *cellular nodules* if there is no evidence of proliferation in the form of mitotic activity. When mitotic activity or other evidence of proliferation (e.g., Ki-67 reactivity) is present, the lesions are termed *cellular and proliferative nodules*. Mitotic activity and

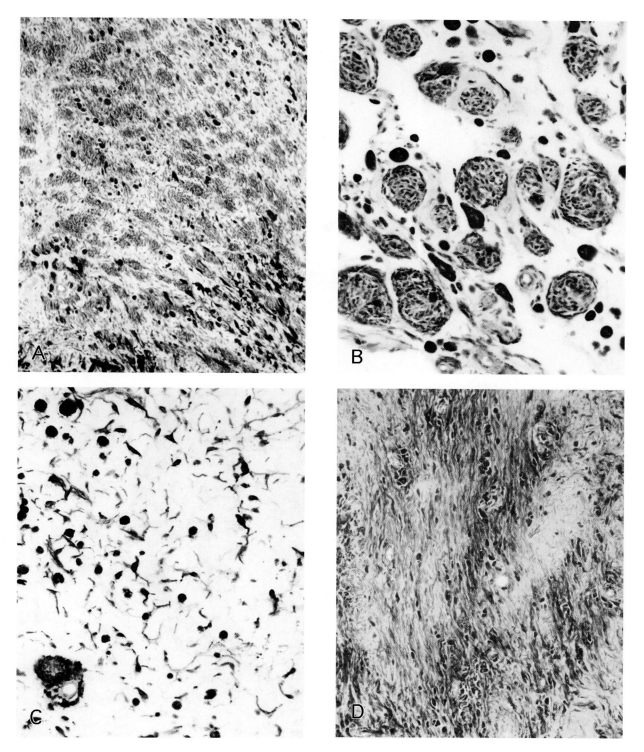

Figure 5-10

GIANT CONGENITAL MELANOCYTIC NEVUS WITH HAMARTOMA-LIKE PATTERNS

There are hamartomatous malformations of the nevoid cells, with unusual palisading patterns reminiscent of neural crest differentiation. This morphology may overlap with that of so-called neurocristic hamartoma.

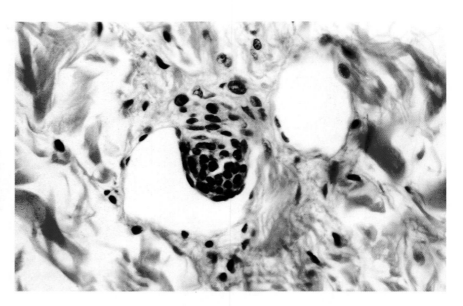

Figure 5-11

CONGENITAL MELANOCYTIC NEVUS WITH LYMPHATIC BUDDING

Nevus cells invaginate the endothelium of this lymphatic channel. This phenomenon may be seen in acquired nevi as well, and is not indicative of malignancy.

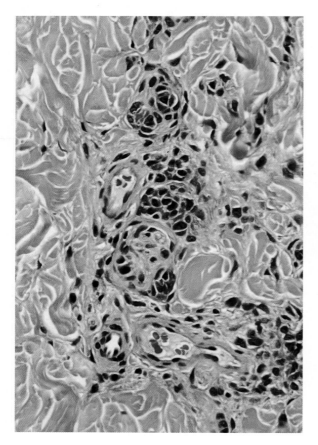 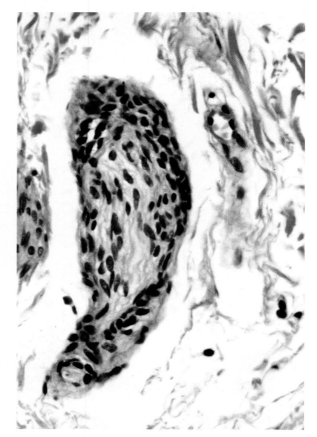

Figure 5-12

CONGENITAL MELANOCYTIC NEVUS WITH NERVE INVOLVEMENT

Nevus cells involving the perineurium or even the endoneurium of peripheral nerves are not indicative of malignancy in a congenital nevus. A similar phenomenon is also seen in blue nevi including cellular blue nevi.

cytologic atypia in these lesions should both be minimal, however, and if not, the lesions are termed *melanocytic tumors of uncertain malignant potential*. Cellular and proliferative nodules may simulate the rare nodular melanoma occurring in the dermal component of a nevus.

Clinical Features. Although cellular and proliferative nodules that develop in congenital nevi typically affect neonates, nodular areas present at birth or during later life in a congenital nevus (usually of the giant type) can pose extremely difficult diagnostic problems (48). Occasionally, clinical or parental concern is prompted by keratin granuloma formation around occluded or cystic hair follicles. In other cases, however, true nodular proliferations of melanocytes are observed. In the most usual presentation in neonates, these nodules are small, less than 5 mm in diameter, although they often grow rapidly, a potential cause of alarm for the observer. They may appear similar to a papular compound nevus, except for their location in the larger background lesion. Sometimes these small nodules are multiple. Their surface is smooth but not usually shiny or ulcerated, and their color is often jet black or dark brown. The lesions typically do not grow progressively, and with the passage of time, some lesions become softer, less pigmented, and smaller until after some years they blend imperceptibly into the background nevus.

Microscopic Findings. Histologically, there is a nodular cluster of cells in the dermis that is more cellular than the background lesion, with somewhat larger and sometimes more heavily pigmented epithelioid and often spindle-shaped cells (figs. 5-13–5-18). These features suggest malignancy at scanning magnification. More definitive indicators of malignancy should then be sought at higher power, including evidence of mitotic activity, uniform high-grade nuclear atypia, necrosis or ulceration, apparent destructive growth with obliteration of local structures, and an abrupt interface with the surrounding benign nevic cells. Benign nodules, in contrast, lack necrosis, frequent mitoses, and high-grade atypia, and at their periphery the lesional cells of the nodule appear to "blend" with or transition to the surrounding nevus cells. We interpret this blending pattern as indicative of maturation of the cells in the nodule, and a strong indicator that the lesion is likely to be benign (see Table 5-1).

Several studies of these cellular and proliferative nodules in congenital nevi have been published (51–53). In an immunohistochemical study of 30 lesions from 78 patients, the nodules and their parent nevi similarly expressed most melanocytic, lymphocytic, and cell cycle/proliferative and apoptotic markers. Interestingly, however, a greater proportion of the nodules were reactive for p53 (67 versus 30 percent, P <0.0098) and c-kit (97 versus 3 percent, P <0.0001) than the parent nevus. The expression of c-kit in nearly all of the nodules and its absence in nearly all of the nevi may be potentially useful for recognition of these nodules.

An early study of the cell biology of two lesions from neonates found that the cells from the nodules did not form permanent cell lines, were nontumorigenic in nude mice, and had a normal karyotype (54). More recently, Bastian and colleagues (55) used comparative genomic hybridization to analyze chromosomal aberrations in different types of proliferations arising in congenital nevi, and found that seven of nine cases of "a proliferation simulating nodular melanoma" showed aberrations. These aberrations were defined histologically as "nodular proliferations of high cellularity, nuclear atypia, and markedly increased proliferation rate," and therefore differ, at least in degree, from most of the lesions under discussion in this section. Six of the seven cases had numerical aberrations of whole chromosomes exclusively, a pattern that differed significantly from the findings in melanoma (either within or independent of congenital nevi), in which only 5 percent showed numerical changes only. The authors concluded that their findings identify these nodules as clonal neoplasms with a form of genomic instability consistent with a mitotic spindle checkpoint defect. These differences, compared to the aberration pattern found in most melanomas, may explain their more benign clinical behavior and may be of diagnostic value in ambiguous cases (55).

Addressing the biologic potential of cellular nodules, Xu et al. (53) provided a follow-up study of 26 patients, 16 of whom were followed for an average of 5 years, without any evidence of recurrence or metastasis. Features useful in differentiating the cellular nodules from melanoma included: 1) lack of high-grade uniform

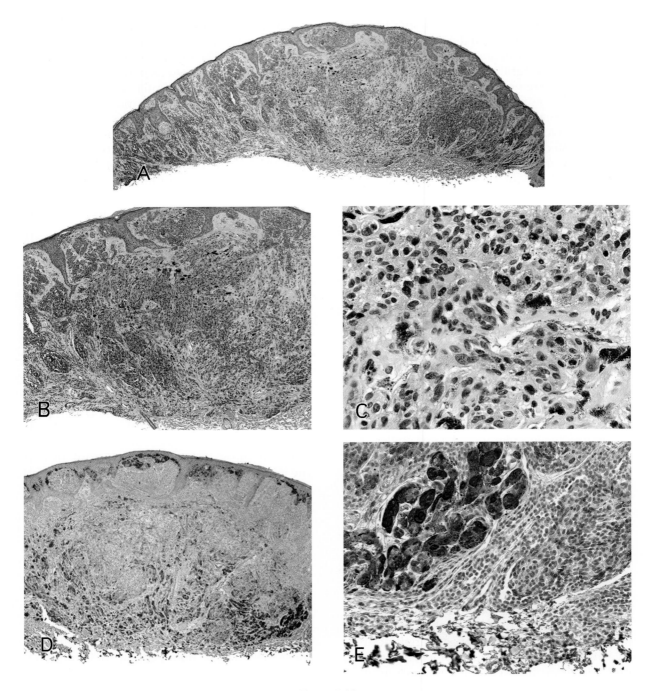

Figure 5-13

CELLULAR NODULE IN A CONGENITAL PATTERN NEVUS

A: At scanning magnification, there is an ill-defined area of increased cellularity and a small to intermediate-sized congenital nevus from a 20-year-old patient.

B: At higher magnification, the cells in the nodule blend with those of the surrounding nevus, without forming a distinct zone of demarcation.

C: The cells have large nuclei but regular nuclear membranes and clear chromatin.

D,E: An HMB45 stain highlights the cells in the nodule, perhaps indicative of some degree of immaturity; however, there were no mitoses. Therefore, this nodule is termed cellular, but not proliferative.

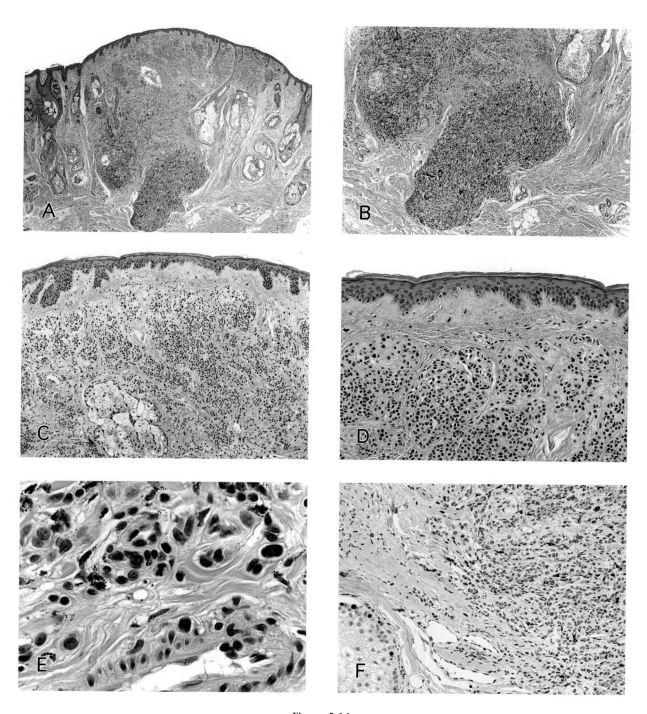

Figure 5-14

CELLULAR NODULE IN A CONGENITAL PATTERN NEVUS

A,B: This cellular nodule occurring in a small congenital nevus in a 47-year-old man mimics a cellular blue nevus, which might be a reasonable alternative interpretation of it.

C,D: Superficially, the lesion consists of orderly small nevus cells.

E: The cells in the nodule are larger and a rare mitotic figure is present.

F: Ki-67 is essentially negative in the cells of the nodule. Therefore, this nodule is both cellular and weakly proliferative.

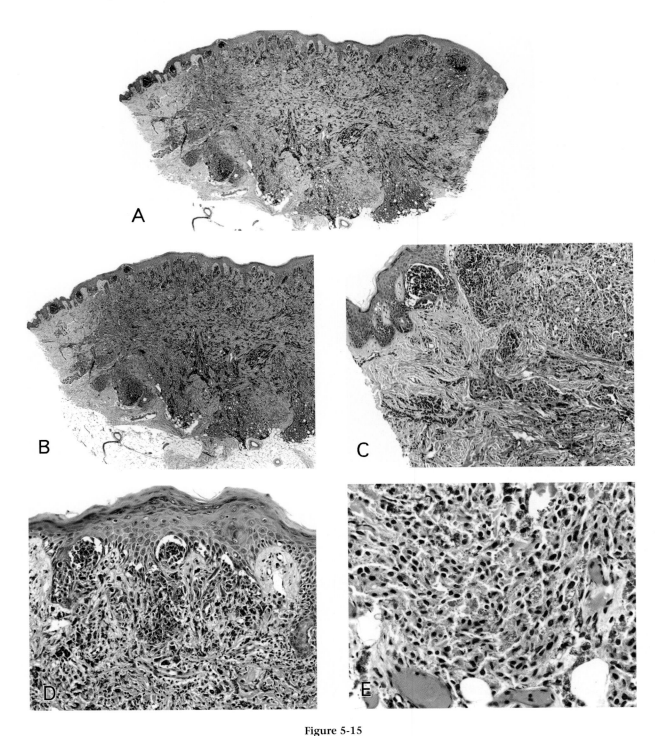

Figure 5-15

**CELLULAR NODULE IN A
CONGENITAL MELANOCYTIC NEVUS**

A–C: The nodule in this biopsy from a 3-year-old patient comprises almost the whole of the nevus, but residual small nevus cells can be seen on the margin at the left.

D: In this case, the cells of the nodule involve the overlying epidermis, an unusual feature.

E: Cytologically, there is no severe atypia and no mitotic activity.

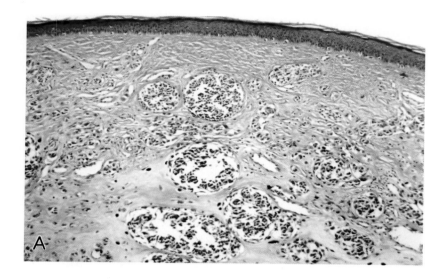

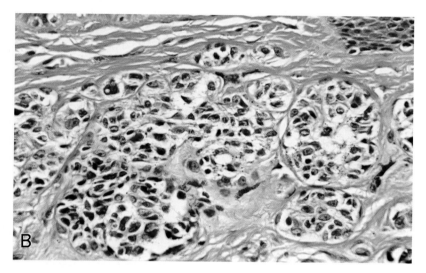

Figure 5-16

**CELLULAR NODULE
IN A CONGENITAL
MELANOCYTIC NEVUS**

A: This lesion occurred in a 49-year-old man who has subsequently been followed for 15 years with no recurrence.

B: Despite the presence of cytologic atypia, mitotic activity was absent.

C: At the periphery, the cells of the nodule blend with those of the surrounding nevus.

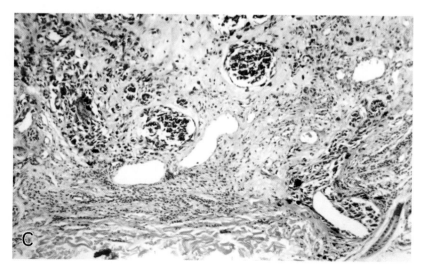

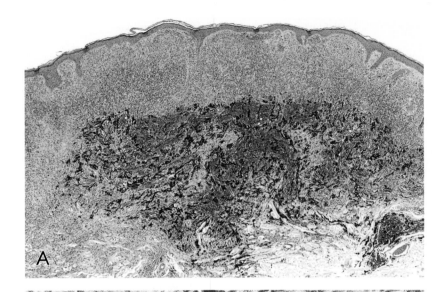

Figure 5-17

CONGENITAL MELANOCYTIC NEVUS WITH CELLULAR NODULE RESEMBLING PIGMENTED EPITHELIOID MELANOCYTOMA

A: This small to intermediate-sized congenital pattern nevus contains a cellular nodule composed of uniformly heavily pigmented spindle to epithelioid melanocytes.

B: At higher magnification, there is a tendency to blending as well as infiltration into the surrounding nevus, the latter being an atypical feature.

C: The cells have open chromatin and regular nuclear membranes; mitotic figures were rare or absent.

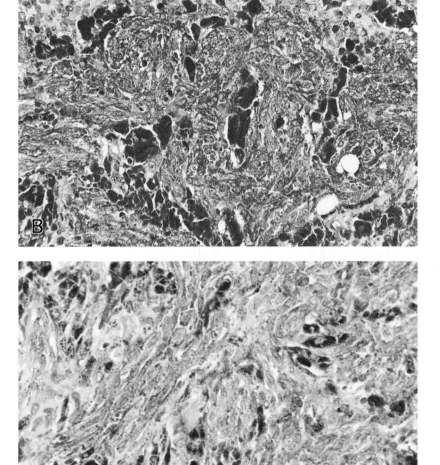

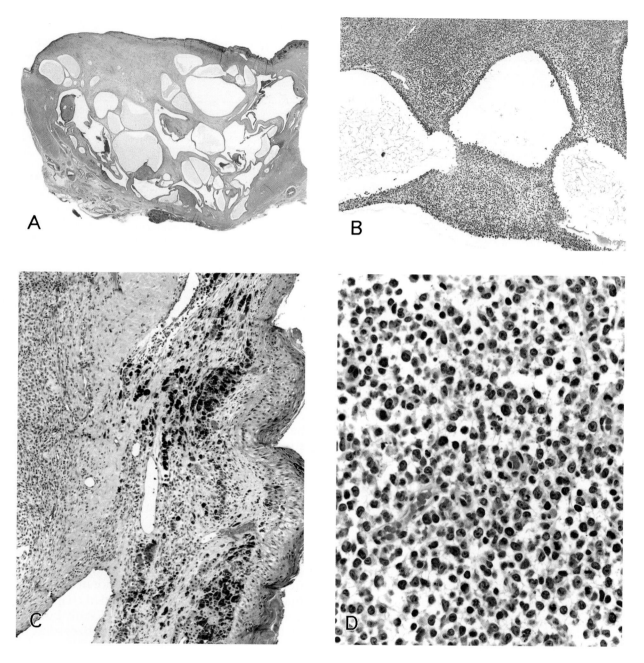

Figure 5-18

CONGENITAL MELANOCYTIC NEVUS WITH MELANOCYTIC TUMOR OF UNCERTAIN MALIGNANT POTENTIAL

A: This highly unusual giant congenital nevus in a neonate contains complex multicystic spaces, reminiscent, perhaps, of peculiar embryonic differentiation.

B: Cytologically, the spaces are outlined by small round "blastic" cells.

C: The small blastic cells blend with adjacent, more characteristic, nevoid melanocytes, some of which are heavily pigmented.

D: Frequent mitotic figures are observed in the small blastic cells. The behavior of lesions such as this is unpredictable. The possibility of neoplastic progression, including metastasis, cannot be ruled out. Lesions with this degree of cellularity and mitotic activity have not always metastasized or progressed, in our experience. This lesion could be considered to overlap histologically with neurocristic hamartoma. (Courtesy of Dr. Edgar Ballard, Cincinnati, OH.)

Table 5-1

FEATURES HELPFUL IN DIFFERENTIATING CELLULAR NODULES AND MELANOMA FORMING IN CONGENITAL NEVI[a]

	Cellular Nodule	Melanoma
Clinical Features		
Rapid growth	Present	May be insidious
Age of onset	Neonatal period	Childhood and adulthood
Architecture		
Diameter	Usually <5 mm	Often >5 mm
Blending with adjacent nevus cells	Gradual transitions present	Abrupt demarcation
Focality	May be multifocal	Unifocal
Ulceration	Absent	May be present
Expansile/destructive growth	Absent	Present
Cytology		
High-grade atypia	Absent	Present
Mitoses	Absent or few	Often many
Necrosis	Absent	Often present

[a]Lesions with intermediate features are best regarded as atypical proliferative nodules and warrant complete excision and close follow-up.

cellular atypia; 2) lack of necrosis within the nodule; 3) rarity of mitoses; 4) evidence of maturation in the form of blending or transitional forms between the cells in the nodule and the adjacent nevus cells; 5) lack of pagetoid spread into the overlying epidermis; and 6) no destructive expansile growth.

If all or most of the indicators of malignancy described above (i.e., severe cellular atypia, high mitotic activity, necrosis, a loss of maturation, and a destructive growth pattern) are present in a lesion in a patient beyond the neonatal period, and especially if the nodule is larger than a few millimeters, the lesion is likely to be malignant, and may be signed out as malignant melanoma arising in the dermal component of a congenital nevus. In such cases, the traditional microstaging attributes developed for use in common forms of melanoma may have little predictive value. In our experience and that of others, the prognosis tends to be better than expected by thickness alone. In particular, nodular proliferative lesions occurring within congenital nevi in neonates seem to behave in a benign fashion almost without regard to their histology (56), although there are rare exceptions to this rule, and a cautious approach to management is clearly warranted (57–63).

Because of the rarity of mitoses or Ki-67-labeled cells in many of these nodular lesions, we consider the term "cellular nodule" to be preferable to "proliferative nodule" (53). The degree of proliferation if any, can then be estimated separately in terms of mitotic activity and/or Ki-67 staining. For example, there may be a cellular nodule without proliferation or a cellular nodule with varying degrees of proliferation ("cellular and proliferative nodule"). Nodular dermal lesions in congenital nevi that lack mitoses and severe atypia, and whose component cells appear to blend with the surrounding benign nevic tissue without evidence of destructive expansile growth, behave in a benign fashion in our experience and that of others and should be interpreted as benign cellular and/or proliferative nodules. If only a few of the changes mentioned above are noted, and if they are present only focally or subtly, the lesion will most likely behave in a benign fashion, and may be classified descriptively as an "atypical cellular and proliferative nodule in a giant congenital nevus," or as a "melanocytic tumor of uncertain malignant potential," as discussed in chapter 10. Some such lesions have recurred locally but not metastasized (27). Table 5-1 summarizes some of the features that assist in differentiating cellular and/or proliferative nodules from melanoma developing in congenital nevi.

Superficial Atypical Melanocytic Proliferations in Congenital Nevi

Lesions with atypical features that simulate melanoma histologically but not clinically have been associated with some congenital nevi shortly after birth (figs. 5-19–5-21). Large epithelioid nevus cells are found at all levels of the

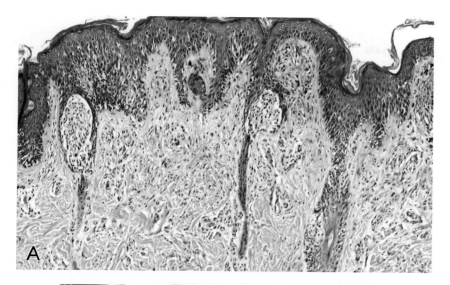

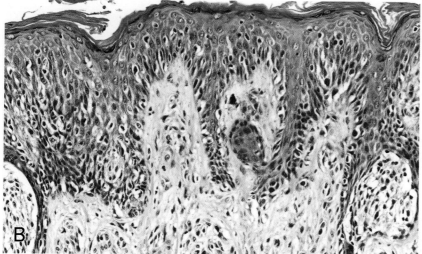

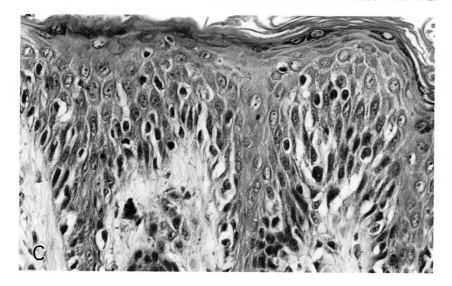

Figure 5-19

**CONGENITAL NEVUS WITH
SUPERFICIAL ATYPICAL
MELANOCYTIC PROLIFERATION
OF UNCERTAIN
SIGNIFICANCE (SAMPUS)**

A: This lesion, in a 1-year-old child, shows pagetoid extension of nevoid to epithelioid melanocytes into the epidermis, predominantly not beyond the middle third.

B,C: There is no high-grade or uniform atypia. Although these changes may suggest evolving melanoma in situ, the same lesional cells appear to undergo maturation upon descent into the dermis, and our admittedly limited and anecdotal experience has shown that such proliferations, in young individuals close to the time of birth, are not usually accompanied by aggressive behavior or progression. (Courtesy of Dr. T. Ferringer, Danville, PA.)

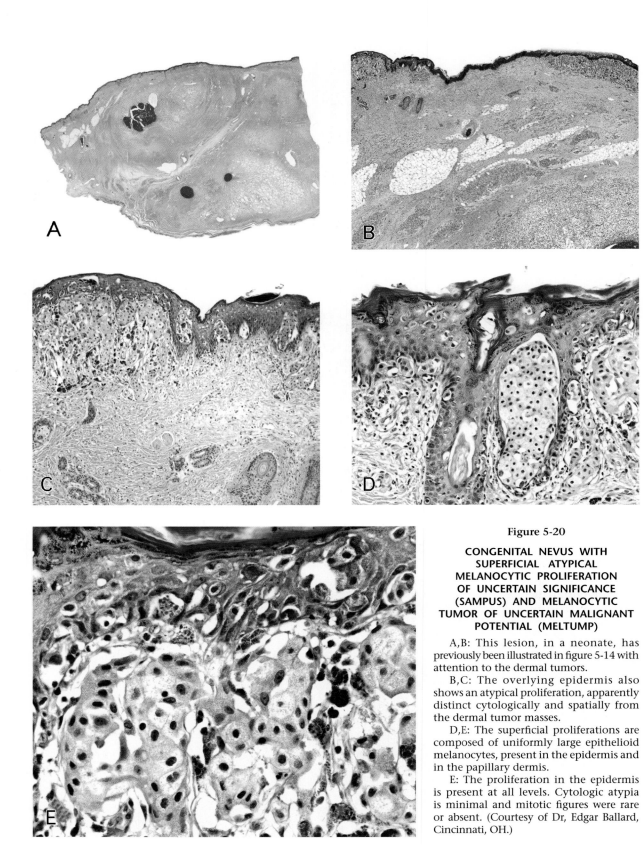

Figure 5-20

CONGENITAL NEVUS WITH SUPERFICIAL ATYPICAL MELANOCYTIC PROLIFERATION OF UNCERTAIN SIGNIFICANCE (SAMPUS) AND MELANOCYTIC TUMOR OF UNCERTAIN MALIGNANT POTENTIAL (MELTUMP)

A,B: This lesion, in a neonate, has previously been illustrated in figure 5-14 with attention to the dermal tumors.

B,C: The overlying epidermis also shows an atypical proliferation, apparently distinct cytologically and spatially from the dermal tumor masses.

D,E: The superficial proliferations are composed of uniformly large epithelioid melanocytes, present in the epidermis and in the papillary dermis.

E: The proliferation in the epidermis is present at all levels. Cytologic atypia is minimal and mitotic figures were rare or absent. (Courtesy of Dr. Edgar Ballard, Cincinnati, OH.)

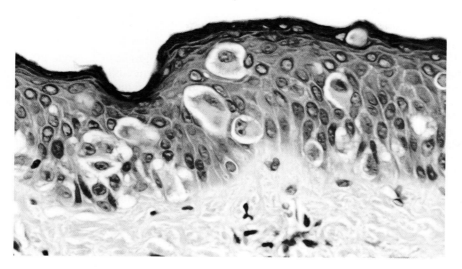

Figure 5-21

PAGETOID PROLIFERATION OF EPITHELIOID MELANOCYTES IN A CONGENITAL NEVUS

A finding such as this should be interpreted in the context of the whole lesion. This field could be a component of a melanoma arising in a congenital nevus or an atypical proliferation in a neonate.

epidermis, simulating a pagetoid pattern. The nuclei are usually regular in configuration, without macronucleoli and with few if any mitoses; severe cellular atypia is not seen. The diagnosis of congenital nevus may be made with confidence if the characteristic features of congenital nevus are observed in the dermis, or by clinicopathologic correlation. The atypical findings just described may be mentioned in a descriptive note, indicating that their biologic significance appears to be benign, although follow-up of the patient is appropriate, as is true for most patients with congenital nevi. In patients beyond the neonatal period, authentic superficial spreading melanomas may occur. Although this phenomenon is extraordinarily rare in childhood, it is the most common pathogenesis of melanoma that occurs in congenital melanocytic nevi in adults. The pathology of the lesions is indistinguishable from that of the common forms of melanoma and is described in chapter 8.

In our experience, all of the atypical proliferations (nodular and intraepidermal) that we have seen in congenital nevi of neonates and in infants in the first few months of life have had a benign course, irrespective of histology. While this generalization may not hold up in every case (and there have been rare reports of aggressive and even fatal melanomas presenting within giant congenital nevi in neonates [57,60,62]), it is our view that the diagnosis of melanoma arising in a congenital nevus should never be made in this age group without qualification that the behavior of such lesions in neonates is unpredictable but is likely to be benign.

Occasional, usually low-level (below the stratum granulosum) intraepidermal pagetoid spread of melanocytes occurs in a variety of nevus types in addition to congenital nevi in neonates; these include Spitz nevi, pigmented spindle cell nevi, acral nevi, genital nevi, and recurrent nevi. Such proliferations, termed *pagetoid melanocytosis* by Stern and Haupt (64,65), are generally separable from melanoma in situ by the focality, banal cytology, and lack of lateral growth beyond a nevic dermal component.

REFERENCES

1. Bauer J, Curtin JA, Pinkel D, Bastian BC. Congenital melanocytic nevi frequently harbor NRAS mutations but no BRAF mutations. J Invest Dermatol 2007;127:179-182.

2. Castilla EE, Da Graca Dutra M, Orioli-Parreiras IM. Epidemiology of congenital pigmented naevi: I. Incidence rates and relative frequencies. Br J Dermatol 1981;104:307-315.

3. Kroon S, Clemmensen OJ, Hastrup N. Incidence of congenital melanocytic nevi in newborn babies in Denmark. J Am Acad Dermatol 1987;17:422-426.

4. Bittencourt FV, Marghoob AA, Kopf AW, Koenig KL, Bart RS. Large congenital melanocytic nevi and the risk for development of malignant melanoma and neurocutaneous melanocytosis. Pediatrics 2000;106:736-741.

5. Lorenz S, Maier C, Segerer H, Landthaler M, Hohenleutner U. [Skin changes in newborn infants in the first 5 days of life]. Hautarzt 2000;51:396-400. [German]

6. Zaenglein AL, Heintz P, Kamino H, Zisblatt M, Orlow SJ. Congenital Spitz nevus clinically mimicking melanoma. J Am Acad Dermatol 2002;47:441-444.

7. Harris MN, Hurwitz RM, Buckel LJ, Gray HR. Congenital spitz nevus. Dermatol Surg 2000;26:931-935.

8. Palazzo JP, Duray PH. Congenital agminated Spitz nevi: immunoreactivity with a melanoma-associated monoclonal antibody. J Cutan Pathol 1988;15:166-170.

9. Micali G, Innocenzi D, Nasca MR. Cellular blue nevus of the scalp infiltrating the underlying bone: case report and review. Pediatr Dermatol 1997;14:199-203.

10. Busam KJ, Lohmann CM. Congenital paucimelanotic cellular blue nevus. J Cutan Pathol 2004;31:312-317.

11. Rose C, Kaddu S, El Sherif TF, Kerl H. A distinctive type of widespread congenital melanocytic nevus with large nodules. J Am Acad Dermatol 2003;49:732-735.

12. Martinez-Barba E, Polo-Garcia LA, Ferri-Niguez B, Ruiz-Macia JA, Kutzner H, Requena L. Congenital giant melanocytic nevus with pigmented epithelioid cells: a variant of epithelioid blue nevus. Am J Dermatopathol 2002;24:30-35.

13. Alla P, Carsuzaa F, Fesselet J, et al. [Blue nevus of the scalp associated with a meningeal melanocytoma]. Ann Dermatol Venereol 1998;125:129-131. [French]

14. Gunduz K, Shields JA, Shields CL, Eagle RC Jr. Periorbital cellular blue nevus leading to orbito-palpebral and intracranial melanoma. Ophthalmology 1998;105:2046-2050.

15. Hofmann UB, Ogilvie P, Mullges W, Brocker EB, Hamm H. Congenital unilateral speckled lentiginous blue nevi with asymmetric spinal muscular atrophy. J Am Acad Dermatol 1998;39:326-329.

16. Bennaceur S, Buisson T, Levan P, Fraitag S, Chretien-Marquet B. [Congenital giant blue nevus. Apropos of a case]. Rev Stomatol Chir Maxillofac 1997;98:275-276. [French]

17. Pearson JP, Weiss SW, Headington JT. Cutaneous malignant melanotic neurocristic tumors arising in neurocristic hamartomas. A melanocytic tumor morphologically and biologically distinct from common melanoma. Am J Surg Pathol 1996;20:665-677.

18. Rhodes AR, Slifman NR, Korf BR. Familial aggregation of small congenital nevomelanocytic nevi. Am J Med Genet 1985;22:315-326.

19. Rivers JK, MacLennan R, Kelly JW, et al. The Eastern Australian Childhood Nevus Study: prevalence of atypical nevi, congenital nevus-like nevi, and other pigmented lesions. J Am Acad Dermatol 1995;32:957-963.

20. Rhodes AR. Congenital nevomelanocytic nevi. Histologic patterns in the first year of life and evolution during childhood. Arch Dermatol 1986;122:1257-1262.

21. Maize JC, Ackerman AB. Pigmented lesions of the skin. Clinicopathologic correlations. Philadelphia: Lea & Febiger; 1987.

22. Kaddu S, Smolle J, Zenahlik P, Hofmann-Wellenhof R, Kerl H. Melanoma with benign melanocytic naevus components: reappraisal of clinicopathological features and prognosis. Melanoma Res 2002;12:271-278.

23. Rhodes AR, Silverman RA, Harrist TJ, Melski JW. A histologic comparison of congenital and acquired nevomelanocytic nevi. Arch Dermatol 1985;121:1266-1273.

24. Rhodes AR, Sober AJ, Day CL, et al. The malignant potential of small congenital nevocellular nevi. An estimate of association based on a histologic study of 234 primary cutaneous melanomas. J Am Acad Dermatol 1982;6:230-241.

25. Clemmensen OJ, Kroon S. The histology of "congenital features" in early acquired melanocytic nevi. J Am Acad Dermatol 1988;19:742-746.

26. Barnhill RL Fleischli M. Histologic features of congenital melanocytic nevi in infants 1 year of age or younger. J Am Acad Dermatol 1995;33:780-785.

27. Reed RJ, Ichinose H, Clark WH Jr, Mihm MC Jr. Common and uncommon melanocytic nevi and borderline melanomas. Semin Oncol 1975;2:119-147.

28. Stenzinger W, Suter L, Schumann J. DNA aneuploidy in congenital melanocytic nevi: suggestive evidence for premalignant changes. J Invest Dermatol 1984;82:569-572.

29. Everett MA. Histopathology of congenital pigmented nevi. Am J Dermatopathol 1989;11:11-12.

30. Kopf AW, Levine LJ, Rigel DS, Friedman RJ, Levenstein M. Prevalence of congenital-nevus-like nevi, nevi spili, and cafe au lait spots. Arch Dermatol 1985;121:766-769.

31. Cribier BJ, Santinelli F, Grosshans E. Lack of clinical-pathological correlation in the diagnosis of congenital naevi. Br J Dermatol 1999;141:1004-1009.

32. Clark WH Jr, Elder DE, Guerry D 4th, Epstein MN, Greene MH, Van Horn M. A study of tumor progression: the precursor lesions of superficial spreading and nodular melanoma. Hum Pathol 1984;15:1147-1165.

33. Betti R, Inselvini E, Vergani R, Crosti C. Small congenital nevi associated with melanoma: case reports and considerations. J Dermatol 2000;27:583-590.

34. Massi D, Carli P, Franchi A, Santucci M. Naevus-associated melanomas: cause or chance? Melanoma Res 1999;9:85-91.

35. Smolle J, Kaddu S, Kerl H. Non-random spatial association of melanoma and naevi—a morphometric analysis. Melanoma Res 1999;9:407-412.

36. Harley S, Walsh N. A new look at nevus-associated melanomas. Am J Dermatopathol 1996;18:137-141.

37. Marghoob AA, Dusza S, Oliveria S, Halpern AC. Number of satellite nevi as a correlate for neurocutaneous melanocytosis in patients with large congenital melanocytic nevi. Arch Dermatol 2004;140:171-175.

38. Illig L, Weidner F, Hundeiker M, et al. Congenital nevi less than or equal to 10 cm as precursors to melanoma. 52 cases, a review, and a new conception. Arch Dermatol 1985;121:1274-1281.

39. Sahin S, Levin L, Kopf AW, et al. Risk of melanoma in medium-sized congenital melanocytic nevi: a follow-up study. J Am Acad Dermatol 1998;39:428-433. Comment in J Am Acad Dermatol 1999;41:131-132.

40. Watt AJ, Kotsis SV, Chung KC. Risk of melanoma arising in large congenital melanocytic nevi: a systematic review. Plast Reconstr Surg 2004;113:1968-1974.

41. Egan CL, Oliveria SA, Elenitsas R, Hanson J, Halpern AC. Cutaneous melanoma risk and phenotypic changes in large congenital nevi: a follow-up study of 46 patients. J Am Acad Dermatol 1998;39:923-932.

42. DeDavid M, Orlow SJ, Provost N, et al. A study of large congenital melanocytic nevi and associated malignant melanomas: review of cases in the New York University Registry and the world literature. J Am Acad Dermatol 1997;36:409-416.

43. Marghoob AA, Schoenbach SP, Kopf AW, Orlow SJ, Nossa R, Bart RS. Large congenital melanocytic nevi and the risk for the development of malignant melanoma. A prospective study. Arch Dermatol 1996;132:170-175.

44. Swerdlow AJ, English JS, Qiao Z. The risk of melanoma in patients with congenital nevi: a cohort study. J Am Acad Dermatol 1995;32:595-599.

45. Shpall S, Frieden I, Chesney M, Newman T. Risk of malignant transformation of congenital melanocytic nevi in blacks. Pediatr Dermatol 1994;11:204-208.

46. Lorentzen M, Pers M, Bretteville-Jensen G. The incidence of malignant transformation in giant pigmented nevi. Scand J Plast Reconstr Surg 1977;11:163-167.

47. Berg P, Lindelof B. Congenital melanocytic naevi and cutaneous melanoma. Melanoma Res 2003;13:441-445.

48. Reed WB, Becker SW Sr, Becker SW Jr, Nickel WR. Giant pigmented nevi, melanoma, and leptomeningeal melanosis: a clinical and histopathologic study. Arch Dermatol 1965;91:100-119.

49. Hendrickson MR, Ross JC. Neoplasms arising in congenital giant nevi: morphologic study of seven cases and a review of the literature. Am J Surg Pathol 1981;5:109-135.

50. Dasu MR, Barrow RE, Hawkins HK, McCauley RL. Gene expression profiles of giant hairy naevi. J Clin Pathol 2004;57:849-855.

51. Herron MD, Vanderhooft SL, Smock K, Zhou H, Leachman SA, Coffin C. Proliferative nodules in congenital melanocytic nevi: a clinicopathologic and immunohistochemical analysis. Am J Surg Pathol 2004;28:1017-1025.

52. Leech SN, Bell H, Leonard N, et al. Neonatal giant congenital nevi with proliferative nodules: a clinicopathologic study and literature review of neonatal melanoma. Arch Dermatol 2004;140:83-88.

53. Xu X, Bellucci KS, Elenitsas R, Elder DE. Cellular nodules in congenital pattern nevi. J Cutan Pathol 2004;31:153-159.

54. Mancianti ML, Clark WH Jr, Hayes FA, Herlyn M. Malignant melanoma simulants arising in congenital melanocytic nevi do not show experimental evidence for a malignant phenotype. Am J Pathol 1990;136:817-829.

55. Bastian BC, Xiong J, Frieden IJ, et al. Genetic changes in neoplasms arising in congenital melanocytic nevi: differences between nodular proliferations and melanomas. Am J Pathol 2002;161:1163-1169.

56. Clark WH Jr, Elder DE, Guerry D 4th. Dysplastic nevi and malignant melanoma. In: Farmer ER, Hood AF, eds. Pathology of the skin. New York: Appleton & Lange; 1990:684-756.

57. Carroll CB, Ceballos P, Perry AE, Mihm MC Jr, Spencer SK. Severely atypical medium-sized congenital nevus with widespread satellitosis and placental deposits in a neonate: the problem of congenital melanoma and its simulants. J Am Acad Dermatol 1994;30:825-828.

58. de Vooght A, Vanwijck R, Gosseye S, Bayet B. Pseudo-tumoral proliferative nodule in a giant congenital naevus. Br J Plast Surg 2003;56:164-167.

59. Benoit-Durafour F, Michel JL, Godard W, et al. [Neonatal melanoma arising in a giant congenital nevus]. Ann Dermatol Venereol 1999;126:813-816. [French]

60. Shermak MA, Perlman EJ, Carson BS, Dufresne CR. Giant congenital nevocellular nevus overlying an encephalocele. J Craniofac Surg 1996;7:376-383.

61. Naraysingh V, Busby GO. Congenital malignant melanoma. J Pediatr Surg 1986;21:81-82.

62. Ahmed R. Congenital malignant melanoma in a newborn. Indian Pediatr 1979;16:723-725.

63. Sweet LK, Connerty HV. Congenital melanoma. Am J Dis Child 1941;62:1029-1040.

64. Stern JB, Haupt HM. Pagetoid melanocytosis: tease or tocsin? Semin Diagn Pathol 1998;15:225-229.

65. Haupt HM, Stern JB. Pagetoid melanocytosis: histologic features in benign and malignant lesions. Am J Surg Pathol 1995;19:792-797.

6 DYSPLASTIC MELANOCYTIC NEVI

Dysplastic variants of benign acquired nevi are large, clinically atypical nevi found in families in which at least two members have been affected by melanoma (familial melanoma kindreds) (1–4). Histologically, they are characterized by two general features that together constitute melanocytic dysplasia: immature lentiginous and nested architectural patterns of melanocytic proliferation in the epidermis (architectural disorder) and cytologic atypia. The lentiginous pattern is termed "immature" because it recapitulates the architecture of lentigo simplex, the smallest and earliest identifiable melanocytic tumor. An alternative histologic term is "nevus with architectural disorder and cytologic atypia," which may be cumbersome but describes well the essential cellular features of these lesions although it does not address the typical stromal features that accompany this entity.

These lesions are also known clinically as *familial atypical multiple mole–melanoma nevi* (FAMMM nevi) (5), or more simply as *atypical nevi* (6,7). Many nevi other than dysplastic nevi, however, may be described as "atypical" so in our opinion this term lacks specificity. A 1992 National Institutes of Health (NIH) consensus conference proposed the terminology "nevus with architectural disorder with a statement regarding cytologic atypia," implying that atypia, while it may be present, is not a criterion for the diagnosis (4). Therefore, this term cannot be considered to be synonymous with the term "dysplastic nevus" which requires both architectural disorder and cytologic atypia. The term *Clark nevus* (8) also does not require cytologic atypia and is not synonymous with dysplastic nevus as discussed here. Despite some variation, the term dysplastic nevus is currently the most commonly used diagnostic appellation for these lesions (9). The combination of an immature architectural pattern with cytologic atypia is similar to dysplastic lesions in other organ systems such as the oral mucosa or the uterine cervix.

NATURE AND SIGNIFICANCE OF DYSPLASTIC NEVI

Like other benign nevi, dysplastic nevi are significant almost exclusively in relation to melanoma. They are an important phenotypic risk marker of individuals who are at increased risk of developing melanoma; they are significant as potential precursors of melanoma (even though the vast majority of dysplastic nevi are stable lesions that will never progress); and they are significant in a model of tumor progression that may be of assistance in elucidating the developmental biology of melanoma. Most importantly, dysplastic nevi are highly significant as simulants of melanoma, both clinically and histologically. Histology is the "gold standard" for making the clinically critical distinction between a dysplastic nevus (or any other melanoma simulant) and a melanoma, and this subject is extensively discussed in this section. Dysplastic nevi were first defined clinically, and "clinically dysplastic nevi" constitute the single strongest risk markers for melanoma.

Clinical Features of Dysplastic Nevi

Dysplastic nevi are, by definition, larger than common acquired nevi: by currently accepted definitions, they are larger than 5 mm (10). They are mottled brown, symmetric lesions with ill-defined indefinite or "fuzzy" borders (2,11).

There are two distinct morphologic patterns, which may reflect two pathways of evolution. In the first pattern, the lesions are entirely flat or slightly elevated, with a fuzzy indefinite and slightly irregular border, and slight to moderate pigmentary variegation. In the second pattern, the same type of slightly variegated, irregular flat plaque surrounds a central papular elevation, forming a concentric lesion like a target (fig. 6-1). A mature dermal or compound nevus is often seen in this area of central elevation, suggesting that the dysplastic changes arose at the periphery of a preexisting benign nevus. The entirely flat lesions are presumably de novo lesions, without a detectable antecedent papular

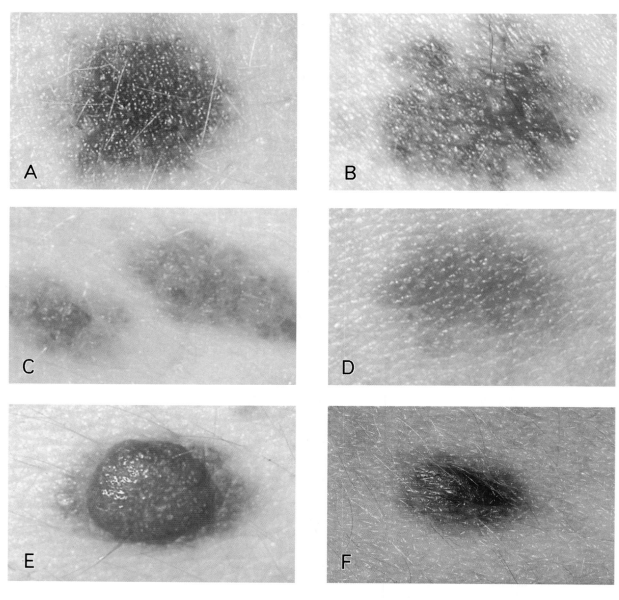

Figure 6-1

DYSPLASTIC NEVI

The attributes of dysplastic nevi illustrated here include the highly characteristic "fuzzy" or "hazy" indefinite border (A), slight to moderate border irregularity (B,D), focal areas of erythema (B,C), pigmentary variegation (B,C), and an ill-defined tannish pink hyperpigmentation with indefinite borders that characterizes epithelioid cell "de novo" dysplasia (D). In E and F, macular dysplasia is seen surrounding a preexisting papular compound nevus. For comparison, G shows an early lesion of melanoma (nontumorigenic, Clark level II, Breslow thickness 0.37 mm) that exhibits somewhat greater pigmentary variegation, with black areas and a discrete rather than indefinite border. (Figs. A–F from Plate IV, Fascicle 2, Third Series.)

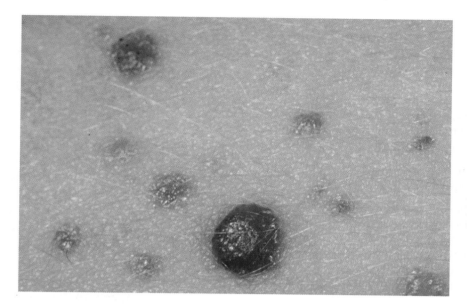

Figure 6-2

MULTIPLE NONDYSPLASTIC NEVI

For comparison with the dysplastic nevi illustrated in the previous figure, this group of nevi ranges from small lentiginous junctional lesions to a papular compound nevus at the upper left and a papular dermal nevus at the bottom center.

nevus. Even the apparently flat lesions are usually slightly raised to side-lighting, but they may be completely impalpable. Nondysplastic nevi, if larger than 3 mm, are compound nevi that are papules, with raised palpable borders, sharp edges, and uniform pigment (fig. 6-2).

Dysplastic nevi usually develop from about the time of puberty into young adulthood; although a few new lesions continue to appear throughout life, this is uncommon enough that such lesions in an adult should be excised to rule out melanoma. Although they are more likely than ordinary nevi to occur on usually covered skin (e.g., buttock, breast in women), dysplastic nevi are preferentially distributed on sun-exposed surfaces, consistent with the idea that they are induced by ultraviolet light (12,13).

Evolving dysplastic nevi grow for a time, but once fully evolved, they are usually stable lesions. Any lesions that show progressive changes in size, shape, or color should be excised to rule out melanoma. Serial follow-up of patients with dysplastic nevi has demonstrated that such changing lesions are rare; indeed, the most common change in a dysplastic nevus is in the direction of less atypia (14). The plaques of junctional or compound dysplastic nevi share many of the clinical features of plaque stage or patch stage melanoma but to a lesser degree. When color variegation is marked in large lesions, especially when there are focal black or very dark areas, dysplastic nevi may be difficult to distinguish

Table 6-1
CRITERIA FOR THE CLINICAL DIAGNOSIS OF DYSPLASTIC NEVUS[a]
Acquired pigmented cutaneous lesions, appear first in adolescence, rare in prepubertal children
Diameter greater than 5 mm, usually less than 12–15 mm
A macular component is present by definition
A papular component may be present, often in the center of the macule
Color slightly variegated: tan to dark brown often on a pink background
Border slightly irregular, ill-defined and impalpable

[a]Data from references 10 and 20.

from early melanomas, and such lesions should be excised to rule out melanoma (fig. 6-1G).

The histologic diagnosis of dysplastic nevi, in our opinion, should be based on the histologic examination of a clinically atypical nevus, and when this is done with agreed upon criteria, the reproducibility of diagnosis is good (15,16). Since most studies that have correlated melanoma risk with dysplastic nevus status have been based on clinical criteria, it is not essential to biopsy a nevus to confirm dysplasia, if melanoma is not suspected clinically. Histologic dysplasia, however, correlates with melanoma risk (17,18), so a biopsy may provide helpful information relating to the need for follow-up and its frequency. Nevi less than 3 to 4 mm in diameter may have "dysplastic features" both clinically and histologically, but are difficult to distinguish from common nevi. Nevertheless, such morphologically dysplastic but small nevi may be associated with increased melanoma risk (10), and may show histologic abnormalities similar to larger dysplastic nevi (19). Table 6-1 summarizes the clinical criteria for the diagnosis of a dysplastic nevus (10,20).

Significance of Common and Dysplastic Nevi as Markers of Melanoma Risk

Epidemiologic studies have identified a number of genetic, phenotypic, and behavioral traits that are indicators of increased risk for melanoma. Genetic melanoma risk factors include a family history of melanoma, and phenotypic and behavioral factors include attributes related to sunlight sensitivity and exposure, the total number of nevi and dysplastic nevi, the presence of poorly tanning skin with a propensity to sunburn, the individual's sun exposure history, and phenotypic indicators of sun exposure such as freckles and actinic skin damage (10,21–23). The presence of melanocytic nevi is among the strongest of the known risk markers, and clinically recognized dysplastic nevi are especially important as risk markers and potential precursors of melanoma (2,10,24). Histologic melanocytic dysplasia has also now been clearly shown to correlate with melanoma risk (17,18).

Dysplastic nevi were first identified in members of many (but not all) familial melanoma kindreds. Soon after, it was realized that dysplastic nevi are also common in patients with melanoma who have no family history (3), and are also present in some members of the general population (21,22).

The significance of a dysplastic nevus in a particular patient varies greatly, depending especially on the family and personal history of melanoma, and also, although to a lesser extent, on the individual phenotypic and behavioral risk factors listed above. In members of hereditary melanoma kindreds, dysplastic nevi are associated with a markedly increased risk for malignant melanoma approaching 100 percent over a lifetime (2,25,26). This risk is analogous to the up to 100 percent lifetime risk for colon cancer in patients with familial multiple polyposis. In contrast to the extremely high risk in hereditary melanoma

kindreds, dysplastic nevi found in members of the general public are associated with less (but still substantial) melanoma risk (27).

Clinically Dysplastic Nevi as Melanoma Risk Markers in Familial Melanoma Kindreds

In a prospective surveillance study of 401 members of 14 hereditary melanoma kindreds, Greene et al. (2) found 39 newly diagnosed melanomas in family members with dysplastic nevi, but none in their unaffected blood relatives. Carey et al. (26) confirmed similar findings in a study of more than 200 families. Since in this study, as in others, some melanomas occurred in patients who lacked dysplastic nevi, these lesions cannot be considered perfect markers of risk status in these kindreds.

The inheritance pattern of dysplastic nevi appears to be complex. Linkage analyses of 19 cutaneous malignant melanoma/dysplastic nevi (CMM/DN) kindreds showed significant evidence of heterogeneity and linkage to both chromosomes 1p and 9p (28). Subsequent studies, using a two-trait locus, two-marker locus linkage method suggested that a chromosome 1p locus (or loci) contributed to both CMM and CMM/DN, whereas a 9p locus contributed to CMM alone (29,30). Other studies, however, have found no consistent genetic linkage (31–33). The differences in study results are likely due to diagnostic and genetic heterogeneity in different populations.

Clinically Dysplastic Nevi as Melanoma Risk Markers in Random Populations

A strong association of dysplastic nevi with melanoma risk has also been described in random population members, without a confirmed family history of melanoma. Nordlund et al. (6) were the first to quantify this risk, in a case-control study in an Australian population.

Although the risk for patients with dysplastic nevi who lack a personal or family history of melanoma is less than that in hereditary melanoma kindreds, it is clinically significant, especially in clinic-based series. Halpern et al. (14), in a clinic-based cohort study, described very high melanoma risk indices in patients with dysplastic nevi, increasing from an annual rate of 154/100,000 patient years and a 16-fold relative risk in patients with no history of melanoma to relative risks of 100-fold in those with a personal history and more than 1000-fold in individuals with a family history of melanoma. Marghoob et al. (34) described similar findings in clinic-based patients with florid dysplastic nevi (termed by them the "classic" atypical mole syndrome [CAMS]). Thirty-two of 118 patients with CAMS and 18 of 173 controls, each with a history of melanoma, developed a second primary melanoma, for a cumulative 10-year lifetime risk of 35.5 percent and 17.0 percent, respectively (P <0.0001). Rigel et al. (35) following patients with dysplastic nevi but no family or personal history of melanoma, found a relative risk of about 16 compared to population incidence data. In the same study, patients with dysplastic nevi who had prior melanoma expressed a relative risk of about 35. The highest reported risk in a cohort study was a greater than 1,000-fold excess risk in patients with dysplastic nevi and a family as well as a personal history of melanoma (14). The melanomas discovered in these and in other reported surveillance programs for dysplastic nevus cases were for the most part diagnosed at a biologically early stage, when a high cure rate can be expected (14,26,36–38).

These clinic-based follow-up studies of high-risk populations have established very high risk indices for melanoma in patients followed because of a combination of risk factors, often including large numbers of nevi and dysplastic nevi, a family history of melanoma, or a personal history of melanoma. These studies likely provide an upper estimate because of the concentration of risk factors in these highly selected patient groups.

Case-control studies, especially if population based, may give a truer picture of the public health significance of dysplastic nevi because the bias of a clinic-based series toward the more florid clinical phenotypes is avoided. In case-control studies of random populations, the risk is somewhat lower than in some of the clinic-based series, but still highly significant. In multiple studies of such populations, the relative risk for melanoma in patients with "sporadic" dysplastic nevi increased up to 12-fold after adjustment for other known risk factors including sun sensitivity, indicators of sun exposure, freckles, and total nevus number

(6,7,10,22,39–42). In these nonfamilial, or sporadic, cases of dysplastic nevi, the risk appears to increase progressively with increasing number of dysplastic nevi (10,22,27). This finding of a positive "dose-response" relationship between the risk for melanoma and an increasing number of dysplastic nevi in several of these studies (10,22,39) adds additional credence to the validity of the association. A recent meta-analysis of these studies has provided an excellent summary of the data (43). In this analysis it was concluded that the number of common nevi and of dysplastic ("atypical") nevi were both important melanoma risk factors, with relative risks of 6.89 for 101 to 120 nevi compared with less than 15, or 6.36 for 5 versus 0 dysplastic nevi. It was also emphasized that the study characteristics significantly influenced the estimates, with case-control studies presenting lower and more precise estimates than cohort studies (43).

In the largest case-control study to date (10), the risk for melanoma strongly related to the number of small nevi, large nondysplastic nevi, and clinically dysplastic nevi. In the absence of dysplastic nevi, increased numbers of small nevi were associated with an approximately two-fold risk, and increased numbers of both small and large nondysplastic nevi were associated with a four-fold risk. One clinically dysplastic nevus was associated with a two-fold risk (95 percent confidence interval, 1.4 to 3.6), while 10 or more conferred a 12-fold increased risk. Clinically "congenital pattern" nevi were not associated with increased risk of melanoma. It was concluded that clinically dysplastic nevi confer a substantial risk for melanoma, while nondysplastic nevi confer a small risk. Interestingly, although the criteria for a clinically dysplastic nevus in this study included a size over 5 mm, morphologically dysplastic nevi smaller than this size were also associated with risk, which was greater than that associated with small or large nondysplastic nevi. In this study, there was also a statistically significant association of risk with even a single dysplastic nevus, although the magnitude of the risk (two-fold) was small and similar to that associated with red hair or freckles. Based on these findings, it is clear that clinicians can identify a population at high risk of developing melanoma on the basis of nevus number and type. At least in members of melanoma-prone families, it has been demonstrated that surveillance of high-risk individuals can lead to earlier diagnosis and a lower predicted mortality rate (26,38,44).

The risk of a second (or subsequent) primary melanoma is greatly increased in patients with a first primary melanoma and dysplastic nevi. In a case-control study, patients with first primary melanoma and histologic dysplastic nevi were at increased risk for a second primary melanoma (odds ratio, 6.2; 95 percent confidence interval, 1.2 to 33.4) (45). In the same study, patients with two or more clinically atypical nevi also had an elevated risk for a second primary (odds ratio, 8.8; 95 percent confidence interval, 1.0 to 80.7). Odds ratios for the association of histologic dysplastic nevi in this study varied from 6.1 to 10.4 when adjusting singly for pigmentary and sun exposure variables. In a two-factor model that included histologic and clinical dysplastic nevi, both variables retained a marginally significant statistical association with multiple primary melanoma. These results indicate that dysplastic nevi are markers of increased risk for multiple primary melanoma and suggest that melanoma patients with histologic or clinical evidence of dysplastic nevi should be followed closely for the development of additional primaries (46). Similar findings were also reported in the cohort studies of Carey et al. (26) and Halpern et al. (14).

Histologically Dysplastic Nevi as Melanoma Risk Markers

Relating histologic dysplasia to melanoma risk has been difficult because in case-control studies biopsies from controls are often not available in sufficient numbers. The question was addressed in a 1991 study by Augustsson (46), who studied 121 prevalent melanoma cases and 378 randomly selected controls. The mean total body nevus count was 115 in the melanoma cases and 67 in the controls. Fifty-six percent of the melanoma cases and 18 percent of the controls had clinical dysplastic nevi. The corresponding figures for histologically diagnosed dysplastic nevi were 40 percent and 8 percent, respectively, indicating a relative risk increase of about five-fold for patients with histologic dysplasia (13,47). Indirect evidence in support of the relationship between histologic dysplasia and risk came from a clinicopathologic correlative study, which found that nuclear and architectural histologic dysplasia on biopsy of the most atypical pigmented lesions correlated with observations regarding total number of nevi, which in turn correlated with melanoma risk (48). Also, as reviewed above, the presence of histologic dysplasia in a nevus associated with a first primary melanoma confers approximately a six-fold increased risk of a second primary (45)

A population-based study of observer reproducibility of diagnosis in biopsies of nevi from patients with melanoma and controls also provided evidence for an association of histologic dysplasia with melanoma risk (48). According to kappa statistics, reproducibility among six observers was substantial, and interobserver concordance was fair, despite differences in published criteria. For three of the observers, there was a difference in the frequency of dysplasia in melanoma cases compared to controls, consistent with a relative risk for melanoma of approximately three-fold in patients with histologic dysplasia.

An important recent contribution to this issue is the study of Arumi-Uria, McNutt, and Finnerty (17). They divided 4,481 patients with 6,275 lesions that were diagnosed as nevi with architectural disorder and melanocytic atypia ("a.k.a. dysplastic nevi") into those whose worst atypia was mild (2,504 lesions), moderate (1,657 lesions), or severe (320 lesions). Review of accession data revealed that a personal history of melanoma was present in 5.7 percent of 2,504 patients with mild, 8.1 percent of 1,657 patients with moderate, and 19.7 percent of 320 patients with severe atypia. Family histories of melanoma were not considered. The odds ratios as a measure of the association between atypical nevi and a personal history of melanoma were 4.1 for patients with severe versus mild atypia, 2.8 for severe versus moderate atypia, and 1.4 for moderate versus mild atypia. The design of this study did not permit the comparison of risk between patients with any dysplasia versus those with no dysplasia in their biopsy. These data show that the probability of a patient having a personal history of melanoma correlates with the grade of dysplasia in a nevus biopsy (fig. 6-3), and that the risk of melanoma is greater for those with nevi with high-grade atypia. The study also provides an evidence-based set of criteria for grading of melanocytic dysplasia.

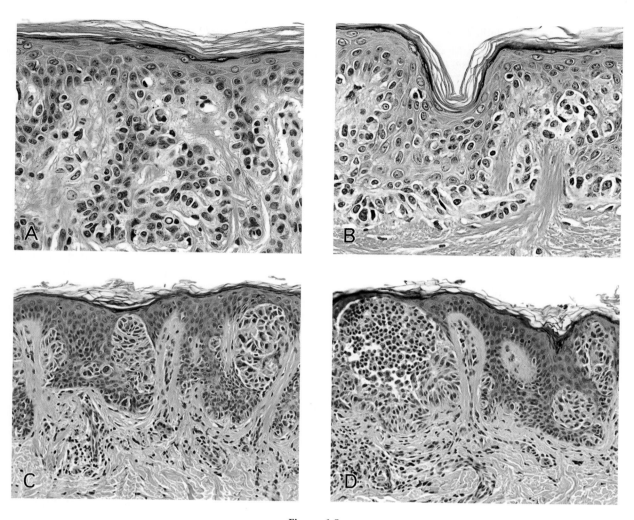

Figure 6-3

MILD, MODERATE, AND SEVERE DYSPLASIA

There is a gradation of architectural disorder and cytologic atypia from the nevi in A and B through the nevi in C and D (see also figs. 6-4–6-13). The number of enlarged hyperchromatic nuclei increases, and also the size and variability of the nests.

A case control study of melanoma risk in relation to histologic dysplasia was presented by Shors et al. (49). The clinically most atypical macular nevus was biopsied from 80 patients with newly diagnosed melanoma and from spouse controls. Histologic dysplasia was assigned a grade on a subjective 0 to 4 point scale by a 13-member panel of dermatopathologists from the North American Melanoma Study Group. Subjects with panel average ratings over 1 (i.e., moderate dysplasia or worse) had an increased relative risk of melanoma, with an odds ratio after adjustment for confounders of 3.99, with 95 percent confidence interval of

1.02 to 15.71. The kappa statistic was 0.28 for the panel histologic diagnoses, indicating poor interobserver reproducibility. The observers had not agreed on criteria prior to the study, but now have the opportunity to re-study the cases with consensus criteria which best predict risk, and thus provide an evidence-based set of refined criteria for grading histologic dysplasia.

In our opinion, this and the other studies reviewed above conclusively indicate that histologically defined melanocytic dysplasia, like clinical dysplasia or atypia, is significantly associated with melanoma risk. A pathology finding of a dysplastic nevus, or of a nevus with

Table 6-2
RISK-BASED CLASSIFICATION OF PATIENTS WITH DYSPLASTIC NEVI[a]
Low prospective risk for melanoma (<10% lifetime risk)
Few dysplastic nevi and no family or personal history of melanoma
High prospective risk for melanoma (up to 100% lifetime risk)
Florid dysplastic nevi (more than 10 to hundreds of dysplastic nevi)
Any dysplastic nevi and a personal or family history of melanoma

[a]Data from reference 20.

dysplastic features, should initiate an evaluation of the patient's total risk profile for melanoma, and a consideration of surveillance. A nevus biopsy should primarily be done to rule out melanoma in a clinically suspicious lesion. The grade of the dysplasia in a nevus biopsy has now been demonstrated to correlate with risk (17,18). These findings provide evidence in support of the common practice of biopsying nevi to assess atypia as a guide to recommendations for nevi surveillance. These studies also provide the capacity to develop evidence-based histologic criteria for the diagnosis and grading of melanocytic dysplasia as a melanoma risk marker.

Risk-Based Classification of Dysplastic Nevus Cases

The classification of patients with dysplastic nevi into low- and high-risk groups proposed by the 1984 National Institutes of Health (NIH) Consensus Conference on Precursors to Melanoma considered family and personal history of melanoma as added risk factors (20). In addition, the number of dysplastic nevi is also a risk factor. A classification based on these considerations is presented in Table 6-2.

Significance of Dysplastic Nevi as Potential Precursors of Melanoma

The development of cytologic abnormalities, coupled with atypical patterns of growth in dysplastic nevi, is consistent with a model of tumor progression whereby a tumor may evolve from a melanocyte to a fully malignant melanoma through intermediate steps including a dysplastic nevus. The most direct evidence that dysplastic nevi may be potential precursors of melanoma

(in addition to being markers for risk of melanoma) is provided by the serendipitous observation of a change in a previously photographed and initially stable dysplastic nevus. We and others have made this observation often enough to suggest something more than a chance association, but rarely enough to confirm the statistical inference that progression to melanoma is likely to be an infequent event in any given prospectively followed dysplastic nevus (45).

Additional evidence that dysplastic nevus is a melanoma precursor is provided by the finding that a putative precursor dysplastic nevus is contiguous with a melanoma in about 30 percent or more of cases (50–55). In one large study from Western Australia (55), a nevus was associated with melanoma in 51 percent of cases (n = 147). Of these, 82 (56 percent) were dysplastic nevi, 61 (41 percent) were common acquired nevi, and 4 (3 percent) were congenital nevi. Lentiginous melanocytic proliferation was present in the epidermis adjacent to 219 melanomas (75 percent) and in 44 percent of these cases (n=97), a coexisting nevus was also present. In a more recent study from Austria of 667 consecutive cases of primary cutaneous melanoma, 22.1 percent had an associated nevus; of these nevi, 55 percent were dysplastic nevi, 40 percent were congenital pattern nevi, and only 5 percent were considered to be banal nevi (56). Generally, melanomas containing benign nevus components are thinner than melanomas without benign nevi but the prognosis is the same when stratified by tumor thickness. This study also suggests a more important role for superficial congenital nevi as precursor lesions of nevus-associated melanomas than presently recognized.

Although they are regarded as potential precursors of melanomas, the majority of dysplastic nevi are stable lesions (57). This paradox may be explained by the fact that dysplastic nevi are much more common than melanomas in the population. In a population of 100 million individuals, similar to the white population of the United States, the prevalence of dysplastic nevi is 5 percent and the average number of lesions per affected individual is two: such a population has at least 10 million dysplastic nevi. If the incidence of melanoma is 20 per 100,000, then 20,000 melanomas occur in that population per year. If 50 percent of the melanomas develop in a preexisting dysplastic nevus, then 10,000 melanomas develop in the 10 million dysplastic nevi, or 1/1,000 dysplastic nevi per year. This is an upper estimate, as the assumptions listed above are conservative. In addition, there is evidence that many melanomas arise de novo. In a cohort follow-up study, Kelly et al. (44) found that 13 of 20 newly diagnosed melanomas arose as new lesions and only 3 (15 percent) from dysplastic nevi. Thus, even in patients at increased risk for melanoma because of dysplastic nevi, the most common pathway of evolution of a melanoma does not include a clinically or histologically detectable dysplastic nevus precursor. Therefore, melanoma could not be prevented by the wholesale excision of dysplastic nevi in these patients.

The suggestion that benign nevi may be precursors of melanoma and not just chance associations is supported by recent molecular studies of mutations in the oncogenes *BRAF* or *NRAS*. In melanomas with an associated nevus, the mutation was either present (with occasional exceptions) in both the underlying nevus cells and the melanoma cells or both lesions were negative for the mutation, supporting the theory of clonal progression of the nevus into a malignant melanoma (58,59).

DYSPLASTIC NEVI IN A MODEL OF TUMOR PROGRESSION

Because dysplastic nevi are important precursors, risk markers, and simulants of melanoma, understanding their biology may provide clues to the mechanisms involved in melanoma development.

Cell Biology of Dysplastic Nevi

The molecular basis of the susceptibility to melanoma that characterizes patients with dysplastic nevi may relate to increased sensitivity to the mutagenic effects of ultraviolet (UV) light. Some of these patients have evidence of chromosomal instability (60,61). Patients with dysplastic nevi have an increased frequency of random chromosomal abnormalities in their circulating lymphoid cells (60,61), and the cells of dysplastic nevi themselves also have chromosomal abnormalities in about one third of cases studied (62). These defects are apparently associated with abnormal DNA repair in the early period (first hour) after UV light-induced injury. Lymphoblastoid cells from patients with dysplastic nevi, mostly members of hereditary melanoma kindreds, are abnormally sensitive to UV damage in the premitotic G2 phase of the cell cycle (63), and exhibit an increased frequency of mutations after UV exposure (64). Fibroblasts from such patients exhibit delayed removal of UV-induced thymidine dimers when studied 30 to 60 minutes after UV injury (65). In another study, however, DNA repair synthesis following irradiation with UV light was not diminished in fibroblasts from patients with dysplastic nevi. These variations in results are probably a consequence of diagnostic heterogeneity (66). Another study demonstrated that abnormalities of DNA repair may contribute to the melanoma risk in patients with dysplastic nevi (67). Ultraviolet B (UVB)-induced DNA damage was determined in pigment cells derived from foreskin, common melanocytic nevi, and dysplastic nevi. The nevus cells originating from dysplastic nevi showed the highest sensitivity to UVB irradiation: 65 percent higher induction of DNA damage compared to the induction in foreskin melanocytes. Common melanocytic nevus cells were most resistant and showed a 30 percent lower induction of DNA damage in comparison to foreskin melanocytes.

In further support of the hypothesis that dysplastic nevi result in part from abnormalities of DNA repair, studies found that the expression of DNA mismatch repair proteins and of growth arrest DNA damage (*GADD*) genes was significantly lower in dysplastic nevi than in nondysplastic nevi (68,69). The absence or decrease of *GADD* gene expression in these nevi was thought to be consistent with a potential for malignant transformation. In another study of mismatch repair genes, there was a gradual decrease in immunohistochemical staining values during the progression from nondysplastic nevi to dysplastic nevi to melanomas (70). Once the lesions evolve, it is possible that continuing exposure to sunlight results in the accumulation of additional mutations, perhaps accounting for the cytologic atypia that characterizes these lesions and distinguishes them from common nevi.

In support of the idea that cytologic atypia in dysplastic nevi reflects damage to the cellular DNA, a study found that 87 percent of markedly atypical dysplastic nevi but only about 40 percent of the mildly atypical lesions had abnormal DNA histograms (71). Further, in studies of microsatellite instability, deficient DNA repair was found with increased frequency in dysplastic nevi and melanomas but not in benign melanocytic nevi (72,73). In addition, there was a statistically significant correlation between the degree of atypia and the frequency of microsatellite instability in dysplastic nevi (73). In a similar study, there was a lower frequency of microsatellite instability in common nevi; dysplastic nevi were again intermediate between melanomas and common nevi (74).

These abnormalities may be especially pronounced in members of hereditary melanoma kindreds. Using a shuttle vector plasmid, Moriwaki et al. (75) found evidence of post-UV plasmid hypermutability in members of melanoma-prone families with dysplastic nevi, with or without a history of melanoma. This finding demonstrates that patients with familial melanoma have a defective mechanism for handling UV-induced DNA damage. These patients may have not only increased sensitivity to UV damage, but also deficient DNA repair mechanisms.

These findings have now been extended to the population level. In a 2002 study, DNA repair capacity was determined for 132 patients with incident melanoma and for 145 control subjects (41). The DNA repair capacity strongly influenced melanoma risk in individuals with a low tanning ability or with dysplastic nevi. For the latter group, the odds ratio of risk was increased 6.7-fold for individuals lacking dysplastic nevi and having a low repair capacity, compared to individuals without dysplastic nevi and with a high repair capacity. Subjects with dysplastic nevi and a high repair capacity had an intermediate risk.

The data reviewed above are consistent with the hypothesis that UV-induced damage to DNA plays a role in the pathogenesis and evolution of dysplastic nevi, and that many but probably not all patients with dysplastic nevi have an abnormality of DNA repair that may represent a single-gene defect in a repair enzyme. This enzyme could be encoded by a "melanoma susceptibility gene" such as the putative susceptibility gene(s) discussed in the previous section, or alternatively, the trait could be polygenic.

In addition to the DNA repair abnormalities discussed above, there is evidence that the lesional cells themselves are more susceptible to DNA damage from exposure to the sun. Sun sensitivity in dysplastic nevus cells appears to be enhanced by the relative overexpression of red-brown pheomelanin pigment compared to the darker brown eumelanin pigment in these cells. Pheomelanin may not only be a poor sunscreening agent, but also may release reactive oxygen species during UV exposure, which could damage and potentially mutate cellular DNA (76). Salopek et al. (76) found that dysplastic nevi contain significantly higher amounts of pheomelanin than either common melanocytic nevi or normal skin. According to the hypothesis of Jimbow et al. (77), altered melanin synthesis may profoundly affect carcinogenesis in malignant melanoma. Pheomelanin is increased in malignant melanoma and dysplastic nevi, but not in normal skin and common nevi; pheomelanin and its precursors could aid the malignant transformation of melanocytes through the generation of mutagenic UV photoproducts in dysplastic nevi. It is possible that increased pheomelanin and perhaps other abnormalities of melanin precursors enhance oxidative DNA damage, promoting mutations and other DNA abnormalities, and leading to the dysplastic nevus phenotype (78). The changes in nitrous oxide metabolism that have been documented in dysplastic nevi may be related to this (79). The mutations attributable to such mechanisms would not be limited to the thymidine dimer formation that characterizes UV-related mutations, which have been identified in some but not in all melanomas (80).

The involvement of the RAF/RAS/MAP kinase pathway in common nevi has already been discussed in chapter 2. The incidence of mutations in *BRAF* and *NRAS* oncogenes appears to be similar in common nevi and dysplastic nevi, indicating that these genes are not responsible for the development of atypia in nevi (58,59,81). Nor are they likely to represent a direct causal factor in the progression of nevi to melanoma, although they undoubtedly play a critical permissive role.

Although the critical genetic events that may be pathogenic for dysplastic nevi have not been identified, a study of loss of heterozygosity

(LOH) in nevi and melanomas found evidence of hemizygous deletion (LOH) in seven of nine (78 percent) dysplastic nevi at one or more loci for p16; no LOH was detected in any of the benign intradermal nevi studied (82). In another such study, LOH at the p16 locus was discovered in 64 percent of dysplastic nevi and 50 percent of benign nevi; homozygous deletion of p16 was found in 29 percent (4 of 14) of dysplastic nevi but in no benign nevi (83). The p16 molecule is a tumor suppressor that is lost either through genetic or epigenetic mechanisms in most melanoma lesions, contributing to loss of cell cycle control in these tumors. These data suggest that deletion of p16 may play an important role in the development of dysplastic nevus as an early event and that the changes may represent an early event in the development of malignant melanoma (82).

The dysplastic nevus trait itself appears to be independent of the *CDKN2A* locus where p16 resides, but may add to the risk in individuals with inherited abnormalities of *CDKN2A*. In a study of five Swedish familial melanoma kindreds characterized by germline mutations in *CDKN2A* and dysplastic nevi, there were significant correlations between dysplastic nevus phenotype and melanoma, and between mutation status and the presence of dysplastic nevi (84). In *CDKN2A* mutation carriers, all early-onset melanomas occurred in dysplastic nevi, and the mean age at melanoma diagnosis was significantly lower in individuals with dysplastic nevi than in those without a confirmed dysplastic nevus phenotype. These results were considered to be consistent with the hypothesis that germline *CDKN2A* mutations and dysplastic nevi both contribute to the predisposition to melanoma and may lead to the development of early-onset melanoma when present in the same individual.

The evidence from these studies shows that patients with dysplastic nevi may be abnormally susceptible to UV-induced damage, perhaps by a mechanism involving reactive oxygen species, and that their ability to repair such damage may be deficient. These abnormalities may result in somatic genetic alterations of precursor melanocytes, leading to the development of nevi, dysplastic nevi, and, ultimately, melanomas. Gain of oncogenic mutations in genes such as

BRAF and *NRAS*, and loss of suppressor genes such as *p16*, appear to be critical events. These genetic changes result not only in increased risk of progression, but also in morphologic alterations of lesional cells reflecting changes associated with progression that are of diagnostic and prognostic utility.

Cellular and Molecular Markers of Progression in Dysplastic Nevi

The cells of dysplastic nevi tend to be intermediate in melanocytic tumor progression between those of common nevi and melanomas as measured by morphologic, immunohistochemical, and molecular techniques. Although resembling nevi with most markers, dysplastic nevi tend to share other features with melanomas. Studies show three groups of markers that distinguish dysplastic nevi as intermediate lesions: in the first group, dysplastic nevi tend to resemble radial growth phase melanomas in terms of marker expression; in a second group, the marker studies demonstrate greater similarities to common nevi; and in the third group, there are no consistent differences among the three categories.

One early study showed how dysplastic nevi tend to differ from common nevi and to resemble radial growth phase melanoma (85). HMB45 antigen reactivity (a feature more commonly associated with melanoma cells in the dermis) was found in the dermal nevus cells of moderately and severely dysplastic nevi. This antigen did not react with the dermal cells of common nevi, and the findings in this study were considered to support the concept of dysplastic nevi as precursor lesions of melanoma with undetermined biologic potential. Another study used a panel of 16 monoclonal antibodies against antigens including epidermal growth factor (EGF) receptor, GD2 and GD3 gangliosides, human leukocyte antigen (HLA)-DR, nerve growth factor (NGF)-receptor, and melanoma-associated proteoglycan as well as six unknown antigens to distinguish between radial and vertical growth phase melanomas, but not between dysplastic nevi and radial growth phase melanoma (86). In a study of the expression of cathepsin D, this protease was expressed in all of 10 dysplastic nevi and 21 primary and metastatic melanomas tested but in only 18 percent of nevocellular nevi (5 of 27), while normal melanocytes showed no expression (87). In a study of the neuropeptide/mast cell secretagogue, substance P, this potentially angiogenic and fibrogenic peptide was frequently expressed in melanomas and dysplastic nevi, as well as in Spitz nevi, but was not detected in any acquired benign melanocytic nevi (P <0.05) (88). In yet another study, the expression of a high molecular weight chondroitin sulfate proteoglycan, versican, was negative in benign melanocytic nevi, weakly to strongly positive in dysplastic nevi, and intensely positive in primary malignant melanomas and metastatic melanomas (89).

Some markers that are differentially expressed in nevi and dysplastic nevi show a gradation with increasing atypia of dysplastic nevi. In a study that evaluated the activation of the cell signaling molecule Akt using an antibody specific for phospho-Akt, normal and slightly dysplastic nevi exhibited no significant expression, in marked contrast to dramatic Akt immunoreactivity seen in severely dysplastic nevi and melanomas (66.3 percent positive) (90). This molecule is thought to be important in the activation of the transcription factor NF-kappaB which is seen in most melanomas.

In other marker studies, dysplastic nevi have reacted intermediate between mature nevi and melanomas. Some of these studies are related to the oxygen metabolism in nevi, reviewed in the previous section. For example, it was demonstrated nearly two decades ago that dysplastic nevi contain significantly higher amounts of pheomelanin than either common melanocytic nevus or normal skin (76). It was suggested that pheomelanin and its precursors could aid the malignant transformation of melanocytes through the generation of mutagenic UV photoproducts in patients with familial dysplastic nevus syndrome (77). Pavel et al. (78) have recently confirmed and extended these findings. They found a significantly higher content of pheomelanin in melanosomes from dysplastic nevus cells and melanoma cells when compared with normal melanocytes and banal nevi. They also demonstrated that dysplastic nevus cells exhibit higher concentrations of radical oxygen species than normal skin melanocytes. These authors proposed that increased pheomelano-genesis in dysplastic nevus cells is connected with oxidative imbalance, which is reflected by increased intracellular concentrations of reactive oxygen species. The metabolic alterations in dysplastic nevus cells resemble those found in melanoma cells, and are considered by the authors to provide support for the idea that dysplastic nevi are true precursor lesions of melanoma (91).

Studies possibly related to abnormal oxygen metabolism have included measurements of lipoxygenase and nitric oxide synthase in nevi and melanomas (79,92). The expression of 12-lipoxygenase (12-LOX) was determined in normal human skin melanocytes and in melanocytes of compound nevi, dysplastic nevi, and melanomas. Expression was unchanged in compound nevi and was increased in dysplastic nevi and melanomas compared with normal skin melanocytes. Melanomas had higher levels of expression compared with dysplastic nevi. These data suggest that 12-LOX may be an important novel marker for cancer progression within the melanoma system, and therefore could be a useful biomarker and therapeutic target for melanoma chemoprevention (92). In a study of the expression of nitric oxide synthase in paraffin sections of melanocytic lesions, dysplastic nevi and melanomas showed increased immunoreactivity compared to common acquired nevi (79). This enzyme can generate toxic nitric oxide, which is a reactive molecule that may enhance tumor progression and metastasis. It was postulated by these authors that the frequent expression of nitric oxide synthase in the junctional part of dysplastic nevi may be responsible for their particular histologic features.

Among other studies that have demonstrated the intermediate character of dysplastic nevi, a study of the cell signaling receptor, endothelin B, showed a significant increase in intensity of its expression from common nevi over dysplastic nevi and primary melanoma to metastatic melanoma (93). In addition, two polymerase chain reaction (PCR)-based studies have demonstrated that telomerase activity increases from benign melanocytic nevi to atypical (dysplastic) nevi and further to malignant melanoma and metastatic melanoma cells, suggesting that telomerase may play a role in tumor initiation and progression, and suggesting the future utility of this marker as a diagnostic and possible prognostic tool (94,95).

Quantitative cell cycle and nuclear morphometric studies have also tended to demonstrate findings intermediate between common nevi and melanomas for dysplastic nevi. In melanocytic lesions studied with an antibody to the cell cycle marker proliferating cell nuclear antigen (PCNA)/cyclin, positive tumor cells increased in number and staining intensity according to the following progression: common melanocytic nevi, dysplastic nevi, primary melanomas, and metastatic melanomas (96). Nucleolar organizer regions (AgNORs), which have been associated with dysplastic lesions in other systems, were studied by Fogt et al. (97) and found to increase progressively from nevi to dysplastic nevi to radial and vertical growth phase melanomas. It was concluded that stepwise increases in cellular AgNORs paralleled the melanocytic progression model and thereby corroborated the intermediate nature of the dysplastic nevus. In an analysis of melanocytic lesions by DNA image cytometry, a "distinctly aneuploid histogram" was not identified in low-grade lesions, but was observed in 2 of 9 dysplastic nevi with moderate atypia and 6 of 8 with severe atypia, and in 7 of 11 melanomas (98). It was concluded that dysplastic nevi exhibit a spectrum of abnormal DNA content intermediate between banal nevi and melanomas, and that DNA content generally correlates with the age of patients and degree of atypia in melanocytic nevi. Consistent with these observations of DNA abnormalities, studies of microsatellite instability, mismatch repair proteins, and loss of heterozygosity (reviewed in more detail in the previous section) have more or less uniformly shown dysplastic nevi to be intermediate between common nevi and melanomas (70,72–74,99).

The studies reviewed in this section, taken together, strongly support the concept that dysplastic nevi occupy a position intermediate between common nevi and early melanoma in melanocytic tumor progression. While some of these markers may be of value for clinical diagnosis, studies of their sensitivity, specificity, and predictive value in routine and difficult cases are lacking, so that their routine use cannot be recommended except as an adjunct to more traditional diagnostic tools.

Critiques of the Concept of Melanocytic Dysplasia

The concept of melanocytic dysplasia has been controversial, as discussed in a thoughtful critique by Piepkorn (100), who noted that the original studies of dysplastic (atypical) nevi described a clinical trait, as described above. Controversies about the nature, definition, and clinical significance of dysplastic nevi have arisen from disputes about the definition of the lesions and the reproducibility of the diagnosis, and have resulted in large measure from a lack of control data regarding the histology of clinically typical nevi from subjects not at risk for melanoma. Piepkorn himself has begun to address these questions in his ground-breaking case-control study of nevi in melanoma patients and spouse controls (48).

A major source of disagreement has been the use by different investigators of different sets of criteria for the diagnosis of melanocytic dysplasia. In some of these criteria sets, cytologic atypia, which was considered necessary in the original descriptions, is not thought to be of importance in making the diagnosis. Even when the criteria used appears to be similar as viewed in written form, they may be very different in practice. Thus, in a large interobserver and intraobserver agreement study using population-based nevus samples from the University of Utah (48), there was variation among observers such that the prevalence of "dysplasia" in the dataset ranged from 7 to 32 percent! Despite this graphic demonstration of interobserver variation, this study found good intraobserver agreement when the slides were recirculated, indicating that the source of the disagreement was the use of different criteria.

It has been argued by Ackerman (101) that there has been a failure "to define meaningfully melanocytic dysplasia, dysplastic nevus, and dysplastic nevus syndrome." Yet, as was pointed out in a response by McNutt (101a) to this assertion, "the definitions and illustrations in eight current textbooks on dermatopathology are in remarkable agreement about the main features of the lesions to which these terms pertain." Also, as demonstrated in the Utah study reviewed above (48), there is direct experimental evidence that the use of different criteria results in failure to agree about the diagnosis, and thus the significance, of these lesions.

As also pointed out by Piepkorn (100), controlled analyses that relate histologic criteria with objective biologic markers are necessary to determine the significance of histologically dysplastic nevi. Many such studies have been reviewed above, in the section on the significance of these lesions in a biologic model of tumor progression. In terms of clinical phenotypes and risk, Piepkorn accepts in his critique that correlations, "albeit not strong," exist between the histologic assessment of atypia and the clinical parameters of nevus number and size, parameters that in turn are associated with melanoma risk. Beyond that, since this critique was published in 2001, two studies discussed earlier in the section on histologically dysplastic nevi as markers of melanoma risk have established more directly that there is a correlation between histologic atypia in dysplastic nevi and melanoma. In the correlation study of Arumi-Uria et al. (17), it was demonstrated that individuals whose nevi exhibit more severe atypia have a higher risk of melanoma than those with lesser atypia. Similarly, in Piepkorn's own 2005 study (102), it was demonstrated for the first time in a case-control format adjusted for confounders that patients whose nevi demonstrated atypia beyond a mild degree had an almost four-fold increased risk of melanoma compared to the baseline patients with either mild or no atypia. Histologically atypical or dysplastic nevi, especially when the dysplasia is severe, are clearly markers of individuals at increased risk for melanoma, just as is the case for clinically atypical or dysplastic nevi.

PATHOLOGY OF JUNCTIONAL AND COMPOUND DYSPLASTIC NEVI

Microscopic Features

Histologically, dysplastic nevi differ from common nevi in their size, architectural features, cytologic features, and stromal features (11,103).

Architectural Features. Important architectural features of dysplastic nevi are the size of the lesion and the presence of a sizable macular or plaque component, either comprising the entirety of the lesion or located at the periphery or "shoulder" of a preexisting papule. At scanning magnification, dysplastic nevi are broad lesions whose size can be estimated microscopically and should be taken into account in making the diagnosis. *Junctional dysplastic nevi* are characterized by a flat lentiginous component (clinically, a barely elevated plaque or occasionally, a perfect macule), with no associated papular compound nevus. *Compound dysplastic nevi* most often combine a central collection of nevus cells (sometimes forming a papule) with a peripheral lentiginous plaque component, located at the shoulder of the papule (figs. 6-4, 6-5).

Histologically, the central papule may have features of a banal compound nevus, presumably a preexisting lesion, at the periphery of which dysplasia has developed as a secondary phenomenon (the "nevus with dysplasia"). In other cases, the cells of the dermal component resemble those of the junctional dysplastic component except that they have undergone maturation to a smaller cell type (fig. 6-4). Another category of compound dysplastic nevus includes lesions that are mostly flat and clinically indistinguishable from junctional dysplastic nevus, or that have a slightly "pebbly" quality to their surface topography. The pebbles seem to represent small groups of cells that have migrated into the dermis at many points of the undersurface of a predominantly junctional lesion. In these cases, the cells in the dermis may be immature like those in the epidermis (dermal and epidermal dysplasia), and a discrete papule of mature dermal nevic cells is not observed.

The macular component is recognized histologically as a pattern of delicate, fairly uniformly elongated rete ridges, with an increased number of nested and single nevus cells in the basal epidermis, the latter forming a pattern that is termed *lentiginous proliferation* (figs. 6-4–6-13). Typically, the nests of nevus cells are only slightly variable in size and shape, and often oriented with their long axis parallel to the surface of the skin. Some of the nests appear to "bridge" or coalesce between adjacent rete ridges, and there are nests at the tips and on the sides of the rete (1,3,11,15,16). In addition to the nested melanocytes, there are single cells as well. Unlike normal melanocytes, these single cells tend to be in contact with one another rather than being separated by keratinocytes. They are typically present at the sides and tips of the rete,

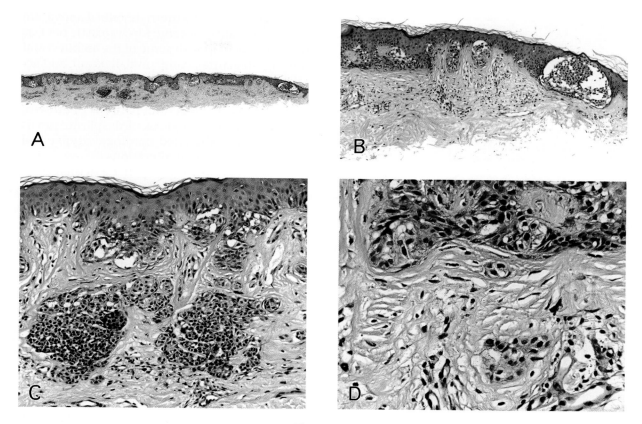

Figure 6-4

COMPOUND NEVUS WITH MODERATE DYSPLASIA (COMPOUND DYSPLASTIC NEVUS, MODERATE)

A: At scanning magnification, this is a broad, moderately cellular lesion, with the dermal component in the center and a junctional component forming "shoulders" at each side.

B: Higher magnification shows an increased number of predominantly nested melanocytes, mostly near the dermal-epidermal junction, with some nests bridging between adjacent elongated rete ridges. In the dermis, there is well-developed lamellar fibroplasia and a patchy perivascular lymphocytic infiltrate.

C: High magnification shows orderly nevus cells extending from the epidermis into the dermis, cytologically continuous with the cells in the epidermis and maturing to a smaller cell type at the base.

D: Scrutiny of the "fibroblasts" in the plates of lamellar fibroplasia reveals that they contain melanin pigment, indicating that they are of melanocytic derivation.

but not along the suprapapillary plate region of the epidermis. Thus, there is "contiguous" but not "continuous" or "confluent" proliferation of the nevus cells (figs. 6-4–6-13).

The rete ridge and melanocytic patterns together are termed lentiginous because they recapitulate the architecture of a lentigo simplex, the simplest and smallest melanocytic tumor (104). The term lentiginous, however, pertains to proliferations of melanocytes within the basal cell layer in the absence of elongation or prominence of rete ridges (as in the case of certain lentiginous variants of melanoma in situ). The persistence of this pattern, particularly beyond the dermal

component to form a junctional "shoulder," may be regarded as an immature form of growth because in normal nevi it is the rule for junctional proliferations to undergo a process of maturation that results in the formation of an entirely papular compound nevus. Because dysplastic nevi share many elements in common with simple lentigines, and because lentigines may give rise to melanocytic nevi with persistent lentiginous components in the absence of dysplasia, it is appropriate to diagnose histologic dysplasia with caution in lesions smaller than 3 to 4 mm, especially if the lesion in question constitutes the single clinically most "atypical" lesion in a

177

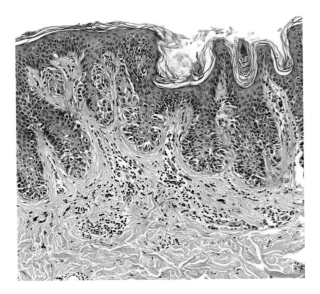

Figure 6-5

COMPOUND NEVUS WITH SEVERE DYSPLASIA (COMPOUND DYSPLASTIC NEVUS, SEVERE)

This lesion is highly cellular, and single cells predominate over nests. The cells are arranged mainly at the tips and sides of elongated rete ridges, however, without continuous proliferation between the rete, and without extensive pagetoid involvement of the epidermis. These findings constitute severe architectural disorder (architectural atypia). Cytologic atypia is present but is generally moderate and confined to randomly scattered lesional cells (random cytologic atypia).

particular patient. Studies, however, have demonstrated that small (less than 5 mm) nevi with either clinically atypical features (10) or with histologic architectural disorder and cytologic atypia (19) may have the same significance as larger ones, since cytologic atypia has been shown to correlate with a patient's risk of developing a melanoma in a dataset that did not use size as an explicit criterion (17). In case of doubt, a descriptive diagnosis can be issued, along with a recommendation for clinicopathologic correlation, with a complete assessment of the patient's risk factors for the development of melanoma.

The junctional nests of dysplastic nevi, especially those forming the shoulder of the lesion, differ from those of nondysplastic nevi by originating at the rete edges and inter-rete spaces, coalescing across adjacent rete ridges ("bridging"), and forming nonuniform enlarged nests occasionally exhibiting internal dyshesion. These architectural features, along with the lentiginous growth pattern described above, are not in themselves specific for dysplastic nevi, as they may overlap with some of the architectural findings in genital, congenital, flexural, and acral nevi (nevi of special sites) and occasionally with the junctional components above dermal nevic cells with congenital patterns of growth. Accordingly, the diagnosis of dysplastic nevus also requires associated cytologic atypia and characteristic stromal alterations.

Cytologic Features. Whether a dermal component is present or not, the prototypic and diagnostic changes of melanocytic dysplasia are found in the junctional compartment of the lesion (figs. 6-4, 6-5). Melanocytic dysplasia may extend into the epidermis above a papular dermal compartment, but most characteristically is found in the epidermis, extending in a compound lesion at least two to three rete ridges and usually much more beyond the most lateral dermal nevus cells. In a junctional dysplastic nevus, the changes are entirely intraepidermal. The predominant background cell type in most lesions is similar to that of banal nevi, namely, a small round cell having relatively sparse but identifiable cytoplasm, scanty coarse melanin pigment, and, often, a degree of cytoplasmic retraction artifact comparable to that observed in normal melanocytes.

In addition to these banal nevus cells, another cell type is present in dysplastic nevi. These cells, usually a minority of the total population but occasionally tending to predominate (fig. 6-3C,D), are larger than most common nevus cells, with more abundant cytoplasm, i.e., they are frankly epithelioid cells. The cytoplasm may contain sparse, finely divided, "dusty" (also termed dirty, muddy, smoky, or finely divided) melanin pigment (dysplastic nevi are not heavily pigmented lesions as a rule). It is of interest that although the character of cytoplasmic melanization does not in itself constitute cytologic dysplasia, it is a marker even at scanning magnification that assists in identifying these cells that ultimately will be confirmed to contain dysplastic nuclei. It may be that this marker correlates with the phenomenon of preferential expression of pheomelanin rather than eumelanin, which in turn may correlate with an increased susceptibility to oxidative damage to DNA and increased mutagenesis, as discussed earlier. The nuclei of these epithelioid cells are more variable than those in the banal nevic cells. Some are quite small and pyknotic; others are larger, with somewhat irregular and angulated, often geometric nuclear membranes; yet others have prominent large eosinophilic or amphophilic nucleoli. These cells have been termed giant basal and epithelioid melanocytes (105). Although they are benign nevus cells, they share some immunohistochemical and ultrastructural markers with the epithelioid cells of melanomas in the epidermis (106). In an ultrastructural comparison of the cytology of the cells of dysplastic nevi with those of superficial spreading melanoma and common nevi, it was concluded by Langer et al. (107) that "dysplastic nevi fill the biological gap between benign nevocellular nevi and malignant melanomas."

Dermal Component. As noted above, small collections of dermal nevus cells may be seen at multiple points across the breadth of an otherwise predominantly junctional dysplastic nevus. When these are present, they tend to resemble the cells of the junctional component, sometimes with obvious random nuclear atypia, but never with mitotic activity or other evidence of tumorigenicity. The cells of the papular component, in those compound dysplastic nevi that exhibit this feature, are usually similar in arrangement and cytology to those of a common acquired nevus, presenting aggregated nests and loosely cellular sheets of banal nevus cells that form a localized cluster in the papillary dermis and occasionally extend into the reticular dermis.

Some examples of dysplastic nevi with reticular dermal involvement represent instances of congenital pattern nevi with dysplasia (108). The dermal component of a large series of nevi with junctional dysplasia was studied by Toussaint and Kamino (109). They observed the histopathologic changes previously described in dysplastic melanocytic nevi in association with a dermal component characteristic of other types of melanocytic nevi or overlapping with features of other varieties of nevi. Among 2,164 compound dysplastic melanocytic nevi, about 8 percent showed a dermal component with a congenital pattern, 3 percent demonstrated epidermal and dermal characteristics of Spitz nevus, while less than 1 percent each had features of a combined blue nevus, a halo phe-

nomenon, or a neurotized dermal (neuronevus). The biologic significance of these variants, if any, remains to be established.

The dermal nevus cells of a dysplastic nevus usually do not show significant atypia when located in a papule, but by comparison with common acquired nevi, the papules may appear somewhat more cellular, and pigment production may extend deeper into the lesion. By contrast, flat compound dysplastic nevi often show atypia of both dermal and epidermal components (dermal and epidermal dysplasia, fig. 6-4), and these dermal cells may be HMB45 positive, unlike the cells of common nevi (85). In differentiating between atypical dermal nevus cells and small melanoma cells, the presence of maturation and the lack of mitotic figures in the dermis are important, as is the character of any contiguous intraepidermal proliferation. This important differential diagnosis is discussed in more detail in chapter 9.

Stromal Features and Host Responses. The stromal changes of dysplastic nevi are characteristic but not diagnostic. A lymphocytic infiltrate is almost always present, often with some degree of associated melanin pigment incontinence, and the diagnosis should be made with caution, if at all, in the absence of lymphocytes. The lymphocytes are distributed about vessels of the superficial plexus in a patchy pattern. In contrast, a dense band-like infiltrate in a melanocytic plaque lesion is suggestive of in situ or microinvasive melanoma, especially when it is associated with irregular thickening of the epidermis rather than the more regular rete ridge elongation that characterizes dysplastic nevi.

Also seen in most dysplastic nevi is a pattern of condensed collagen about the elongated rete, termed *concentric eosinophilic fibroplasia* (fig. 6-6). This pattern is not specific, being observed in some other lentiginous lesions. However, prominent concentric eosinophilic fibroplasia as a dominant stromal feature is uncommon except in a dysplastic nevus. Some nontumorigenic melanoma compartments may exhibit this feature focally, a pattern that may suggest "cancerization" of a preexisting dysplastic nevus component. The other pattern of fibroplasia seen in dysplastic nevi is less common, and is termed *lamellar fibroplasia*. In this pattern, plates of lamellar collagen and fibroblast-like

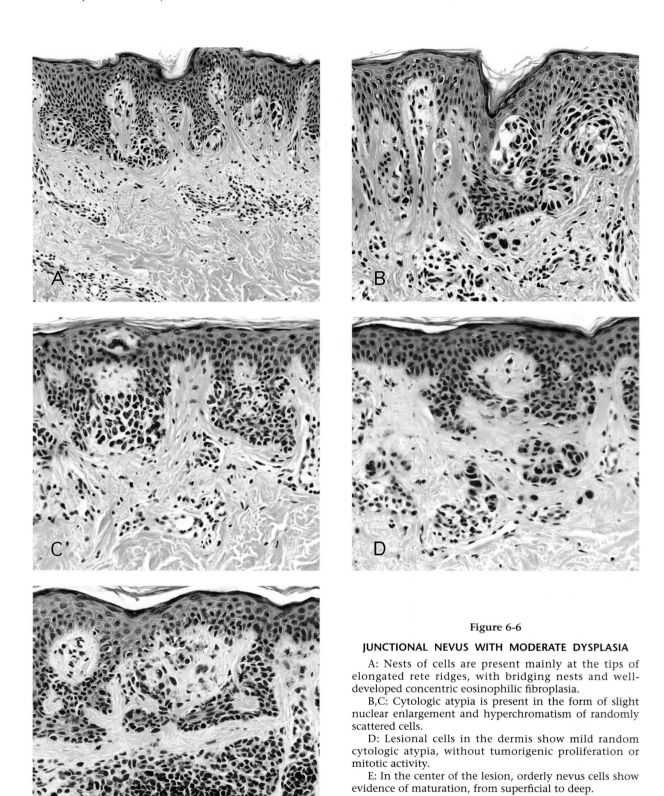

Figure 6-6

JUNCTIONAL NEVUS WITH MODERATE DYSPLASIA

A: Nests of cells are present mainly at the tips of elongated rete ridges, with bridging nests and well-developed concentric eosinophilic fibroplasia.

B,C: Cytologic atypia is present in the form of slight nuclear enlargement and hyperchromatism of randomly scattered cells.

D: Lesional cells in the dermis show mild random cytologic atypia, without tumorigenic proliferation or mitotic activity.

E: In the center of the lesion, orderly nevus cells show evidence of maturation, from superficial to deep.

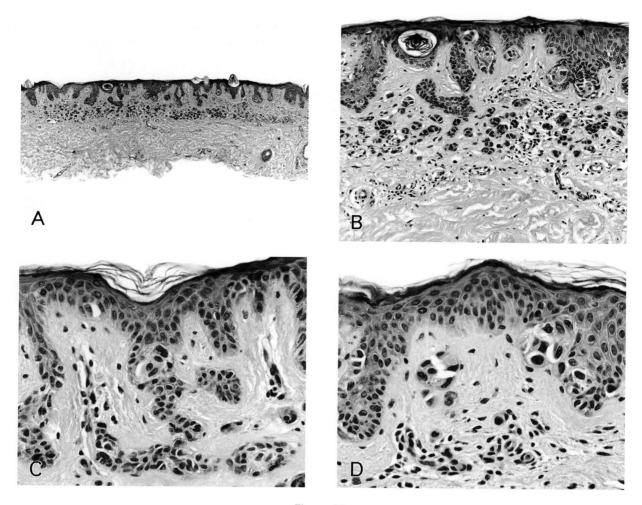

Figure 6-7

COMPOUND NEVUS WITH SEVERE DERMAL AND EPIDERMAL MELANOCYTIC DYSPLASIA

A: At scanning magnification, a dermal component and an adjacent junctional shoulder are seen.

B: Lesional cells in the dermis resemble those in the epidermis and show at least some tendency to maturation along nevoid lines. There is no pagetoid or continuous proliferation in the epidermis.

C,D: There is moderate to severe enlargement, irregularity, and hyperchromatism of scattered lesional cell nuclei. Similar atypia is present in the dermis, however, there is no mitotic activity or tumorigenic proliferation there (D). This lesion shows severe cytologic atypia, but the architectural changes are those of a nevus and do not support a diagnosis of melanoma.

cells extend down from the tip of an elongated rete ridge (figs. 6-4–6-10). In the epidermis at the tip of the rete, the nevus cells may show transitional forms, from round cells to spindle cells in the plate of lamellar collagen. These spindle cells may react with melanocytic markers such as S-100 protein, and in occasional lesions they are pigmented (fig. 6-4). These observations suggest that lamellar fibroplasia may represent a process of neuroid differentiation of nevus cells rather than a proliferation of true fibroblasts.

The stromal reactions of melanocytic neoplasms were classified in detail by Clark et al. (110). Dysplastic nevi are characterized by concentric eosinophilic fibroplasia and lamellar fibroplasia, while fibroplasia with a plaque-like lymphocytic infiltrate and diffuse eosinophilic fibroplasia are noted in radial growth phase melanoma (fig. 6-11) and much less often in nevi (fig. 6-12). Fibroplasia with angiogenesis or an absence of evidence for parenchymal stromal reciprocal interactions

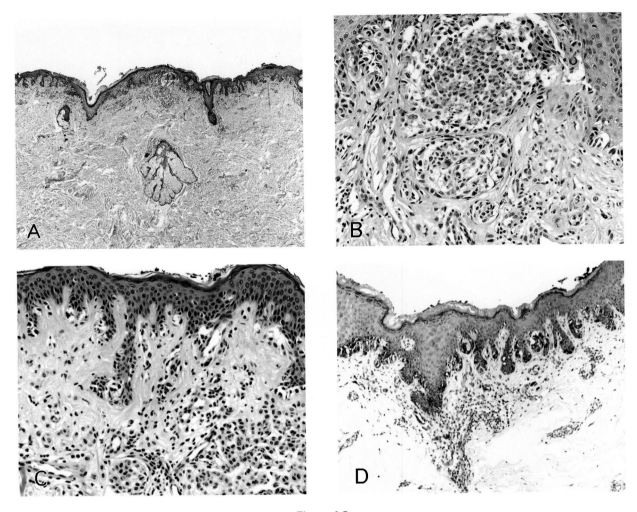

Figure 6-8

COMPOUND NEVUS WITH SEVERE DERMAL AND EPIDERMAL DYSPLASIA

A: Scanning magnification shows regular elongation of the rete ridges at the left, with an area of an irregular epidermal thickening and thinning in the center.

B: In this central area, there is uniform atypia and a large nest, however, the same cells seem to mature along nevic lines upon descent into the dermis.

C: At the periphery, there are smaller cells with mild random atypia located in the tips and sides of elongated rete ridges and there are mature nevoid cells in the dermis.

D: A Melan-A stain highlights the cells in the nests and demonstrates the lack of continuous proliferation between the rete ridges on the right, with a suggestion of continuous proliferation on the left. These changes were interpreted as possible evolving melanoma in situ in a dysplastic nevus (SAMPUS).

mark thick or deeply invasive vertical growth phase melanomas.

Histologic Criteria for Diagnosis

Many studies have examined criteria for the histologic diagnosis of dysplastic nevi in series of clinically characterized cases. In a semiquantitative histologic study, Steijlen et al. (111) examined the histopathologic criteria that resulted in "reasonable diagnostic efficiency" for dysplastic nevi, and found that the presence of dust-like melanin, irregular nevoid nests, markedly increased junctional activity (high lesional cellularity), melanocytic nuclei greater or equal in size to neighboring keratinocytes, and a lymphocytic infiltrate were significant

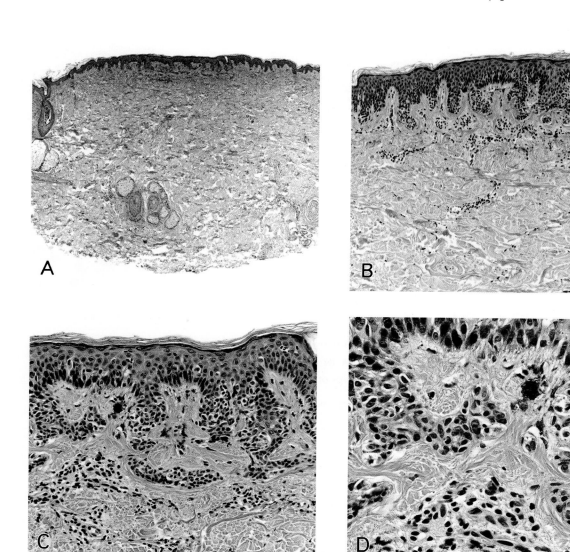

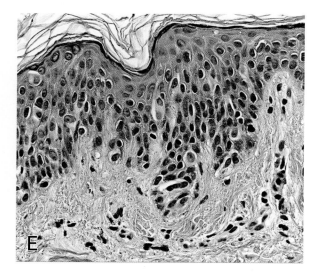

Figure 6-9

DYSPLASTIC NEVUS WITH
EVOLVING MELANOMA IN SITU

A: This lesion, in a 21-year-old patient, shows uniform elongation of the rete ridges at scanning magnification.

B,C: Higher power shows predominantly nested melanocytes, mostly near the tips of elongated rete ridges, with bridging nests. Closer examination shows a few single cells between the rete ridges, some of them extending slightly above the dermal-epidermal junction.

D: Cytologically, there is mild nuclear enlargement with fairly prominent nucleoli. This atypia involves a majority of the lesional cells (uniform atypia).

E: Focally in the epidermis, pagetoid proliferation of mildly, albeit uniformly atypical cells, extends to the stratum granulosum.

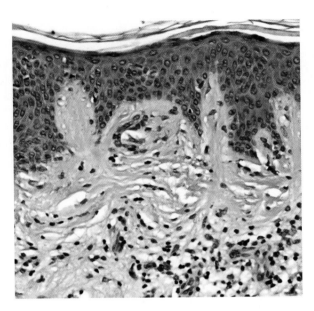 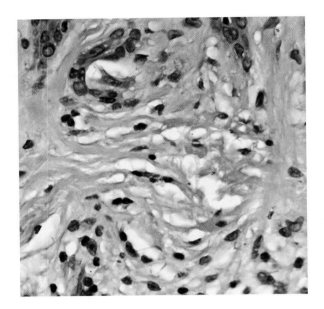

Figure 6-10

LAMELLAR FIBROPLASIA IN A DYSPLASTIC NEVUS

Left: The plates of fibroplasia extend down from the tips of the rete ridges and are probably the result of facultative fibroblastic activity by lesional melanocytes.

Right: High magnification shows scant pigment in the cytoplasm of one of the cells, supporting this hypothesis.

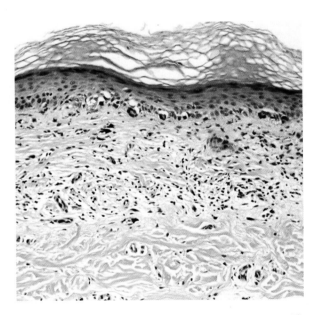 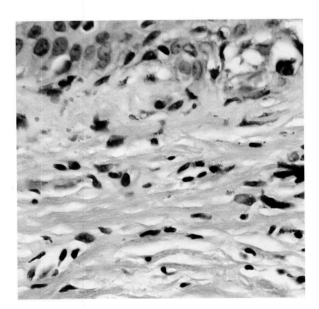

Figure 6-11

DIFFUSE FIBROPLASIA IN A MELANOMA

Left: The epidermal rete ridge pattern is effaced and there is a partly continuous proliferation of atypical melanocytes along the junction. The papillary dermis is widened and expanded by diffuse fibroplasia, tending to be oriented parallel to the surface.

Right: High magnification shows fibroblasts in the area of diffuse fibroplasia, with scattered melanophages. Compare with figure 6-10.

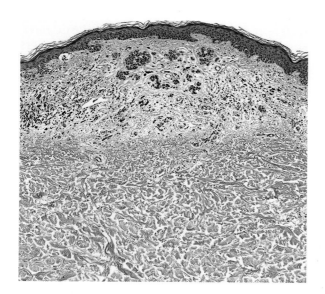 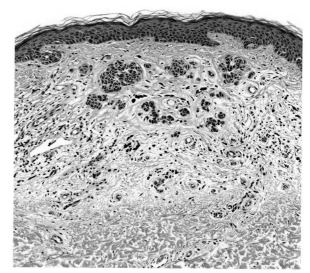

Figure 6-12

ATYPICAL NEVUS WITH FIBROPLASIA

This lesion shows some features of a dysplastic nevus in the epidermis at the left of the left figure, with mature nevus cells in the dermis in the center. The unusual feature is the widening of the papillary dermis with diffuse fibroplasia (both figures). This feature is more characteristic of melanomas than of nevi. It is not clear whether it represents a regression reaction or a stromal response. The architectural and cytologic features of this lesion are suggestive, but not diagnostic, of melanocytic dysplasia. Cytologic atypia is minimal, fibroplasia is essentially absent, and the cellularity of the junctional component is very low. We would interpret a lesion such as this as a compound nevus with atypical features, raise a differential diagnosis of melanocytic dysplasia, and suggest evaluation of the patient's phenotypic risk factors for melanoma.

in a discriminant analysis. To these criteria, we would add lesional size and architectural pattern features as discussed above.

Rivers et al. (112) attempted to quantify the histologic features of 100 consecutively accessioned clinically and histologically characteristic dysplastic nevi. They considered that the important diagnostic features included a central dermal nevocytic component with a peripheral extension of a junctional component, bridging of nests of melanocytes at the dermoepidermal junction, nests of melanocytes at the sides of rete ridges as well as at their bases, and concentric eosinophilic fibrosis. These authors considered the cytologic features of melanocytes to be less valuable than the architectural features in classifying these lesions. In a study by Shea et al. (113) of 166 consecutive Clark nevi, the degree of architectural disorder (assessed in terms of circumscription, symmetry, cohesiveness of nests, suprabasal melanocytes, confluence, and single cell proliferation), correlated with the degree of cytologic atypia (round/euchromatic nuclei, nuclear enlargement, cell enlargement,

and prominent nucleoli). Because some cases displayed a high score for one parameter but a low score for the other, it was felt that quantification of both parameters permits a more complete histopathologic evaluation of these lesions and may provide additional information for their clinical management.

In a conference sponsored by the World Health Organization (WHO), seven pathologists evolved the following mutually acceptable criteria for the diagnosis of dysplastic nevi (15). The major criteria were: basilar proliferation of atypical nevomelanocytes extending at least three rete ridges beyond a dermal nevocellular nevus and lentiginous or epithelioid cell pattern of the atypical intraepidermal melanocytic proliferation. The minor criteria included two or more of the following: concentric eosinophilic fibrosis or lamellar fibroplasia, neovascularization, dermal inflammatory host response, and fusion of rete ridges. Using these histologic criteria, coupled with standard clinical criteria, five pathologists from three countries were able to achieve diagnostic concordance in the

Table 6-3

HISTOLOGIC CRITERIA FOR THE DIAGNOSIS OF DYSPLASTIC NEVUS

Architecture
Size usually greater than 4 mm; not less than 2 mm; dysplastic nevi cannot be reliably recognized when <4 mm
Superficial plaque only (junctional); or plaque surrounds papule (compound)
"Lentiginous" elongation of rete ridges
Anastomosis of rete ridges
Nests bridge rete ridges
Nests at tips and sides of rete ridges
Few single cells between nests
Little or no continuous proliferation between rete ridges
Little or no pagetoid intraepidermal spread
Few if any mitoses

Host Responses
Patchy lymphocytes: "band-like" response suggests melanoma
Concentric eosinophilic fibroplasia
Lamellar fibroplasia (uncommon)
Prominent vessels sometimes

Cytology
"Random" slight to moderate atypia
Occasional macronucleoli
Scattered epithelioid nevus cells
Scattered cells with "dusty" melanin pigment

90 percent range for common nevi, dysplastic nevi, and melanomas circulated among their laboratories (15,114). These and other criteria are summarized in Table 6-3.

REPRODUCIBILITY AND CONTROVERSY REGARDING THE DIAGNOSIS OF HISTOLOGIC DYSPLASIA

A cause of controversy regarding the significance of dysplastic nevi has been the failure to adopt uniform criteria, despite the clear descriptions of these criteria in many peer-reviewed publications, textbooks, reviews, and consensus conferences. Using a histologic definition of dysplastic nevi that did not require either clinical criteria or cytologic atypia for diagnosis (relying instead on the lentiginous pattern), a prevalence of 62 percent was found for "dysplastic nevi" in a population of spouses of melanoma patients (115,116). In a subsequent study in which six pathologists reviewed material from the same population-based series of cases and controls, the prevalence estimates ranged from 7 to 32 percent (48). In that study, the pathologists had

different published criteria for dysplastic nevi, some requiring cytologic atypia while others did not. In addition, there was variation in the use of lesional size as a criterion. In reproducibility studies it was found, according to kappa statistics, that intraobserver reproducibility was substantial, while interobserver concordance was fair, even despite the differences in criteria. Further, ignoring the one outlier observation of 32 percent, the range of prevalence estimates was 7 to 19 percent, much closer to the prevalence found in clinical studies. In a more recent study in which criteria were agreed upon and photographically defined, the reproducibility was substantial to excellent (117).

Lesions defined histologically but without consideration of cytologic atypia as a diagnostic criterion have been said to be the most common nevi with an epidermal component seen in a dermatopathology practice (118). This finding may to some extent have to do with referral bias (dermatologists are more likely to biopsy atypical nevi), but especially with the sensitivity of the architectural criteria used for diagnosis. In a study of the histology of macular or nearly macular nevi selected for their lack of clinically atypical features, Klein and Barr (119) selected 75 lesions that were 5 mm or less in diameter, symmetric, round or slightly oval, with uniform pigmentation, distinct and regular margins, and no erythema. The lesions were evaluated for histologic pattern atypia, cytologic atypia, and host response. These three features of histologic dysplasia were found together in 29.3 percent of the lesions, "albeit minimally." These minimal changes, in our opinion, do not meet an appropriate threshold for melanocytic dysplasia in small lesions, particularly since there is evidence for a gradation of risk from mild through moderate to severe histologic dysplasia (17,18).

In another classification scheme proposed by Ackerman (8), a lesion termed Clark nevus was defined in terms of architectural pattern criteria only as follows: "melanocytes arranged mostly in nests, confined to the dermo-epidermal junction and papillary dermis. The junctional component tends to extend a few rete ridges beyond the intradermal component. As a rule, there is no atypia." This definition does not consider either size or cytologic atypia, and would include myriads of small lentiginous junctional nevi that are present in members of the normal population studied in case-control series (1,10). Such lesions are undoubtedly very common in the community, but their definition is not synonymous with Clark's dysplastic nevi as defined here and originally by Clark (1). These considerations emphasize the importance of adherence to the commonly agreed and widely published criteria in the diagnosis of any disease marker, including dysplastic nevi.

In our view, both cytologic atypia and architectural atypia are necessary for the accurate and reproducible diagnosis of dysplastic nevi (120,121). In a study that attempted to quantify architectural features and to correlate them with cytology, several particular architectural and cytologic variables showed significant interdependence, but some cases displayed a relatively high score for one parameter but a low score for the other (113). It was considered that quantification of both parameters might permit a more complete histopathologic evaluation of these lesions. In the NIH criteria, cytologic atypia was considered to be "usually present but not essential" (20). In our own definition of histologic dysplasia, we require random cytologic atypia of at least a few of the lesional cells (121). This requirement for cytologic atypia in dysplastic nevi can be compared to that for a Reed-Sternberg cell in Hodgkin disease. Just as Reed-Sternberg cells may be difficult to find in some cases of authentic Hodgkin disease, so may the randomly scattered "atypical" cells with their slight to moderate nuclear and cytoplasmic changes be sparsely distributed in dysplastic nevi. If no atypia is demonstrated in a lesion that otherwise has some or many of the pattern features of a dysplastic nevus, we believe that the lesion should be classified descriptively, for example, as a lentiginous (nondysplastic, junctional, or compound) nevus. The term "nevus with architectural disorder" may also be used (122). These lesions with architectural but no cytologic atypia are generally smaller and less cellular than classic dysplastic nevi. Their clinical significance, if any, remains to be discovered.

GRADING OF DYSPLASTIC NEVI

Melanocytic dysplasia is defined in terms of both architectural and cytologic features. Cytologic atypia alone may be seen in other melanocytic nevi and is not necessarily synonymous with dysplastic nevi. Atypia in dysplastic nevi can readily be placed along a spectrum from mild to severe (117,123,124). In most studies, there is better discrimination of severe dysplasia than of the other two grades, suggesting that "moderate" and "severe" dysplasia are the two most meaningful categories (125). Grading of dysplastic nevi has taken on greater importance since the studies of McNutt's group have clearly demonstrated a relationship between the degree of atypia in a dysplastic nevus and the patient's melanoma risk (17). These studies have also provided biologic validation of their grading scheme, as described and illustrated in their seminal publication.

Low-grade atypia (in many studies graded as mild, or mild to moderate) consists of increased nuclear size (similar to a basal keratinocyte), with mild but definite pleomorphism of the nuclei and condensed chromatin with sometimes striking hyperchromasia (fig. 6-3). It is important to recall that the nuclei of normal melanocytes tend to be uniformly hyperchromatic, albeit round to ovoid in contour. The larger nuclei of mildly atypical dysplastic nevus cells show similar uniform hyperchromasia, but their contours tend to be less rounded and uniform, with slight angulation of the nuclear membrane. In general, cytologic atypia in low-grade dysplasia affects less than 10 percent of the junctional component of the dysplastic nevus.

High-grade atypia (in many studies graded as severe, or moderate to severe) is associated with progressively larger nuclei (larger than a basal keratinocyte) and more striking pleomorphism, markedly angulated irregular nuclei, and eosinophilic nucleoli in occasional severely atypical cells. Importantly, the chromatin pattern tends not to be uniformly hyperchromatic, as is the case in normal melanocytes and mildly atypical ones, but rather is more "open," with a coarsely-clumped, "vesicular" pattern. The nuclear membrane, perhaps owing to aggregation of chromatin along its inner surface, may also appear to be irregularly thickened. The cells may have more prominent cytoplasm, reminiscent of melanoma cells, but there is little or no upward pagetoid spread. Such lesions generally show cytologic atypia affecting more than 10 percent (often 50 percent) of the junctional nevus cells, and unlike mild atypia, which is low grade, is considered to constitute high-grade atypia. Indeed, lesions with a dominant pattern of severe atypia may suggest early evolution in the direction of melanoma in situ, and we frequently document such changes in a comment subsidiary to the primary diagnosis. Mitoses (which in our experience are present in about 30 percent of melanomas in the epidermis) are rare in the junctional or dermal components of dysplastic nevi (usually absent and never present in numbers greater than one or two mitotic figures in multiple sections of a particular specimen).

As atypia increases, the cellularity also often increases, as does the proportion of the lesional cells that can be characterized as atypical. In melanomas, these atypical cells predominate in a monotonous, apparently clonal proliferation in the epidermis and papillary dermis (uniform cytologic atypia) (51). In a morphometric study, significant differences were observed in nuclear area and standard deviation of nuclear area between melanoma and dysplastic nevi with severe atypia, and between dysplastic nevi with severe atypia and all other categories of nevi (126). No differences in nuclear area were found among dysplastic nevi with moderate or slight atypia, nevi with features of dysplasia, and typical nevi. These results were considered to demonstrate an objective distinction of low-grade (slight-moderate atypia) and high-grade or severe atypia from each other and from melanoma.

As noted above, low- and high-grade melanocytic dysplasia is defined in terms of both architectural and cytologic features. Like cytologic atypia, the architectural features can also be placed on a spectrum of increasing abnormality. When nuclear atypia of even moderate degree is associated with architectural features suggestive, but not diagnostic, of possible progression to melanoma, such as focally continuous proliferation along the dermal-epidermal junction or a tendency to pagetoid intraepidermal spread that does not extend above the lower two thirds of the epidermis (and if there are no other indicators of malignancy), we use the term *severe melanocytic dysplasia* as an indication that the lesion has some features suggestive of incipient progression to melanoma (figs. 6-8–6-10). It may also be appropriate to include a descriptive note indicating that such lesions may be in transition to mela-

noma in situ or have significant precursor potential for its formation. In these circumstances, a conservative reexcision is generally appropriate if the original biopsy has narrow margins (123). When such pagetoid changes extend as far as the granular layer and stratum corneum or when the atypia is uniform (involving a majority of the lesional cells) and especially when mitoses are present in lesional cells, melanoma in situ is usually the most appropriate diagnosis.

In a recent British study of 123 atypical melanocytic nevi (dysplastic nevi), the lesions were evaluated as mild, moderate, or severe based on histologic variables that included junctional and dermal symmetry, lateral extension, cohesion and migration of epidermal melanocytes, maturation, regression, nuclear features, nuclear grade, melanin deposition, inflammatory infiltrate location, and fibroplasia (125). The severe category correlated with three or more nuclear abnormalities (especially pleomorphism, heterogeneous chromatin, and prominent nucleolus) and on the architectural features of absence of regression, mixed junctional pattern, and suprabasal melanocytes on top of lentiginous hyperplasia. The diagnostic accuracy for severe dysplasia was 99.5 percent using these criteria. In contrast, no architectural features distinguishing mild from moderate dysplasia were selected as significant by the discriminant analysis. It was concluded that histologic criteria can reliably distinguish severe dysplasia but fail to differentiate mild from moderate dysplasia. This suggests that mild and moderate dysplasia should be categorized together as low-grade dysplasia, with severe dysplasia constituting a high-grade category, for which complete excision and consideration of follow-up (depending on other risk factors) may be suggested (123). Grading criteria adapted from several published studies are presented in Table 6-4 (16,17,125,127,128). As in other systems, such as that for dysplasia of the uterine cervix, architectural features are as important if not more important than cytologic atypia in the grading of histologic melanocytic dysplasia.

CLINICOPATHOLOGIC CORRELATION OF MELANOCYTIC DYSPLASIA

Several studies have correlated the clinical and histologic features of melanocytic dysplasia (129–131). In an interesting study of 150 lesions

Table 6-4

CRITERIA FOR LOW-GRADE AND HIGH-GRADE DYSPLASIA

	Low-Grade Dysplasia (Mild to Moderate Dysplasia)	High-Grade Dysplasia (Severe Dysplasia)
Architecture		
Diameter	May be <4 mm	Usually >4 mm
Symmetry	Usually present	May be flawed
Rete ridges	Uniformly elongated	More irregular or focally effaced
Junctional proliferation	Discontinuous	May be focally continuous
Pagetoid spread	Absent	Absent or focal, low level
Pigment distribution	Diffuse	Diffuse
Maturation in dermis	Present	May be incomplete
Cytology		
Distribution of atypia	Minority of cells (random)	Often >10% of cells
Nuclear shape	Irregular, often polyhedral	Irregular, often marked angulation
Chromatin pattern	Densely hyperchromatic	Some with clumped chromatin
Nucleoli	Smaller	Larger, more irregular
Membrane irregularity	Fairly regular	Some cells markedly irregular
Mitoses	Absent	Absent or rare
Necrosis	Absent	Often present
Single cells at base	Present	Absent

selected as the most clinically atypical lesion in a given patient, the histologic diagnosis of a dysplastic nevus was strongly associated with the total number of palpable arm nevi, any arm nevi, nevi on any body type, and clinically atypical nevi on the body (correlation coefficients, 23.2 percent to 30.4 percent with P <0.01 in each instance) (48). Thus, in this study, the histologic features of a single nevus were predictive of melanoma risk factors at about the same level of risk as demonstrated by clinical examination of the whole subject. There was also a strong correlation between the numbers of nevi and certain types of architectural histologic features, including fusion (bridging of junctional nests), lymphocyte response, and fibroplasia of the papillary dermis. In other studies, the association of histologic and clinical atypia was more limited (132) or poor (133); in the latter study, histologic dysplasia was found in some nevi that had no clinically atypical characteristics. In contrast, another study demonstrated that the absence of a macular component in melanocytic nevi in a person with fewer than 13 total body nevi accurately predicts the absence of melanocytic dysplasia on histologic examination (131).

In a recent study, it was concluded that dermoscopy using pattern analysis showed better results than clinical examination for the noninvasive detection of nevi with architectural disorder, with or without cytologic atypia (134). The dermoscopic features that best predicted histologic atypia in nevi were regression-related structures (white scar-like areas or peppering), irregular vascular pattern, and gray-blue areas (positive predictive values, 83 percent, 83 percent, and 73 percent, respectively). It was concluded that dermoscopy by means of pattern analysis enhances the diagnostic accuracy of the prediction of histologic atypia in melanocytic nevi compared with clinical examination alone. There seems to be a correlation between histologic and clinical features, and this correlation is likely to be more profound for architectural than cytologic features. Thus, a diagnosis based on a combination of clinical and histologic features, as discussed above, is likely to be more specific in identifying lesions associated with clinical risk.

Because most of the studies that have correlated risk with dysplastic nevi have been based on clinical criteria, it seems best to us to take clinicopathologic criteria into account when making a diagnosis histopathologically. The WHO "Blue Book" published in 1996 defined a dysplastic nevus based on clinicopathologic criteria as follows: "A variant of an acquired nevus *that is clinically atypical* and characterized histologically by the combination of an immature (lentiginous) architectural pattern of melanocytic proliferation in the epidermis and cytologic atypia" (135) (italics added). These considerations suggest that the diagnosis should be made with caution in small lesions, and probably not at all in lesions smaller than 3 to 4 mm (measured on a histologic slide). In case of doubt, a descriptive diagnosis may be rendered, an approach fortified by evidence that even very small nevi with dysplastic features may correlate with increased melanoma risk (10). In this situation, the presence of "dysplastic features" can be noted, and a recommendation can be made for clinicopathologic correlation with evaluation of the patient's entire risk profile.

DIFFERENTIAL DIAGNOSIS

Dysplastic nevi have significance as simulants of melanoma and as risk markers for melanoma, and their differential diagnosis is thus considered in terms of malignant melanoma and benign conditions that are not risk markers. Malignant lesions that simulate dysplastic nevi include the variants of radial growth phase melanomas, including superficial spreading melanoma, lentigo maligna melanoma, and acral-lentiginous melanoma. Although these radial growth phase lesions are biologically incapable of metastasis, they have locally recurring potential. We have seen a number of such cases that have been inappropriately diagnosed as dysplastic nevi followed by persistence, recurrent growth, and sometimes by progression to vertical growth phase and metastatic disease.

When the atypical epithelioid cell type becomes prominent, there may be difficulty in distinguishing between a dysplastic nevus and the radial growth phase of superficial spreading melanoma in the epidermis. Indeed, such lesions may represent examples of dysplasia in the process of evolution to melanoma in situ. Unless the criteria for melanoma are met in full, we sign such lesions out as severe melanocytic dysplasia, sometimes with a note that the changes are histologically borderline and that consideration of additional excision may be appropriate. It is also important to take into account patient age, as a superficial epithelioid cell component in a dysplastic nevus with low-grade atypia is more likely to be a biologically different lesion in a 14-year-old prone to such age-related cytologic changes than a similar lesion in a 64-year-old,

where epithelioid cell changes tend to indicate high-grade dysplasia or in situ malignancy. Cases like these may be difficult even for experts to interpret (136,137). Patients can be reassured that these histologically borderline lesions have no capacity for metastasis.

When junctional nests are present, lentigo maligna and lentigo maligna melanoma, as well as the recently described lentiginous pattern melanoma that occurs in nonatrophic epidermis (138), can sometimes simulate dysplasia. Despite this occasional morphologic overlap, it is likely that lentigo maligna and dysplastic nevi represent different pathways of melanoma progression, with a different genetic basis (139). Lentigo maligna virtually always occurs in moderately to severely sun-damaged skin. The lesions are often larger than all but a few dysplastic nevi, and cytologic atypia is often more severe and more uniform. The cells are more likely to prominently involve skin appendages, but this phenomenon may also be seen in dysplastic nevi. Of considerable importance in this differential diagnosis, the rete ridge pattern in lentigo maligna is effaced in striking contrast to the regular rete ridge elongation of dysplastic nevi. Occasional lesions of lentiginous radial growth phase melanoma, however, may involve the acral and truncal skin of older individuals without evidence of associated epidermal atrophy (as is generally present in lentigo maligna involving sun-damaged facial skin). Such lesions may resemble dysplastic nevi, especially when represented partially in small biopsies where the distinction between continuous and noncontinuous lentiginous proliferation and assessment of the uniformity of cytologic atypia may be difficult or impossible to assess. Accordingly, careful clinicopathologic correlation and recommendation for complete excision are generally required for most accurate diagnoses of such lesions. The differential diagnosis of acral-lentiginous melanoma and dysplastic nevus is discussed in a later chapter. In general, it appears that dysplastic nevi are uncommon on acral skin.

Difficulty may also be encountered in distinguishing atypical cells in the dermal component of a dysplastic nevus from small melanoma cells. Findings useful for distinguishing benign nevi include small and uniform nests, absence of dermal mitotic activity, a gradual continuum of

Table 6-5

FEATURES HELPFUL IN DIFFERENTIATING PAPULAR COMPOUND NEVUS AND DYSPLASTIC NEVUS

Papular Compound Nevus	Dysplastic Nevus
Architectural Features	
Usually less than 10 mm in diameter	Greater than 4 mm (histologic), may be greater than 10–12 mm
A wholly papular lesion	Either wholly macular, or macular component surrounds papule
Symmetric	Symmetric
No lentiginous compartment	Entirely lentiginous, or lentiginous compartment at shoulders of papule
No elongation, bridging, or anastomosing rete at shoulders of dermal compartment	Uniform slight elongation of rete in lentiginous compartment at shoulders with bridging nests anastomosing rete
Nests uniform in size, shape, and distribution	Nests uniform in size, shape, and distribution
Host Responses	
Lymphocytes absent except in halo nevi	Patchy lymphocytes in dermis
Eosinophilic and lamellar fibroplasia absent	Eosinophilic fibroplasia usually present; lamellar fibroplasia occasionally present
Little or no vascular proliferation or endothelial hypertrophy in papillary dermis	May be moderate hypertrophy of endothelial cells and slight increase in vessels
Cytologic Features	
Nuclear size smaller than basal keratinocytes	Randomly scattered larger nuclei
No atypical nevus cells in epidermis	Moderate "random" cytologic atypia in epidermis
Macronucleoli absent or rare	Macronucleoli frequently present in a minority of the lesional cells in the epidermis
Epithelioid cells with finely divided cytoplasmic pigment usually absent	Scattered atypical epithelioid cells with dusty melanin pigment, nucleoli, anisokaryosis
Mitoses absent in dermis and epidermis	Mitoses rare in epidermis, absent in dermis
Pigment in dermis usually superficial only	Pigment may be superficial and deep in dermal nevus cells

evolution ("maturation") from a dysplasia pattern with larger epithelioid cells in the epidermis to a smaller cell type with descent into the dermis, absence of prominent macronucleoli in a majority of the lesional cells, and absent mitoses. Any mitoses at all in the dermal component of a putative dysplastic nevus should prompt serious consideration of melanoma, especially when combined with severe atypia, apparent expansile growth in the dermis, or pagetoid growth of similar cells in the overlying epidermis. One or two mitoses in the epidermis may be acceptable in an otherwise benign lesion, but these should not be frequent or associated with pagetoid intraepidermal spread of large epithelioid cells. This important differential diagnosis is discussed in more detail in chapter 8.

In addition to their importance as simulants of melanoma, dysplastic nevi are significant risk markers for melanoma. It is important, especially in members of hereditary melanoma kindreds, to recognize affected individuals so that surveillance and educational intervention can be offered to them, but it is also important to avoid overdiagnosis and overtreatment of individuals who are not at increased risk. The important differential diagnosis of compound nevi and dysplastic nevi has been discussed extensively above and is summarized in Tables 6-5 and 6-6. As with melanoma, especially melanomas that are in situ or microinvasive, the diagnosis of a dysplastic nevus depends on a synthesis of multiple criteria and no one criterion can be considered diagnostic. We do not feel that a lesion should be termed dysplastic in the absence of the characteristic slightly to moderately atypical epithelioid nevus cell. As previously discussed, this cell is considered analogous to the Reed-Sternberg cell, which, by definition, is required for the diagnosis of Hodgkin disease but is diagnostic only in an appropriate background as it may also be seen in other conditions. In the same way, at least low-grade cellular atypia in a dysplastic nevus is necessary for the diagnosis, but is sufficient for the diagnosis only when seen in the appropriate architectural pattern of lentiginous proliferation and host response in a lesion of sufficient size.

Table 6-6

FEATURES HELPFUL IN DIFFERENTIATING LENTIGINOUS JUNCTIONAL NEVUS AND JUNCTIONAL DYSPLASTIC NEVUS

Lentiginous Junctional Nevus	Junctional Dysplastic Nevus
Architectural Features	
Usually less than 4 mm in diameter	Greater than 4 mm (histologic), may be greater than 10–12 mm
Symmetric	Symmetric
Small round nests	Larger ovoid nests
Uniformly elongated rete ridges (shorter)	Uniformly elongated rete ridges (longer)
Little dyshesion of cells in nests	Dyshesion often present
Few bridging nests	More numerous bridging nests
Nests at tips of rete	Nests at tips and sides of rete
Nests uniform in size, shape, and distribution	Nests uniform in size, shape, and distribution
Host Responses	
Lymphocytes absent/minimal	Patchy lymphocytes in dermis
Eosinophilic and lamellar fibroplasia absent/minimal	Eosinophilic fibroplasia usually present; lamellar fibroplasia occasionally present
Little or no vascular proliferation or endothelial hypertrophy in papillary dermis	May be moderate hypertrophy of endothelial cells and slight increase in vessels
Cytologic Features	
No atypical nevus cells in epidermis	"Random" cytologic atypia in epidermis
Macronucleoli absent or rare	Macronucleoli frequently present in a minority of the lesional cells in the epidermis
Epithelioid cells with finely divided cytoplasmic pigment usually absent	Scattered atypical epithelioid cells with dusty melanin pigment, nucleoli, anisokaryosis
Mitoses rare, usually absent	Mitoses rare, usually absent

Particular variants of melanocytic nevi may resemble dysplastic nevi in one or more of their special attributes. Congenital nevi may have lentiginous patterns of growth in the epidermis that are suggestive of dysplasia. Since congenital nevi, like dysplastic nevi, are potential precursors of melanoma, some such lesions may be best regarded as congenital nevi with dysplasia if cytologic atypia is also present. Most of these lesions, however, lack the stromal response and melanocytic atypia that characterize the usual acquired dysplastic nevi. Even if cytologic atypia is observed, many of these congenital lesions are clinically solitary, and do not seem to carry the connotation of a systemic abnormality as may be the case when multiple dysplastic nevi are present in a given individual. Nevi of genital skin may also be associated with lentiginous patterns and enlarged melanocytes in the epidermis, but these changes are observed above the dermal component of the nevus, without extending into the epidermis at its shoulder. The diagnosis of a dysplastic nevus should be made with caution in the palms and soles, because acral nevi may be associated with a lentiginous proliferation of

nevus cells in the epidermis (acral lentiginous nevi). Usually the stromal changes associated with dysplasia in the dermis are lacking, but even if there is some fibroplasia, the diagnosis of dysplasia should not be made unless the population of randomly scattered epithelioid melanocytes with slight to moderate nuclear atypia and dusty cytoplasmic pigment that characterizes dysplastic nevi is observed.

The pigmented spindle cell nevus of Reed is another nevoid lesion that may show a predominant lentiginous pattern associated with some nuclear atypia. Clinically, these are symmetric, uniformly dark lesions that may suggest melanoma because of their black color, but they do not significantly resemble dysplastic nevi and they are often seen in people who do not have obvious dysplastic nevi elsewhere. Histologically, they are composed of a more uniform spindle cell population than is seen in dysplastic nevi where spindle cells, if present at all, are a minority population. Some junctional Spitz nevi may overlap with dysplastic nevi, although their uniformly large spindle or epithelioid cell type and the presence of Kamino bodies usually allow a distinction to be made.

Some apparently benign melanocytic and nevoid lesions may show more of the changes that have just been described in dysplastic nevi, or in other nevoid variants, but cannot be assigned to a specific category. Urso (140) studied the distribution and relationships of six atypical histologic features: dimension greater than 5 mm, lentiginous proliferation, disordered nested pattern, melanocytic dyskaryosis, dermal lymphocytic infiltrate, and suprabasal melanocytes. One or more of the features was found in 72 percent of nevi, either singly or in variable combinations. There appeared to be a histologic lesional spectrum showing a progressively increasing incidence of atypical features rather than two discrete classes (common and dysplastic nevi). Thus, there are many lesions that cannot easily be assigned to one of two discrete classes. For these lesions, descriptive terminology may be used.

Lesions that appear to exhibit some architectural and cytologically atypical features but do not meet stringent criteria for melanocytic dysplasia may be signed out descriptively as "nevi with dysplastic features," or the more cumbersome descriptive terminology proposed by a 1989 NIH consensus conference, "nevus with architectural disorder and cytologic atypia" with a statement as to the severity of the atypia (141). This is not an endorsement on our part of this terminology as a surrogate for a true dysplastic nevus, but rather recognition that this less specific descriptor may be useful for certain lesions that do not rigorously fulfill all architectural, cytologic, and stromal features of authentic dysplastic nevi. Nevi with lentiginous architectural features but without cytologic atypia may be characterized as lentiginous melanocytic nevi. These lentiginous nevi no doubt constitute a heterogeneous group of lesions whose significance, if any, remains to be discovered (figs. 6-12, 6-13).

ROLE OF THE PATHOLOGIST IN DIAGNOSIS OF DYSPLASTIC NEVI

Because most of the studies that have related risk of melanoma to the presence of dysplastic nevi have relied on a clinical definition of these lesions, it follows that risk assessment for melanoma should be a primarily clinical exercise. Although dysplastic nevi are important

contributors to melanoma risk, other factors reviewed above must also be assessed in context. In patients who are thought to be at increased risk for melanoma, biopsies of lesions should be done if necessary to rule out melanoma; a secondary purpose may be the assessment of the degree of histologic atypia (low versus high grade) if desired for use as a guide to the intensity of surveillance. Because clinical and histologic dysplasia are not well correlated in individual lesions, a biopsy negative for dysplasia does not indicate that melanoma risk is not increased in a patient with clinically dysplastic nevi, and melanoma risk assessment in this situation should be based on the clinical findings (133).

Conversely, melanocytic dysplasia is frequently found in a biopsy that has been submitted without a specific indication. In these circumstances, the finding of histologic dysplasia can contribute to patient and family management by prompting an assessment of other risk factors. Patients with a nevus with dysplastic features, like those with a more definitively diagnosed dysplastic nevus, should have a clinical assessment of their melanoma risk factors and should be managed according to these clinical findings. As noted above, the most important role of pathology in the assessment of clinically atypical lesions is to rule in or out the diagnosis of melanoma. In lesions that are not melanoma, the identification of histologically dysplastic features can lead to the recognition of individuals at increased risk for melanoma. The risk associated with a single clinically dysplastic nevus is relatively small, of the order of two-fold, comparable to having red hair or freckles. Patients with multiple dysplastic nevi, however, especially if associated with a family or personal history of melanoma, have a dramatically increased risk for melanoma (58). Individuals with atypical or dysplastic features in a nevus biopsy should be assessed clinically, and follow-up (if necessary) should be based on the overall risk profile. In our practice, we commonly add a comment to the report of a histologically dysplastic nevus, or of a nevus with some "dysplastic features," to the effect that additional evaluation and possible surveillance may be indicated, especially if the patient has other clinically atypical or dysplastic nevi, or a family or personal history of melanoma.

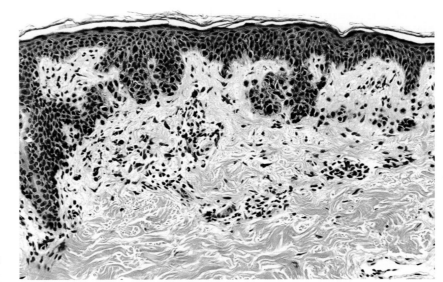

Figure 6-13

ATYPICAL NEVUS

This lesion has some "dysplastic features" but these are insufficient, in our opinion, for a diagnosis of a dysplastic nevus. We would interpret such a lesion descriptively, with a suggestion for examination of the patient for other possible melanoma risk factors.

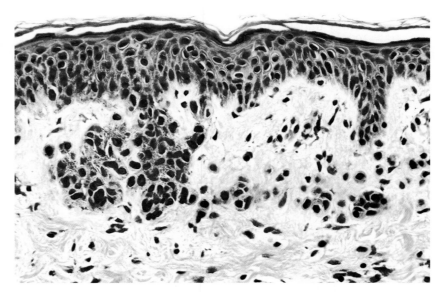

Murphy and Mihm (128) provided a simple checklist to assist in the discrimination of dysplastic from common acquired nevi: 1) Is the lesion clinically atypical (large, variegated, indefinite edge)? 2) Does the lesion have architectural disorder such as bridging nests, nests between or at edges of rete ridges? 3) Are stromal alterations present (concentric fibroplasia, lymphocytes, melanophages, prominent vessels)? and 4) Is there random or more uniform (diffuse) cytologic atypia? As noted by these authors, a diagnosis of dysplastic nevus clearly does not indicate that a patient is fated to develop a melanoma. It should, however, alert the clinician that such patients ought to be questioned concerning the family and environmental history, and should have a comprehensive skin examination. Patients who do not have multiple dysplastic nevi may be reassured and educated as to avoidance of risk factors and self or possible physician surveillance. Patients with multiple clinically dysplastic nevi will likely require physician monitoring. In these high-risk individuals, the pathologist's recognition of "dysplastic features" or frank dysplasia in a nevus biopsy could have life-saving importance (128). These features are summarized in Tables 6-5 and 6-6.

REFERENCES

1. Clark WH Jr, Reimer RR, Greene MH, Ainsworth AM, Mastrangelo MJ. Origin of familial malignant melanomas from heritable melanocytic lesions. 'The B-K mole syndrome'. Arch Dermatol 1978;114:732-738.
2. Greene MH, Clark WH Jr, Tucker MA, et al. Acquired precursors of cutaneous malignant melanoma. The familial dysplastic nevus syndrome. N Engl J Med 1985;312:91-97.
3. Elder DE, Goldman LI, Goldman SC, Greene MH, Clark WH Jr. Dysplastic nevus syndrome: a phenotypic association of sporadic cutaneous melanoma. Cancer 1980;46:1787-1794.
4. NIH consensus conference. Diagnosis and treatment of early melanoma. JAMA 1992;268:1314-1319.
5. Fusaro RM, Lynch HT. The FAMMM syndrome: epidemiology and surveillance strategies. Cancer Invest 2000;18:670-680.
6. Nordlund JJ, Kirkwood J, Forget BM, et al. Demographic study of clinically atypical (dysplastic) nevi in patients with melanoma and comparison subjects. Cancer Res 1985;45:1855-1861.
7. Bataille V, Bishop JA, Sasieni P, et al. Risk of cutaneous melanoma in relation to the numbers, types and sites of naevi: a case-control study. Br J Cancer 1996;73:1605-1611.
8. Ackerman AB, Briggs PL, Bravo F. Dysplastic nevus, compound type vs. Clark's nevus, compound type. In: Ackerman AB, Briggs PL, Bravo F, eds. Differential diagnosis in dermatopathology III. Philadelphia: Lea & Febiger; 1993:158-161.
9. Shapiro M, Chren MM, Levy RM, et al. Variability in nomenclature used for nevi with architectural disorder and cytologic atypia (microscopically dysplastic nevi) by dermatologists and dermatopathologists. J Cutan Pathol 2004;31:523-530.
10. Tucker MA, Halpern A, Holly EA, et al. Clinically recognized dysplastic nevi. A central risk factor for cutaneous melanoma. JAMA 1997;277:1439-1444.
11. Friedman RJ, Heilman ER, Rigel DS, Kopf AW. The dysplastic nevus. Clinical and pathologic features. Dermatol Clin 1985;3:239-249.
12. Kopf AW, Lindsay AC, Rogers GS, Friedman RJ, Rigel DS, Levenstein M. Relationship of nevocytic nevi to sun exposure in dysplastic nevus syndrome. J Am Acad Dermatol 1985;12:656-662.
13. Augustsson A. Melanocytic naevi, melanoma and sun exposure. Acta Derm Venereol Suppl (Stockh) 1991;166:1-34.
14. Halpern AC, Guerry D 4th, Elder DE, Trock B, Synnestvedt M. A cohort study of melanoma in patients with dysplastic nevi. J Invest Dermatol 1993;100:346S-349S.
15. Clemente C, Cochran A, Elder DE, et al. Histopathologic diagnosis of dysplastic nevi: concordance among pathologists convened by the World Health Organization Melanoma Programme. Hum Pathol 1991;22:313-319.
16. Duncan LM, Berwick M, Bruijn JA, Byers HR, Mihm MC, Barnhill RL. Histopathologic recognition and grading of dysplastic melanocytic nevi: an interobserver agreement study. J Invest Dermatol 1993;100:318S-321S.
17. Arumi-Uria M, McNutt NS, Finnerty B. Grading of atypia in nevi: correlation with melanoma risk. Mod Pathol 2003;16:764-771.
18. Shors AR, Kim S, White E, et al. Dysplastic naevi with moderate to severe histological dysplasia: a risk factor for melanoma. Br J Dermatol 2006;155:988-993.
19. Braun-Falco M, Hein R, Ring J, McNutt NS. Histopathological characteristics of small diameter melanocytic naevi. J Clin Pathol 2003;56:459-464.
20. Consensus conference: precursors to malignant melanoma. JAMA 1984;251:1864-1866.
21. Crutcher WA, Sagebiel RW. Prevalence of dysplastic naevi in a community practice. Lancet 1984;1:729.
22. Holly EA, Kelly JW, Shpall SN, Chiu SH. Number of melanocytic nevi as a major risk factor for malignant melanoma. J Am Acad Dermatol 1987;17:459-468.
23. Rhodes AR, Weinstock MA, Fitzpatrick TB, Mihm MC Jr, Sober AJ. Risk factors for cutaneous melanoma. A practical method for recognizing predisposed individuals. JAMA 1987;258:3146-3154.
24. Goldstein AM, Tucker MA, Crutcher WA, Hartge P, Sagebiel RW. The inheritance pattern of dysplastic naevi in families of dysplastic naevus patients. Melanoma Res 1993;3:15-22.
25. Kraemer KH, Greene MH, Tarone R, Elder DE, Clark WH Jr, Guerry D 4th. Dysplastic naevi and cutaneous melanoma risk. Lancet 1983;2:1076-7.
26. Carey WP Jr, Thompson CJ, Synnestvedt M, et al. Dysplastic nevi as a melanoma risk factor in patients with familial melanoma. Cancer 1994;74:3118-3125
27. Roush GC, Nordlund JJ, Forget B, Gruber SB, Kirkwood JM. Independence of dysplastic nevi from total nevi in determining risk for nonfamilial melanoma. Prev Med 1988;17:273-279.
28. Bale SJ, Dracopoli NC, Tucker MA, et al. Mapping the gene for hereditary cutaneous malignant melanoma-dysplastic nevus to chromosome 1p. N Engl J Med 1989;320:1367-1372.
29. Goldstein AM, Dracopoli NC, Engelstein M, Fraser MC, Clark WH Jr, Tucker MA. Linkage of cutaneous malignant melanoma/dysplastic nevi to chromosome 9p, and evidence for genetic heterogeneity. Am J Hum Genet 1994;54:489-496.

30. Goldstein AM, Goldin LR, Dracopoli NC, Clark WH Jr, Tucker MA. Two-locus linkage analysis of cutaneous malignant melanoma/dysplastic nevi. Am J Hum Genet 1996;58:1050-1056.

31. Cannon-Albright LA, Goldgar DE, Wright EC, et al. Evidence against the reported linkage of the cutaneous melanoma-dysplastic nevus syndrome locus to chromosome Ip36. Am J Hum Genet 1990;46:912-918.

32. Gruis NA, Bergman W, Frants RR. Locus for susceptibility to melanoma on chromosome 1p. N Engl J Med 1990;322:853-854.

33. Nancarrow DJ, Palmer JM, Walters MK, et al. Exclusion of the familial melanoma locus (MLM) from the PND/D1S47 and MYCL1 regions of chromosome arm 1p in 7 Australian pedigrees. Genomics 1992;12:18-25.

34. Marghoob AA, Slade J, Kopf AW, Salopek TG, Rigel DS, Bart RS. Risk of developing multiple primary cutaneous melanomas in patients with the classic atypical-mole syndrome: a case-control study. Br J Dermatol 1996;135:704-711.

35. Rigel DS, Rivers JK, Kopf AW, et al. Dysplastic nevi: markers of increased risk for melanoma. Cancer 1989;63:386-389.

36. Vasen HF, Bergman W, Van Haeringen A, Scheffer E, Van Slooten EA. The familial dysplastic nevus syndrome. Natural history and the impact of screening on prognosis. A study of nine families in the Netherlands. Eur J Cancer Clin Oncol 1989;25:337-341.

37. Rivers JK, Kopf AW, Vinokur AF, et al. Clinical characteristics of malignant melanomas developing in persons with dysplastic nevi. Cancer 1990;65:1232-1236.

38. Masri GD, Clark WH Jr, Guerry D 4th, Halpern A, Thompson CJ, Elder DE. Screening and surveillance of patients at high risk for malignant melanoma result in detection of earlier disease. J Am Acad Dermatol 1990;22:1042-1048.

39. MacKie RM, Freudenberger T, Aitchison TC. Personal risk-factor chart for cutaneous melanoma. Lancet 1989;2:487-490.

40. Fargnoli MC, Piccolo D, Altobelli E, Formicone F, Chimenti S, Peris K. Constitutional and environmental risk factors for cutaneous melanoma in an Italian population. A case-control study. Melanoma Res 2004;14:151-157.

41. Landi MT, Baccarelli A, Tarone RE, et al. DNA repair, dysplastic nevi, and sunlight sensitivity in the development of cutaneous malignant melanoma. J Natl Cancer Inst 2002;94:94-101.

42. Halpern AC, Guerry D 4th, Elder DE, et al. Dysplastic nevi as risk markers of sporadic (nonfamilial) melanoma. A case-control study. Arch Dermatol 1991;127:995-999.

43. Gandini S, Sera F, Cattaruzza MS, et al. Meta-analysis of risk factors for cutaneous melanoma: I. Common and atypical naevi. Eur J Cancer 2005;41:28-44.

44. Kelly JW, Yeatman JM, Regalia G, Mason G, Henham AP. A high incidence of melanoma found in patients with multiple dysplastic naevi by photographic surveillance. Med J Aust 1997;167:191-194.

45. Titus-Ernstoff L, Duray PH, Ernstoff MS, Barnhill RL, Horn PL, Kirkwood JM. Dysplastic nevi in association with multiple primary melanoma. Cancer Res 1988;48:1016-1018.

46. Augustsson A, Stierner U, Rosdahl I, Suurkula M. Common and dysplastic naevi as risk factors for cutaneous malignant melanoma in a Swedish population. Acta Derm Venereol 1991;71:518-524.

47. Roush GC, Barnhill RL. Correlation of clinical pigmentary characteristics with histopathologically-confirmed dysplastic nevi in nonfamilial melanoma patients. Studies of melanocytic nevi IX. Br J Cancer 1991;64:943-947.

48. Piepkorn MW, Barnhill RL, Cannon-Albright LA, et al. A multiobserver, population-based analysis of histologic dysplasia in melanocytic nevi. J Am Acad Dermatol 1994;30:707-714.

49. Shors AR, Kim S, White E, et al. Dysplastic naevi with moderate to severe histological dysplasia: a risk factor for melanoma. Br J Dermatol 2006;155:988-993.

50. McGovern VJ. Melanoma. Histologic diagnosis and prognosis. New York: Raven Press; 1983:3-24.

51. Clark WH Jr, Elder DE, Guerry D 4th, Epstein MN, Greene MH, Van Horn M. A study of tumor progression: the precursor lesions of superficial spreading and nodular melanoma. Hum Pathol 1984;15:1147-1165.

52. Rhodes AR, Harrist TJ, Day CL, Mihm MC Jr, Fitzpatrick TB, Sober AJ. Dysplastic melanocytic nevi in histologic association with 234 primary cutaneous melanomas. J Am Acad Dermatol 1983;9:563-574.

53. McGovern VJ, Shaw HM, Milton GW. Histogenesis of malignant melanoma with an adjacent component of the superficial spreading type. Pathology 1985;17:251-254.

54. Gruber SB, Barnhill RL, Stenn KS, Roush GC. Nevomelanocytic proliferations in association with cutaneous malignant melanoma: a multivariate analysis. J Am Acad Dermatol 1989;21:773-780.

55. Skender-Kalnenas TM, English DR, Heenan PJ. Benign melanocytic lesions: risk markers or precursors of cutaneous melanoma? J Am Acad Dermatol 1995;33:1000-1007.

56. Kaddu S, Smolle J, Zenahlik P, Hoffmann-Wellenhof R, Kerl H. Melanoma with benign melanocytic naevus components: reappraisal of clinicopathological features and prognosis. Melanoma Res 2002;12:271-278.

57. Halpern AC, Guerry D, Elder DE, Trock B, Synnestvedt M, Humphreys T. Natural history of dysplastic nevi. J Am Acad Dermatol 1993;29:51-57.

58. Yazdi AS, Palmedo G, Flaig MJ, Kutzner H, Sander CA. Different frequencies of a BRAF point mutation in melanocytic skin lesions. Pigment Cell Res 2003;16:580.

59. Demunter A, Ahmadian MR, Libbrecht L, et al. A novel n-ras mutation in malignant melanoma is associated with excellent prognosis. Cancer Res 2001;61:4916-4922.

60. Caporaso N, Greene MH, Tsai S, Pickle LW, Mulvihill JJ. Cytogenetics in hereditary malignant melanoma and dysplastic nevus syndrome: is dysplastic nevus syndrome a chromosome instability disorder? Cancer Genet Cytogenet 1987;24:299-314.

61. Jaspers NG, Roza-de Jongh EJ, Donselaar IG, et al. Sister chromatid exchanges, hyperdiploidy and chromosomal rearrangements studied in cells from melanoma-prone individuals belonging to families with the dysplastic nevus syndrome. Cancer Genet Cytogenet 1987;24:33-43.

62. Parmiter AH, Balaban G, Clark WH Jr, Nowell PC. Possible involvement of the chromosome region 10q24-q26 in early stages of melanocytic neoplasia. Cancer Genet Cytogenet 1988;30:313-317.

63. Sanford KK, Tarone RE, Parshad R, Tucker MA, Greene MH, Jones GM. Hypersensitivity to G2 chromatid radiation damage in familial dysplastic naevus syndrome. Lancet 1987;2:1111-1116.

64. Perera MI, Um KI, Greene MH, Waters HL, Bredberg A, Kraemer KH. Hereditary dysplastic nevus syndrome: lymphoid cell ultraviolet hypermutability in association with increased melanoma susceptibility. Cancer Res 1986;46:1005-1009.

65. Roth M, Boyle JM, Muller H. Thymine dimer repair in fibroblasts of patients with dysplastic naevus syndrome (DNS). Experientia 1988;44:169-171.

66. Thielmann HW, Popanda O, Edler L, Boing A, Jung EG. DNA repair synthesis following irradiation with 254-nm and 312-nm ultraviolet light is not diminished in fibroblasts from patients with dysplastic nevus syndrome. J Cancer Res Clin Oncol 1995;121:327-337.

67. Noz KC, Bauwens M, Van Buul PP, et al. Comet assay demonstrates a higher ultraviolet B sensitivity to DNA damage in dysplastic nevus cells than in common melanocytic nevus cells and foreskin melanocytes. J Invest Dermatol 1996;106:1198-1202.

68. Korabiowska M, Brinck U, Ruschenburg I, Dengler H, Droese M, Berger H. Expression of DNA mismatch repair genes in naevi. In Vivo 1999;13:251-254.

69. Korabiowska M, Brinck U, Betke H, Droese M, Berger H. Growth arrest DNA damage gene expression in naevi. In Vivo 1999;13:247-250.

70. Hussein MR, Roggero E, Sudilovsky EC, Tuthill RJ, Wood GS, Sudilovsky O. Alterations of mismatch repair protein expression in benign melanocytic nevi, melanocytic dysplastic nevi, and cutaneous malignant melanomas. Am J Dermatopathol 2001;23:308-314.

71. Bergman W, Ruiter DJ, Scheffer E, van Vloten WA. Melanocytic atypia in dysplastic nevi. Immunohistochemical and cytophotometrical analysis. Cancer 1988;61:1660-1666.

72. Palmieri G, Ascierto PA, Cossu A, et al. Assessment of genetic instability in melanocytic skin lesions through microsatellite analysis of benign naevi, dysplastic naevi, and primary melanomas and their metastases. Melanoma Res 2003;13:167-170.

73. Hussein MR, Sun M, Tuthill RJ, et al. Comprehensive analysis of 112 melanocytic skin lesions demonstrates microsatellite instability in melanomas and dysplastic nevi, but not in benign nevi. J Cutan Pathol 2001;28:343-350.

74. Birindelli S, Tragni G, Bartoli C, et al. Detection of microsatellite alterations in the spectrum of melanocytic nevi in patients with or without individual or family history of melanoma. Int J Cancer 2000;86:255-261.

75. Moriwaki SI, Tarone RE, Tucker MA, Goldstein AM, Kraemer KH. Hypermutability of UV-treated plasmids in dysplastic nevus/familial melanoma cell lines. Cancer Res 1997;57:4637-4641.

76. Salopek TG, Yamada K, Ito S, Jimbow K. Dysplastic melanocytic nevi contain high levels of pheomelanin: quantitative comparison of pheomelanin/eumelanin levels between normal skin, common nevi, and dysplastic nevi. Pigment Cell Res 1991;4:172-179.

77. Jimbow K, Salopek TG, Dixon WT, Searles GE, Yamada K. The epidermal melanin unit in the pathophysiology of malignant melanoma. Am J Dermatopathol 1991;13:179-188.

78. Pavel S, Smit NP, Van der Muelen H, et al. Homozygous germline mutation of CDKN2A/p16 and glucose-6-phosphate dehydrogenase deficiency in a multiple melanoma case. Melanoma Res 2003;13:171-178.

79. Ahmed B, Van den Oord JJ. Expression of the neuronal isoform of nitric oxide synthase (nNOS) and its inhibitor, protein inhibitor of nNOS, in pigment cell lesions of the skin. Br J Dermatol 1999;141:12-19.

80. Eskandarpour M, Hashemi J, Kanter L, Ringborg U, Platz A, Hansson J. Frequency of UV-inducible NRAS mutations in melanomas of patients with germline CDKN2A mutations. J Natl Cancer Inst 2003;95:790-798.

81. Uribe P, Wistuba II, Gonzalez S. BRAF mutation: a frequent event in benign, atypical, and malignant melanocytic lesions of the skin. Am J Dermatopathol 2003;25:365-370.

82. Park WS, Vortmeyer AO, Pack S, et al. Allelic deletion at chromosome 9p21(p16) and 17p13(p53) in microdissected sporadic dysplastic nevus. Hum Pathol 1998;29:127-130.

83. Tran TP, Titus-Ernstoff L, Perry AE, Ernstoff MS, Newsham IF. Alteration of chromosome 9p21 and/or p16 in benign and dysplastic nevi suggests a role in early melanoma progression (United States). Cancer Causes Control 2002;13:675-682.

84. Hashemi J, Linder S, Platz A, Hansson J. Melanoma development in relation to non-functional p16/INK4A protein and dysplastic naevus syndrome in Swedish melanoma kindreds. Melanoma Res 1999;9:21-30.

85. Smoller BR, McNutt NS, Hsu A. HMB-45 staining of dysplastic nevi. Support for a spectrum of progression toward melanoma. Am J Surg Pathol 1989;13:680-684.

86. Elder DE, Rodeck U, Thurin J, et al. Antigenic profile of tumor progression stages in human melanocytic nevi and melanomas. Cancer Res 1989;49:5091-5096.

87. Podhajcer OL, Bover L, Bravo AI, et al. Expression of cathepsin D in primary and metastatic human melanoma and dysplastic nevi. J Invest Dermatol 1995;104:340-344.

88. Khare VK, Albino AP, Reed JA. The neuropeptide/mast cell secretagogue substance P is expressed in cutaneous melanocytic lesions. J Cutan Pathol 1998;25:2-10.

89. Touab M, Villena J, Barranco C, Arumi-Uria M, Bassols A. Versican is differentially expressed in human melanoma and may play a role in tumor development. Am J Pathol 2002;160:549-557.

90. Dhawan P, Singh AB, Ellis DL, Richmond A. Constitutive activation of Akt/protein kinase B in melanoma leads to up-regulation of nuclear factor-kappaB and tumor progression. Cancer Res 2002;62:7335-7342.

91. Pavel S, van Nieuwpoort F, Van der Muelen H, et al. Disturbed melanin synthesis and chronic oxidative stress in dysplastic naevi. Eur J Cancer 2004;40:1423-1430.

92. Winer I, Normolle DP, Shureiqi I, et al. Expression of 12-lipoxygenase as a biomarker for melanoma carcinogenesis. Melanoma Res 2002;12:429-434.

93. Demunter A, Wolf-Peeters C, Degreef H, Stas M, van den Oord JJ. Expression of the endothelin-B receptor in pigment cell lesions of the skin. Evidence for its role as tumor progression marker in malignant melanoma. Virchows Arch 2001;438:485-491.

94. Glassl A, Bosserhoff AK, Buettner R, Hohenleutner U, Landthaler M, Stolz W. Increase in telomerase activity during progression of melanocytic cells from melanocytic naevi to malignant melanomas. Arch Dermatol Res 1999;291:81-87.

95. Miracco C, Pacenti L, Santopietro R, Laurini L, Biagioli M, Luzi P. Evaluation of telomerase activity in cutaneous melanocytic proliferations. Hum Pathol 2000;31:1018-1021.

96. Takahashi H, Strutton GM, Parsons PG. Determination of proliferating fractions in malignant melanomas by anti-PCNA/cyclin monoclonal antibody. Histopathology 1991;18:221-227.

97. Fogt F, Vortmeyer AO, Tahan SR. Nucleolar organizer regions (AgNOR) and Ki-67 immunoreactivity in cutaneous melanocytic lesions. Am J Dermatopathol 1995;17:12-17.

98. Schmidt B, Weinberg DS, Hollister K, Barnhill RL. Analysis of melanocytic lesions by DNA image cytometry. Cancer 1994;73:2971-2977.

99. Rubben A, Bogdan I, Grussendorf-Conen EI, Burg G, Boni R. Loss of heterozygosity and microsatellite instability in acquired melanocytic nevi: towards a molecular definition of the dysplastic nevus. Recent Results Cancer Res 2002;160:100-110.

100. Piepkorn M. Whither the atypical (dysplastic) nevus? Am J Clin Pathol 2001;115:177-179.

101. Ackerman AB. Dysplastic nevus. Am J Surg Pathol 2000;24:757-758.

101a. McNutt NS. Dysplastic nevus. [Letter]. Am J Surg Pathol 200;24:758.

102. Piepkorn MW. A case control study of histological dysplasia in melanocytic nevi. 40. 2005. Vancouver, BC Canada, 6th World Conference on Melanoma.

103. Elder DE. The dysplastic nevus. Pathology 1985;17:291-297.

104. Elder DE, Greene MH, Bondi EE, Clark WH Jr. Acquired melanocytic nevi and melanoma: the dysplastic nevus syndrome. In: Ackerman AB, ed. Pathology of malignant melanoma. New York: Masson; 1981:185-216.

105. Aronson PJ, Ito K, Fukaya T, Hashimoto K, Mehregan AH. Monoclonal antibody (AFH1) immunoreactive on morphologically abnormal basal melanocytes within dysplastic nevi, nevocellular nevus nests, and melanoma. J Invest Dermatol 1988;90:452-458.

106. Rhodes AR, Seki Y, Fitzpatrick TB, Stern RS. Melanosomal alterations in dysplastic melanocytic nevi. A quantitative, ultrastructural investigation. Cancer 1988;61:358-369.

107. Langer K, Rappersberger K, Steiner A, Konrad K, Wolff K. The ultrastructure of dysplastic naevi: comparison with superficial spreading melanoma and common naevi. Arch Dermatol Res 1990;282:353-362.

108. Sagebiel RW, Banda PW, Schneider JS, Crutcher WA. Age distribution and histologic patterns of dysplastic nevi. J Am Acad Dermatol 1985;13:975-982.

109. Toussaint S, Kamino H. Dysplastic changes in different types of melanocytic nevi. A unifying concept. J Cutan Pathol 1999;26:84-90.

110. Clark WH Jr, Hood AF, Tucker MA, Jampel RM. Atypical melanocytic nevi of the genital type with a discussion of reciprocal parenchymal-stromal interactions in the biology of neoplasia. Hum Pathol 1998;29(Suppl 1):S1-S24.

111. Steijlen PM, Bergman W, Hermans J, Scheffer E, Van Vloten WA, Ruiter DJ. The efficacy of histopathological criteria required for diagnosing dysplastic naevi. Histopathology 1988;12:289-300.
112. Rivers JK, Cockerell CJ, McBride A, Kopf AW. Quantification of histologic features of dysplastic nevi. Am J Dermatopathol 1990;12:42-50.
113. Shea CR, Vollmer RT, Prieto VG. Correlating architectural disorder and cytologic atypia in Clark (dysplastic) melanocytic nevi. Hum Pathol 1999;30:500-505.
114. Christensen WN, Friedman KJ, Woodruff JD, Hood AF. Histologic characteristics of vulval nevocellular nevi. J Cutan Pathol 1987;14:87-91.
115. Meyer LJ, Piepkorn MW, Seuchter SA, et al. Genetic and epidemiologic evaluation of dysplastic nevi. Pigment Cell Res 1988;7(Suppl 1):144-151.
116. Piepkorn M, Meyer LJ, Goldgar D, et al. The dysplastic melanocytic nevus: a prevalent lesion that correlates poorly with clinical phenotype. J Am Acad Dermatol 1989;20:407-415.
117. Weinstock MA, Barnhill RL, Rhodes AR, Brodsky GL. Reliability of the histopathologic diagnosis of melanocytic dysplasia. The Dysplastic Nevus Panel. Arch Dermatol 1997;133:953-958.
118. Maize JC, Ackerman AB. Pigmented lesions of the skin. Clinicopathologic correlations. Philadelphia: Lea & Febiger; 1987.
119. Klein LJ, Barr RJ. Histologic atypia in clinically benign nevi. A prospective study. J Am Acad Dermatol 1990;22:275-282
120. Clark WH Jr, Ackerman AB. An exchange of views regarding the dysplastic nevus controversy. Semin Dermatol 1989;8:229-250.
121. Clark WH Jr, Elder DE, Guerry D 4th. Dysplastic nevi and malignant melanoma. In: Farmer ER, Hood AF, eds. Pathology of the skin. New York: Appleton & Lange; 1989:684-756.
122. NIH consensus conference. Diagnosis and treatment of early melanoma. JAMA 1992;268:1314-1319.
123. Tong AK, Murphy GF, Mihm MC Jr. Dysplastic nevus: a formal histogenetic precursor of malignant melanoma. Monogr Pathol 1988;(30):10-18.
124. Rhodes AR, Mihm MC Jr, Weinstock MA. Dysplastic melanocytic nevi: a reproducible histologic definition emphasizing cellular morphology. Mod Pathol 1989;2:306-319.
125. Pozo L, Naase M, Cerio R, Blanes A, Diaz-Cano SJ. Critical analysis of histologic criteria for grading atypical (dysplastic) melanocytic nevi. Am J Clin Pathol 2001;115:194-204.
126. Bruijn JA, Berwick M, Mihm MC Jr, Barnhill RL. Common acquired melanocytic nevi, dysplastic melanocytic nevi and malignant melanomas: an image analysis cytometric study. J Cutan Pathol 1993;20:121-125.
127. Smoller BR, Egbert BM. Dysplastic nevi can be diagnosed and graded reproducibly: a longitudinal study. J Am Acad Dermatol 1992;27:399-402.
128. Murphy GF, Mihm MC. Recognition and evaluation of cytological dysplasia in acquired melanocytic nevi. Hum Pathol 1999;30:506-512.
129. Roush GC, Dubin N, Barnhill RL. Prediction of histologic melanocytic dysplasia from clinical observation. J Am Acad Dermatol 1993;29:555-562.
130. Barnhill RL, Roush GC. Correlation of clinical and histopathologic features in clinically atypical melanocytic nevi. Cancer 1991;67:3157-3164.
131. Barnhill RL, Roush GC. Histopathologic spectrum of clinically atypical melanocytic nevi: II. Studies of nonfamilial melanoma. Arch Dermatol 1990;126:1315-1318.
132. Meyer LJ, Piepkorn M, Goldgar DE, et al. Interobserver concordance in discriminating clinical atypia of melanocytic nevi, and correlations with histologic atypia. J Am Acad Dermatol 1996;34:618-625.
133. Annessi G, Cattaruzza MS, Abeni D, et al. Correlation between clinical atypia and histologic dysplasia in acquired melanocytic nevi. J Am Acad Dermatol 2001;45:77-85.
134. Carli P, De Giorgi V, Massi D, Giannotti B. The role of pattern analysis and the ABCD rule of dermoscopy in the detection of histological atypia in melanocytic naevi. Br J Dermatol 2000;143:290-297.
135. Heenan PJ, Elder DE, Sobin LH. Histologic typing of skin tumors, 2nd ed. New York: Springer-Verlag; 1996.
136. Wiecker TS, Luther H, Buettner P, Bauer J, Garbe C. Moderate sun exposure and nevus counts in parents are associated with development of melanocytic nevi in childhood: a risk factor study in 1,812 kindergarten children. Cancer 2003;97:628-638.
137. Schmoeckel C. How consistent are dermatopathologists in reading early malignant melanomas and lesions "precursor" to them? An international survey. Am J Dermatopathol 1984;6:13-24.
138. King R, Page RN, Googe PB, Mihm MC. Lentiginous melanoma: a histologic pattern of melanoma to be distinguished from lentiginous nevus. Mod Pathol 2005;18:1397-1401.
139. Curtin JA, Fridlyand J, Kageshita T, et al. Distinct sets of genetic alterations in melanoma. N Engl J Med 2005;353:2135-2147.
140. Urso C. Atypical histologic features in melanocytic nevi. Am J Dermatopathol 2000;22:391-396.
141. National Institutes of Health summary of the Consensus Development Conference on Sunlight, Ultraviolet Radiation, and the Skin. Bethesda, Maryland, May 8-10, 1989. Consensus Development Panel. J Am Acad Dermatol 1991;24:608-612.

7 COMBINED NEVI

Although symmetry and uniformity from side to side characterize most benign nevi, there are some lesions that combine features of two or more types of nevi, leading to an unusual appearance that can simulate a melanoma.

A *combined nevus* is a melanocytic nevus that combines features of two or more types of benign nevi. In the most common type, dermal nevus cells of the usual sort have pigmented spindle cells "placed" between collagen bundles, as seen in blue nevi. The common nevus cells are superficial to the blue nevus component and admixed with it, so that the predominant clinical morphology is that of a common acquired nevus (1,2). Other combinations of benign nevi are occasionally observed, and these may be classified descriptively. For example, a spindle and epithelioid cell (Spitz) nevus may be combined with a common nevus (3). A recent study discussed 49 nevi in this general category as *biphenotypical nevi* or *nevi with phenotypical heterogeneity*, including nevi with atypical dermal nodules and nevi with a focal atypical epithelioid cell component. Although combinations of other types of nevi (for example, a congenital pattern dermal nevic component) may be seen with dysplastic nevi, the interpretation of an atypical dermal component in association with junctional atypia should be made with great caution. The worrisome histology of these lesions may result in a wrong diagnosis of malignancy (4); however, care should be taken not to underdiagnose a malignant melanoma.

CLINICAL FEATURES

Combined nevi are often excised incidentally or because of focally increased pigmentation, but they are usually considered clinically to represent banal nevi. The lesions may occur anywhere on the skin, but are most common on the face, and appear to be somewhat more common in young adult women (1). A typical lesion is a dark blue-black, small (4 to 10 mm), slightly raised papule with a regular, well-defined border, resembling a common nevus (fig. 7-1). Most are stable lesions, with no history of change or growth, but some lesions are excised because of the appearance of a focal black area within a preexisting banal papular compound nevus. There is no evidence of any significant propensity for malignant change. Ulceration, even after trauma, is rare.

MICROSCOPIC FINDINGS

The usual combined nevus exhibits features of blue nevus and congenital pattern or common acquired nevus (1,2,5). The key feature of such a combined nevus at scanning magnification is the presence of pigmented cells in the dermis, mixed with or focally replacing dermal nevus cells of the ordinary sort arranged in the architectural pattern of a banal or congenital pattern nevus (figs. 7-2–7-6). Most often, the pigmented cells resemble the dendritic or spindle cells that characterize blue nevi and

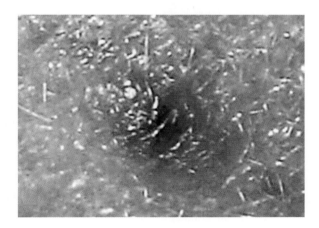

Figure 7-1

COMBINED NEVUS

This lesion is similar to a papular compound nevus, but the "two-tone" blue-black component results from a focal blue nevus-like component in the dermis. (Fig. E from Plate II, Fascicle 2, Third Series.)

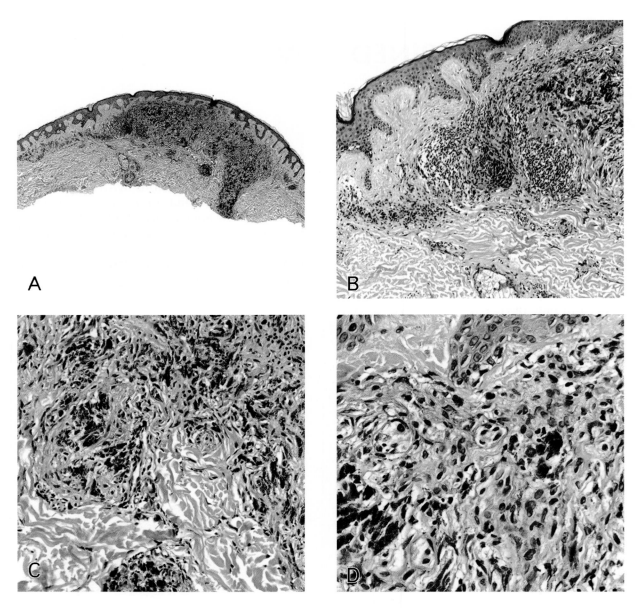

Figure 7-2

COMBINED NEVUS

A: Scanning magnification shows a heavily pigmented spindle cell component occurring within a congenital pattern nevus in the upper dermis to the left and right of the image.

B: Higher power shows blending of the congenital pattern nevus and the blue nevus-like component.

C: The pigmented spindle cells form an ill-defined nodule, overlapping morphologically with cellular nodule, cellular blue nevus, and, perhaps, pigmented epithelioid melanocytoma. These distinctions are somewhat arbitrary.

D: Importantly, cytologic atypia is minimal, there is no necrosis, and there are no mitoses.

their variants. Sometimes, however, they are more epithelioid in character, like the cells of a spindle and epithelioid cell (Spitz) nevus, or are composed of fusiform nonpigmented cells infiltrating coarse collagen bundles, as seen in the

sclerosing variants of a Spitz nevus. In the latter cases, the diagnosis of combined Spitz and common acquired nevus may be appropriate (1,3). In some combined nevi, there is an organized blue nevus component, with spindle/dendritic

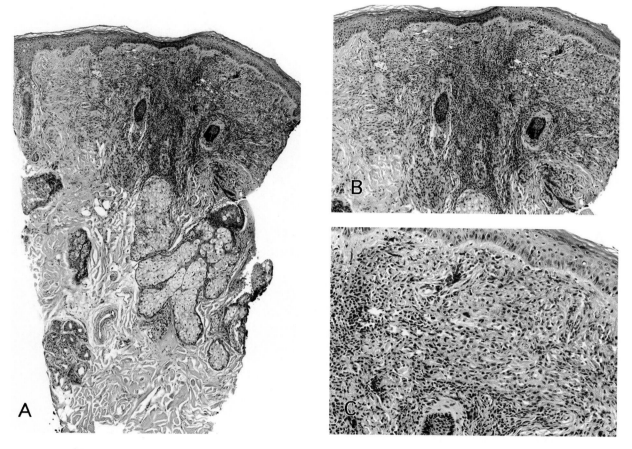

Figure 7-3

COMBINED NEVUS

In this lesion, from the nose of a 40-year-old woman, there is a blue nevus-like proliferation of pigmented spindle cells to the right and center (A–C), blending with an adjacent more ordinary congenital pattern nevus component (B). The differential diagnosis for this lesion might include a cellular nodule or a cellular blue nevus.

pigmented cells that are "placed" between dermal collagen bundles around the edges of a banal dermal nevic component. As in benign blue nevi, the pigmented spindle cells may be seen in nerves and in blood vessel walls. Most combined nevi show a fairly intimate admixture of common nevus cells and dendritic/spindled nevus cells, and forms transitional between the two cell types may be observed.

The pigmented cellular component, especially in epithelioid cell combined nevi, is sometimes focal within an otherwise banal compound or dermal nevus, explaining the clinical observation of focal dark brown-black pigmentation (fig. 7-5). Because of this focal appearance of a novel cell type, these lesions

have also been known as "clonal nevi." In one study of 72 such lesions, immunostains identified increased staining for p53 protein in 50 percent of the dermal "clones" but not in ordinary nevus cells adjacent to the clones (6). There is also overlap between these clonal nevi and nevi with cellular or proliferative nodules (discussed in chapter 5). Although the focal pigment in combined or clonal nevi may be newly evolved by history, indicating some propensity for growth or proliferation, mitotic figures are absent. Importantly, there is no evidence of expansile, nodular, or destructive growth of the pigmented cell population; there is no spontaneous necrosis; and there are no mitoses except perhaps in a few combined nevi with

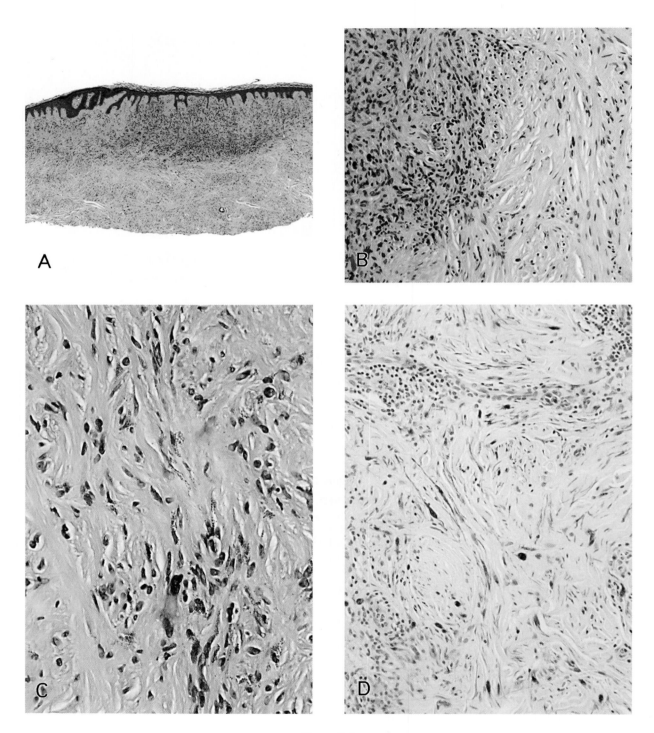

Figure 7-4

COMBINED NEVUS, WITH CONGENITAL PATTERN AND AMELANOTIC BLUE NEVUS COMPONENTS

A: Scanning magnification shows a congenital pattern nevus overlying an area of dermal sclerosis.

B,C: In the area of sclerosis, spindle-shaped to nevoid melanocytes are placed among the collagen bundles. Although the lesion is mostly amelanotic, focal spindle cells contain melanin pigment.

D: The spindle cells are clearly labeled with S-100 protein.

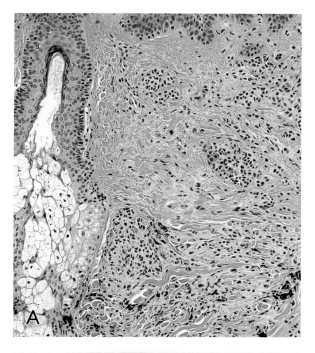

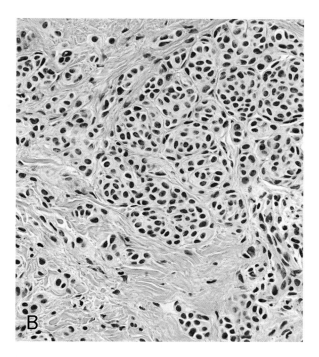

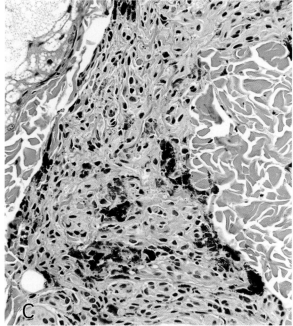

Figure 7-5

COMBINED NEVUS CLONAL PATTERN

In a small congenital pattern nevus (A,B), there is a "clonal" focus of hyperpigmented epithelioid to spindle-shaped melanocytes (C).

features of Spitz nevus (1). In a study of the immunophenotypic profile of nevi with a focal atypical epithelioid cell component or dermal nodules, the large polygonal cells expressed gp100, S-100 protein, tyrosinase, and Melan-A, but no immunoreactivity for the Ki-67 (MIB-1) proliferation marker (4).

The deep penetrating (plexiform spindle cell) nevus has also been described as a frequent participant in combined nevus (7). These lesions are often associated with a junctional component which could be interpreted either as a combined common compound nevus or as a combined compound nevus and deep penetrating nevus. In

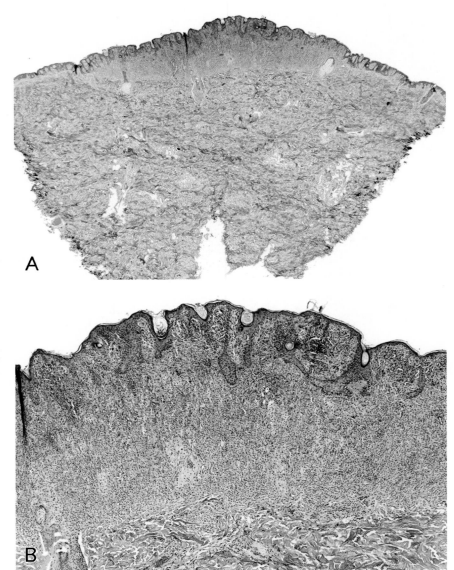

Figure 7-6

MILD HISTOLOGIC DYSPLASIA COMBINED WITH A DERMAL NEVUS WITH CONGENITAL FEATURES

A: Although not necessarily thought of as a combined nevus, dysplastic features may be seen in association with a congenital pattern dermal nevic component, as here.

B: The central nevic component shows orderly nevus cells extending into the reticular dermis and around skin appendages.

another category of combined nevus, lesions with features of deep penetrating nevi and/or Spitz nevi have been described in association with epithelioid blue nevi of the type seen with the Carney complex (8). Finally, histologic melanocytic dysplasia associated with a congenital pattern nevus could be regarded as a form of combined nevus. It is not certain whether the significance of dysplasia in this situation carries the same significance as a melanoma risk marker (fig. 7-6).

Because certain variants of combined nevus produce the impression of inversed maturation, with larger, more pigmented cells deep to smaller, less pigmented cells, some may be erroneously interpreted as so-called inverted type A nevi. This latter designation is best reserved for those nevi that simply show ordinary type A nevus nests below type B nests, producing an inversion of the normal pattern of downward differentiation within an otherwise banal acquired nevocellular nevus.

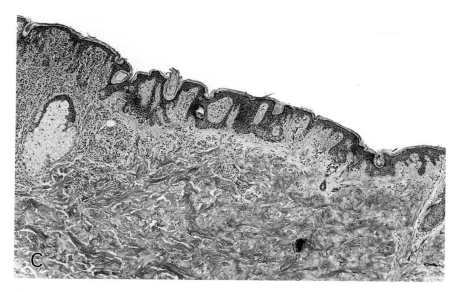

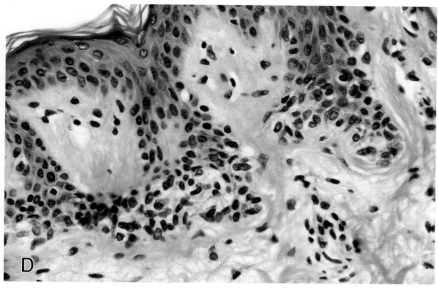

Figure 7-6 (Continued)

C,D: Changes of dysplasia are seen in the adjacent epidermis at the shoulder. There is mild random cytologic atypia with bridging nests. In our experience, dysplasia such as this in association with a congenital nevus is often minimal to mild in degree, and may not necessarily be associated with dysplastic nevi elsewhere on the patient's skin.

REFERENCES

1. Pulitzer DR, Martin PC, Cohen AP, Reed RJ. Histologic classification of the combined nevus: analysis of the variable expression of melanocytic nevi. Am J Surg Pathol 1991;15:1111-1122.

2. Fletcher V, Sagebiel RW. The combined nevus: mixed patterns of benign melanocytic lesions must be differentiated from malignant melanomas. In: Ackerman AB, ed. Pathology of malignant melanoma. New York: Masson; 1981:273-283.

3. Jin ZH, Kumakiri M, Ishida H, Kinebuchi S. A case of combined nevus: compound nevus and spindle cell Spitz nevus. J Dermatol 2000;27:233-237.

4. Winnepenninckx V, van den Oord JJ. Immunophenotype and possible origin of nevi with phenotypical heterogeneity. Arch Dermatol Res 2004;296:49-53.

5. Aroni K, Georgala S, Papachatzaki E, Liossi A, Davaris P. Coexistence of plaque-type blue nevus and congenital melanocytic nevi. J Dermatol 1996;23:325-328.

6. Ball NJ, Golitz LE. Melanocytic nevi with focal atypical epithelioid cell components: a review of seventy-three cases. J Am Acad Dermatol 1994;30:724-729.

7. Cooper PH. Deep penetrating (plexiform spindle cell) nevus. A frequent participant in combined nevus. J Cutan Pathol 1992;19:172-180.

8. Groben PA, Harvell JD, White WL. Epithelioid blue nevus: neoplasm Sui generis or variation on a theme? Am J Dermatopathol 2000;22:473-488.

8

MALIGNANT TUMORS (MELANOMAS AND RELATED LESIONS)

TUMOR PROGRESSION PHASES AND CLASSIFICATION

The epidemiology of malignant melanoma has undergone striking and important changes since the early seminal descriptions by Hutchinson (1) and Dubreuilh (2). These changes have affected our understanding of the frequency and pattern of melanoma in populations. Especially over the last 50 years, the most important change has been the recognition of most melanomas in their early stages of development, or "progression," when they are more likely to be curable. Thus, while the incidence of melanoma has been steadily rising, the mortality rate has risen at a slower pace, and the case-fatality rate has fallen over this period.

The incidence of melanoma began to rise rapidly about the beginning of the last century in most Western countries (3). The incidence in whole populations rose at an annual rate sufficient to double the incidence each decade (4), but in the groups of people at highest risk, it may be presumed to have risen even faster. Melanoma, once a rare disease, has become a significant public health problem in many communities (5,6). The trends may reflect increased sun exposure, with variation among different populations and age groups and between the sexes (7). The rising incidence has affected a population of young, middle-class men and women who, in general, work indoors but go outdoors for their recreation, tend to have skin that is susceptible to sunburn, and often were heavily exposed to the sun in childhood. As discussed in an earlier section of this Fascicle, individuals at particular risk include those with dysplastic nevi or multiple large nevi (8,9), those with fair skin that burns readily (10), and those with a family history of skin cancer (9). Other risk factors include evidence of solar injury in the form of freckles or actinic skin damage and a history of intermittent sun exposure (9). The only consistently documented environmental

risk factor is exposure to sunlight, particularly exposures causing sunburn in childhood. Recreational activity leading to sunburn in adulthood is also associated with risk (11). A recent meta-analysis of 57 studies concluded that the relationship between sun exposure and melanoma risk was complex, including variation with country and latitude (12). The analysis suggested that "well-conducted" studies supported the intermittent sun exposure hypothesis by a positive association for intermittent sun exposure, while there was a suggestion of an inverse association with a continuous pattern of sun exposure, except perhaps in older age groups.

The incidence of melanoma is rare in childhood and increases dramatically with age, although perhaps because of cohort effects, melanoma disproportionately affects a younger age group than most other major solid tumors. Recent data are beginning to indicate that in high-risk populations, such as in Australia and New Zealand, the incidence rates for melanoma, especially in the younger cohorts, may be beginning to stabilize and decrease (11,13). It has been concluded that melanoma incidence may continue to rise in the United States, at least until the majority of the current population in the middle-age group becomes the oldest population. In recent years, the incidence of thin tumors (under 1 mm) has been rising faster than that of thick tumors (over 4 mm), except in men aged 60 years or older (14,15).

At the same time that the incidence and total mortality rates of patients with malignant melanoma have been rising, the mortality rate for individual patients has been falling. In the first quarter of this century, the 5-year survival rate at a major treatment center was a dismal 12.5 percent (16). Today, the survival rate is about 90 percent (17–22). Since there has been little or no significant therapeutic innovation for metastatic melanoma in the last half century, this improving survival rate is likely due to

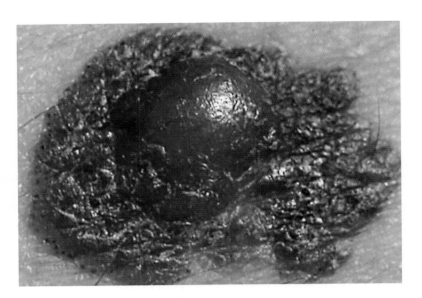

Figure 8-1

MALIGNANT MELANOMA

A tumorigenic vertical growth phase nodule is present within a nontumorigenic radial growth phase plaque. Note the tendency to symmetry of the vertical growth phase, and the difference in pigment content compared to the more heavily pigmented radial growth phase. (Fig. D from Plate V, Fascicle 2, Third Series.)

earlier diagnosis, which may in part be due to educational programs designed to improve the early detection of melanoma (11,22–25).

The decrease in the thickness of melanomas and the increasing proportion of thin melanomas at diagnosis support the importance of earlier diagnosis (25). Published descriptions of melanoma in the early literature emphasized the late stage of the disease that is characterized by a large tumor nodule (vertical growth phase), often associated with satellite metastases. Not until the descriptions of Allen (26), Clark (27), McGovern (28), Mihm et al. (29), and others over the last 40 years or so was it recognized that most malignant melanomas proceed through a variable but often prolonged radial growth phase, or plaque stage, during which time they are readily curable in most patients by simple surgical techniques. Importantly, such lesions tend to be easily diagnosed because of their relatively large radial diameter, irregular borders, and strikingly variegated colors. Unlike most other potentially life-threatening cancers, malignant melanomas, because of their superficial location, are visible from their earliest evolutionary stages and do not require expensive or invasive tests to make the diagnosis of a primary lesion. While melanomas in their radial growth phase are easily recognized and cured, when left untreated, they are at high risk of eventual progression to the vertical growth phase, a stage where prognosis has changed little, if at all, from that of 50 years ago.

Malignant melanoma can be defined quite simply as a malignant neoplasm of melanocytes. There are, however, many heterogeneities among individual cases that can be recognized clinically, histologically, and epidemiologically. These differences have been cataloged in various classification schemes, the best known of which is that of Wallace H. Clark Jr. (27). This classification, which is based on clinical as well as histologic observations, was the first to employ a clear concept of tumor progression. Clark recognized that melanomas often evolve through a phase during which they are predominantly flat and their net direction of growth clinically is along the radii of an imperfect circle (fig. 8-1). This phase is termed the *radial growth phase* of melanoma tumor progression. To the histologist, the "radial" proliferation, as viewed clinically, may appear more "horizontal." Radial growth phase melanomas have the capacity for local persistence, recurrence, and progression if not excised.

In the next phase of progression, a nodule forms, usually within the confines of a preexisting radial growth phase tumor. The nodule results in a net direction of growth perpendicular to the radial or horizontal growth phase and has therefore been termed the *vertical growth phase*. Vertical growth phase melanomas may metastasize as well as locally recur.

The Clark classification scheme of progression phases was seminal in leading to the recognition that melanomas could be diagnosed at a stage when cure was likely to be the rule

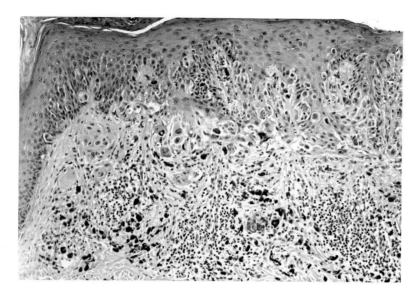

Figure 8-2

INVASIVE NONTUMORIGENIC MELANOMA (RADIAL GROWTH PHASE MELANOMA)

Invasive melanoma is characterized by several clusters of uniformly atypical epithelioid melanocytes in the papillary dermis, in relation to a lymphohistiocytic and fibrovascular host response. None of these clusters is larger than the largest cluster in the overlying epidermis. Clusters are irregularly and widely spaced, without forming a papule, as in the example of "accretive" vertical growth (fig. 8-5).

rather than the exception. Prior to the recognition of the radial growth phase as an early stage of tumor progression in most melanomas, most descriptions of melanoma had emphasized vertical growth phase nodules, and the diagnosis of melanoma was commonly not made until the lesion was clinically advanced and the prognosis grim. The concept of the radial growth phase is of paramount importance because this is a stage of tumor progression in which cure is practically assured after complete excision.

RADIAL AND VERTICAL GROWTH PHASES (NONTUMORIGENIC AND TUMORIGENIC) MELANOMAS

The essential biologic characteristic of *radial growth phase melanoma* is the slow but more or less inexorable proliferation of atypical cells in the epidermis. This may or may not be accompanied by atypical cell migration into the papillary dermis, where the cells do not proliferate to form a tumor, and may either undergo regression or persist in the dermis as relatively stable cells. They differ from benign nevus cells (which also proliferate in the epidermis and migrate into the dermis) in that the proliferation in the epidermis does not appear to be self-limited. The radial growth phase cells, in vivo, exhibit the property of inexorable growth, and clinically, they may recur locally if incompletely excised. For these reasons, these nontumorigenic neoplastic cells are judged by most observers to qualify as cancer cells or "melanoma cells."

The capacity to migrate into the dermis is considered to be a form of invasion across the basement membrane. The radial growth phase cells that accomplish this, however, do not proliferate in the dermis to form a tumor mass, and they do not compress or obliterate preexisting structures there. Consistent with this, it has been demonstrated recently that melanoma cells in the epidermal compartment of radial growth phase melanomas express relatively high levels of the proliferation marker Ki-67 (MIB-1), while the level of proliferation in the dermal compartment is very low, comparable to that in benign nevi (30). In addition, lesional cell mitoses may be seen in the epidermis, but not in the dermal compartment of a radial growth phase melanoma (31).

Recognizing that "invasion" in these lesions is superficial, nondestructive, and not associated with dermal proliferation or tumor nodule formation, the term *microinvasive melanoma* has been suggested (32). A microinvasive melanoma is a neoplasm that has invaded the dermis but has not formed a tumorigenic nodule (or papule) (fig. 8-2). As in other tumor systems, such as for example the dysplasia-squamous cell carcinoma sequence in the uterine cervix, this microinvasive stage of melanoma is characterized clinically by excellent survival. Although we have seen rare exceptions to this rule, the disease-free survival rate approaches 100 percent in our experience with prospectively studied invasive stage I radial growth phase melanoma

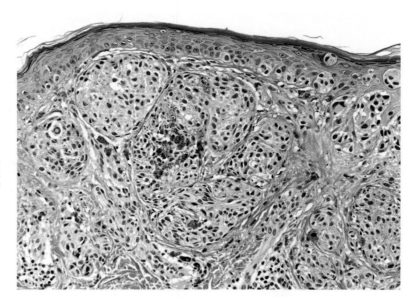

Figure 8-3

MELANOMA WITH EARLY TUMORIGENIC VERTICAL GROWTH PHASE

There are several clusters of cells in the papillary dermis that are clearly larger than the largest clusters in the overlying (or nearby) junctional component.

cases followed for 8 years or more (33,34). This excellent survival rate for a large group of patients with "invasive" melanomas may initially seem surprising. However, mortality from melanoma as from any other cancer is usually due to metastases, which are tumor masses established at a location remote from that of the primary neoplasm. On reflection, it seems reasonable to suppose that a radial growth phase melanoma cell that does not have the capacity to form a mass in the presumably favorable microenvironment of its primary location would not have that ability at a distant location either.

The radial growth phase is characterized histologically by a proliferation of melanocytes in the epidermis, with or without neoplastic melanocytes in the superficial papillary dermis as single cells or small clusters of cells without the formation of a tumor nodule (fig. 8-2). Thus, these lesions may be termed *nontumorigenic melanomas*, a term that we favor as being clearer than the synonymous term "microinvasive." The concept of invasive but nontumorigenic melanoma is related to the Breslow thickness and Clark level, either of which can define a very low risk population of patients, but are not synonymous. Because radial growth phase melanoma, when invasive, is by definition nontumorigenic, theoretically there is no essential limit to the thickness that a radial growth phase melanoma can attain. Because thickness, according to Breslow, is measured from the top of

the granular layer to the deepest invasive tumor cell, if there is 1 mm of epidermal hyperplasia, even a single cell could account for a melanoma of greater than 1 mm in total Breslow thickness while being nontumorigenic and nonmitogenic and conferring a very good prognosis. Similarly, most nontumorigenic melanomas are Clark level II; however, it is theoretically possible for a small group of nontumorigenic cells to have entered Clark level IV, or for a very small cluster to have expanded and filled an unusually thin papillary dermis, qualifying as level III (see Clark Levels of Invasion, Table 8-8).

Tumor nodule formation is the essential feature of the next stage of progression, termed the vertical growth phase because the net direction of growth clinically and/or histologically is now "vertically" into or out from the skin, perpendicular to the direction of growth of the radial growth phase (see fig. 8-1). Histologically, a true tumor nodule is present in the dermis. Vertical growth phase is not considered simply synonymous with invasion, but refers to the development of a new pattern of nodular or tumorigenic growth. Specifically, this concept relates to the formation of an intradermal nodule of melanoma cells that exceeds in diameter that of any nest of similar cells along the dermal-epidermal junction, a pattern that heralds the development of a clone capable of expansile growth (fig. 8-3). Molecular evidence supports the notion that the cells of the vertical growth phase are clonally derived from cells of

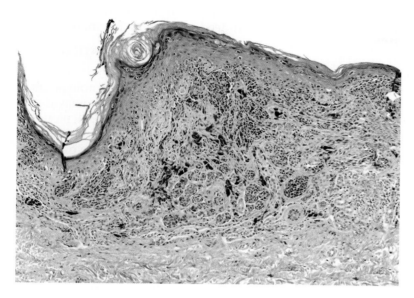

Figure 8-4

INVASIVE MELANOMA WITH ACCRETIVE NONTUMORIGENIC VERTICAL GROWTH

A papule of melanoma fills and expands the papillary dermis (Clark level III). The papule is formed of clusters of cells, none of which is larger than the largest intraepidermal cluster of lesional cells. The lesional cells are cytologically continuous with the melanoma cells in the overlying epidermis, despite a tendency to nevoid maturation, and they show only mild to moderate cytologic atypia. More than five clusters of such cells are present in a close array, constituting a well-developed area of accretive vertical growth.

the radial growth phase (35,36), and also from an associated nevus when this is present (37).

Prior to the onset of tumorigenic growth (as defined above), there may be a phase of so-called *variant,* or *accretive, vertical growth.* Neoplastic melanocytes extend as single cells or as small clusters into the papillary dermis, sometimes forming a tumor-like mass by the accretion of clusters, much as a brick wall is built to a considerable height from individual bricks. This process was originally defined by Richard Reed (38,39). Reed described the "dysplasia-melanoma sequence" (DMS), which Tuthill (40) has recently emphasized as an alternative to the commonly espoused carcinoma-like "in situ-invasive" model of tumor progression in melanoma. The DMS begins as a nevo-melanocytic lesion in which it is considered normal for melanocytes to move across the basement membrane into the superficial dermis (as in a compound nevus), and in some cases to even migrate into the mid and deep reticular dermis (as in a Spitz nevus). In this model, according to Tuthill, melanoma arises from dysplasia not once but as a series of steps of evolving melanomatous vertical growth, which is most likely to arise in relation to severe dysplasia and/or radial growth phase melanoma (which is considered in the model to be a form of high-grade dysplasia). Thus, this model defines at least two different patterns of melanomatous vertical growth: accretive and tumorigenic (or expansile) (38–40).

In the minimal case, accretive vertical growth is defined as the presence of at least five nests of cells in the dermis forming a nodule (fig. 8-4) (38,39). The individual nests do not show evidence of expansile growth as in tumorigenic vertical growth (fig. 8-3).

Gimotty et al. (30) have recently studied patterns of proliferation of melanoma cells in the dermis using the proliferation marker Ki-67. The mean Ki-67 expression rate was 13.9 percent in tumorigenic dermal vertical growth phase cells, 9.6 percent in accretive dermal vertical growth phase melanoma cells, and only 3.5 percent in radial growth phase melanoma cells in the dermis, while the corresponding mitotic rates were 1.4, 0.5, and 0 (P <.001). Intradermal melanoma cell Ki-67 positivity was lower than intraepidermal melanoma cell Ki-67 positivity in most of the radial growth phase lesions, with a mean difference between epidermal and dermal Ki-67 expression of 14.8 percent (P <.001). These results demonstrate that intradermal proliferation rates are higher in vertical than in radial growth phase lesions, and that accretive vertical growth phase cells are intermediate between radial growth phase and tumorigenic vertical growth phase cells in the dermis in terms of their proliferation index.

The above descriptions of the vertical and radial growth phases of malignant melanoma can be applied to almost all examples of primary melanoma, although, as already noted, not all melanomas exhibit each of these lesional compartments. About 45 percent of new cases, in our experience, are entirely in the radial growth phase, 10 percent present in vertical growth phase alone, and the remaining 45 percent present with a vertical growth phase tumor nodule surrounded by a radial growth phase plaque. In this latter situation, it is assumed that the plaque preceded the onset of the nodule, an assumption that is typically supported by the clinical history and occasionally by family photographs. This assumption of progression from a nontumorigenic plaque to a tumorigenic nodule that may have competence for metastasis has obvious implications for control of mortality from melanoma, since it suggests that progression may be prevented by removal of melanomas in the radial growth phase, when the lesions clinically are nontumorigenic plaques and histologically are either in situ or microinvasive.

The 10 percent of melanomas that present with a tumorigenic vertical growth phase nodule and no evident radial growth phase plaque in the adjacent epidermis and papillary dermis appear to represent tumorigenic melanoma from close to their inception, although it is likely that most of them do have an epidermal origin. There may be a clinically inapparent short-lived in situ or microinvasive phase that is obliterated by the rapidly proliferating tumorigenic nodule (41). In any event, such lesions, classically termed *nodular melanomas*, are more difficult to diagnose at an early low-risk stage, since the vertical growth phase nodules do not present many of the clinical features that characterize the radial growth phase and account for its clinically disturbing appearance.

A series of cases considered to represent primary dermal melanomas has been described (42). These were large, usually well-circumscribed, dermal-based tumors with, by definition, no epidermal or follicular connections and no evidence of ulceration, regression, or a preexisting nevus. Obvious malignant cytologic features were present in all of the lesions, with frequent mitoses and necrosis. Our impression of these lesions is that they are indistinguishable from metastases. Nevertheless, workup showed no evidence of a primary elsewhere, and the survival rate was good at 92 percent over an average of 44 months follow-up, suggesting that it is appropriate to manage these lesions, after a full clinical workup, as if they were indeed primary melanomas.

HISTOGENETIC CLASSIFICATION OF MELANOMAS

Considering the clinical and histologic morphology of a series of primary melanomas as well as the prior literature, Clark (27,29,43,44) proposed a clinicopathologic classification scheme that was based first on the presence or absence of a radial growth phase, and then on the clinical and histologic morphology of the lesion. At about the same time, McGovern (45) proposed a similar primarily histologic classification. The classification was further developed in two international conferences (46,47), and its continued use has subsequently been recommended (48,49).

Melanomas with tumorigenic nodular growth that lack a radial growth phase are classified as nodular melanomas, while those with a radial growth phase are classified on the basis of the morphology of the radial growth phase. Initially two major clinicopathologic variants of the radial growth phase were defined, termed *superficial spreading melanoma* (or *pagetoid melanoma* in the Australian classification), and *lentigo maligna* and *lentigo maligna melanoma* (the former originally called *Hutchinson melanotic freckle*) (46,50). Two additional radial growth phase variants, *acral-lentiginous* and *mucosal-lentiginous melanomas*, were later described by other observers (Table 8-1; fig. 8-5) (51). The existence of morphologic overlap among these various histogenetic types has been emphasized (52).

Molecular studies have demonstrated fundamental differences among melanomas classified by site (36,53,54) or by histogenetic type (35,36), and the morphologic subtypes likely are a reflection of these genetic differences. For example, acral melanomas differ significantly from superficial spreading melanomas in the pattern of their chromosomal amplifications (55). Additionally, in one study of *BRAF* mutation frequency, 50 percent of superficial spreading melanomas and 33 percent of acral lentiginous melanoma had the mutation, in contrast to none in the other types studied (nodular, lentigo maligna, and mucosal melanomas) (55). In another study, the *BRAF* mutation was present in 64 percent of cutaneous melanomas, but in only 1 of 25 mucosal melanomas; these authors concluded

Table 8-1

CLASSIFICATION OF MELANOMA[a]

Radial Growth Phase Variants	Tumorigenic Melanomas
In situ	(all are invasive by definition)
Invasive	
nontumorigenic (no VGP[b])	**Melanoma Without Radial Growth Phase**
with tumorigenic VGP	Nodular melanoma
Superficial spreading melanoma	
(Pagetoid melanoma)	**Vertical Growth Phase Variants**
Lentigo maligna melanoma	(with or without an associated radial growth phase)
(Hutchinson melanotic freckle)	Usual vertical growth phase
Acral-lentiginous melanoma	Epithelioid cells predominating
Mucosal-lentiginous melanoma	Spindle cells predominating
	Mixed and other cell types – small, blastic, signet cell, rhabdoid
	Desmoplastic melanoma
	Neurotropic melanoma
	Nevoid melanoma (minimal deviation, "spitzoid")
	Malignant blue nevus
	Other unusual variants and melanocytic tumors of uncertain potential

[a]The classification presented above is similar but not identical to the current WHO classification of melanoma, published recently and based on the work of an international committee (60). In this classification, the radial growth phase variants are separated in a manner similar to the scheme above, and a few special variants are added.
[b]VGP = vertical growth phase.

that "this finding additionally supports the view that the various subtypes of melanoma are not equivalent and that distinct genetic alterations may underlie well-recognized differences in risk factors and behavioral patterns" (56).

More recently, Curtin et al. (57) presented evidence for genetic variation among melanomas classified by the presence or absence of severe solar damage, one of the histologic hallmarks of the lentigo maligna subtype of melanoma: 81 percent of melanomas on skin without chronic sun-induced damage (the most common melanomas) had mutations in *BRAF* or *NRAS*, while the majority of the rarer melanomas from chronically sun-exposed or -unexposed sites had mutations in neither gene, providing additional support for the intermittent-exposure hypothesis reviewed above (57). Many (about one third) of these latter melanomas contained mutations of the oncogene *KIT* (58). In subsequent work, the same group demonstrated that superior prediction of mutation status can be achieved using factors already in use for melanoma subclassification, namely, a combination of histologic and clinical parameters such as high nesting and scatter, low age, and large cell size. A tree-based algorithm was developed which involves an initial separation based on nesting and scatter, and then additional separation based

on cell size and age. These authors concluded that these routinely available parameters allow good prediction of *BRAF* mutation status, which will no doubt be useful in stratifying patients for targeted therapies. In addition, they argue that "the strong association between genetic alterations and morphological findings further supports the existence of biologically distinct melanoma types, and the use of genetic factors to develop and clarify improved clinically applicable classification systems" (59).

The classification scheme that we currently use is presented in Table 8-1. The more or less distinctive radial growth phase pattern defines a subclassification of melanomas that is presented in the left-hand column. These lesions may be confined to the radial growth phase or they may present with a focal tumorigenic vertical growth phase and an adjacent radial growth phase lesion. As discussed above, these radial growth phase variants tend to correlate with site, age, actinic skin damage, and other attributes often associated with patterns of sun exposure. Other forms of melanoma that are more or less distinctive are variants of the vertical growth phase or tumorigenic melanoma compartment; these include desmoplastic and neurotropic melanomas, nevoid and minimal deviation melanomas, and certain unusual malignant

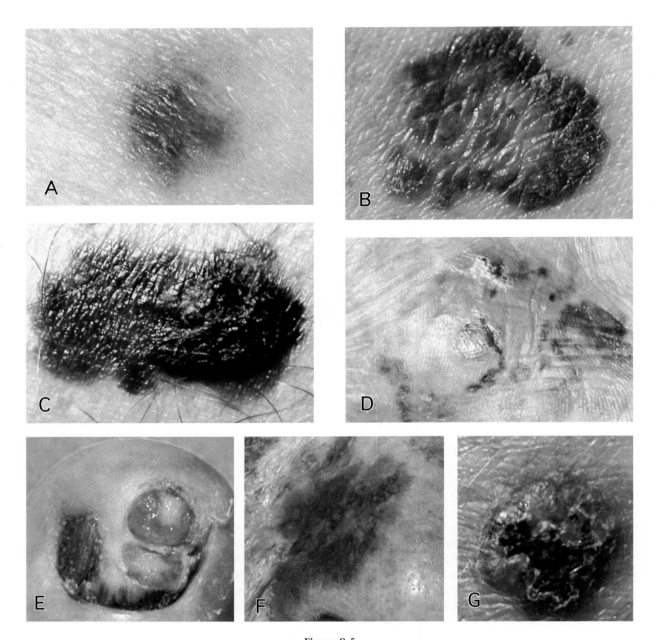

Figure 8-5

HISTOGENETIC SUBTYPES OF MALIGNANT MELANOMA

A through C are melanomas of the superficial spreading type.

A: An early radial growth phase melanoma, Clark level II, Breslow thickness 0.42 mm. The differential diagnosis includes a dysplastic nevus, but the variegation of colors with blue-black is more suggestive of a melanoma.

B: A more obvious nontumorigenic radial growth phase melanoma exemplifies the ABCD criteria: asymmetry, border irregularity, color variegation (with a gray area of regression), and diameter greater than 6 mm.

C: A black tumorigenic vertical growth phase nodule is present in a tan radial growth phase background.

D: A large acral-lentiginous melanoma, most of which is "broken up" by extensive radial growth phase regression.

E: A subungual melanoma, in which the radial growth phase is just beginning to spread onto the cuticle (an early Hutchinson sign, see chapter 10).

F: A large but predominantly in situ radial growth phase lentigo maligna melanoma from the nose of an elderly woman.

G: A pure tumorigenic or nodular melanoma, dark blue-black in color, with an area of surface ulceration. (Figs. A–D are figs. A, B, C, and F from Plate V, Fascicle 2, Third Series; E-G are figs. A, B, and E from Plate VI, Fascicle 2, Third Series.)

melanocytic neoplasms that may arise in relation to congenital nevi, blue nevi, and dermal melanocytoses. These are listed in the right-hand column. Histopathology is the "gold standard" in the diagnosis of malignant melanoma, and knowledge of the morphologic variation among the subtypes of melanoma is important to facilitate accurate histologic diagnosis.

The classification presented above is similar but not identical to the current World Health Organization (WHO) classification of melanoma, published recently and based on the work of an international committee (60). In this classification, the radial growth phase variants are separated in a manner similar to the scheme above, and a few special variants are added (Table 8-2).

There has been discussion and controversy regarding the importance of these classification schemes, which are descendants of the original "Sydney Classification" of 1973 (46). Arguments against an important general clinical role for classification include the failure of histogenetic type to associate with survival independent of other prognostic factors, and the finding in formal studies that the interobserver reproducibility of the histogenetic classification is "modest" (61). Reproducibility was highest in nodular melanoma and was of a moderate level for superficial spreading or lentigo maligna melanoma. Certainly, there is morphologic overlap among the various histogenetic types (52). Furthermore, as earlier lesions are removed and submitted for histopathologic diagnosis, the features are likely to be more subtle, rendering the classification more difficult. For clinical purposes, a diagnosis of malignant melanoma (not otherwise classified) is usually sufficient, as long as relevant prognostic ("microstaging") factors are also included.

The classification into types of radial growth phase has some slight prognostic significance for survival in established lesions. Multivariable modeling studies do not demonstrate independent significance of histogenetic type for survival (34,62–64). However, Cochran et al. (62) demonstrated in a multivariable modeling study based on 1,042 patients that the probability of recurrence (but not survival) was related to melanoma subtype, as well as other factors. Nodular and acral-lentiginous melanomas were

Table 8-2
WHO HISTOLOGIC CLASSIFICATION OF MALIGNANT MELANOMA
Superficial spreading melanoma
Nodular melanoma
Lentigo maligna
Acral melanoma
Desmoplastic melanoma
Melanoma arising from blue nevus
Melanoma arising in a giant congenital nevus
Melanoma of childhood
Nevoid melanoma
Persistent melanoma

most likely to recur, lentigo maligna intermediate, and superficial spreading type least likely. Sagebiel (65), in a review, concluded that variants of melanoma exist as in other neoplasms, and that they are of epidemiologic and therapeutic importance. He also added that "until further data are available or networked, database analysis should use microstage measurements in the common forms of superficial spreading and nodular melanomas only, and approach the unusual variants separately and cautiously."

Outside the realm of prognosis, there are important differences in the epidemiology, developmental biology, diagnostic criteria, and differential diagnosis of the lesions. The solar etiologic hypothesis for superficial spreading melanoma is not likely to be valid for mucosal- or acral-lentiginous melanomas, and most clinicians believe that the pace of evolution of superficial spreading melanoma is more rapid than that of lentigo maligna melanoma, which may persist as an indolently expanding patch in the skin for many years before progressing to the vertical growth phase. The histogenetic types of melanoma also differ substantially in terms of their precursor lesions; in one study, the incidence of a contiguous precursor (benign or dysplastic) nevus in superficial spreading melanomas was 22 times that in lentigo maligna melanomas, and histogenetic type was the only variable that was independently predictive of the existence of a precursor lesion, results that were considered to support the concept of the heterogeneity of melanoma histogenesis (66).

Table 8-3

DIFFERENCES AMONG MAJOR CLINICOPATHOLOGIC SUBTYPES OF MELANOMA

Feature	Nodular Melanoma	Superficial Spreading	Lentigo Maligna	Acral-Lentiginous
Growth phase	Vertical only (tumorigenic)	Radial always, +/- vertical	Radial always, +/- vertical	Radial always, +/- vertical
Predominant RGP[a] pattern	NA[b]	Pagetoid	Lentiginous	Lentiginous
Predominant cell type in RGP	NA	Large, epithelioid	Small, nevoid to epithelioid	Variable size, often dendritic
Predominant cell type in VGP	Large, epithelioid	Large, epithelioid	Small epithelioid, often spindled	Small epithelioid, often spindled
Associated nevus	Occasional	Frequent	Occasional	Unusual
Location (sun exposure)	Back, limbs (intermittent sun)	Back, limbs (intermittent sun)	Head and neck (chronic sun)	Acral skin (sun protected)
Clinical morphology	Papule or nodule	Well-circumscribed plaque, +/- nodule	Poorly circumscribed plaque, +/- nodule	Poorly circumscribed plaque, +/- nodule

[a]RGP = radial growth phase; VGP = vertical growth phase.
[b]NA = not available.

Table 8-4

DIFFERENTIAL DIAGNOSIS OF MELANOMA

Melanoma with Pagetoid Radial Growth Phase
Spindle and epithelioid cell (Spitz) tumor, plaque variants
Pigmented spindle cell tumor
Dysplastic nevus
Halo nevus
Recurrent nevus
Epidermotropic metastatic melanoma
Mycosis fungoides
Paget disease
Pagetoid squamous cell carcinoma (Bowen disease)
Sebaceous carcinoma, pagetoid variants
Merkel cell carcinoma, pagetoid variants

Melanoma with Lentiginous Radial Growth Phase
Dysplastic nevus
Pigmented spindle cell tumor
Pigmented actinic keratosis
Lentiginous junctional or compound nevus
Atypical fibroxanthoma (tumorigenic lesions)
Spindle cell squamous carcinoma (tumorigenic lesions)

Melanoma with No Radial Growth Phase (Nodular Melanoma)
Dysplastic nevus
Spindle and epithelioid cell (Spitz) tumor, nodular variants
Metastatic melanoma
Histiocytoid hemangioma
Kaposi sarcoma (nodular stage)
Fibrous histiocytoma
Merkel cell carcinoma
Desmoplastic Spitz tumor
Blue nevus
Neurothekeoma (nerve sheath myxoma)
Malignant peripheral nerve sheath tumor
Cellular blue nevus

Additionally, vertical growth phase tumors associated with particular patterns of radial growth phase tend to differ, and this may affect diagnostic criteria and differential diagnosis. Neurotropism and spindle cell morphology, for example, are much more common in lentiginous melanoma than in superficial spreading melanoma. This controversy will likely be laid to rest as genetic profiling identifies subsets of melanomas that broadly correlate with the traditional clinicopathologic subsets under discussion here (59), providing the opportunity to refine and extend this classification, as molecular targets as selective inhibitors of oncogenic pathways are developed and introduced into practice. Differences among the clinicopathologic subtypes are presented in Table 8-3.

The differences in the differential diagnosis of the different clinicopathologic variants of melanoma constitute another reason to preserve the classification scheme, as also pointed out by Mackie (49). Barnhill and Mihm (67) discussed the differential diagnosis of melanoma in terms of the classification scheme just described, as presented in modified form in Table 8-4.

Despite the importance of the concepts it expresses, the practical application of this classification system is sometimes confusing. For example, one problem in terminology is that the term "nodular melanoma" is reserved for cases of vertical growth phase without a radial growth phase component. However, similar nodules may be seen within plaques of radial growth phase, and the survival of patients with such nodules is the same, when thickness and other prognostic variables are controlled (68). The terms "radial" and "vertical" refer to clinically defined directions of enlargement of the lesions, which are not always intuitively obvious to pathologists. This is because terms that were developed to be descriptive of clinical phenomena are defined in terms of microscopic morphology. In a histologic preparation, the vertical growth phase, which is actually an imperfect sphere, may appear to be more or less circular when cut in cross section. The radial growth phase, which is actually a plaque, may appear more or less linear. Thus, the vertical growth phase may present histologically as a circle with readily apparent radii, while the radial growth phase is a horizontal line. In consequence, the term "horizontal growth phase" has greater intuitive value than the term "radial growth phase" for pathologists.

An additional problem is that the term "radial" growth is often mistakenly considered to be synonymous with a lack of invasion; however, lesions in the radial growth phase may be in situ or superficially invasive. The key feature of the vertical growth phase that is lacking in the superficially invasive component of radial growth phase lesions is the property of expansile, preferential growth in the dermis forming a mass or "tumor"—a swelling in the classic terminology of pathology.

A final consideration is that the term "phase" of tumor progression has temporal implications but its spatial implications are unclear. For example, it is sometimes incorrectly assumed that the vertical growth phase replaces and supplants the radial phase throughout the substance of the lesion. In most lesions, however, the radial and vertical growth phases appear to represent separate "compartments" of the lesion, and the behavior of each is independent of the other. Thus, it is not uncommon for a rapidly growing vertical growth phase nodule to appear within the confines of a radial growth phase lesion that has been clinically stable or very indolent, or that has even been undergoing partial regression.

For these reasons and others, alternate systems have been proposed by some observers to describe these phenomena of tumor progression. Ackerman (69), for example, proposed the terms "plaque stage" and "nodule stage." Although these terms are clinically intuitive and aptly describe the clinical phenomenon of tumor progression for most cases of melanoma, they do not provide a rigorous histologic definition of the nodule stage. Furthermore, the term "plaque" does not have a clear histologic connotation for many pathologists, and some lesions considered to be in the vertical growth phase by the Clark criteria may, confusingly, have a plaque-like rather than nodular configuration clinically and histologically. Acral-lentiginous melanomas, in particular, may be deeply invasive and yet almost completely macular clinically.

A more appropriate terminology to describe the pathology of melanoma might be based primarily on the most essential histologic characteristics of the two phases, or compartments, of tumor progression (32). In such a scheme, which we consider to have descriptive as well as prognostic value, the vertical growth phase in most cases is characterized histologically as well as clinically by the phenomenon of focal swelling or tumor formation, and is therefore termed the "tumorigenic" compartment of the lesion. Because growing intradermal tumoral nodules often exhibit evidence of active cell proliferation (e.g., mitotic figures), the term "mitogenic" also may be a surrogate for the presence of tumorigenic growth potential. The radial growth phase is termed "nontumorigenic," and is divided into in situ and microinvasive categories, recalling that the superficially invasive components of true radial growth phase melanomas neither form expansile nodules nor do they exhibit mitotic activity.

NONTUMORIGENIC MELANOMA (RADIAL GROWTH PHASE)

Most cutaneous melanomas evolve from an initial proliferation of neoplastic melanocytes in the epidermis, as previously discussed. While confined to the epidermis, the proliferation is termed in situ. Just as the nevus cells of a junctional nevus may migrate from the epidermis, so may the neoplastic melanocytes of an in situ melanoma migrate into the papillary dermis. Although this migration of neoplastic melanocytes into the dermis is often termed invasion, it is not necessarily accompanied by acquisition of the capacity to survive, proliferate, or invade vessels or stroma. When the neoplastic melanocytes of a melanoma are present in the dermis, but have not acquired the capacity for proliferation, a tumor or mass lesion is not formed in the dermis, and the lesion may be termed invasive but nontumorigenic, or microinvasive. These nontumorigenic melanomas, with only rare exceptions, are not associated with competence for metastasis. In some rare cases of metastasizing radial growth phase melanomas, additional sections have revealed the presence of a small vertical growth phase, indicating the need for adequate block sampling (70). In other cases, regression has been present and a small tumorigenic or mitogenic focus may have been present in the area of regression (31). The presence of a tumorigenic component, even in a thin melanoma, predicts the existence of some degree of statistical probability of metastasis, the likelihood of which depends also on additional prognostic factors, reviewed in the sections following (31,33,34,71,72). The discussion that follows here of nontumorigenic melanoma also pertains to the nontumorigenic compartment ("adjacent component") of a complex primary melanoma that also has a tumorigenic compartment (vertical growth phase).

Definition. A *nontumorigenic melanoma* is an evolving malignant melanoma that initially presents clinically as a lesion that grows indolently but progressively as a spreading tan, brown, or black patch or plaque in the skin. The lesional cells may be confined to the epidermis (*in situ melanoma* [fig. 8-6]), or they may invade the papillary dermis (*microinvasive melanoma* [fig. 8-7]), but by definition there is no evidence of proliferation in the dermis or of tumor formation. In situ and microinvasive melanomas together constitute the nontumorigenic melanomas. These lesions are also termed *radial growth phase melanomas* (27,44) because in this stage they present clinically as a patch or plaque in the skin which expands more or less along the radii of an imperfect circle (fig. 8-8). When a melanoma progresses to become tumorigenic, the tumorigenic compartment appears as a focal swelling or nodule within the antecedent nontumorigenic compartment, which in general retains its morphologic characteristics, except for the presence of the nodule.

Other terms that have been applied to this stage of melanoma evolution include *precancerous melanosis* (2), *atypical melanocytic hyperplasia* (73), *plaque stage melanoma* (73), *intraepithelial melanocytic neoplasia* or *intraepithelial atypical melanocytic proliferation* (74,75), *melanocytic intraepidermal neoplasia* (76), and *nontumorigenic in situ* or *microinvasive melanoma* (77). Present usage overwhelmingly favors the term *melanoma in situ* for a melanoma that is confined to the epidermis. The most appropriate terminology for lesions that involve the epidermis and dermis has not been agreed upon. Lesions that involve the superficial dermis but do not exhibit tumorigenic proliferation have little or no capacity for metastasis. The existence of a prolonged, readily treatable phase of radial nontumorigenic growth in populations at increased risk for the disease offers a potent rationale for efforts at early diagnosis and treatment of melanoma.

Biologic Behavior. Patterns of proliferation in melanocytic tumors were studied by Carey et al. (78). Using an antibody directed against a paraffin-reactive epitope of the cell cycle (proliferation) marker Ki-67, it was demonstrated that the percentage of reactive lesional melanocytes was very low in the epidermal and dermal compartments of compound melanocytic nevi, but higher in melanomas. Similar findings have been reported by others (79–86). In situ and microinvasive melanomas (radial growth phase) demonstrate substantial numbers of reactive lesional cells within the epidermal compartment. In contrast, the microinvasive cells in the dermis demonstrate low levels of Ki-67 reactivity, similar to nevi. In tumorigenic melanomas, the cells in the dermis often exhibit very high levels of proliferation, and similar high levels are also seen in metastases (78,80,86,87). These data demonstrate that tumorigenic melanomas exhibit evidence of proliferative capacity in the dermis, while proliferation in in situ and microinvasive melanomas is confined to lesional cells in the epidermal compartment. These findings suggest that the phenomenon of microinvasion in melanoma is more closely related to the migration of nevus cells from the

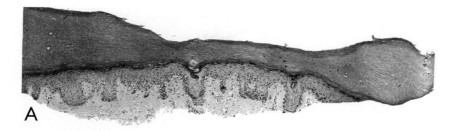

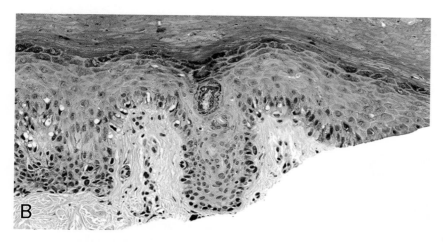

Figure 8-6

MELANOMA IN SITU, ACRAL-LENTIGINOUS TYPE

A,B: Scanning magnification shows a moderately cellular, partly continuous proliferation of nevoid to epithelioid melanocytes along with a dermal-epidermal junction extending to a specimen margin.

C: At higher magnification, the lesional cells show mild to moderate but uniform cytologic atypia in the form of nuclear enlargement and slight hyperchromatism. A few lesional cells extend up into the epidermis in a pagetoid pattern, focally to the stratum corneum. In addition, pigment is present in the keratinocytes in the epidermis and in the stratum corneum.

D: A Melan-A stain demonstrates continuous proliferation of all melanocytes along the dermal-epidermal junction, supporting the diagnosis of melanoma in situ.

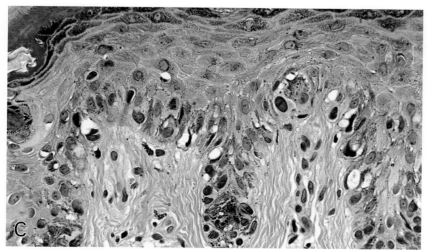

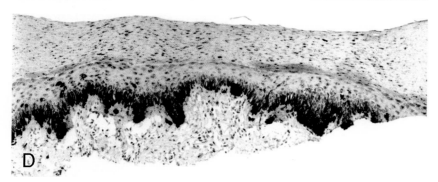

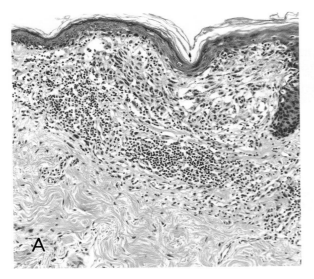

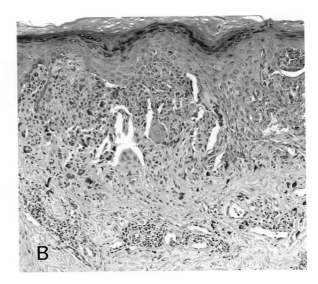

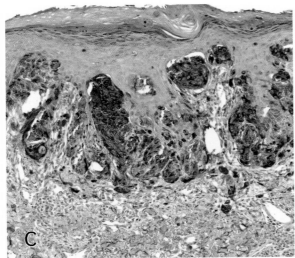

Figure 8-7

**MALIGNANT MELANOMA,
SUPERFICIAL SPREADING TYPE**

A,B: The melanoma is invasive but not tumorigenic, Clark level II, Breslow thickness approximately 0.5 mm.

C: A Melan-A stain shows the cellular proliferation in the epidermis, nests that vary in size and shape, the tendency to pagetoid extension into the epidermis including single cells in the stratum corneum, and the small foci of invasive but nontumorigenic melanoma in the dermis.

Figure 8-8

**NONTUMORIGENIC
MELANOMA
WITH REGRESSION**

The term radial growth phase describes a model of development of a plaque of melanoma which enlarges along radii of an imperfect circle. This lesion is partially "broken up" by regression of the radial growth phase. There is no tumorigenic vertical growth phase nodule.

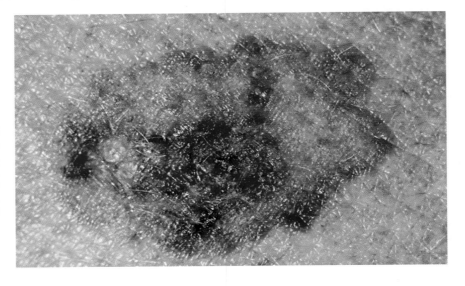

epidermis into the dermis than to the property of destructive and infiltrative invasion as seen in most fully malignant neoplasms. Stated differently, it would appear that radial growth phase melanoma cells are biologically different than vertical growth phase cells, thus accounting for their different patterns of biologic behavior within the dermal layers. Although studies are needed to adequately evaluate the sensitivity, specificity, and predictive value of diagnostic and prognostic testing based on Ki-67, this marker can provide a useful test for potentially tumorigenic melanomas.

Interesting recent work by Lee et al. (88) has demonstrated a significant difference between the intraepidermal components of in situ and invasive melanomas in terms of the prevalence of increased copy numbers of chromosome 1 as determined by interphase cytogenetic studies. The in situ melanomas were similar in copy numbers to nevi and dysplastic nevi, while the intraepithelial components of invasive melanomas showed levels comparable to that of the dermal components and to metastases. These findings suggest that interphase cytogenetics (fluorescent in situ hybridization [FISH]) could be used to identify those in situ melanomas with greater risk of progression. The findings were also considered to support the concept of clonal expansion giving rise to the vertical growth phase lesion.

The phenomenon of invasion of melanoma cells from the epidermis into the dermis was studied in vitro in epidermal reconstructs by Hsu et al. (89). Epidermal reconstructs are created by applying a layer of cultured keratinocytes to a substrate of collagen containing an admixture of fibroblasts. The cultured keratinocytes spread over the substratum and spontaneously differentiate to form stratified squamous epithelium. When neoplastic melanocytes from a radial growth phase-like cell line were admixed with the keratinocyte culture, they proliferated exclusively in the epidermal layer of the reconstruct, without invading the underlying dermis. Based on evidence that the integrin subunit, beta3, is overexpressed in tumorigenic melanoma (vertical growth phase), compared to nontumorigenic (radial growth phase) melanoma (90), the same radial growth phase-like (weakly tumorigenic) cell line was then transfected with the beta3

integrin gene using an adenovirus vector. When the transfected melanoma cells were admixed with the keratinocyte cell line and applied to the artificial epidermis, they proliferated extensively within the artificial epidermis but also invaded and proliferated within the artificial dermis. The integrin dimer alphavbeta3 has previously been shown in vitro to have the property of protecting cells against programmed cell death (apoptosis) when bound to an appropriate cell matrix ligand. Partially hydrolyzed collagen fibers (like certain other cell matrix molecules such as vitronectin) can provide an appropriate ligand. The melanoma cells proliferating in the artificial skin reconstruct were then evaluated by an in situ test for apoptosis (in situ end labeling [ISEL]). In the untransfected cell line, the lesional cells underwent apoptosis upon entering the dermis. In the same cell line after beta3 transfection, the lesional cells in the artificial dermis showed no evidence of apoptosis and survived to infiltrate the dermal collagen. These findings are consistent with the hypothesis that protection from apoptosis plays a permissive (perhaps necessary, but not sufficient) role in the process of microinvasion.

In this and other studies, it has been demonstrated that overexpression of functional alphavbeta3 in radial growth phase primary melanoma cells: 1) promotes both anchorage-dependent and -independent growth; 2) initiates invasive growth from the epidermis into the dermis in three-dimensional skin reconstructs; 3) prevents apoptosis of invading cells (91); 4) increases tumor growth in vivo (89); and 5) activates proteases (92,93). Thus, it may be concluded that alphavbeta3 serves diverse biologic functions during the progression from the nontumorigenic radial growth phase to the tumorigenic and invasive vertical growth phase primary melanoma. Beta3 integrin expression could have some potential utility as a diagnostic test for tumorigenic melanoma. However, some tumorigenic melanomas are negative and a few nontumorigenic melanomas are positive for this antigen, and in addition, Spitz nevi are commonly reactive (90,94). Thus, beta3 integrin does not in itself provide a perfect marker for tumorigenicity. It does, however, provide a molecular basis for the more pragmatic diagnostic concepts of tumorigenic and nontumorigenic melanoma, and the experimental findings are consistent with the notion that transition of radial growth phase to vertical growth phase melanoma cells involves clonal evolution to a more aggressive molecular phenotype.

Clinical Features and Gross Findings. Four major clinical characteristics have been described as the "ABCD" criteria for melanoma diagnosis. These apply in particular to the superficial nontumorigenic phase of melanoma growth (figs. 8-2, 8-5, 8-8) (95). The features are typically best developed in microinvasive radial growth phase melanomas, but also are seen in some in situ melanomas as well.

"A" Stands for Asymmetry. Melanomas are not symmetric about any axis, in contrast to most benign lesions, which are round or oval. Melanomas have an irregular map-like configuration, like the contour of a small island.

"B" Stands for Border Irregularity. The "coastline" of the lesion is conspicuously irregular and indented. A "notch" in the border is often seen. In some lesions, especially lentigo maligna melanomas and acral-lentiginous melanomas (see sections following), the margin is indefinite or "hazy," but the most common form of melanoma (superficial spreading melanoma) has a sharply demarcated, slightly raised edge.

"C" Stands for Color Variegation. Unlike many benign lesions, most melanomas are composed of more than one color, including light brown, tan, dark brown, and, most importantly, black and blue-black attributable to melanin pigment located high in the epidermis (black) or the dermis (blue-black). In addition, areas of erythema and of gray-white scale may be observed due to associated inflammation, and gray or slate-blue may be seen in areas of partial regression (leading to the frequently observed and classic "red, white, and blue" colors of melanoma).

"D" Stands for Diameter. Melanomas are larger, on average, than common acquired nevi and dysplastic nevi, although there is some overlap in size, especially with the latter. Melanoma is not often recognized when less than 4 mm in diameter, and most lesions, including in situ melanomas, are larger than 10 mm. Smaller lesions are currently being excised and are challenging both clinically and histologically (96,97). Nevi, and especially dysplastic nevi, overlap with radial growth phase melanoma

not only in terms of size but also in many of the other morphologic criteria discussed here.

To the ABCD criteria, Fitzpatrick added *"E"* for *elevation* (98). Although melanomas in situ may be impalpable and completely flat to side-lighting, the process of invasion into the dermis usually imparts some degree of thickening to the lesion, so that invasive radial growth phase melanomas are almost always at least slightly raised. Perhaps an additional and even more relevant meaning for the letter E would be "evolution," as malignant lesions, unlike benign ones, tend to change over time. For observers not familiar with the significance of the ABCD signs, or for lesions that occasionally do not fully adhere to these trends, clinical recognition of change as an indicator of inexorable progression may be life-saving. More recently, the concept of the "ugly duckling", or of a mole that is "out of step" with a patient's other moles, has been emphasized for lay persons and also for professionals. A recent publication demonstrated promising agreement among observers for this sign (99).

It is generally believed that a large but unknown percentage of in situ melanomas grow inexorably and progress to the microinvasive radial growth phase. It is also possible that a significant but unknown percentage of these lesions do not progress (100). In situ and microinvasive melanomas in the radial growth phase are rendered biologically benign upon complete excision in the sense that they generally are incapable of metastasis (72,101). Similarly, it is likely, although not proven, that most microinvasive melanomas ultimately progress further to tumorigenic vertical growth phase melanoma, with the focal emergence of a nodule in the plaque lesion and, potentially, the acquisition of competence for metastasis. Such progression may be delayed for many months or, commonly, years. When a nodule does emerge, however, its subsequent enlargement and progression may be rapid. In this regard, it is of interest that although melanoma in the radial phase of growth provides ample clinical clues (the ABCD, as discussed above) over considerable intervals of time as to its biologic potential, onset of vertical growth in untreated lesions even of the size of a split pea may portend mortality for some patients.

It is possible that some radial growth phase melanomas would never progress to vertical growth phase, even if their natural history had not been interrupted by excision (100,102). Because in situ melanomas are not associated with metastases (with vanishingly rare and controversial exceptions), we use the diagnostic term "melanoma in situ" rather than "malignant melanoma in situ," and distinguish these lesions carefully from the more dangerous tumorigenic and potentially malignant melanomas that enter the vertical growth phase. Invasive lesions that lack the tumorigenic vertical growth phase exhibit favorable prognostic characteristics similar to melanoma in situ, and for this reason they are termed microinvasive melanomas. By analogy with other tumor systems, such as carcinoma of the uterine cervix (103), these lesions, although invasive, are considered to share the same highly favorable prognosis as the more strictly in situ lesions.

Melanomas in situ usually exhibit some of the ABCD criteria, but the appearances are often considerably more subtle than those of invasive radial growth phase lesions, and may overlap with junctional dysplastic nevi. Most of these in situ lesions are asymptomatic, with no history of change, and they are commonly found incidentally in the course of examination for other conditions. Although change cannot always be documented, a history of change, when present, is often the only feature that calls attention to a possible in situ melanoma. Without historic or photographic documentation of change, the diagnosis may be impossible except by excision and histologic examination. Many microinvasive melanomas are also asymptomatic, with no history of change, and like the in situ melanomas, may be diagnosed incidentally by an alert physician or acquaintance. Lesions are often called to the attention of physicians because the patient has noticed a change in one or all of the parameters described above—with a lesion becoming more irregular, darker and/or more variegated, or larger. The lesion appears different from a patient's other moles, a phenomenon that has been called the "ugly duckling" sign (99). Occasionally, the lesion becomes pruritic. Although the absence of change or other symptomatology does not rule out melanoma, a history of changing size, shape, color, or sensation in a pigmented lesion should never be ignored.

Although the clinical appearance may be highly characteristic, radial growth phase in situ or microinvasive melanoma can be diagnosed with certainty only by an adequate biopsy, which is required as well for accurate microstaging and prognostication. Optimally, a complete excisional biopsy should be done for diagnosis and microstaging, and this should be planned to permit re-excision later, if necessary, for definitive treatment. A punch biopsy is acceptable in lesions that are very large, in cosmetically sensitive areas, or near important organs, and should be done in the thickest or darkest areas of a flat lesion. Curettage and superficial shave biopsy generally do not preserve anatomic relationships sufficiently to permit accurate microstaging, and should be avoided if possible in situations where a diagnosis of melanoma is suspected; a deep shave biopsy can be completely satisfactory.

Microscopic Findings. The diagnosis of primary malignant melanoma depends on the assessment of both architectural and cytologic features. The architectural changes involve not only the lesional cells, but also neighboring cells, including both epidermal keratinocytes and dermal stromal cells. The latter include lymphocytes and other inflammatory cells, fibroblasts, and endothelial cells. The architectural features are best appreciated at scanning magnification, which typically shows a broad, asymmetric lesion with changes confined to the epidermis or papillary dermis. A pattern of somewhat irregular (asymmetric) epithelial thickening and thinning, in conjunction with a band-like lymphocytic infiltrate and fibroplasia in the papillary dermis, is highly characteristic of microinvasive melanoma. In situ melanomas may show a similar epidermal reaction, but there may be little or no host response or other alteration in the dermis. In a recent study of the efficacy of histologic criteria in melanoma based on metastasizing cases compared to control nevi, cytologic atypia, dermal lymphocytic infiltrate, asymmetry, size greater than 6 mm, and absence of maturation were highly sensitive features (present in over 90 percent of melanomas), while absence of maturation, mitoses, necrosis, asymmetric melanin, suprabasal melanocytes, and melanin in deep cells were highly specific (absent in over 90 percent of benign nevi) (104).

Most, but not all, melanomas are characterized by a relatively large lesional diameter. In the original presentation of the ABCD criteria, the letter D stood for size greater than 6 mm (95). Although large size is still the rule, melanomas today are commonly diagnosed when less than 6 mm in diameter (97,105). Lesions larger than 1 cm in diameter are likely to be either dysplastic nevi, congenital pattern nevi, or melanomas. Paradoxically, thicker melanomas that are entirely in the tumorigenic vertical growth phase (nodular melanomas) may be smaller than thinner lesions in the nontumorigenic radial growth phase because lateral or horizontal spread is a characteristic primarily of the nontumorigenic radial growth phase compartment. The size of any given lesion is primarily a clinical attribute. An impression of size, however, can also be gleaned from the microscopic sections, although many ovoid lesions are sectioned across their short axes, thus providing a minimal estimate of lesional diameter based on the tissue profile alone.

A tendency to asymmetry characterizes most nontumorigenic melanomas (tumorigenic melanomas may be as symmetric as any benign lesion). Asymmetry is present when half of the lesion to one side of an imaginary line formed at the center and perpendicular to the epidermis is not a mirror image of the other half (fig. 8-9) (106). This asymmetry may be at the level of the silhouette of the entire lesion, or it may be at the cytologic level. For example, the cells may be smaller in some areas of the lesion than in others. Commonly, the presence of a focus of invasion, with or without tumorigenic proliferation, contributes to an asymmetric appearance in an otherwise in situ or microinvasive lesion. Asymmetry of melanin distribution is a readily recognized and highly sensitive criterion for melanoma (104). Asymmetry of the immune response, including regression, may also be observed. The earliest, predominantly in situ lesions may not exhibit substantial asymmetry. In addition, as Okun (107) has emphasized, many melanomas may appear quite symmetric in particular section planes. In our experience, many benign lesions, such as cellular blue nevi and some Spitz nevi, may lack symmetry at

the silhouette level although less often at the cytologic level.

The *pagetoid* and *lentiginous patterns* of proliferation constitute two major distribution patterns of melanoma cells in the epidermis; many melanomas exhibit mixed features. At the periphery of a plaque of melanoma, the lesional cells may be mainly basal, especially in the lentiginous variant of melanoma (lentigo maligna and acral lentiginous melanoma). The lentiginous pattern is characterized by uniformly atypical, basally located melanocytes arranged in contiguity with one another, constituting a pattern termed "continuous" or "confluent" uniform cytologic atypia (figs. 8-9, 8-10). In most melanomas, however, there is some evidence of extension into the epidermis in a "pagetoid" pattern centrally, and this is especially marked in melanomas of the superficial spreading type (fig. 8-11).

In the epidermis of a predominantly pagetoid melanoma, even at scanning magnification, there is an increased number of considerably enlarged, rather pale melanocytes, arranged singly and in small groups near the dermal-epidermal junction, and extending upward into the epidermis, usually into the stratum corneum. This pattern is termed pagetoid because of its resemblance to mammary or extramammary Paget disease (27). Distinguishing features of the pagetoid pattern were discussed more than 20 years ago by Clark (27) and McGovern (28). Clark and Mihm (50) clearly described the lentiginous patterns of lentigo maligna melanomas. The cytologic attributes of lentiginous and pagetoid melanomas were also discussed by Mishima (108), who noted structural and other similarities between the lesional cells of lentiginous melanomas and melanocytes (both variably dendritic), while relating the cells of pagetoid melanomas to nevus cells (both more rounded to epithelioid).

Pagetoid melanocytic proliferation is defined as an upward extension of melanocytes, singly or in groups, into the epidermis (fig. 8-11) (109). Such proliferation may be seen in melanomas or in nevi. In melanoma, the pagetoid proliferation is composed of uniformly atypical melanocytes. It is characterized in terms of its height of extension into the epidermis (high level or lower level), and in terms of its extent across the breadth of the lesion. In our practice, we consider a high

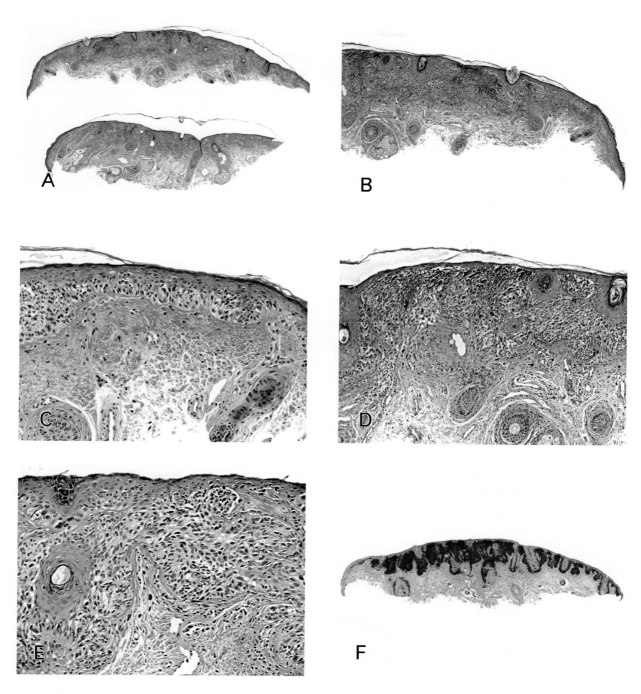

Figure 8-9

MALIGNANT MELANOMA, LENTIGO MALIGNA TYPE

A,B: This lesion, from the cheek of a 48-year-old man, is characterized at low power by asymmetric proliferations of melanocytes and reactive keratinocytes.

C: Higher magnification shows areas of basal proliferation of single cells.

D,E: Other more cellular and confluent areas are seen.

F: A stain for the melanocytic markers Melan-A and tyrosinase highlights these features.

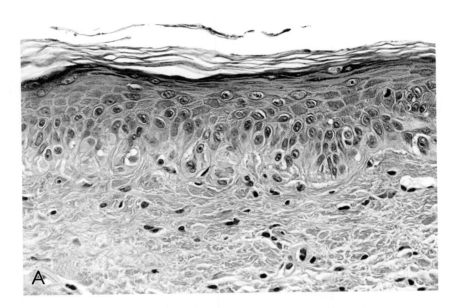

Figure 8-10

MELANOMA IN SITU, LENTIGINOUS PATTERN, WITH CONTINUOUS BASAL PROLIFERATION (LENTIGO MALIGNA MELANOMA)

A: The hematoxylin and eosin (H&E) stain shows an increased number of uniformly although moderately atypical melanocytes along the dermal-epidermal junction.

B,C: Distinction between atypical melanocytes and reactive or dysplastic basal keratinocytes may be difficult. Melan-A stain demonstrates continuous proliferation along the junction, extending close to the margin (C).

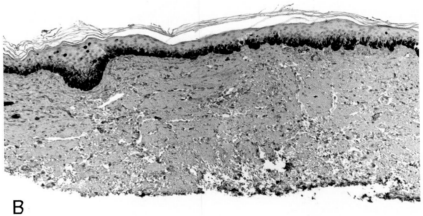

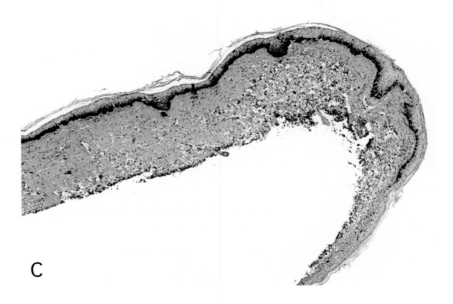

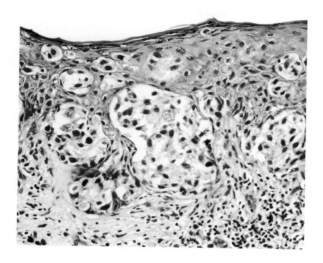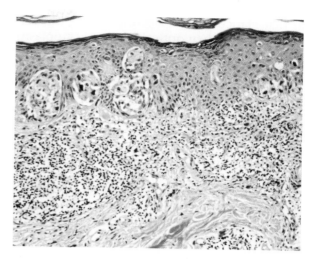

Figure 8-11

MALIGNANT MELANOMA, PAGETOID PATTERN (SUPERFICIAL SPREADING MELANOMA)

Left: There is an increased number of uniformly atypical epithelioid melanocytes, arranged singly and in nests. High magnification demonstrates the uniform atypia of the lesional cells. The atypia is mild to moderate in this example. Pagetoid proliferation is extensive within this high power field, and it extends to a high level of the epidermis, the stratum granulosum in this example.

Right: A few similar cells are present in the dermis in relation to a dense lichenoid lymphocytic infiltrate.

level and extensive pagetoid proliferation of uniformly atypical melanocytes to be a strong indicator of melanoma. High level extension is defined as extension into the stratum granulosum or especially into the stratum corneum. Extensive pagetoid proliferation is defined as the presence of melanocytes that extend into the epidermis over one high-power field or more within the lesion. Pagetoid proliferation of the epidermis by melanocytes, also termed "buckshot scatter," is regarded by some as being essential for the confident histopathologic diagnosis of primary cutaneous melanoma, but it is neither perfectly sensitive, nor perfectly specific. Fallowfield and Cook (110) found conspicuous pagetoid infiltration in 32.1 percent of 340 melanomas, while occasional melanocytes were observed within the stratum spinosum in a further 23.5 percent of cases. No pagetoid infiltration, however, could be seen in 44.4 percent. The finding of pagetoid infiltration of the epidermis was most common within in situ or thin horizontal growth phase melanomas, and was conspicuous in only one third of cases. While its presence is useful in the diagnosis of melanoma, its absence should not preclude it.

Pagetoid melanocytic proliferation (generally low level and generally not extensive)

can be seen in benign lesions, especially Spitz nevi, often but not exclusively in children, and in acral nevi (111–114). Nonmelanocytic neoplasms that sometimes mimic melanoma include mammary and extramammary Paget disease, pagetoid squamous cell carcinoma, clear cells of Toker and pagetoid dyskeratosis (which represent pale and vacuolated keratinocytes, respectively), clear cell papulosis (which is a rare childhood condition characterized by multiple white papules in which the pagetoid cells may react in marker studies similarly to those of Paget disease but are cytologically benign), sebaceous carcinoma, Merkel cell carcinoma, eccrine porocarcinoma, cutaneous T-cell lymphoma, and histiocytosis X. These can be recognized by the associated morphology of the respective conditions, if necessary with the aid of immunohistochemical findings as summarized recently by Kohler et al. (115). Staining with syndecan-1, a cell surface proteoglycan cell-cell and cell-matrix adhesion molecule which labels cells of Paget disease and of pagetoid squamous cell carcinoma in situ but not those of melanoma in situ, has recently been suggested as a discriminatory marker (116). Glycogenated keratinocytes appear as cells with a perinuclear clear space surrounded by a mantle of cytoplasm, and thus at first glance mimic pagetoid cells. However, the latter owe their optical clarity to cytoplasm that intimately surrounds the nucleus, not to artifactual cytoplasmic retraction. Finally, even normal basally located melanocytes may appear pagetoid when rete ridges are cut tangentially or section orientation deviates from true perpendicular sections.

As already noted, pagetoid proliferations must be interpreted with caution. In a study of the short-term effects of UV light on melanocytic nevi, increased melanocytes above the dermal-epidermal junction were observed in 7 of 12 nevi, simulating a melanoma in 3 nevi (117). In addition, UV irradiation of nevi may induce increased expression of HMB45, an activation marker for melanocytes; increased expression of proliferation markers including Ki-67 and topoisomerase II alpha; and occasional mitotic figures. In addition, there is increased expression of p21 and p53, probably related to growth control and DNA repair. Thus, irradiated nevi may express a number of markers of melanoma in situ, suggesting that pagetoid proliferation, even when associated with mitotic activity and Ki-67 expression, should be interpreted with caution, especially when there is a possibility of recent sun exposure. Haupt and Stern (112,118) have concluded that factors favoring melanoma in a pagetoid melanocytic proliferation include diffuse and dense extension over a wide area, prominent melanocytic atypia, and pagetoid melanocytic proliferation without an underlying junctional melanocytic component ("free-floating pagetoid melanosis"). These authors concluded, and we agree, that pagetoid melanocytic proliferation should alert the pathologist to the possibility of melanoma but does not of necessity require a malignant interpretation. The final interpretation of a melanocytic lesion requires evaluation of all the pertinent histologic and clinical findings.

The origin of the term lentiginous melanocytic proliferation has been discussed previously (see Lentigo Simplex, chapter 2). Briefly, the term lentiginous is derived from the clinical appearance of simple lentigines as small ovoid or lens-like lesions. This clinical impression of a lens or perhaps of a lentil-like seed has been transformed rather nonintuitively into a histologic appearance that, to some extent, recapitulates

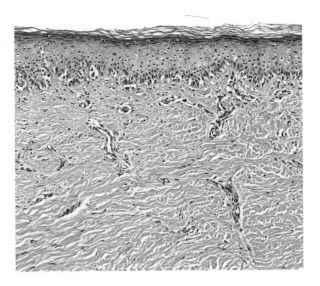

Figure 8-12

MELANOMA IN SITU, LENTIGINOUS PATTERN

There is an increased number of uniform, although mildly atypical, melanocytes forming a line along the dermal-epidermal junction. The cells are "contiguous" with one another, and the proliferation is "continuous."

that of the simple lentigo, the most primitive melanocytic lesion. The basic characteristic of the lentiginous pattern is the proliferation of single melanocytes along the dermal-epidermal junction, more or less replacing the basal layer of keratinocytes (fig. 8-12) (109). This proliferation may be "contiguous" (cells are in contact) or "noncontiguous" (they are separated by keratinocytes). The proliferation may also be "continuous" along the dermoepidermal junction, or "noncontinuous." In a simple lentigo, there is associated elongation of the rete ridges, but this rete ridge elongation is not seen in all lentiginous lesions. The proliferation in a simple lentigo is contiguous near the tips and sides of the elongated rete, but is typically not continuous from one rete to the next, usually sparing the suprapapillary plate region. In an actinic lentigo, the proliferation is usually noncontiguous, and noncontinuous. In contrast, the epidermal rete ridge pattern is typically effaced in lentigo maligna melanoma, a prototypic form of lentiginous melanoma, and the proliferation is both contiguous and continuous. In acral-lentiginous melanoma the epidermis is usually irregularly thickened, with contiguous and continuous

Table 8-5

PAGETOID AND LENTIGINOUS MELANOMAS: NONTUMORIGENIC COMPARTMENT

Attribute	Pagetoid Melanoma	Lentiginous Melanomas
Clinical/pathologic variants	SSM[a]	LMM, ALM, MLM
Border of lesion	Often palpable	Often impalpable
Cell size	Large, abundant cytoplasm	Smaller, nevoid, dendritic
Pigment	Scant, "dusty"	Often abundant, coarse granules
Cell arrangement	Pagetoid, scattered in epidermis	Contiguous and continuous, basal
Nuclear atypia	Moderate to severe	Often mild to moderate
Dermal component	Often epithelioid, sometimes nevoid	Usually epithelioid, often nevoid
Associated nevus	Frequent	Uncommon

[a]SSM = superficial spreading melanoma; LMM = lentigo maligna melanoma; ALM = acral-lentiginous melanoma; MLM = mucosal-lentiginous melanoma.

lentiginous melanocytic proliferation along the dermal-epidermal junction. A continuous and contiguous proliferation of melanocytes along the junction is often referred to as a "confluent proliferation" and is an important sign of melanoma in situ (figs. 8-6, 8-9, 8-10, 8-12). Often, particularly in regions where the melanoma is invasive, there will be foci of pagetoid proliferation in an otherwise lentiginous melanoma. The lentiginous pattern is usually best seen at the periphery of the lesion. Some differences between pagetoid and lentiginous melanomas are summarized in Table 8-5.

As was emphasized by Maize and Ackerman (119), single cells usually predominate over nests in the epidermal component of small (presumably early) melanomas, while nests predominate in larger, more fully evolved lesions. These authors have also emphasized the "poor circumscription" of melanomas in the epidermis, meaning that the last lesional cells at the borders are arranged as single cells rather than as nests. Okun (120) has emphasized, however, that many melanomas do not satisfy this criterion, and poor circumscription was not a specific or sensitive finding in a recent diagnostic study (104).

Cytologic Findings. Cytologic features in terms of the architecture of their distribution, in our opinion, are of critical importance for the accurate diagnosis of melanoma.

Presence of Uniformly (Monotonously) Atypical Melanocytes. At high magnification, lesional melanocytes (melanoma cells) are enlarged and often have abundant rounded or polygonal epithelioid cytoplasm containing finely divided "dusty" or "cloudy" melanin pigment, especially in the most common of the variant patterns of melanoma, the superficial spreading variant. In contrast to the random cytologic atypia that characterizes dysplastic nevi (see chapter 7), in our experience melanomas are characterized by uniform atypia, which we define as cytologic atypia involving 50 percent or more of the lesional cells (it is often considerably greater). The cells that do not meet the threshold of atypia nevertheless tend to resemble the more atypical cells in their overall nuclear and cytologic characteristics, as if they are part of the same neoplastic clone.

Cytologic atypia is defined as in dysplastic or other atypical nevi in terms of the following nuclear features: nuclear enlargement by comparison with basal keratinocytes, nuclear membrane irregularity in contour or caliber, nuclear hyperchromatism, clumping or irregularity of nuclear chromatin, and eosinophilic or amphophilic macronucleoli. These nuclei may also be described as pleomorphic, in that there tends to be variation in size, shape, and chromatin pattern. The term "uniform" thus does not indicate uniformity of shape, but rather a monotonous single population of atypical cells within which there is variation (pleomorphism) in the context of sufficient overall similarity to indicate that this is a single cell population. The lesional cells are pleomorphic, but they are uniformly, or monotonously, so, in contrast to the randomly scattered atypical cells that may be seen in some benign conditions, especially the random atypia that characterizes dysplastic nevi (figs. 8-13, 8-14).

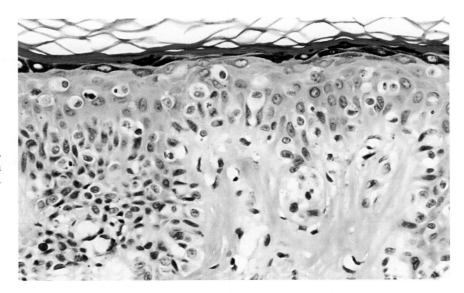

Figure 8-13

MELANOMA IN SITU, PAGETOID PATTERN

Pagetoid melanocytic pro-liferation with moderate uniform atypia (melanoma in situ, superficial spreading type).

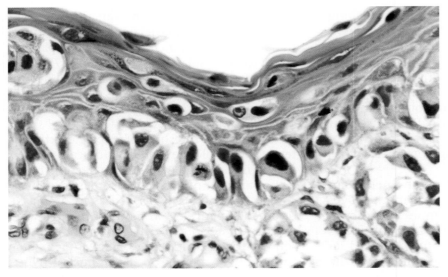

Figure 8-14

MELANOMA IN SITU, PAGETOID PATTERN

Pagetoid melanocytic prolif-eration with severe uniform atypia and intraepidermal lesion-al cell mitosis (melanoma in situ, superficial spreading type).

Contiguous Proliferation in the Epidermis of Uniformly Atypical Melanocytes (Melanoma Cells). Contiguous proliferation (also referred to as confluent proliferation or fusion of nests) is defined as the presence of melanocytes whose cell bodies are in contiguity, or touching one another. This important property differentiates benign and malignant melanocytic neoplasms from normal melanocytes and melanocytic hyperplasia. Contiguous proliferation may be present in nevi and melanomas, but is more prominent in the latter, wherein the prolifera-tion is not only contiguous but also continuous (see next paragraph). Especially prominent in

lentiginous melanomas, contiguous prolifera-tion is present when the uniformly atypical le-sional melanocytes defined above are in contact with one another (figs. 8-9, 8-10, 8-12).

Continuous Proliferation of Melanoma Cells. In nevi, the contiguous proliferation tends to be discontinuous, typically present at the tips and sides of rete ridges, but sparing the epidermis above the dermal papillae (see figs. 6-3, 6-4, 6-6). In melanomas, the proliferation is continuous over much of the breadth of the lesion, i.e., the proliferation tends to be both contiguous (or confluent) and continuous (figs. 8-9, 8-10, 8-12). Contiguous and continuous proliferation along the dermal-epidermal junction for several rete ridges or more is considered to be a very strong indicator of evolving or established melanoma in situ. Along with high-level and extensive pagetoid proliferation, extensive continuous basal proliferation of atypical melanocytes is one of the two fundamental architectural patterns that differentiate nevi from melanomas.

Mitotic Activity of Lesional Melanocytes in the Epidermis. Based on our unpublished experience, mitotic figures are seen within the epidermal compartment in approximately one third of in situ or microinvasive (radial growth phase) melanomas (fig. 8-14). Mitotic figures in the epidermis may also be seen in some nevi, notably Spitz nevi and pigmented spindle cell nevi (Reed nevi). When present in the dermis in a melanoma, mitotic figures, by definition, indicate the presence of at least an early vertical growth phase compartment. Again, however, dermal mitoses may be seen in Spitz nevi and less often in other benign nevi. Mitotic figures in the dermis are absent in most nontumorigenic melanomas, and when present, are indicative of the presence of nontumorigenic (mitogenic) vertical growth phase.

Lack of Maturation. The lack of maturation of invasive melanoma cells with vertical descent within the dermis is of considerable value in diagnosis. In contrast to the dermal cells of compound nevi, the cells in melanomas tend to resemble the cells in the epidermis, and do not undergo maturation or reduction in size upon descent into the dermis. Thus, they exhibit uniform cytologic atypia in terms of cellular and nuclear enlargement as discussed above in relation to the junctional component (fig. 8-15). Such absence of maturation is generally present in both nontumorigenic and tumorigenic melanomas.

Characteristic Epidermal and Stromal Features of Nontumorigenic Melanomas. An epidermal reaction is usually present in melanomas of the superficial spreading type, resulting in irregular thickening and thinning of the epidermis, associated with the presence of a variably cellular proliferation of uniformly atypical lesional melanocytes and asymmetrically distributed stromal responses (fig. 8-16). Similar appearances are seen in acral-lentiginous and mucosal-lentiginous melanomas. In lentigo maligna melanoma, by contrast, the initially atrophic epidermis

within which these lesions occur tends not to be altered by the presence of the melanoma. In more advanced lesions, however, there may be progression to a larger melanoma cell type, with pagetoid proliferation in the epidermis and often with at least microinvasive extension into the dermis. In such lesions, the epidermis often becomes irregularly hyperplastic. The epidermal layer may also be thickened in certain nevi, such as Spitz nevi. It has recently been emphasized that melanoma cells tend to replace, efface, and "consume" the lowermost layers of the thickened epidermis, whereas Spitz nevus cells do not (fig. 8-17) (121). Basal proliferation of neoplastic melanocytes with replacement of the basal layer and its attachments to the dermis may account for another abnormality at the dermal-epidermal junction often observed in nontumorigenic melanoma, namely that of clefting artifact, which also may be observed in predominantly in situ proliferations as well as in tumorigenic melanomas (fig. 8-17) (122).

Characteristic Stromal Changes of Invasive Melanoma. The stroma of melanoma in situ may be completely unaltered compared to adjacent uninvolved skin. However, especially when microinvasion is present, and also in some apparently strictly in situ lesions, there may be a vigorous response in the papillary dermis characterized by diffuse fibroplasia, with a patchy to band-like lymphocytic response and scattered melanophages. The patterns of stromal response were characterized by Clark as "fibroplasia with a plaque-like lymphocytic infiltrate" (fig. 8-18), and "diffuse eosinophilic fibroplasia" (fig. 8-19) (123). The lymphocytic response may disrupt the basal lamina and obscure the lesional melanocytes, especially in mucosal and acral melanomas, so that a diagnosis of a lichenoid keratosis or other dermatosis may be mistakenly made.

Regression of Melanoma. A common and fascinating feature of melanoma that is of diagnostic and prognostic importance is the frequent finding of partial or complete immunologic regression (124). Clinically, regression usually occurs in the radial growth phase and results in the appearance of irregular geographic areas where pigment is lost clinically. In these areas, the brown-black color of the evolving neoplasm is replaced by red colors signifying inflammation,

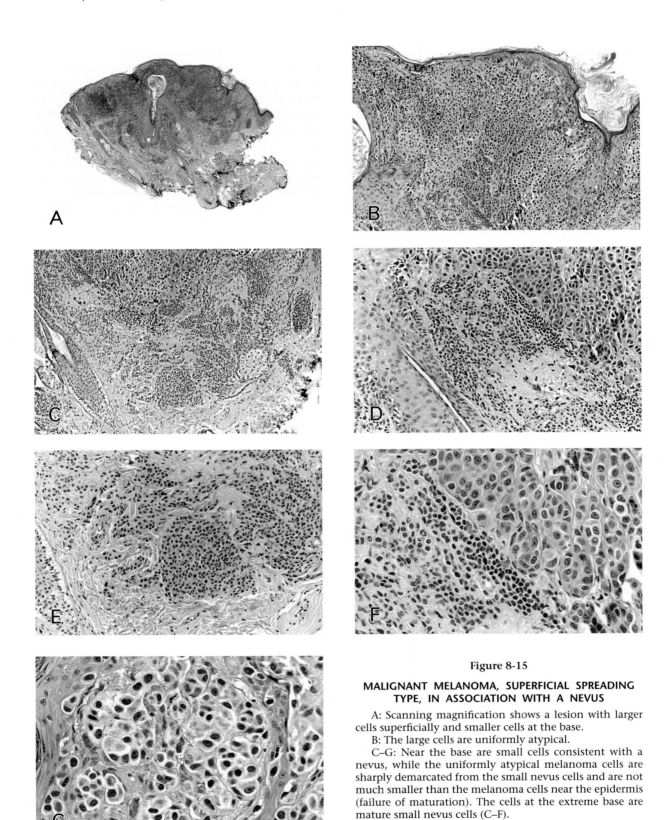

Figure 8-15

MALIGNANT MELANOMA, SUPERFICIAL SPREADING TYPE, IN ASSOCIATION WITH A NEVUS

A: Scanning magnification shows a lesion with larger cells superficially and smaller cells at the base.

B: The large cells are uniformly atypical.

C–G: Near the base are small cells consistent with a nevus, while the uniformly atypical melanoma cells are sharply demarcated from the small nevus cells and are not much smaller than the melanoma cells near the epidermis (failure of maturation). The cells at the extreme base are mature small nevus cells (C–F).

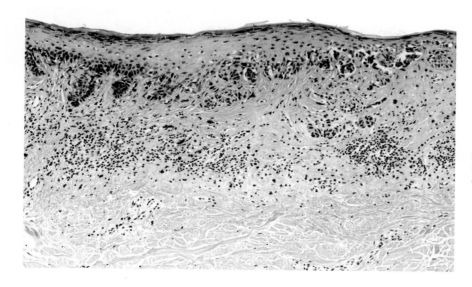

Figure 8-16

EPIDERMAL REACTION IN A MELANOMA

Irregular thickening and thinning of the epidermis in a superficial spreading melanoma occurring in a 72-year-old man.

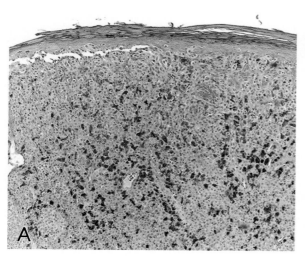

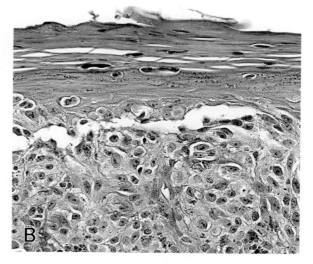

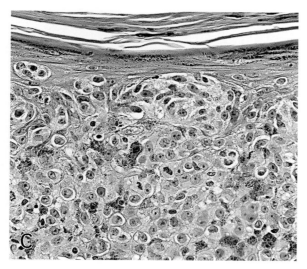

Figure 8-17

"CONSUMPTION OF THE EPIDERMIS" AND CLEFTING IN A MELANOMA

A,B: At the left of the field there is clefting artifact between the epidermis and the dermal tumor. At the right of A, there is thinning of the epidermis with attenuation of the basal and suprabasal layers.

C: There is a loss of rete ridges in an area of direct contact with the neoplastic melanocytes.

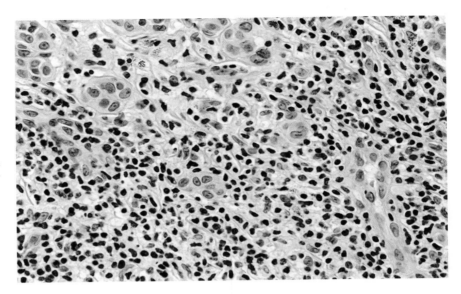

Figure 8-18

**REGRESSION IN
A MELANOMA**

This melanoma exhibits a plaque-like lymphocytic infiltrate.

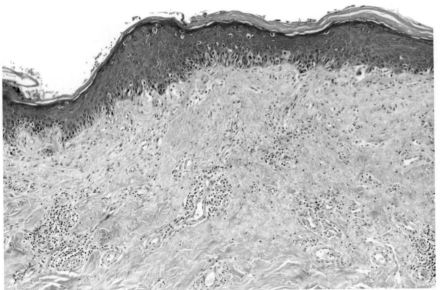

Figure 8-19

**DIFFUSE EOSINOPHILIC
FIBROPLASIA IN
A MELANOMA**

There is a stromal response of diffuse eosinophilic fibroplasia in a melanoma. The differential diagnosis could include a scar from a prior biopsy.

white and gray-blue hues signifying dermal fibrosis and pigmentary incontinence, and later by a seeming return toward normal flesh tones and textures. The areas of regression account in good measure for the play of colors ("red, white, and blue") that form an important part of the diagnostic criteria for radial growth phase melanoma. Patients who observe these changes may erroneously feel that their lesion is "breaking up and going away" (fig. 8-20). Unfortunately, it seems that the appearance of regression in the radial growth phase is often accompanied by progression elsewhere in the lesion, sometimes with

the evolution of a vertical growth phase nodule. Regression has paradoxically been determined to be an adverse prognostic variable in some studies, although not in all (34). This attribute may be significant even in melanomas that appear to lack a vertical growth phase (31), perhaps because there was a small vertical growth phase that metastasized before it regressed. In cases with a vertical growth phase, the regression is typically confined to the nontumorigenic radial growth phase compartment, while the tumorigenic compartment continues to progress unaffected by the process of regression.

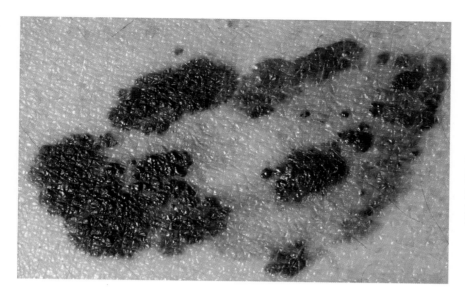

Figure 8-20

REGRESSION IN A SUPERFICIAL SPREADING MELANOMA

The lesions typically begin as a more homogeneous expanding plaque that appears to be "breaking up and going away" in some foci of regression, while progression typically continues in other foci.

Histologically, locally complete regression appears as an area without melanoma cells, but where the papillary dermis is widened by fibrosis and contains a variably dense infiltrate of lymphocytes and melanophages, often with an increased number of dilated and thick-walled blood vessels (fig. 8-21). Typically, there is residual in situ or microinvasive melanoma to one side or both sides of the area of regression. These changes appear to represent the residual stromal "footprint" of the regressed portion of the melanoma—the stromal "fibroplasia with a plaque-like lymphocytic infiltrate and diffuse eosinophilic fibroplasia" of Clark et al. (123, 125). When a vertical growth phase is present in a radial growth phase melanoma that has undergone partial regression, it is often located within or adjacent to the area of regression. A portion of the neoplasm, often including the vertical growth phase, may become separated from the remainder of the radial growth phase as a result of this regression. Occasionally, this phenomenon leads clinicians and pathologists alike into the mistaken belief that this separated tumorigenic vertical growth phase nodule is a satellite metastasis. True satellites, however, are separated from components of the primary tumor by a region of normal stroma.

These are occasional examples of lesions that appear to represent completely regressed melanomas, and sometimes these lesions are discovered as a result of finding metastatic melanoma in a regional lymph node. We have also observed similar lesions in patients who have not had metastases, but it is difficult in these circumstances to differentiate a putative regressed primary melanoma from a regressed benign lesion or from a patch of postinflammatory hyperpigmentation. In some of these cases, the patients have described clearly an irregular, asymmetric, brown-black lesion that became fragmented and then disappeared. This history, in combination with the histologic findings discussed above, is virtually diagnostic of regressed melanoma in our opinion. Unless residual melanoma cells are found focally, however, the differential diagnosis could include other regressed pigmented lesions, including dysplastic nevi and pigmented keratoses, or possibly a postinflammatory pigmentary alteration. We have prospectively diagnosed and followed several patients with such lesions, and their clinical courses have been benign in most cases. Occasional patients do develop metastases in prospective follow-up of these putative regressed primary melanomas. This may suggest that a small tumorigenic component was present in the area of regression, and that it had metastasized before the regression occurred. It is possible, indeed likely, that there may be many cases of regressed melanoma that never come to the attention of patients or physicians, but there is no evidence either for or against this speculation.

The examples mentioned above represent apparent partial or complete regression of the nontumorigenic radial growth phase compartment

Melanocytic Tumors of the Skin

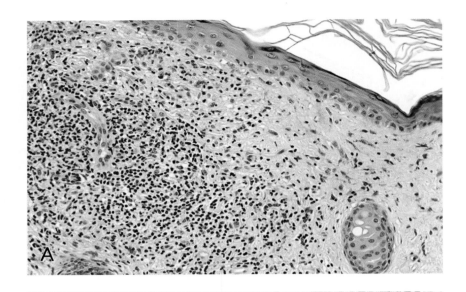

Figure 8-21

REGRESSION IN A MELANOMA

A: There is diffuse fibroplasia with a dense lymphocytic response in the dermis in this melanoma from the arm of a 49-year-old woman.

B: At top left are a few neoplastic melanocytes in a plaque-like lymphocytic infiltrate with diffuse fibroplasia.

C: An area from the same lesion shows more complete cell-poor ("burned-out") regression, with the absence of melanoma cells and the presence in the dermis of pigmented melanophages, indicating that a pigment-synthesizing process had been present in the area.

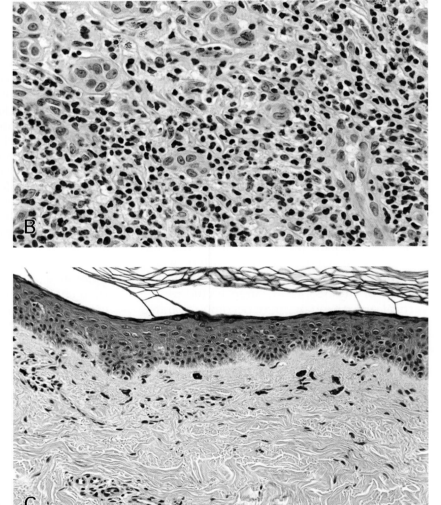

Table 8-6

FEATURES HELPFUL IN DIFFERENTIATING NONTUMORIGENIC MELANOMAS AND DYSPLASTIC NEVI

Feature	Nontumorigenic Melanoma	Dysplastic Nevus
Lesional Features		
Size	Larger	Smaller
Symmetry	Poor	Good
Epidermal Features		
Epidermal keratinocytes	Irregular thickening and thinning	Uniform elongated rete ridges
Lentiginous proliferation	Continuous lentiginous basal proliferation	Nested and discontinuous lentiginous basal proliferation
Pagetoid proliferation	High level and extensive	Focal, low level, minimal
Nuclear features	Uniform moderate to severe atypia-enlargement, irregularity, hyperchromatism, nucleoli	Random mild to moderate atypia
Mitoses	Present in about 1/3 of cases	Almost always absent
Dermal Features		
Maturation	Fail to mature	Mature with descent
Papillary dermis collagen	Diffuse fibroplasia	Eosinophilic concentric and lamellar fibroplasia
Lymphocytes	Bandlike, lichenoid	Patchy, perivascular
Regression	Frequent, may be extensive	Rare, minimal

of melanomas, although as speculated above, it is possible that there had been a focus of tumorigenic proliferation in some of them. Occasional examples of partial or apparently complete regression of tumorigenic vertical growth phase or of metastatic nodules are observed. In these cases, the footprint of the regressed tumorigenic melanoma has the silhouette of a tumor nodule, but is composed of stromal cells, including fibroblasts, lymphocytes, and melanophages. In partially regressed cases, this stromal response is present in a portion of the tumor nodule, while residual melanoma cells are present in the other portions of the nodule. The pathology of regression is discussed further in the section on prognostic features of melanoma.

These and other useful criteria for the recognition of early nontumorigenic melanoma are summarized in Table 8-6, which compares superficial spreading melanoma with a dysplastic nevus, a common differential diagnostic problem.

Variant patterns of radial growth phase include those described as superficial spreading, lentigo maligna, mucosal-lentiginous, and acral-lentiginous melanomas. These are described in sections following.

Differential Diagnosis. As discussed above, the most common pattern of melanoma in the epidermis, seen in the radial growth phase of superficial spreading melanomas, is pagetoid

growth, so named because of its resemblance to mammary or extramammary Paget disease. In a poorly pigmented lesion this distinction may be difficult. The basal nests in pagetoid melanomas tend (like normal melanocytes) to be in direct contact with the basement membrane, while in Paget disease there is often a rim of keratinocytes between the lowest pagetoid cells and the papillary dermis. Mucicarmine or periodic acid–Schiff (PAS) stains may identify mucin in Paget cells, and their immunohistochemical profile is typically keratin and carcinoembryonic antigen (CEA) positive, S-100 protein and HMB45 negative, different from that of melanoma (see sections following) (126–129). Occasional examples of Paget disease can be S-100 protein positive and the lesional cells may contain melanin pigment, presumably synthesized and transferred by reactive benign melanocytes. Pagetoid squamous cell carcinoma is distinguished from melanoma and Paget disease by the recognition of the desmosomal "bridges" between the atypical cells, and by its immunohistochemical profile (positive for keratin, but negative for CEA, S-100 protein, HMB45, and mucin) (128,130). Postinflammatory hyperpigmentations, characterized by pigmentary incontinence with melanophages and lymphocytes in the papillary dermis, may occasionally simulate melanomas clinically. The histologic distinction is not usually difficult, although if there is also fibroplasia of the papillary dermis it may not be possible to rule out the possibility of regressed melanoma.

The most important differential diagnosis is between radial growth phase melanoma and melanocytic dysplasia, already discussed in the section on dysplastic nevi in chapter 7. Key features in making this distinction at scanning magnification include the patterns of the epidermal and lymphocytic responses as well as the arrangement of the lesional cells in the dermis and epidermis. At higher power, the lesional cytology is also important. In melanomas, the epidermis is irregularly thickened or thinned, in contrast to the fairly regular rete ridge elongation that characterizes most dysplastic nevi. The lymphocytic response in the dermis of invasive radial growth phase melanoma is often band-like and lichenoid, a pattern that is not often seen in a dysplastic nevus, where the response is patchy and sparse. In the dermis, microinvasive and some in situ melanomas are characterized by diffuse eosinophilic fibrous thickening of the papillary dermis, with plaque-like lymphocytes and melanophages often associated with areas of regression. These changes are not generally present in dysplastic nevi where the pattern of fibroplasia is concentric, either eosinophilic and homogeneous or lamellar.

Cytologically, the cells of melanomas are relatively uniform in size (although individual cells are pleomorphic) compared to dysplastic nevi in which the atypical (pleomorphic) cell population is a minority of the whole (random atypia). At high magnification, the nuclei of the melanoma cells are clearly enlarged compared to those of nevus cells (including most of the cells of dysplastic nevi) or of keratinocytes and there may be relatively conspicuous nucleoli, which are typically present only in a minority of the cells of a dysplastic nevus. Large eosinophilic or amphophilic nucleoli, common in radial and especially in vertical growth phase and metastatic melanomas, are not conspicuous in dysplastic nevi except occasionally in a minority of the cells. Similarly, many, although certainly not all, radial growth phase melanomas have at least a few mitoses in the epidermis (mitoses in the dermis by definition are indicative of vertical growth phase). In contrast, few dysplastic nevi have mitoses.

A pagetoid pattern of lesional cells in the epidermis is highly characteristic of melanomas and most unusual in dysplastic nevi. As noted above, single cells above the dermal-epidermal junction tend to predominate over groups in the epidermis in early melanomas, while the reverse tends to be true in nevi, where the cells and nests are predominantly basal. Focal extension of lesional cells into the lower third of the epidermis may be seen in a few difficult lesions that lack most other features of melanoma. Such lesions may be best interpreted as examples of focally severe or florid melanocytic dysplasia. Thus, particularly when atypia is only slight to moderate and does not involve more than 50 percent of the lesional cells, we do not consider a focal, partially pagetoid pattern to be diagnostic of melanoma in the epidermis. Features that should suggest the diagnosis of melanoma include: 1) the presence of uniform atypia involving more than 50 percent of the cells, 2) mitoses, 3) extensive pagetoid proliferation that extends more than the breadth of a high-power field, and especially 4) high-level pagetoid proliferation with cells extending into the stratum granulosum and stratum corneum.

Even with the rigorous application of existing criteria, it is not always possible to definitively separate some atypical, unusual, or severely dysplastic nevi from melanomas, and accordingly, complete excision is appropriate for these problematical lesions. Periodic follow-up may also be appropriate, especially if there is a family or personal history of melanoma, or if there are other clinically atypical nevi.

It is appropriate to point out in pathology reports and to emphasize to affected patients that nontumorigenic early melanomas, whether in situ or microinvasive, are likely to be biologically benign and incapable of metastasis (with rare exceptions) as long as there is no vertical growth phase tumor in the dermis, no regression, and the lesions are entirely eradicated by surgical excision.

Using the criteria presented here, most dysplastic nevi can be reliably and reproducibly classified. In one early study, slides were circulated among a panel of seven pathologists convened by the WHO in 1985 (131). The concordance rate for the distinction between radial growth phase melanoma and either dysplastic or common nevi was 95 percent. Several other studies have found similar concordance rates (132–136); in other studies, agreement has been less substantial or poor (137). In one where the participants had not agreed upon criteria, concordance was poor among the observers, but the diagnostic reproducibility was good for individual observers (138). Two studies have evaluated observer agreement in the distinction between nontumorigenic and tumorigenic melanomas (radial and vertical growth phase), and both found acceptable agreement for use in clinical practice (139,140). The features that we use to distinguish between nontumorigenic melanomas and dysplastic nevi are summarized in Table 8-6, and the diagnosis of tumorigenic melanoma is discussed in the following sections.

TUMORIGENIC MELANOMA (VERTICAL GROWTH PHASE)

Definition. *Vertical growth phase*, or *tumorigenic, melanoma* is a stage in the evolution of a malignant melanoma when, often after a period of indolent but progressive growth as a spreading tan, brown, or black plaque of nontumorigenic radial growth phase, it acquires competence in one or more focal areas of tumorigenic growth in the dermis. The vertical growth phase, unlike the radial growth phase, is associated with a statistical chance for distant metastasis, even in a "thin" (American Joint Committee on Cancer [AJCC] stage I) melanoma (31,33,34,71,72). The probability of metastasis depends on features of the tumor and the host, discussed below as prognostic features.

During the vertical growth phase, clinical growth tends to result in a papular or nodular elevation of the skin surface, invasion of the dermis vertically, or as an imperfectly formed sphere, in contrast to the horizontal enlargement of the more or less circular radial growth phase plaque. The usual clinical result is a frank tumor nodule, and this stage has thus been termed the *nodule stage of melanoma*. Nodular melanomas (those with nodule stage growth de novo) have been recently identified as an important subset because of their propensity for rapid growth to a dangerous thickness in a short period of time (141). Clinical nodules are not always evident in lesions that satisfy histologic criteria for vertical growth phase (in deeply

invasive endophytic lesions, for example, especially in certain acral-lentiginous lesions and in many desmoplastic melanomas, where vertical tumorigenic invasion may occur while the skin surface remains flat).

Clinical Features. The ABCD criteria of asymmetry, border irregularity, color variegation, and diameter greater than 6 mm for the clinical diagnosis of melanoma (95) apply only to the plaques and patches of radial growth phase melanoma. In contrast, tumorigenic nodules of vertical growth phase melanoma are often not asymmetric, irregularly contoured, variegated, or especially large. A vertical growth phase tumor may evolve either de novo (from apparently normal skin) or from an antecedent radial growth phase plaque. Those melanomas that evolve directly to vertical growth phase with no detectable antecedent radial phase are termed *nodular melanomas*. A nodular melanoma may present as a symmetric round or ovoid mass of variable, sometimes large size but often considerably less than 1 cm in greatest dimension, with obliterated overlying skin marking patterns, a smooth surface, and a discrete regular border (fig. 8-22). The nodule is usually at least partly pigmented, but occasionally it is clinically amelanotic, presenting as a pink nodule. Usually, at least a few flecks of pigment are present on hand lens inspection. These features may not strongly suggest malignancy until the biologically late symptoms of ulceration and bleeding occur.

Most vertical growth phase tumor nodules (about 90 percent) evolve within the confines of a radial growth phase (nontumorigenic) plaque. A patient who may or may not have been aware of a slowly spreading, flat, variegated, irregular plaque may then notice an initially small but quite rapidly enlarging nodule (sometimes misinterpreted as a "blister") within it, signaling that the melanoma has progressed from an entirely nontumorigenic to a tumorigenic phase. In contrast to many radial growth phase melanomas, which are often asymptomatic and evolve insidiously, most patients eventually detect evidence of change in vertical growth phase lesions because of their more rapid growth. When ulceration occurs, the lesions may bleed, ooze, and stain clothing. Occasionally (5 percent or less of cases), the presenting symptoms of a vertical growth phase melanoma are due

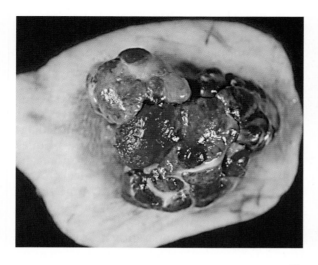 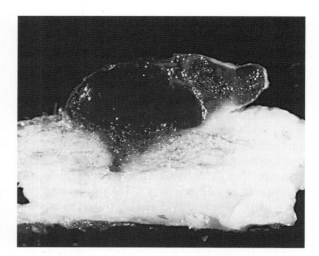

Figure 8-22

MALIGNANT MELANOMA

Left: This bulky, ulcerated, polypoid and tumorigenic vertical growth phase melanoma is arising in a preexisting radial growth phase plaque.

Right: A cross-section of a bulky tumorigenic vertical growth phase melanoma shows invasion through the reticular dermis into the upper panniculus (Clark level V).

to local metastases in the skin (satellites), or to regional nodal or distant (e.g., central nervous system) metastases.

It is likely that most vertical growth phase melanomas grow inexorably, progressively, and increasingly rapidly, often with the development of multiple nodules and the appearance of new populations of cells (clonal heterogeneity or intralesional transformation). As the lesion becomes larger and thicker, the number and severity of risk factors, such as ulceration, level IV or V invasion, high mitotic rate, or microscopic satellites, increase and the prognosis becomes commensurately poorer. Even very small vertical growth lesions (e.g., those the size of a grain of rice) possess the potential to metastasize and result in patient mortality.

Microscopic Findings. The issues of importance in the diagnosis of vertical growth phase melanoma include not only the necessity for accurate diagnosis but also the need for complete and accurate microstaging. The diagnosis in most large lesions is relatively simple because of the presence of cytologic and pattern features that are readily recognized as those of a malignant neoplasm: high-grade nuclear atypia, frequent mitoses, and destructive invasion of surrounding tissues, often with ulceration and

necrosis (figs. 8-22–8-25). Diagnostic difficulties are encountered in some differentiated lesions when a benign common or Spitz nevus is simulated (see Nevoid Melanomas, chapter 10), and in small lesions where the problem is typically whether a melanoma has entered the vertical growth phase or not (discussed below).

The appearance of vertical growth melanomas at scanning magnification depends on whether or not there is an associated antecedent radial growth phase compartment. As already mentioned, lesions that evolve directly from apparently normal skin to vertical growth phase melanoma are termed nodular melanomas, and in these cases, the tumor nodule represents the entire lesion (see Nodular Melanoma). In the more common case of a complex primary melanoma with both radial and vertical growth phases, the vertical growth phase nodule is surrounded by an adjacent, flat peripheral component where the changes are those of radial growth phase melanoma, often with an associated nevus as well (fig. 8-26). In cases where the diagnosis of the vertical growth phase presents some difficulty, such as for example in some desmoplastic melanomas, the presence of a histologically characteristic radial growth phase can be of diagnostic importance. At the same time, it must be remembered that

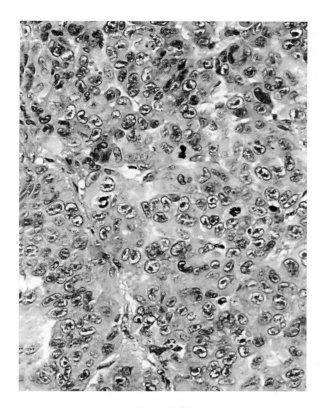

Figure 8-23

TUMORIGENIC MALIGNANT MELANOMA

Frequent mitoses and high-grade nuclear atypia are seen.

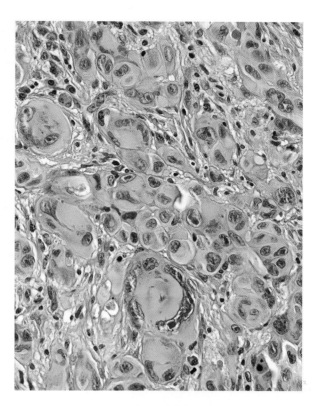

Figure 8-24

**TUMORIGENIC MALIGNANT MELANOMA
WITH ANAPLASTIC TUMOR GIANT CELLS**

This is the upper end of the range of cytologic atypia seen in melanomas.

radial growth phase melanoma can develop in relation to a benign precursor nevus, which may present as a nodule or papule of benign nevus cells located within the confines of the radial growth phase compartment. The criteria we use to distinguish nevus cells from small melanoma cells are summarized in Table 8-7, and illustrated in figures 8-15 and 8-27.

Diagnosis of Vertical Growth Phase in Thin Lesions. Almost all melanomas larger than about 1 mm in thickness, or of Clark level III or beyond, are in the vertical growth phase. Smaller lesions that fail to fill and expand the papillary dermis may be more difficult to recognize as melanomas, and the distinction from radial growth phase melanoma may be difficult (142). The microscopic features of small lesions are similar to those described above (and in more detail below) for larger vertical growth phase nodules, but generally less in degree. Because the invasive component is small, it may be dif-

ficult to distinguish it from a large microinvasive nest. To make this distinction, we use two major criteria and several minor ones. The two major criteria are simple to apply (figs. 8-28, 8-29), and include either the presence of a dermal nest of melanoma cells that is larger than the largest intraepidermal nest, the property of tumorigenicity, or the presence of one or more mitoses in melanoma cells in the dermis, the property of mitogenicity (fig. 8-28).

Either of these findings implies that there has been a proliferation of cells in the dermis, which is the key biologic feature distinguishing the radial and vertical growth phases. Each of these properties has prognostic significance, independent of the other (31). When there is a proliferation of cells in the dermis, the neoplasm potentially exhibits the critical property of tumorigenicity at the local site, which appears to be a necessary (although not sufficient) property

Table 8-7

FEATURES HELPFUL IN DIFFERENTIATING NEVUS CELLS FROM MATURING SMALL MELANOMA CELLS

Nevus Cells	Small Melanoma Cells
Discontinuous with melanoma cells in upper dermis and epidermis	Continuous with melanoma cells in upper dermis and epidermis
Small uniform nests at base	Larger variably sized and shaped nests at base
Little or no pigment, or uniformly distributed mainly coarse pigment	Irregularly scattered pigmented cells at base of lesion; dusty pigment
Absent lymphocytes usually	Lymphocytes present
Single attenuated cells dispersed between reticular dermis collagen bundles at base of lesion	Nests and fascicles rather than single cells in the reticular dermis
Reticulin surrounds individual cells	Reticulin surrounds clusters of cells
Smaller cytologically typical nuclei	Larger cytologically atypical nuclei
No nucleoli at base of lesion (may be seen in upper dermis)	Conspicuous nucleoli
No mitoses	Mitoses sometimes present
Ki-67 (MIB-1) reactivity is low	Ki-67 reactivity may be high

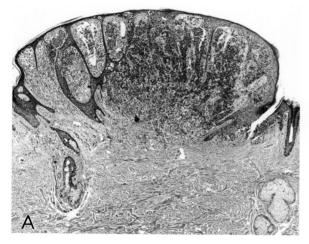

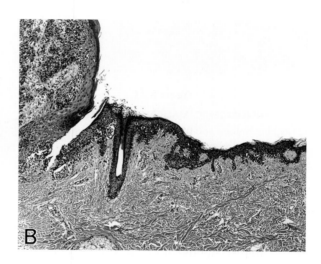

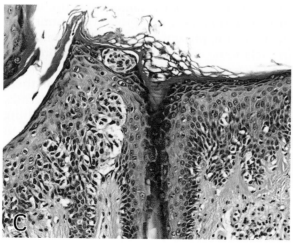

Figure 8-25

MALIGNANT MELANOMA, TUMORIGENIC VERTICAL AND ADJACENT IN SITU RADIAL GROWTH PHASE

A: This tumorigenic nodule in a superficial spreading melanoma shows an area of radial growth phase regression at the left and an area of residual in situ melanoma and associated dysplastic nevus at the right.

B: In situ melanoma and dysplastic nevus are in the adjacent epidermis.

C: In situ melanoma on the left with pagetoid proliferation of uniformly atypical large epithelioid melanocytes.

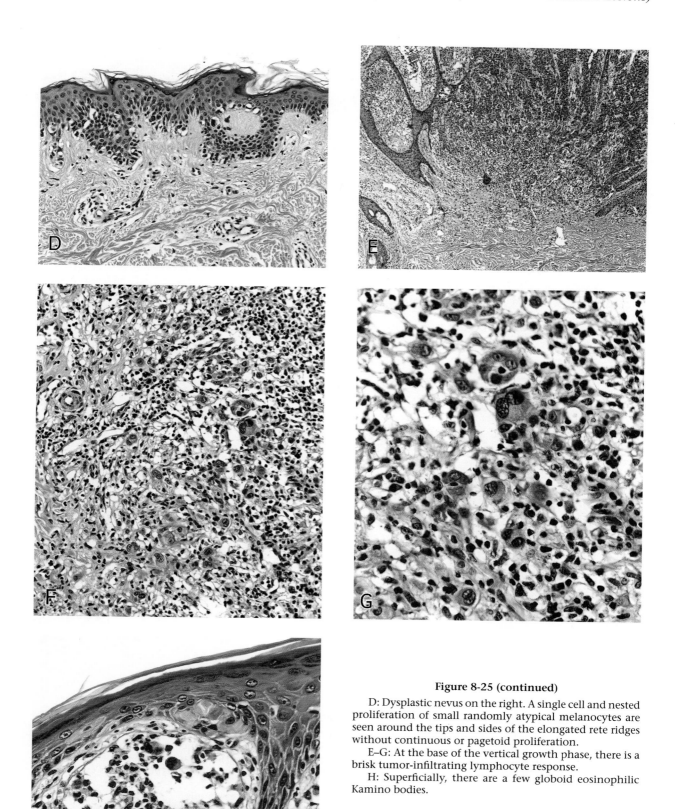

Figure 8-25 (continued)

D: Dysplastic nevus on the right. A single cell and nested proliferation of small randomly atypical melanocytes are seen around the tips and sides of the elongated rete ridges without continuous or pagetoid proliferation.

E–G: At the base of the vertical growth phase, there is a brisk tumor-infiltrating lymphocyte response.

H: Superficially, there are a few globoid eosinophilic Kamino bodies.

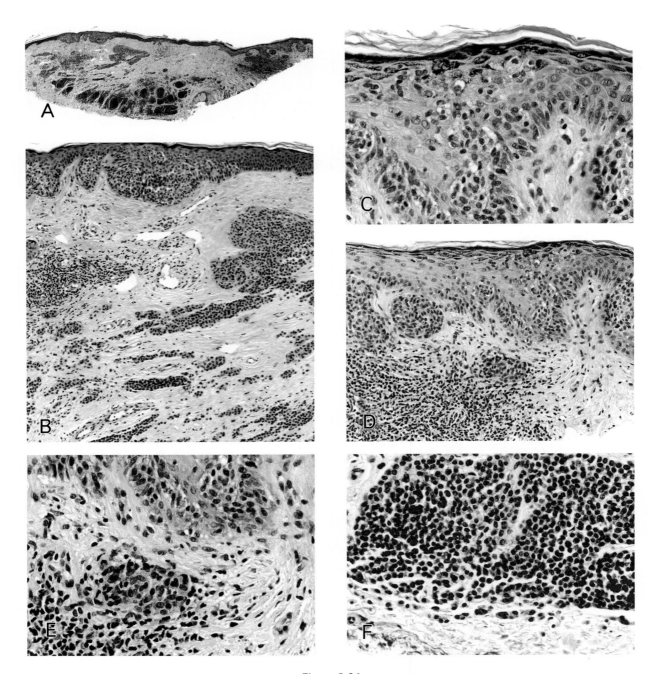

Figure 8-26

MALIGNANT MELANOMA, WITH SMALL CELL NEVOID TUMORIGENIC VERTICAL GROWTH PHASE

A: This lesion, on the back of a 50-year-old man, shows nests of small cells in the dermis that vary greatly in size, shape, and orientation, and an atypical proliferation in the epidermis, which is irregularly thickened and thinned.

B: Higher magnification shows the atypical proliferation in the epidermis. Similar cells are present in the upper dermis in the form of irregular nests. There is maturation from superficial to deep to a smaller cell type, which is cytologically continuous with the overlying atypical proliferation.

C: Pagetoid proliferation of uniformly atypical epithelioid melanocytes in the epidermis.

D,E: Similar atypical cells are in the upper dermis.

F: Nevoid cells at the base of the lesion are considered to be part of the melanoma because of cytologic continuity with the overlying in situ component (seen in B and D).

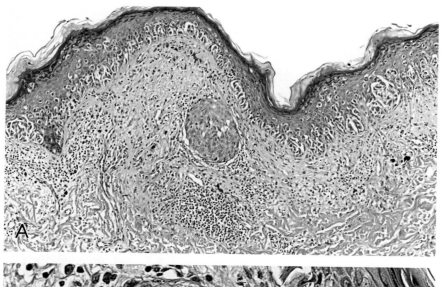

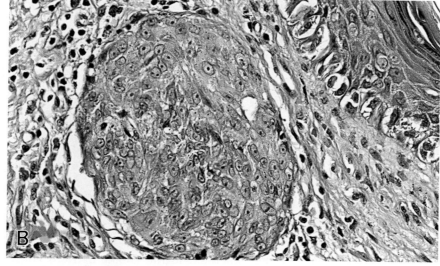

Figure 8-27

MALIGNANT MELANOMA, SUPERFICIAL SPREADING TYPE, WITH TUMORIGENIC AND MITOGENIC VERTICAL GROWTH PHASE

A: A cluster of cells in the dermis is larger than the largest intraepidermal clusters.

B,C: Within this cluster is a cell in mitosis.

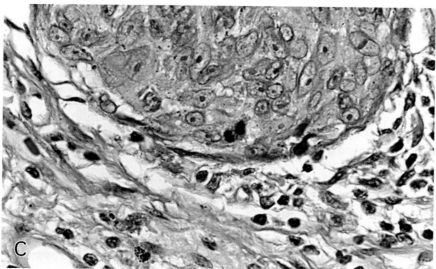

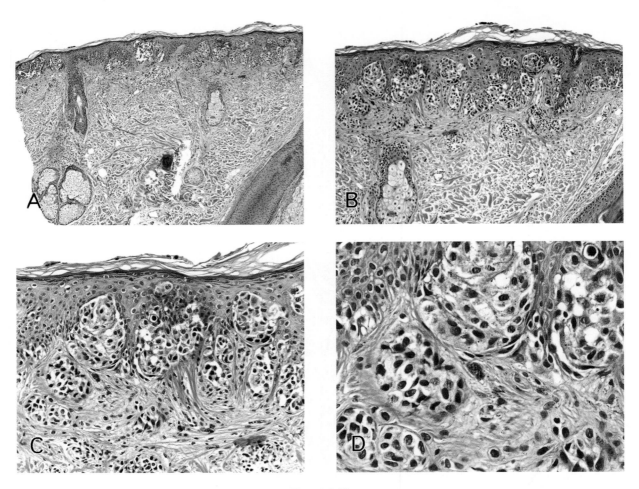

Figure 8-28

MALIGNANT MELANOMA, SUPERFICIAL SPREADING TYPE, INVASIVE NONTUMORIGENIC RADIAL GROWTH PHASE

A: Prominent pagetoid proliferation is seen.

B: Invasive clusters are present at the bottom left.

C: The clusters of cells in the dermis are not larger than the largest intraepidermal clusters.

D: There is severe uniform atypia of the dermal component, resembling that in the epidermal component, and there are no dermal mitoses.

for metastasis (fig. 8-30). Most lesions that are tumorigenic are also mitogenic; however, occasionally mitoses cannot be detected in a lesion judged to represent a tumorigenic melanoma. Although the concept of tumorigenicity is correlated with the Clark level, these terms are not synonymous, as summarized in Table 8-8. Other features that are observed in most vertical growth phase lesions include those listed in Table 8-9. The focal proliferation of cells results in a mass that may, in a small lesion, fail to fill

and expand the papillary dermis (Clark level II), have a "pushing" border that fills and expands the papillary dermis, displacing or compressing surrounding structures (Clerk level III); or have a frankly invasive, destructive border extending into the reticular dermis (Clark level IV).

The vertical growth phase cells appear to have a "selective growth advantage" (143) compared to those of the surrounding radial phase. The cells of the vertical growth phase probably represent a subclone derived by tumor

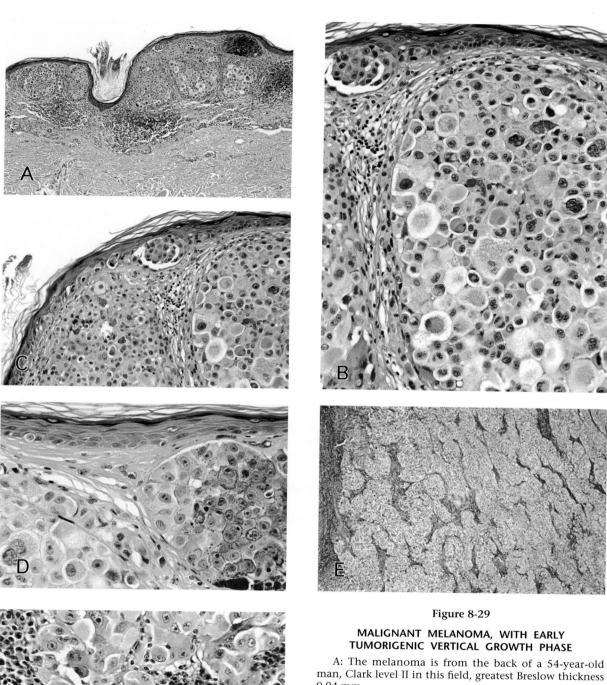

Figure 8-29

MALIGNANT MELANOMA, WITH EARLY TUMORIGENIC VERTICAL GROWTH PHASE

A: The melanoma is from the back of a 54-year-old man, Clark level II in this field, greatest Breslow thickness 0.94 mm.

B,C: There are several clusters of cells in the papillary dermis that are larger than the largest intraepidermal cluster (top left). Dermal mitotic figures were also present (not shown).

D: The lesional cells show severe uniform atypia with irregular nuclear membranes and prominent nucleoli; however, the chromatin pattern is relatively open.

E,F: Metastatic tumor in a regional lymph node occurred after about 3 years of follow-up. The patient was alive and well at 10 years of follow-up.

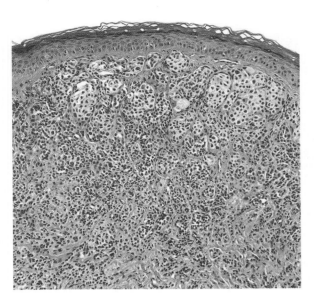 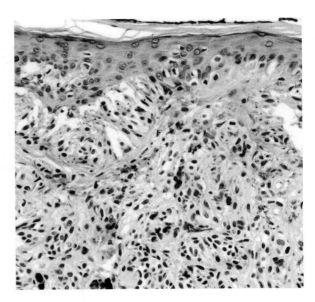

Figure 8-30

TUMORIGENIC MALIGNANT MELANOMA, SHOWING PSEUDOMATURATION

Left: Pseudomaturation from a larger cell type superficially to a smaller cell type at the base. The lesional cells at the base do not disperse as single cells, as is characteristic of benign nevi.

Right: Another example of maturation in a melanoma.

Table 8-8

COMPARISON OF CONCEPTS OF RADIAL AND VERTICAL GROWTH PHASE AND CLARK LEVEL

Classification	Description	Clark Level	Tumorigenicity[a]	Mitogenicity[b]
Clark level I	No invasion of the dermis	I	Never	Never
Clark level II	No tumor that fills and expands the papillary papillary dermis	II	Usually not	Usually not
Clark level III	Tumor fills and expands the papillary dermis	III	Usually	Frequently
Clark level IV	Tumor invades the reticular dermis	IV	Usually	Frequently
Radial growth phase	In situ or invasive but nontumorigenic and nonmitogenic	I or II, rarely III, IV	No by definition	No by definition
Vertical growth phase	Tumorigenic and/or mitogenic	II, III, IV, or V	Yes	Frequently

[a]Defined as formation of invasive nests or micronodules larger than the largest junctional melanoma nest.
[b]Defined as the presence of any mitoses in the dermis.

progression from the radial growth phase, and their morphology usually differs slightly from that of the radial growth phase cells. Often, for example, the vertical growth phase cells have more abundant cytoplasm and less melanin pigment. The lymphocytic response to the vertical growth phase is often conspicuously less than that to the radial phase, and the vertical growth phase often seems to occur in areas of partial regression of the radial growth phase, observa-

tions that suggest the existence of antigenic differences between the two cellular compartments of the melanoma.

The reproducibility of diagnosis in thin vertical phase melanomas has been studied by two groups, both of whom documented acceptable levels of agreement (139,140). McDermott et al. (139), in an Irish study, found that although overall agreement for the growth phase was moderate, agreement between experienced observers was good and

Table 8-9

FEATURES HELPFUL IN DIFFERENTIATING RADIAL GROWTH PHASE FROM VERTICAL GROWTH PHASE MELANOMA

Radial Growth Phase (Invasive)	Vertical Growth Phase
Single cells or small clusters in dermis	Clusters in dermis larger than the largest intraepidermal nest
No mitoses in dermis (mitoses and cell proliferation occur only in epidermis)	Mitoses usually present in dermal vertical growth phase
Cells in dermis resemble those in epidermis (single clone is present)	Dermal cells differ from epidermal cells; less pigment, more compact
Often a brisk lymphocytic response	Lymphocytic response is often less than that to surrounding radial phase
Almost always thinner than 1 mm	Often thicker than 1 mm
Nests in dermis do not compress or distort surrounding tissues	Vertical phase has growth preference over surrounding tissues
Usually Clark level I (in situ) or level II (microinvasive); not fully malignant	Usually Clark level III, IV, or V; frankly tumorigenic fully malignant melanoma
Low Ki-67 (MIB-1) reactivity in dermis	Ki-67 in dermis may be high

equal to the agreement for Breslow thickness. These findings suggested that "if the predictive value of the vertical growth phase proves to be robust, it will be used with an acceptable level of accuracy in routine diagnostic practice."

In some melanomas, the possibility that a small vertical growth phase is present in an otherwise predominantly radial growth phase lesion cannot be ruled out with complete certainty. We label such cases in our laboratory "probable early vertical growth phase," because we believe that it is in the best interests of our patient population to ensure that on the one hand patients and their physicians have the option of treating the probable tumorigenic melanoma according to the "worst-case scenario," and on the other hand that the diagnosis of "pure" radial growth phase melanoma is made as specifically as possible. Generally, these small and diagnostically challenging probable early vertical growth phase tumors are thin, with no mitoses by definition and few if any other adverse prognostic variables (see below). The prognosis of patients with such lesions may be almost as good as that of those with pure radial growth phase melanomas. Although radial growth phase melanomas are generally curable with complete excision, some potential for metastasis exists, as a statistical chance, in all invasive melanomas, especially those that have entered the vertical growth phase.

The presence of vertical growth phase in thin lesions is associated with significant risk for metastasis. Conversely, metastasis is exceedingly rare in melanomas (of any thickness, although most are thin) that lack vertical growth (31,33,71,72,144,145). In a Brazilian study of 77 patients with lesions of 1 mm or less, ulceration (P = 0.019), high mitotic rate (P = 0.008), and vertical growth phase (P = 0.002) were the only factors that positively correlated with micrometastases (144). In a French case-control study of metastasizing thin melanomas, vertical growth phase was the only statistically significant prognostic factor (71). In a Cartesian regression tree analysis, Gimotty et al. (31) recently demonstrated that patients with thin melanoma could be separated into four risk groups whose metastasis rates were 0.5, 4.1, 12.5, and 31.5 percent respectively, based on mitogenicity, tumorigenicity, and gender (reviewed in the section, Staging of Malignant Melanoma). These studies suggest that the presence or absence of vertical growth phase (tumorigenicity and/or mitogenicity) should be taken into consideration in the management of patients with thin (less than 1mm) cutaneous melanomas.

Criteria that we find to be of assistance in making the important distinction between radial and vertical growth phase melanomas include the defining criteria listed above and some additional less specific features listed in Table 8-9.

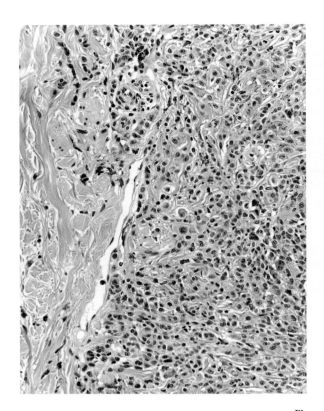 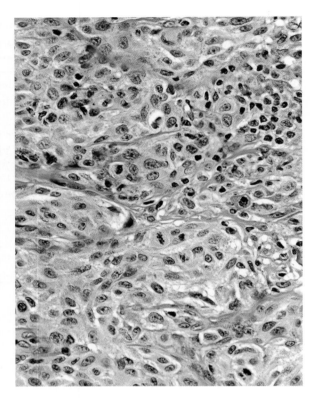

Figure 8-31

MALIGNANT MELANOMA, TUMORIGENIC VERTICAL GROWTH PHASE, WITH PROBABLE VASCULAR INVASION

Left: Scanning magnification shows a bulky, tumorigenic vertical growth phase melanoma. At the base of the tumor (on the left), lesional cells infiltrate among the reticular dermal collagen fibers (Clark level IV), and undermine endothelial cells of a lymphatic vessel, consistent with "uncertain" or "mural" vascular invasion.

Right: There is mitotic activity within the tumorigenic vertical growth phase component (tumorigenic and mitogenic malignant melanoma).

Diagnosis of Vertical Growth Phase in Thick Lesions. Thick melanomas with bulky tumor nodules are usually easily recognized as malignancies, and the prognostically important distinction between radial and vertical phase melanoma is readily made. Problems arise in distinguishing melanoma from a benign simulant nevus (figs. 8-27, 8-31). Criteria that aid in this distinction include those listed in Table 8-10. Many of these criteria, however, also may be seen in benign simulants. In addition, precise, agreed-upon definitions for these criteria are often lacking: the definition of a "high" mitotic rate, for example, may be different for benign simulants and in different age groups.

Architectural Features. The pathology of advanced vertical growth phase melanoma is that of cancer anywhere—a contiguous mass of large,

cytologically atypical, mitotically active cells that tend to exhibit a destructive relationship with the surrounding tissues, may contain areas of spontaneous necrosis (not often extensive in primary melanomas), and may contain areas of surface ulceration (quite common in advanced primary melanomas). Features specific for melanoma, as compared to other malignant tumors, include the presence of a surrounding, diagnostically helpful, radial growth phase plaque compartment and melanin pigment that has been synthesized within neoplastic cells. In an amelanotic lesion lacking a radial growth phase (amelanotic nodular melanoma), the nested pattern of growth and the tendency to biphasic spindle and epithelioid cell differentiation are often helpful in suggesting melanocytic differentiation. Whether it arises in relation to a

Table 8-10

CRITERIA FOR DIAGNOSIS OF BULKY TUMORIGENIC MELANOMA

Criterion	Simulants that May Exhibit Criterion
Large size: >0.5–1.0 cm	Many benign lesions: CBN, DPN, CN, DMN[a]
Invasiveness: infiltrative versus pushing border	Many benign lesions: CBN, DPN, CN, SN
High cellularity: sheetlike as opposed to nested growth	Relatively specific for melanoma if pronounced
Failures of maturation/senescence: smaller cell type at the base	Seen in some melanomas: desmoplastic Absent in some benign lesions: CBN, DPN
High mitotic rate	Relatively specific for melanoma
High-grade cytologic atypia	Relatively specific for melanoma if "uniform" (involving a majority of the lesional cells)
High Ki-67 rate	Relatively specific for melanoma if very high (>30%): cutpoints for most benign lesions are not known
Ulceration	May be seen in benign lesions subjected to trauma
Tumor necrosis	Rare in benign lesions but not often seen in primary melanomas
Lymphovascular invasion	Rare in benign lesions but not often seen in primary melanomas
Perineural invasion	Commonly seen in benign lesions: BN, CBN, DPN
Poor circumscription	Not a useful criterion

[a]CBN = cellular blue nevus; DPN = deep penetrating nevus; CN = compound nevus; DMN = dermal melanocytic nevus; SN = Spitz nevus; BN = blue nevus.

radial growth phase or not, the vertical growth phase typically is a nodular tumor mass that elevates the epidermis, expands and fills the papillary dermis, and sometimes extends into the reticular dermis or the panniculus.

The epidermal reactions to the underlying vertical growth phase tumor are highly variable, ranging from the more common patterns of atrophy with effacement of the rete ridges to the striking verrucous epidermal hyperplasia and hyperkeratosis that occur in a few lesions (146). Perhaps paradoxically in view of their sinister reputation, most vertical growth phase melanoma nodules do not have a strikingly infiltrative relationship with the dermis, although there are certainly many exceptions to this. Perhaps the most common pattern of growth is that of a hemispheric papule or nodule of one to several millimeters or more in greatest diameter and thickness, elevating the epidermis and compressing the interface of the papillary and reticular dermis into a straight deep border. In other melanomas that have a greater capacity for infiltrative growth, the lower border of the neoplasm appears jagged, with tumor cells extending into the reticular dermis or beyond.

When reticular dermal invasion occurs, the tumor cells extend among the coarse, thick, "leathery" collagen bundles of the reticular dermis as tongues or fascicles of cells. In benign nevi including Spitz nevi, by contrast, many or most of the cells at the base of the lesion are single cells or arranged in narrow files. This pattern of single cells predominating over fascicles at the base of the lesion is characteristic of nevi, especially Spitz nevi, but is uncommon in the vertical growth phase of melanomas except in some desmoplastic melanomas. In an elegant series of computer simulation analyses, Smolle et al. (147) have demonstrated that the pattern of invasion at the base of a tumor depends on the balance of the infiltrative and proliferative capacity of the tumor. Lesions with a relatively high infiltrative but comparatively low proliferative capacity, such as Spitz nevi and desmoplastic melanomas, have single cells at the base. Lesions with a greater proliferative capacity, such as melanomas, may initially infiltrate as single cells, but then form contiguous clusters, fascicles, or tongues of cells at the base of the tumor as a result of continuing rounds of cell division (147).

At scanning magnification, vertical growth phase melanoma nodules generally present as a cohesive collection of fairly large epithelioid cells, which are usually cuboidal in shape and have abundant cytoplasm, resembling an epithelial neoplasm. Often, there is a tendency to focal spindle cell differentiation, and there may also be an admixture of smaller cells. Even in a predominantly spindle cell melanoma, there is usually a minor population of epithelioid cells, and this biphasic morphology of a single malignant cell type is a feature that should suggest the possibility of melanocytic differentiation even in an anaplastic, amelanotic tumor (including metastatic tumors). Purely spindle cell melanomas may simulate a sarcoma.

In some lesions that have two cell types, a focal spheroidal mass of cells of one type is surrounded by a larger population of cells of a different type. This phenomenon, which is suggestive of the evolution of a new subclone of cells, has been termed "intralesional transformation" (148). The morphology of the cells in tumorigenic vertical growth phase nodules may be influenced by the type of adjacent radial growth phase, to the extent that there is a tendency to predominance of spindle cells and to neurotropism in the nodules of the lentiginous variants of melanoma. Indeed, neurotropism is common enough in acral-lentiginous melanomas and lentigo maligna melanomas that its presence should be actively sought in lesions of these types that involve the reticular dermis.

A variable lymphocytic response is present in relation to vertical growth phase melanomas. The lymphocytes can be classified as infiltrating (tumor-infiltrating lymphocytes [TIL]), or noninfiltrating lymphocytes (NIL; peritumoral lymphocytes). The tumor-infiltrating lymphocyte response (when "brisk" or "nonbrisk" compared to "absent") has been associated with favorable survival (see Staging of Malignant Melanoma) (fig. 8-32). In a few instances, the lymphocytic response is associated with apparent dissolution of the vertical growth phase, constituting the "vertical growth phase regression" phenomenon (figs. 8-33, 8-34) that is much less common than regression of the nontumorigenic compartment of a melanoma ("radial growth phase regression").

Cytologic Findings. The lesional cells of melanomas tend to be epithelioid (cuboidal), spindled, or mixed in configuration. The epithelioid cell type is highly characteristic of melanomas. These large pale cells typically have dusty melanin pigment in their abundant cytoplasm, with

uniformly atypical nuclei, often with prominent nucleoli (fig. 8-29D). Such epithelioid cells are rarely seen in the dermal component of nevi, except in some combined nevi, although these should lack uniform nuclear atypia upon closer scrutiny. An admixture of smaller cells is commonly also present, and this admixture of small and large cells, typically in an asymmetric pattern of distribution, is helpful in distinguishing melanoma from a Spitz nevus, in which the cell type should be a uniform population (from "side to side") of large spindle and/or epithelioid cells, with gradual maturation from superficial to deep (149). Occasionally, epithelioid lesional cells may gradually give rise to smaller yet still malignant-appearing cells with descent into the dermis. Such lesions that retain other architectural and cytologic features of malignant melanoma are considered to show "pseudomaturation" and must be distinguished from ordinary melanocytic nevi with maturation in the context of other features of benignancy.

The lesional cell nuclei in a tumorigenic melanoma are typically large, with irregular membranes and clumped, hyperchromatic chromatin (fig. 8-33). Especially in the epithelioid cell type, large, often irregular eosinophilic or amphophilic nucleoli are frequently present in vertical growth phase melanomas and in metastases, as are peculiar round intranuclear eosinophilic "pseudoinclusions" that actually represent invaginations of the cell cytoplasm into the nucleus (150). Macronucleoli are usually present in a majority of the lesional cells (fig. 8-29D), but the intranuclear pseudoinclusions are less frequent, especially in primary melanoma. Immunopathologic studies usually permit a specific diagnosis of melanocytic differentiation in primary or metastatic melanoma. These techniques are discussed in a later section. None of the above findings taken in isolation, including immunopathologic differentiation marker studies, are specific for melanoma, however, and may be seen, for example, in Spitz or other types of benign nevi.

Unusual Patterns of Differentiation in Vertical Growth Phase Melanoma. Various unusual differentiation patterns in vertical growth phase melanoma have been described. In a review of 335 malignant melanomas to identify variant morphologic patterns that might be confused with other tumors, 27 predominantly amelanotic

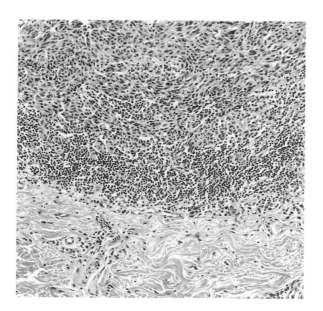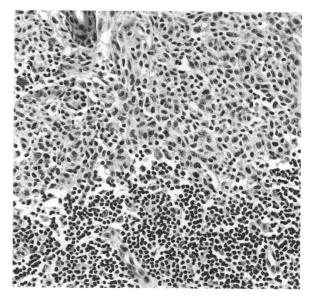

Figure 8-32

TUMOR-INFILTRATING LYMPHOCYTES IN A MELANOMA

Left: A brisk tumor-infiltrating lymphocyte response (brisk, by definition, is a response that extends entirely across the base of the vertical growth phase). Tumor-infiltrating lymphocytes are present, by definition, among the tumor cells.

Right: Those lymphocytes at the base that are not among tumor cells are noninfiltrating lymphocytes.

neoplasms with unusual histologic features were identified (151). These included 9 with an adenoid or pseudopapillary pattern, 7 small cell neoplasms, 5 with prominent myxoid stroma, 4 with a hemangiopericytoma-like appearance, and 2 composed of neoplastic cells with a signet ring configuration. Thus, melanomas can mimic adenocarcinomas, small cell carcinomas, and sarcomas. Osseous and/or cartilaginous (osteocartilaginous) differentiation of malignant melanoma is a rare phenomenon, and only 15 cases having been reported, often subungual or acral in location (152). Other rare cytologic variants seen occasionally include balloon cells (fig. 8-35) (153), signet ring cells (154–156), and rhabdoid cells. The latter have abundant eosinophilic cytoplasm that indents the nucleus, and may lead to diagnostic consideration of nonmelanocytic rhabdoid tumors, which constitute a highly heterogeneous group (157,158). Another variant pattern associated with prominent ground substance production has been described as myxoid melanoma. This pattern may lead to diagnostic confusion in amelanotic lesions (159). In our experience, a prominent mucinous matrix is common as a focal phenomenon in the vertical

growth phase of advanced primary melanomas, especially those composed mainly of spindle cells. Vertical growth phase melanoma cells may also simulate the formation of vascular spaces, and because this may occur in the setting of lentigo maligna melanoma on the head or face of elderly individuals, must be differentiated from angiosarcoma.

Finally, an appearance that may simulate vertical growth phase in previously biopsied melanocytic lesions should be mentioned (160,161). This is the histiocytic reaction to Monsel solution, which is a ferrous styptic agent commonly used by dermatologists after a punch or shave biopsy. The brown ferrous Monsel pigment is taken up by plump reactive histiocytes, which may quite convincingly simulate melanoma cells. In case of doubt, an iron stain easily resolves the problem.

Diagnostic Criteria from the Literature. In 1984, Jones (162) circulated a questionnaire and received 50 distinct criteria for the diagnosis of malignant melanoma from 48 expert pathologists. The five most commonly cited criteria in this survey were cytologic atypia, melanocytes at all levels of the epidermis, mitotic "activity"

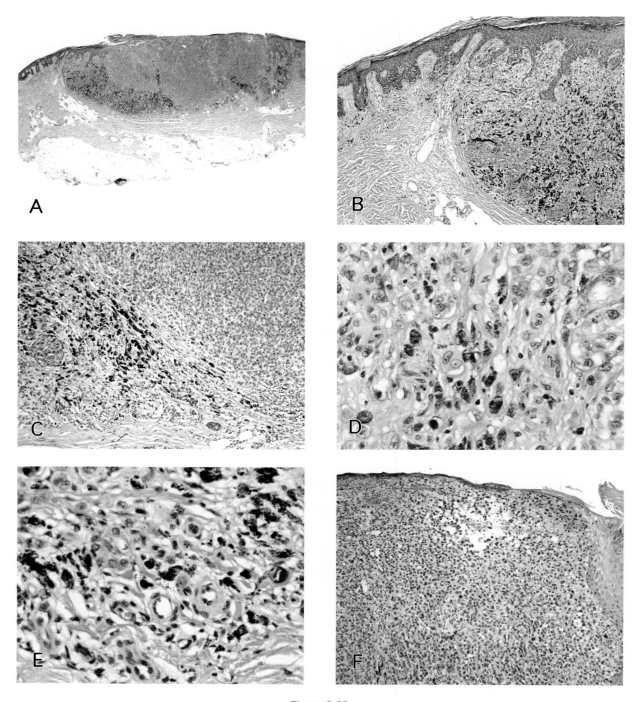

Figure 8-33

**MALIGNANT MELANOMA WITH TUMORIGENIC VERTICAL
GROWTH PHASE AND VERTICAL GROWTH PHASE REGRESSION**

A: This bulky, tumorigenic vertical growth phase melanoma shows a region of infiltration by pigmented melanophages at the left.

B: At higher magnification, macrophages with fibroblasts and vessels appear to be "breaking up" the vertical growth phase.

C–E: In the region of regression, there are melanophages, vessels, and fibroblasts (left of field).

F: In other areas, the vertical growth phase nodule appears intact.

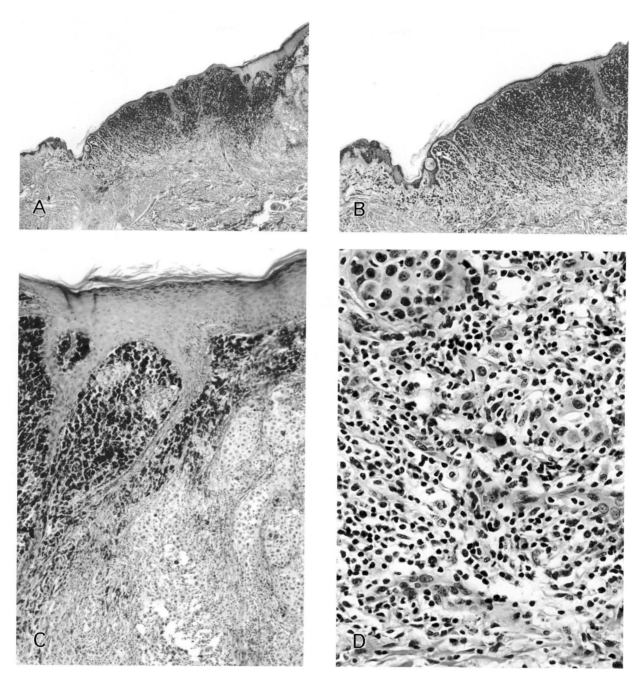

Figure 8-34

**MALIGNANT MELANOMA WITH TUMORIGENIC VERTICAL
GROWTH PHASE AND VERTICAL GROWTH PHASE REGRESSION**

A: There is an area of "tumoral melanosis," representing apparent partial replacement of a vertical growth phase nodule by pigmented macrophages.

B,C: Adjacent to the area of regression, there is an intact vertical growth phase component.

D: At the base of the vertical growth phase, there are tumor-infiltrating lymphocytes, apparently breaking up the tumor and appearing to represent an active phase of vertical growth phase regression.

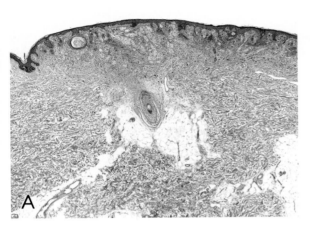

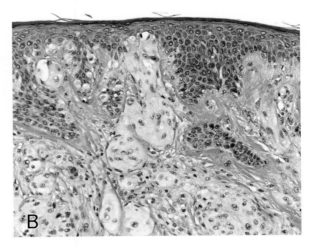

Figure 8-35

MALIGNANT MELANOMA, INVASIVE AND TUMORIGENIC, WITH BALLOON CELL FEATURES

A: This lesion, on the thigh of a 50-year-old woman, shows a cellular and somewhat asymmetric proliferation in the epidermis and dermis.

B: Higher magnification shows cells with abundant cytoplasm forming a tumorigenic dermal component.

C: A dermal mitosis is present, indicating that the lesion is mitogenic.

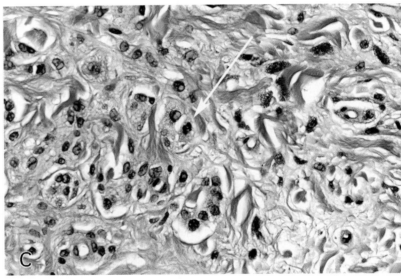

or atypical mitoses, lack of maturation of melanocytes in the deep dermis, and inflammatory reaction in the dermis. Interestingly, these criteria appear to apply mainly to vertical growth phase neoplasms. Stolz et al. (163) studied histologic criteria in 150 melanomas thinner than 1.5 mm, and found that the most sensitive criteria were nuclear atypia (present in 84 percent of the lesions), asymmetry of the lesion (81 percent), and the presence of single cells in the upper layers of the epidermis (80 percent). Two of these three criteria were present in 88 percent of the lesions. The sensitivity of other criteria, including dermal inflammatory response, poor demarcation (circumscription), infiltration of the adnexa, and mitotic activity, ranged downwards from 56 to 33 percent.

In a collection of articles in the journal *Histopathology*, three experts were asked to discuss the issue of whether there are valid morphological criteria which enable reliable distinction between benign and malignant melanocytic lesions. The criteria listed by these experts included the following: 1) clinical history—change in size, shape, or degree of pigmentation; bleeding; irritation (164); 2) low-power architecture—asymmetry is usual in melanomas (164). It was emphasized by Slater (165) that this asymmetry includes melanocytic nests, cytoplasmic and nuclear cytology, cell type, pigmentation, and even the inflammatory response. Okun (107) has cautioned, however, that silhouette symmetry is absent in a significant fraction of melanomas and that

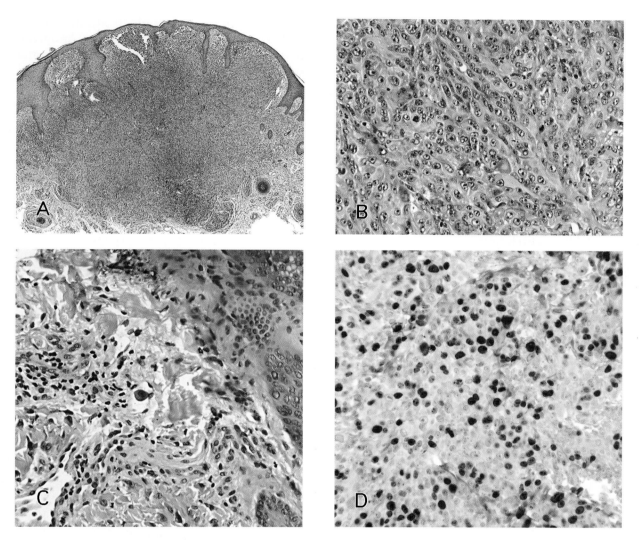

Figure 8-36

TUMORIGENIC MELANOMA, NODULAR TYPE

A: The tumor is in the dermis, with no adjacent in situ component.

B: The tumor is composed of uniformly atypical large epithelioid cells, growing in sheets, with an ill-defined nested and fascicular architecture. Mitotic figures are readily detected.

C: A single tumor cell is seen in the dermal lymphatic space adjacent to the tumorigenic vertical growth phase component.

D: Ki-67 staining reveals a high proportion of reactive cells, indicating a high proliferative fraction in the neoplasm.

over-reliance on this criterion may lead to errors in diagnosis; 3) size of the lesion—melanomas are usually larger than 4 mm (164); 4) cytologic criteria—nuclear and mitotic pleomorphism, eosinophilia, and increase in size of nucleoli (often with change of shape), as well as increased density and thickness of the nuclear membrane (166). In melanoma, the nucleoli are often large and basophilic, with an irregular, often polygonal profile (164). Dusty pigment in the cytoplasm ("dust cells") was considered helpful by two of the experts (165,166); 5) cellularity of the dermal component—an increase favors malignancy, as reported for example in childhood melanoma (111,164,167); 6) mitotic activity (fig. 8-36)—an increase favors melanoma, but absence of mitoses does not exclude it (166). Mitoses in the superficial part of the dermal component are probably less significant than deep mitoses, and the number of mitoses is more significant than their mere presence (164). Intraepidermal mitoses should also raise a question of melanoma, and abnormal mitoses should be considered highly suspicious; 7) distribution of melanocytes in the epidermal component—upward invasion of the epidermis (165,166). Variation in the size of nests and more prominent lentiginous single cell proliferation, pagetoid, or "buckshot" spread of cells into the epidermis were emphasized (164), as well as consideration of the density of intraepidermal spread and its extent in terms of height into the epidermis and lateral extension beyond the main lesion (165); and 8) gradation of nuclear size—decrease in nuclear size with descent or "maturation" was mentioned by all of the authors (165,166), although Kirkham (164) appropriately emphasized that melanomas recapitulate this process of nevoid differentiation to varying degrees, especially in so-called "minimal deviation" or "nevoid" melanomas.

In this interesting series of papers, all authors emphasized that no single feature is diagnostic in itself and that all aspects, including clinical details, should be interpreted together. Okun et al. (166) agreed with others that there are cases of melanoma in which the criteria are so subtle as to circumvent even a differential diagnosis, although they considered that most diagnoses should be made correctly using well-established criteria, as summarized above. Kirkham (164), also favoring the methodical use of criteria, considered that criteria are largely opinion-based rather than evidence-based, but do go beyond mere subjective pattern analysis. In agreement, Slater (165) went further in emphasizing that the interpretation of melanocytic lesions remains predominantly an art that provides a subjective opinion, that there is still a major lack of scientific objectivity, and that pathologists should admit to these difficulties and unashamedly feel free to write "uncertain" in their reports, a conclusion with which we would firmly agree.

Immunohistochemical Findings and Cell Biology. Immunohistochemical markers for melanoma are most applicable to the tumorigenic phase of progression, except for the use of differentiation markers like HMB45 and Melan-A to discriminate among different forms of pagetoid proliferation or to assess contiguous proliferation in possible in situ melanoma versus a lentigo or a dysplastic nevus. Antigenic markers for vertical growth phase melanoma can be used to confirm melanocytic differentiation, and potentially for diagnosis and prognosis (fig. 8-37). These markers can be divided into progression/diagnostic markers, prognostic markers, and differentiation markers.

Progression Markers for Melanoma. Progression markers are potentially very useful if they can discriminate among different stages of disease evolution, such as dysplastic nevus and nontumorigenic melanoma or tumorigenic melanoma. Antigenic differences between radial and vertical growth phase cells have been demonstrated in tissue sections and in vitro using a number of different monoclonal antibodies (78,80,168–172). In general, radial growth phase cells in the dermis react similarly to nevi, especially dysplastic nevi, while vertical growth phase cells react like the cells of metastases. While such markers have some potential as diagnostic tests for vertical growth phase lesions, many of them are limited by their lack of reactivity in paraffin sections. In addition, there is usually sufficient overlap between radial and vertical growth phase melanomas as well as with benign lesions, including for example Spitz nevi and dysplastic nevi, to suggest that the specificity, sensitivity, and predictive value of these markers will be insufficient for diagnostic use in difficult cases.

The Ki-67 proliferation marker has been demonstrated to have diagnostic utility in this and perhaps other diagnostic distinctions (fig. 8-36 and also see figs. 5-5 and 5-14). Kaleem et al. (80) studied Ki-67 (as applied to frozen tissue sections), MIB-1 (as applied to paraffin sections), and p53 immunolabeling in cutaneous melanocytic neoplasia and concluded that these determinants may be used as an adjunct to morphology in the recognition of vertical growth phase melanoma. Using a cutoff of concurrent reactivity for Ki-67 of 10 percent and a 5 percent level for concurrent p53 reactivity, 75 percent of the vertical growth phase tumors were correctly identified, while 8 percent of the radial growth phase tumors were misclassified. The positive predictive value was found to be 83 percent for identification of vertical growth phase tumors. Li et al. (81) also studied Ki-67 expression as a

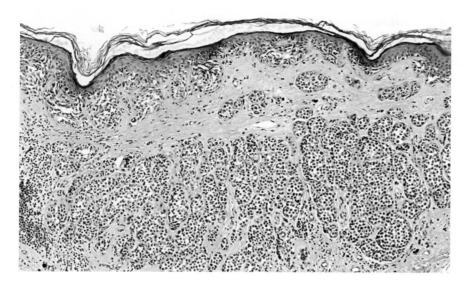

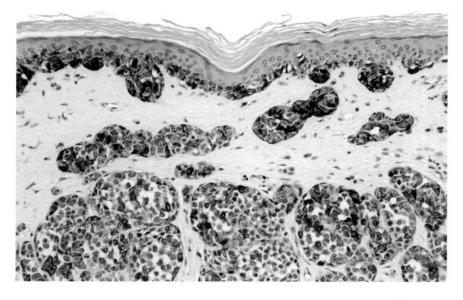

Figure 8-37

TUMORIGENIC MELANOMA

The melanoma (top) stains with HMB45 (bottom).

diagnostic marker and found good discrimination among common nevi, Spitz nevi, and melanomas, as summarized in Table 8-11. These data suggest that a Ki-67 rate of greater than 33 percent focally should be considered diagnostic of melanoma. In our experience of difficult consultation cases, many lesions judged to be vertical growth phase melanomas on other grounds have a Ki-67 rate lower than this, suggesting that this attribute, while likely to be very specific and certainly of diagnostic value when present, has relatively low sensitivity in difficult cases.

Diagnosis of Vertical Growth Phase in Thick Lesions. Thick melanomas with bulky tumor nodules are usually easily recognized as malignancies, and the prognostically important distinction between radial and vertical growth phase melanoma is readily made. Problems occasionally arise in the distinction between melanoma and a benign simulant nevus (figs. 8-26, 8-30). Criteria that aid in this distinction may include those listed in Table 8-12. Many of these criteria may also be seen in benign simulants, however, and in addition, precise, agreed-upon definitions for

Table 8-11

Ki-67 REACTIVITY IN MELANOCYTIC LESIONS[a]

	Compound Nevi	Dysplastic Nevi	Spitz Nevi	Malignant Melanomas
Average % of positive nuclei[b]	0.48 ± 0.10	2.58 ± 0.73	6.92 ± 2.85	23.74 ± 2.21
Maximal % of positive nuclei[c]	0.90 ± 0.19	3.93 ± 1.19	9.93 ± 3.63	32.16 ± 2.21

[a]Data from reference 172.
[b]Average percentage of positive cells based on counting 200 cells across entire lesion.
[c]Average percentage of positive cells based on counting 100 cells from a subjectively determined region of maximal expression ("hot spot").

Table 8-12

CHARACTERISTICS OF VERTICAL GROWTH PHASE PRIMARY MELANOMA (TUMORIGENIC MELANOMA)

Architecture	Nodule <1 mm to a few cm (most melanomas >1 mm thick are tumorigenic)
	Adjacent radial growth phase in 90% of cases
Keratinocytes	Overlying epidermis often compressed or ulcerated
	Hyperkeratosis or scale-crust common over nodule
	Pseudoepitheliomatous hyperplasia sometimes
Pattern of lesional cells	One or more clusters (nests) of cells are present in dermis
	Cluster is larger than largest nest in epidermis (tumorigenicity)
	Papillary dermis usually filled or widened (level III)
	Reticular dermis may be infiltrated (level IV)
	Cluster compresses surrounding tissues (growth advantage)
	Cells do not become smaller with descent into dermis
	Pigment is irregularly distributed within dermal tumor
Host responses	Lymphocytic response often reduced compared to radial phase
	Lymphocytic response at base of lesion is often asymmetrically distributed
Cytology	Cells usually less pigmented, more atypical than radial phase
	Mitoses usually present
	Melanomas with dermal mitoses are tumorigenic by definition (mitogenicity)
Immunopathology	Ki-67 (MIB-1) and p53 reactivity favor vertical growth phase

these criteria are often lacking: the definition of a "high" mitotic rate may be different for different benign simulants and in different age groups.

Other differences observed in vitro between radial and vertical growth phase cells include the difficulty of establishing the radial phase cells as permanent cell lines in tissue culture (173), and a much higher incidence of random and especially of nonrandom chromosomal abnormalities in vertical growth phase cells (30). These differences, unfortunately, are of little use in the diagnosis of small vertical growth phase lesions because the necessary samples are not available and the methods are established only in a few research laboratories. Methods applicable to permanent paraffin sections in routine laboratories would be very valuable for these problem cases.

A number of new progression markers has recently been evaluated. One of interest is the multidrug resistance transporter protein, ABCB5 (174). Antibodies to this epitope have been shown to decorate human melanomas displayed in tissue microarrays in a manner that directly parallels tumor progression from thin to thick primary lesions and finally to metastases (175). This marker also appears to identify a subpopulation of melanoma stem cells capable of initiating and perpetuating tumorigenic growth. Initial attempts in experimental animals to target and destroy ABCB5-expressing cells have been promising, resulting in inhibition of melanoma growth.

Prognostic Markers for Melanoma. Prognostic markers are those features of lesions or patients that may be associated with the metastatic potential of a primary melanoma (143). Prognostic markers are of greatest use in thin AJCC stage I melanomas because therapeutic decisions in thicker melanomas at the present time are more uniformly applied. In future research it will be important to identify by appropriate follow-up, if possible, those seemingly advanced primary melanomas that will not metastasize.

The most useful prognostic markers at the present time are the proliferation markers, of which the best studied is Ki-67 (fig. 8-36). In a recent study, Gimotty et al. (30) characterized three biomarkers of proliferation (Ki-67 expression, mitogenicity [MR >0], and tumorigenicity) in thin (less than 1 mm) primary cutaneous melanomas and examined their association with prognosis (176,177). They used immunohistochemistry to determine Ki-67 expression using the monoclonal antibody MIB-1 in lesions from a prospective cohort that included 396 patients with thin invasive primary melanomas; all were followed for 10 years or more. Associations were discovered with tumor progression and with prognosis. In terms of progression, dermal Ki-67 expression was lower than epidermal Ki-67 expression in 171 radial growth phase melanomas, and dermal Ki-67 expression and mitogenicity were higher in 193 tumorigenic vertical growth phase melanomas compared with radial and nontumorigenic vertical growth phase melanomas. These results were consistent with the model of progression from radial to vertical growth phase tumors while identifying an intermediate subset of nontumorigenic ("accretive" vertical growth phase lesions (discussed later). In terms of prognosis, dermal Ki-67 expression, mitogenicity, growth phase, thickness, ulceration, tumor-infiltrating lymphocytes, and sex were associated with metastasis at 10 years; however, only dermal Ki-67 expression, mitogenicity, and sex were independent prognostic factors. Two high-risk groups were identified: men and women with mitogenic melanomas and dermal Ki-67 expression over 20 percent in tumor cells and men with mitogenicity and Ki-67 expression less than 20 percent, with 10-year metastatic rates of 39 percent and 20 percent, respectively. Patients whose melanomas lacked these attributes enjoyed a much better prognosis. Thus, Ki-67 expression and mitogenicity provide independent prognostic information that can

potentially be used in the risk-based management of patients. It should be emphasized, however, that these data are of value in assessing prognosis for large groups of patients and for recommending therapy, but do not provide any guarantee of outcome (whether favorable or unfavorable) for individual patients.

Differentiation Markers for Melanoma. Especially useful in an amelanotic lesion, immunopathologic markers may help to confirm the diagnosis of melanoma versus another tumor type, but are of no value in assessing malignancy. Most melanomas, including vertical growth phase melanomas, react positively for S-100 protein antigen (178–184). More specific but somewhat less sensitive markers include Melan-A (or MART-1), tyrosinase, and HMB45 antibodies (see fig. 8-9) (185). The diagnosis can be established in a consistent morphologic background by a positive reaction for S-100 protein and one or more of the more specific markers. Melanomas typically are negative with keratin markers, and with epithelial membrane antigen (EMA). If there is a significant question of anaplastic carcinoma, we order several different keratin markers (e.g., AE1/3, CAM5.2, 903), and if the differential diagnosis includes lymphoma, a stain for leukocyte common antigen (LCA) is important. Although instances of keratin-positive melanomas have been described (186), this phenomenon is rare in the experience of most laboratories, including our own, and has been observed for the most part with concentrated antibodies in frozen sections. Ben-Izhak et al. (186) studied epithelial markers in malignant melanoma in routinely processed paraffin sections. Reactivity with polyclonal CEA was observed in 15 (48 percent) of the 31 lesions; 14 were metastatic. No lesion was reactive with monoclonal CEA. Significant cytokeratin (CK) staining was evident in only 3 (9.7 percent) lesions (all metastatic), which also stained specifically with anti-CK18. EMA was observed only focally in 2 (6.5 percent) lesions. All lesions with CK or EMA staining showed concomitant extensive staining for S-100 protein, HMB45, and vimentin. Considering these results and reports of positivity for S-100 protein, vimentin, and HMB45 in epithelial tumors, a wide panel of antibodies was recommended for the study of undifferentiated tumors. Immunohistochemical methods are also discussed in the section on metastatic melanoma.

In a study of the expression of the cellular apoptosis susceptibility protein (CAS), a nuclear transport factor that plays a role in apoptosis and cell proliferation, Boni et al. (187) found that vertical growth phase primary cutaneous melanoma stained stronger than horizontally growing cell clusters, and metastases stained very strongly, while most junctional or dermal nevi were negative. They concluded that CAS staining may be useful for the diagnosis of melanoma and possibly as an immunohistochemical prognostic factor in cutaneous melanocytic lesions.

Morphometric Diagnostic Studies. In a study of 192 lesions in Stockholm, morphometric, DNA, and proliferating cell nuclear antigen (PCNA, a cell cycle marker) measurements were taken of benign melanocytic tumors and malignant melanomas (188). Significant differences among the lesion groups were found in terms of mean nuclear area, coefficient of variation (c.v.) of the nuclear area, c.v. of nuclear shape, nuclear contour index (NCI), DNA content, and PCNA positivity. A logistic regression analysis showed that the c.v. of the nuclear area and the DNA content were significant independent predictors of banal nevi versus primary malignant melanoma. Nuclear polymorphism, i.e., the c.v. of nuclear shape, was greater in metastasizing primary melanomas than in thin nonmetastasizing primary melanomas. PCNA positivity was occasionally increased in keratinocytes adjacent to nevi or melanomas. Higher values for nuclear area, DNA aneuploidy, and PCNA positivity were found in thick malignant melanomas and melanoma metastases than in benign melanocytic lesions and thin malignant melanomas (35,36,189,190). Morphometry, DNA content, and PCNA positivity thus appear to reflect different stages in tumor progression of malignant melanoma, and could potentially provide diagnostic information. The utility of these methods in routine practice has not yet been tested in diagnostically challenging cases, and is limited by the complexity of the analysis procedures.

Molecular Diagnostic Studies. Comparative genomic hybridization (CGH), fluorescence in situ hybridization (FISH) (58,191–196), and RNA expression profiling studies (194,197–200) are newer techniques that are beginning to be applied to the diagnosis of melanoma. In the future, such techniques may supplant or explain some of the present morphologic issues. Aspects of the morphology of tumorigenic melanomas are summarized in Table 8-12.

MANAGEMENT OF "UNCERTAIN" MELANOCYTIC NEOPLASMS: SUPERFICIAL ATYPICAL MELANOCYTIC PROLIFERATIONS OF UNCERTAIN SIGNIFICANCE (SAMPUS) AND MELANOCYTIC TUMORS OF UNCERTAIN MALIGNANT POTENTIAL (MELTUMP)

The topic of "difficult," "uncertain," or "indeterminate" melanocytic tumors is fraught with misunderstanding and controversy (201). Some authorities aver that histologic diagnoses ought to define only what is destined to behave in a consistently benign or potentially malignant manner, while others argue that between these polar extremes there exists a small yet significant continuum where melanocytic tumors possess morphologic attributes that "minimally deviate" from malignancy, or straddle the borderline between indolence and aggressiveness. Introduction of new entities based on biologic uncertainties potentially complicates an already diverse array of melanocytic tumors defined by clinicopathologic characteristics. From an operational point of view, at least, a neoplasm that has been completely excised can only have one of two possible outcomes: it may cause the death of the patient, or not. Yet, in the present state of our knowledge, it is not possible to predict these dichotomous outcomes with certainty, even when there is consensus agreement as to a "malignant" diagnosis.

At least two categories of such uncertain lesions can be identified, with additional "gray zones" between them. In one of these categories, there may be little disagreement about the nosologic category in which a lesion should be placed, but there may be general agreement that the future behavior of this lesion is difficult to predict. These may be termed "biologically borderline" lesions. In another category, there are conflicting diagnostic criteria, and agreement upon a single diagnosis is lacking, even among experts. These lesions may be wholly benign, fully malignant, or "borderline," but current criteria do not allow distinction among these possibilities, and the diagnosis and prognosis remain uncertain. Clearly, there exists a need for pathologists, clinicians, patients, and even litigators to understand the limits of diagnostic certainty as they apply to melanocytic lesions that display histologic characteristics hybrid between nevi and melanoma.

An operational definition of a benign melanocytic tumor is one that 1) grows to a point and then stabilizes or involutes; 2) never spreads beyond its site of origin; and 3) displays well-defined and reproducible histologic characteristics that correlate with its biologic behavior. An example of such a lesion is the ordinary acquired compound melanocytic nevus. For most compound nevi, the diagnosis is both reliably predictive and universally agreed-upon. In contrast, a malignant melanocytic tumor is more difficult to describe. We generally conceive of a malignant melanoma as a tumor that 1) most often grows inexorably if left untreated; 2) has potential over time to metastasize beyond its site of origin; and 3) exhibits histologic features that have predictive value in forecasting these behaviors. However, it is also well recognized that some melanomas actually regress (presumably due to host immune responses); that occasional advanced lesions do not metastasize, while some early lesions do; and that even after metastasis, distant deposits need not grow steadily and inexorably (witness the not uncommon patient who finally develops clinically overt nodal disease many years after complete eradication of the primary tumor).

Thus, even those melanocytic lesions that fully possess architectural and cytologic characteristics of malignancy (Table 8-13) may exhibit diverse biologic potentials. This problem is confounded by the existence of lesions with histologic characteristics intermediate between benignancy and malignancy, where prediction and agreement are both elusive goals.

Historically, recognition of gray-zone melanocytic proliferations dates back three decades to the seminal yet sometimes controversial and misunderstood contribution by Richard Reed and coworkers describing "common and uncommon melanocytic nevi and borderline melanomas" (51). More recent attempts to define and elucidate melanocytic lesions that occupy a gray zone between wholly benign growth and malignant potential, namely those lesions

Table 8-13
GENERIC CHARACTERISTICS OF BENIGN MELANOCYTIC NEVI AND MALIGNANT MELANOMA

	Benign Melanocytic Nevus	Malignant Melanoma
Architecture	Symmetric	Asymmetric
Preexisting structure	Respects	Displaces/infiltrates
Maturation	Present	Absent or defective
Dermal mitoses	Few to absent	Often present
Apoptosis	Absent	Often present
Nuclear atypia	Absent	Present, uniform
Vessel involvement	Absent	May be present
Regression	Rare	Common

for which histopathology fails to predict the odds of biologic outcome with any precision, and where disagreement about the diagnosis prevails, have resulted in multiple categories in which indeterminate lesions may be placed. Nine such categories have recently been proposed for placement of atypical melanocytic lesions with intermediate histologic characteristics that not only are a focus of disagreement and uncertainty, but also could correlate with the potential either to grow inexorably if incompletely excised or to metastasize and be detected even after complete excision (Table 8-14) (201). This proposed classification system is a comprehensive attempt to segregate and separately classify lesions with high-grade (severe) atypia from those deserving of descriptors that imply benignancy (nevus). Moreover, this system emphasizes the complexity and variety of intermediate melanocytic neoplasms as well as the practical necessity for recognition that not all melanocytic proliferations are purely benign or purely malignant.

From a definitional perspective, a benign lesion is one that will grow to a stable volume and that cannot spread beyond the primary site. A malignant lesion, in contrast, is one that if untreated will grow inexorably and that often acquires the capacity to spread beyond the primary site as it enlarges. Thus, malignant lesions may have locally recurring ability, metastasizing ability, or both. An intermediate lesion deviates from a wholly benign process in that it may progress to malignancy. Accordingly, the term

Table 8-14

RECENTLY PROPOSED CATEGORIES FOR INDETERMINATE MELANOCYTIC LESIONS[a]

1. Severely atypical dermoepidermal nevomelanocytic proliferation with borderline features of radial growth phase malignant melanoma

2. Severely atypical dermoepidermal nevomelanocytic proliferation with borderline features of early vertical growth phase melanoma

3. Severely atypical intraepidermal epithelioid cell melanocytic dysplasia mimicking superficial spreading melanoma

4. De novo dermal-based epithelioid melanocytic dysplasia

5. Atypical lentiginous melanocytic proliferation/de novo melanocytic dysplasia mimicking lentigo maligna

6. Severely atypical dermal-based melanocytic proliferation without criteria for nevoid melanoma/minimal deviation melanoma, spitzoid type

7. Severely atypical superficial compound Spitz tumor mimicking superficial spreading melanoma in radial or early vertical growth phase

8. Severely atypical spitzoid proliferation (atypical Spitz tumor) mimicking spitzoid melanoma

9. Borderline lesions mimicking nevoid melanoma

[a]Data from reference 201.

Table 8-15

COMPARISON OF SAMPUS AND MELTUMP LESIONS[a]

Property	SAMPUS	MELTUMP
Local persistence after incomplete excision	Yes	Yes
Local regrowth after incomplete excision	Yes	Yes
Continued progression after incomplete excision	Yes	Yes
Metastases after complete excision	No	Yes

[a]SAMPUS = superficial atypical melanocytic proliferations of uncertain significance; MELTUMP = melanocytic tumors of uncertain malignant potential.

dysplasia connotes a potentially intermediate lesion, especially when severe. Most dysplastic nevi, however, particularly those with random mild atypia, are stable lesions that will never progress, and they do not exhibit the properties of local recurrence or metastasis. In this regard, it is commonly indicated that a characteristic feature of dysplasia is its ability to regress. This is not an exclusive characteristic of dysplasia, however, given the tendency of some benign as well as malignant tumors to regress as well.

In the area of melanocytic biology, there exist two categories of prognostically intermediate lesions, forms related to the concept of radial and vertical growth phase melanomas (202). The first includes nontumorigenic lesions that we descriptively term *superficial atypical melanocytic proliferations of uncertain significance* (SAMPUS). This descriptive term may be applied to lesions that fail to display all the characteristics that permit a diagnosis outright of radial growth phase melanoma, and thus possess indeterminate or uncertain biologic potential to progress inexorably and locally recur (if inadequately excised or "persistent") but not to metastasize (subsequent to adequate excision) (fig. 8-38). The second includes tumorigenic atypical deeper compound and dermal *melanocytic tumors of uncertain malignant potential* (MELTUMP). This term is used for lesions that do not display all of the characteristics that permit a diagnosis of vertical growth phase melanoma, and whose capacity to metastasize is indeterminate or uncertain (fig. 8-39). Both of these categories have risk to progress inexorably upon incomplete excision, however, only the tumorigenic lesions (MELTUMP) have the potential for metastasis after complete excision. These properties are summarized in Table 8-15.

The existence of difficult or uncertain cases, where diagnostic agreement is not likely to be achieved even among experienced observers, suggests a need for a practical means of dealing with these cases in the best interests of the patients. In this regard, we are guided by two main principles: 1) lesions should be managed by means sufficient to provide adequate therapy for the most clinically significant entity in the differential diagnosis of an uncertain neoplasm, and 2) patients and their physicians deserve to know that their lesion cannot be diagnosed specifically with presently available means—uncertainty should not be concealed in a report that provides a false assurance of confidence in any given diagnosis.

In our practices, as in most institutions, slides are routinely reviewed from patients referred from outside institutions or laboratories. In the course of such reviews, a few of the referring diagnoses are revised, in some cases with

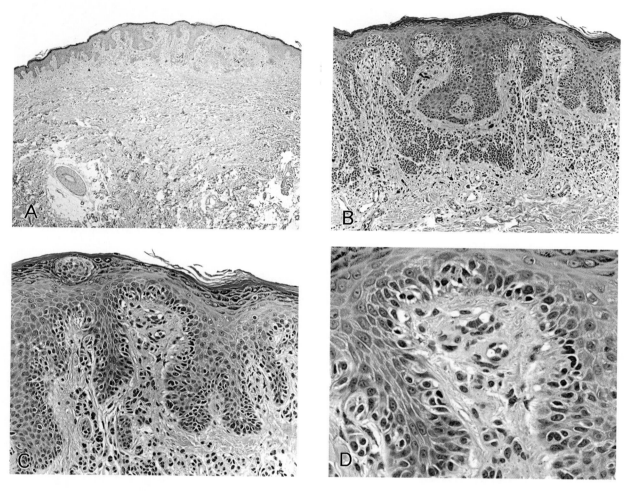

Figure 8-38

**COMPOUND NEVUS WITH SEVERE DYSPLASIA AND POSSIBLE EVOLVING MELANOMA IN SITU
(SUPERFICIAL ATYPICAL MELANOCYTIC PROLIFERATION OF UNCERTAIN SIGNIFICANCE [SAMPUS])**

A: At scanning magnification a fairly broad nevus, with a tendency to focal irregular thickening and thinning of the epidermis, is seen.

B: Orderly nevus cells are present in the dermis, and a few melanocytes extend into the epidermis focally.

C: Mild but relatively uniform nuclear irregularity and hyperchromatism. Several clusters of cells and a few single cells are present in the epidermis.

D: Between the rete ridges is a suggestion of continuous proliferation. These changes were interpreted as those of a compound nevus with severe dysplasia, with a comment that evolving melanoma in situ cannot focally be ruled out.

significant implications for patients (203,204). In some of these cases, the revision involves the reclassification of cases as "tumors of uncertain potential," which have previously been specifically diagnosed as either malignant melanoma or benign nevus. As in the case of usual or more characteristic forms of melanoma, it is helpful to divide these uncertain cases into two catego-

ries, namely superficial and nontumorigenic versus deep and tumorigenic lesions. These are discussed in more detail in later chapters. As time progresses and criteria are refined, including an increasing use of molecular criteria, we expect that cases in this "uncertain" group will diminish.

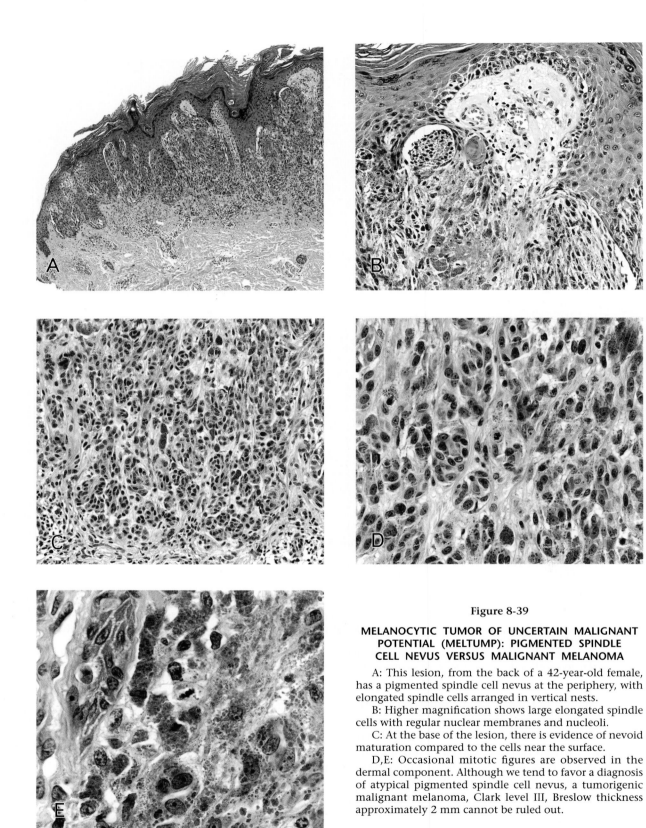

Figure 8-39

MELANOCYTIC TUMOR OF UNCERTAIN MALIGNANT POTENTIAL (MELTUMP): PIGMENTED SPINDLE CELL NEVUS VERSUS MALIGNANT MELANOMA

A: This lesion, from the back of a 42-year-old female, has a pigmented spindle cell nevus at the periphery, with elongated spindle cells arranged in vertical nests.

B: Higher magnification shows large elongated spindle cells with regular nuclear membranes and nucleoli.

C: At the base of the lesion, there is evidence of nevoid maturation compared to the cells near the surface.

D,E: Occasional mitotic figures are observed in the dermal component. Although we tend to favor a diagnosis of atypical pigmented spindle cell nevus, a tumorigenic malignant melanoma, Clark level III, Breslow thickness approximately 2 mm cannot be ruled out.

REFERENCES

1. Hutchinson J. Senile freckles. Arch Surg (London) 1892;3:319.

2. Dubreuilh MW. De la melanose circonscrite precancereuse. Ann Dermatol Syphiligr (Paris) 1912;3:129.

3. Lee JA, Petersen GR, Stevens RG, Vesanen K. The influence of age, year of birth, and date on mortality from malignant melanoma in the populations of England and Wales, Canada, and the white population of the United States. Am J Epidemiol 1979;110:734-739.

4. McCarthy WH, Black AL, Milton GW. Melanoma in New South Wales: an epidemiologic surgery 1970–76. Cancer 1980;46:427-432.

5. Silverberg E, Boring CC, Squires TS. Cancer statistics, 1990. CA Cancer J Clin 1990;40:9-26.

6. Roush GC, Schymura MJ, Holford TR. Risk for cutaneous melanoma in recent Connecticut birth cohorts. Am J Public Health 1985;75:679-682.

7. Severi G, Giles GG, Robertson C, Boyle P, Autier P. Mortality from cutaneous melanoma: evidence for contrasting trends between populations. Br J Cancer 2000;82:1887-1891.

8. Swerdlow AJ, English J, MacKie RM, et al. Benign melanocytic naevi as a risk factor for malignant melanoma. Br Med J 1986;292:1555-1559.

9. Tucker MA, Halpern A, Holly EA, et al. Clinically recognized dysplastic nevi. A central risk factor for cutaneous melanoma. JAMA 1997;277:1439-1444.

10. Green A, Siskind V, Bain C, Alexander J. Sunburn and malignant melanoma. Br J Cancer 1985;51:393-397.

11. Marks R. Campaigning for melanoma prevention: a model for a health education program. J Eur Acad Dermatol Venereol 2004;18:44-47.

12. Gandini S, Sera F, Cattaruzza MS, et al. Meta-analysis of risk factors for cutaneous melanoma: II. Sun exposure. Eur J Cancer 2005;41:45-60.

13. Martin RC, Robinson E. Cutaneous melanoma in Caucasian New Zealanders: 1995-1999. ANZ J Surg 2004;74:233-237.

14. Jemal A, Devesa SS, Fears TR, Hartge P. Cancer surveillance series: changing patterns of cutaneous malignant melanoma mortality rates among whites in the United States. J Natl Cancer Inst 2000;92:811-818.

15. Jemal A, Devesa SS, Hartge P, Tucker MA. Recent trends in cutaneous melanoma incidence among whites in the United States. J Natl Cancer Inst 2001;93:678-683.

16. Pack GT, Gerber DM, Sharnagel IM. End results in the treatment of melanoma: a report of 1190 cases. Ann Surg 1952;136:905-911.

17. Day CL Jr, Lew RA, Mihm MC Jr, et al. The natural break points for primary-tumor thickness in clinical stage I melanoma. N Engl J Med 1981;305:1155.

18. Lemish WM, Heenan PJ, Holman CD, Armstrong BK. Survival from preinvasive and invasive malignant melanoma in Western Australia. Cancer 1983;52:580-585.

19. Silverberg E, Lubera JA. Cancer Statistics, 1989. CA Cancer J Clin 1989;39:3-20.

20. Balch CM, Soong SJ, Gershenwald JE, et al. Prognostic factors analysis of 17,600 melanoma patients: validation of the American Joint Committee on Cancer Melanoma staging system. J Clin Oncol 2001;19:3622-3634.

21. Gatta G, Capocaccia R, Coleman MP, et al. Toward a comparison of survival in American and European cancer patients. Cancer 2000;89:893-900.

22. Giblin AV, Thomas JM. Incidence, mortality and survival in cutaneous melanoma. J Plast Reconstr Aesthet Surg 2007;60:32-40.

23. Little JH, Holt J, Davis N. Changing epidemiology of malignant melanoma in Queensland. Med J Aust 1980;1:66-69.

24. Balch CM, Soong SJ, Milton GW, et al. Changing trends in cutaneous melanoma over a quarter century in Alabama, USA, and New South Wales, Australia. Cancer 1983;52:1748-1753.

25. Beddingfield FC 3rd. The melanoma epidemic: res ipsa loquitur. Oncologist 2003;8:459-465.

26. Allen AC. A reorientation on the histogenesis and clinical significance of cutaneous nevi and melanomas. Cancer 1949;2:28-56.

27. Clark WH Jr. A classification of malignant melanoma in man correlated with histogenesis and biologic behavior. In: Montagna W, Hu F, eds. Advances in the biology of the skin, 6th ed., Vol. 8. The pigmentary system; proceedings the Brown University Symposium on biology of the skin, 1963. New York: Pergamon Press; 1967:621-647.

28. McGovern VJ. The classification of melanoma and its relationship with prognosis. Pathology 1970;2:85-98.

29. Mihm MC Jr, Clark WH Jr, From L. The clinical diagnosis, classification and histogenetic concepts of the early stages of cutaneous malignant melanomas. N Engl J Med 1971;284:1078-1082.

30. Gimotty PA, Van Belle P, Elder DE, et al. Biologic and prognostic significance of dermal Ki67 expression, mitoses, and tumorigenicity in thin invasive cutaneous melanoma. J Clin Oncol 2005;23:8048-8056.

31. Gimotty PA, Guerry D 4th, Ming ME, et al. Thin primary cutaneous malignant melanoma: a prognostic tree for 10-year metastasis is more accurate than American Joint Committee on Cancer staging. J Clin Oncol 2004;22:3668-3676.

32. Clark WH Jr, Elder DE, Guerry D 4th. Dysplastic nevi and malignant melanoma. In: Farmer ER, Hood AF, eds. Pathology of the skin. Norwalk, CT: Appleton & Lange; 1990:684-756.

33. Elder DE, Guerry D 4th, Epstein MN, et al. Invasive malignant melanomas lacking competence for metastasis. Am J Dermatopathol 1984;6:55-62.

34. Clark WH Jr, Elder DE, Guerry D 4th, et al. Model predicting survival in stage I melanoma based on tumor progression. J Natl Cancer Inst 1989;81:1893-1904.

35. Bastian BC, LeBoit PE, Hamm H, Bröcker EB, Pinkel D. Chromosomal gains and losses in primary cutaneous melanomas detected by comparative genomic hybridization. Cancer Res 1998;58:2170-2175.

36. Bastian BC, Kashani-Sabet M, Hamm H, et al. Gene amplifications characterize acral melanoma and permit the detection of occult tumor cells in the surrounding skin. Cancer Res 2000;60:1968-1973.

37. Demunter A, Stas M, Degreef H, Wolf-Peeters C, Van den Oord JJ. Analysis of N- and K-ras mutations in the distinctive tumor progression phases of melanoma. J Invest Dermatol 2001;117:1483-1489.

38. Reed RJ. Minimal deviation melanoma. Monogr Pathol 1988;(30):110-152

39. Reed RJ. Dimensionalities: borderline and intermediate melanocytic neoplasia. Hum Pathol 1999;30:521-524.

40. Tuthill RJ. A new paradigm for melanoma. 19th International Pigment Cell Conference. A focus on human pigmentary diseases. Reston, VA. IPCC Abstracts; 2005:78.

41. Heenan PJ, Holman CD. Nodular malignant melanoma: a distinct entity or a common end stage? Am J Dermatopathol 1982;4:477-478.

42. Cassarino DS, Cabral ES, Kartha RV, Swetter SM. Primary dermal melanoma: distinct immunohistochemical findings and clinical outcome compared with nodular and metastatic melanoma. Arch Dermatol 2008;144:49-56.

43. Clark WH Jr, Elder DE, Guerry D 4th, Epstein MN, Greene MH, Van Horn M. A study of tumor progression: the precursor lesions of superficial spreading and nodular melanoma. Hum Pathol 1984;15:1147-1165.

44. Clark WH Jr, From L, Bernardino EA, Mihm MC Jr. The histogenesis and biologic behavior of primary human malignant melanomas of the skin. Cancer Res 1969;29:705-727.

45. Committee of Australian Pathologists. Moles and malignant melanoma: terminology and classification. Med J Aust 1967;1:123-124.

46. McGovern VJ, Mihm MC Jr, Bailly C, et al. The classification of malignant melanoma and its histologic reporting. Cancer 1973;32:1446-1457.

47. McGovern VJ, Cochran AJ, Van der Esch EP, Little JH, MacLennan R. The classification of malignant melanoma, its histological reporting and registration: a revision of the 1972 Sydney classification. Pathology 1986;18:12-21.

48. Cochran AJ, Bailly C, Cook M, et al. Recommendations for the reporting of tissues removed as part of the surgical treatment of cutaneous melanoma. The Association of Directors of Anatomic and Surgical Pathology. Am J Clin Pathol 1998;110:719-722.

49. MacKie RM. Malignant melanoma: clinical variants and prognostic indicators. Clin Exp Dermatol 2000;25:471-475.

50. Clark WH Jr, Mihm MC Jr. Lentigo maligna and lentigo-maligna melanoma. Am J Pathol 1969;55:39-67.

51. Reed RJ, Ichinose H, Clark WH Jr, Mihm MC Jr. Common and uncommon melanocytic nevi and borderline melanomas. Semin Oncol 1975;2:119-147.

52. Weyers W, Euler M, Diaz-Cascajo C, Schill WB, Bonczkowitz M. Classification of cutaneous malignant melanoma: a reassessment of histopathologic criteria for the distinction of different types. Cancer 1999;86:288-299.

53. Bastian BC, Olshen AB, LeBoit PE, Pinkel D. Classifying melanocytic tumors based on DNA copy number changes. Am J Pathol 2003;163:1765-1770.

54. Bastian BC. Understanding the progression of melanocytic neoplasia using genomic analysis: from fields to cancer. Oncogene 2003;22:3081-3086.

55. Sasaki Y, Niu C, Makino R, et al. BRAF point mutations in primary melanoma show different prevalences by subtype. J Invest Dermatol 2004;123:177-183.

56. Cohen Y, Rosenbaum E, Begum S, et al. Exon 15 BRAF mutations are uncommon in melanomas arising in nonsun-exposed sites. Clin Cancer Res 2004;10:3444-3447.

57. Curtin JA, Fridlyand J, Kageshita T, et al. Distinct sets of genetic alterations in melanoma. N Engl J Med 2005;353:2135-2147.

58. Curtin JA, Busam K, Pinkel D, Bastian BC. Somatic activation of kit in distinct subtypes of melanoma. J Clin Oncol 2006;24:4340-4346.

59. Viros A, Fridyland J, Bauer J, Curtin J, Pinkel D, Bastian BC. Histomorphological signature of mutation status in melanoma. 2007. In: American Association for Cancer Research Annual Meeting: Proceedings; 2007 Apr 14-18; Los Angeles, CA. Philadelphia (PA): AACR; 2007. Abstract nr {154}.

60. de Vries E, Elder DE, Bray F, et al. Malignant melanoma: introduction. In: LeBoit PE, Burg G, Weedon D, Sarasin A, eds. Pathology and genetics of skin tumors. Lyon: IARC Press; 2006:52-65.

61. Heenan PJ, Matz LR, Blackwell JB, et al. Inter-observer variation between pathologists in the classification of cutaneous malignant melanoma in Western Australia. Histopathology 1984;8:717-729.

62. Cochran AJ, Elashoff D, Morton DL, Elashoff R. Individualized prognosis for melanoma patients. Hum Pathol 2000;31:327-331.

63. Barnhill RL, Fine JA, Roush GC, Berwick M. Predicting five-year outcome for patients with cutaneous melanoma in a population-based study. Cancer 1996;78:427-432.

64. Soong SJ, Shaw HM, Balch CM, McCarthy WH, Urist MM, Lee JY. Predicting survival and recurrence in localized melanoma: a multivariate approach. World J Surg 1992;16:191-195.

65. Sagebiel RW. Unusual variants of melanoma: fact or fiction? Semin Oncol 1996;23:703-708.

66. Gruber SB, Barnhill RL, Stenn KS, Roush GC. Nevomelanocytic proliferations in association with cutaneous malignant melanoma: a multivariate analysis. J Am Acad Dermatol 1989;21:773-780.

67. Barnhill RL, Mihm MC Jr. The histopathology of cutaneous malignant melanoma. Semin Diagn Pathol 1993;10:47-75.

68. McGovern VJ, Shaw HM, Milton GW, Farago GA. Prognostic significance of the histological features of malignant melanoma. Histopathology 1979;3:385-393.

69. Roses DF, Harris MN, Ackerman AB. Clinical and histologic features of malignant melanomas. In: Roses DF, Harris MN, Ackerman AB. Diagnosis and management of cutaneous malignant melanoma. Philadelphia: Saunders; 1983:27-76.

70. Abramova L, Slingluff CL Jr, Patterson JW. Problems in the interpretation of apparent 'radial growth phase' malignant melanomas that metastasize. J Cutan Pathol 2002;29:407-414.

71. Lefevre M, Vergier B, Balme B, et al. Relevance of vertical growth pattern in thin level II cutaneous superficial spreading melanomas. Am J Surg Pathol 2003;27:717-724.

72. Guerry D 4th, Synnestvedt M, Elder DE, Schultz D. Lessons from tumor progression: the invasive radial growth phase of melanoma is common, incapable of metastasis, and indolent. J Invest Dermatol 1993;100:342S-345S.

73. Sagebiel RW. Histopathology of borderline and early malignant melanomas. Am J Surg Pathol 1979;3:543-552.

74. Rywlin AM. Malignant melanoma in situ, precancerous melanosis, or atypical intraepidermal melanocytic proliferation. Am J Dermatopathol 1984;6(Suppl):97-99.

75. Rywlin AM. Intraepithelial melanocytic neoplasia (IMN) versus intraepithelial atypical melanocytic proliferation (IAMP). Am J Dermatopathol 1988;10:92-93.

76. Slater DN. Melanocytic intra-epidermal neoplasia (MIN). Histopathology 1997;30:195-197.

77. Elder D. Tumor progression, early diagnosis and prognosis of melanoma. Acta Oncol 1999;38:535-547.

78. Carey WP Jr, Van Belle P, Elder DE. Tumor progression-related reactivity of nevi and melanomas with the MIB-1 (Ki-67) antigen evaluated by streptavidin immunohistochemistry on paraffin sections. Pigment Cell Res 1994;(Suppl 3):18.

79. Bergman R, Malkin L, Sabo E, Kerner H. MIB-1 monoclonal antibody to determine proliferative activity of Ki-67 antigen as an adjunct to the histopathologic differential diagnosis of Spitz nevi. J Am Acad Dermatol 2001;44:500-504.

80. Kaleem Z, Lind AC, Humphrey PA, et al. Concurrent Ki-67 and p53 immunolabeling in cutaneous melanocytic neoplasms: an adjunct to recognition of the vertical growth phase in malignant melanomas? Mod Pathol 2000;13:217-222.

81. Li LX, Crotty KA, McCarthy SW, Palmer AA, Kril JJ. A zonal comparison of MIB1-Ki67 immunoreactivity in benign and malignant melanocytic lesions. Am J Dermatopathol 2000;22:489-495.

82. Korabiowska M, Brinck U, Middel P, et al. Proliferative activity in the progression of pigmented skin lesions, diagnostic and prognostic significance. Anticancer Res 2000;20:1781-1785.

83. Korabiowska M, Brinck U, Mirecka J, Kellner S, Marx D, Schauer A. Antigen Ki-67 and c-myc oncogene as related to histoclinical parameters in pigmented skin lesions. In Vivo 1995;9:433-438.

84. McNutt NS, Urmacher C, Hakimian J, Hoss DM, Lugo J. Nevoid malignant melanoma: morphologic patterns and immunohistochemical reactivity. J Cutan Pathol 1995;22:502-517.

85. Saenz-Santamaria MC, Reed JA, McNutt NS, Shea CR. Immunohistochemical expression of BCL-2 in melanomas and intradermal nevi. J Cutan Pathol 1994;21:393-397.

86. Gimotty PA, Van Belle PA, Elder DE, et al. Biologic and prognostic significance of dermal Ki67 expression, mitoses, and tumorigenicity in thin invasive cutaneous melanoma. J Clin Oncol 2005;23:8048-8456.

87. Soyer HP. Ki 67 immunostaining in melanocytic skin tumors. Correlation with histologic parameters. J Cutan Pathol 1991;18:264-272.

88. Lee JD, Unger ER, Gittenger C, Lee DR, Hebert R, Maize JC. Interphase cytogenetic analysis of 1q12 satellite III DNA in melanocytic lesions: increased aneuploidy with malignant histology. Am J Dermatopathol 2001;23:176-180.

89. Hsu MY, Shih DT, Meier F, et al. Adenoviral gene transfer of beta3 integrin subunit induces conversion from radial to vertical growth phase in primary human melanoma. Am J Pathol 1998;153:1435-1442.

90. Albelda SM, Mette SA, Elder DE, et al. Integrin distribution in malignant melanoma: association of the beta 3 subunit with tumor progression. Cancer Res 1990;50:6757-6764.

91. Montgomery AM, Reisfeld RA, Cheresh DA. Integrin alphavbeta3 rescues melanoma cells from apoptosis in three-dimensional dermal collagen. Proc Natl Acad Sci USA 1994;91:8856-8860.

92. Gouon V, Tucker GC, Kraus-Berthier L, Atassi G, Kieffer N. Up-regulated expression of the beta3 integrin and the 92-kDA gelatinase in human HT-144 melanoma cell tumors grown in nude mice. Int J Cancer 1996;68:650-662.

93. Seftor RE, Seftor EA, Stetler-Stevenson WG, Hendrix MJ. The 72 kDa type IV collagenase is modulated via differential expression of alphavbeta3 and alpha5beta1 integrins during human melanoma cell invasion. Cancer Res 1993;53:3411-3415.

94. Van Belle PA, Elenitsas R, Satyamoorthy K, et al. Progression-related expression of beta3 integrin in melanomas and nevi. Hum Pathol 1999;30:562-567.

95. Friedman RJ, Rigel DS, Kopf AW. Early detection of malignant melanoma: the role of physician examination and self-examination of the skin. CA Cancer J Clin 1985;35:130-151.

96. Bono A, Bartoli C, Baldi M, et al. Micro-melanoma detection. A clinical study on 22 cases of melanoma with a diameter equal to or less than 3 mm. Tumori 2004;90:128-131.

97. Thomas NE, Groben P. Invasive superficial spreading melanomas arising from clinically normal skin. J Am Acad Dermatol 2004;51:466-470.

98. Kibbi AG, Mihm MC Jr, Sober AJ, Fitzpatrick TB. Diagnosis and management of malignant melanoma. Compr Ther 1986;12:23-31.

99. Scope A, Dusza SW, Halpern AC, et al. The "ugly duckling" sign: agreement between observers. Arch Dermatol 2008;144:58-64.

100. Swerlick RA, Chen S. The melanoma epidemic. Is increased surveillance the solution or the problem? Arch Dermatol 1996;132:881-884.

101. Elder DE, Guerry D 4th, Epstein MN, et al. Invasive malignant melanomas lacking competence for metastasis. Am J Dermatopathol 1984;6(Suppl):55-61.

102. Dennis LK. Analysis of the melanoma epidemic, both apparent and real: data from the 1973 through 1994 surveillance, epidemiology, and end results program registry. Arch Dermatol 1999;135:275-280.

103. Winter R. Conservative surgery for microinvasive carcinoma of the cervix. J Obstet Gynaecol Res 1998;24:433-436.

104. Urso C, Borgognoni L, Saieva C, Tinacci G, Zini E. Sensitivity and specificity of histological criteria in the diagnosis of conventional melanoma. Melanoma Res 2008;4:253-258.

105. Bono A, Bartoli C, Moglia D, et al. Small melanomas: a clinical study on 270 consecutive cases of cutaneous melanoma. Melanoma Res 1999;9:583-586.

106. Price NM, Rywlin AM, Ackerman AB. Histologic criteria for the diagnosis of superficial spreading melanoma: formulated on the basis of proven metastatic lesions. Cancer 1976;38:2434-2441.

107. Okun MR. Silhouette symmetry: an unsupportable histologic criterion for distinguishing Spitz nevi and compound nevi from malignant melanoma. Arch Pathol Lab Med 1997;121:48-53.

108. Mishima Y. Melanocytic and nevocytic malignant melanomas. Cellular and subcellular differentiation. Cancer 1967;20:632-649.

109. Clark WH Jr, Evans HL, Everett MA, et al. Early melanoma. Histologic terms. Am J Dermatopathol 1991;13:579-582.

110. Fallowfield ME, Cook MG. Pagetoid infiltration in primary cutaneous melanoma. Histopathology 1992;20:417-420.

111. Busam KJ, Barnhill RL. Pagetoid Spitz nevus. Intraepidermal Spitz tumor with prominent pagetoid spread. Am J Surg Pathol 1995;19:1061-1067.

112. Haupt HM, Stern JB. Pagetoid melanocytosis: histologic features in benign and malignant lesions. Am J Surg Pathol 1995;19:792-797.

113. Mérot Y, Frenk E. Spitz nevus (large spindle cell and/or epithelioid cell nevus). Age-related involvement of the suprabasal epidermis. Virchows Arch A Pathol Anat Histopathol 1989;415:97-101.

114. Boyd AS, Rapini RP. Acral melanocytic neoplasms: a histologic analysis of 158 lesions. J Am Acad Dermatol 1994;31:740-745.

115. Kohler S, Rouse RV, Smoller BR. The differential diagnosis of pagetoid cells in the epidermis. Mod Pathol 1998;11:79-92.

116. Bayer-Garner IB, Reed JA. Immunolabeling pattern of syndecan-1 expression may distinguish pagetoid Bowen's disease, extramammary Paget's disease, and pagetoid malignant melanoma in situ. J Cutan Pathol 2004;31:169-173.

117. Rudolph P, Tronnier M, Menzel R, Moller M, Parwaresch R. Enhanced expression of Ki-67, topoisomerase IIalpha, PCNA, p53 and p21WAF1/Cip1 reflecting proliferation and repair activity in UV-irradiated melanocytic nevi. Hum Pathol 1998;29:1480-1487.

118. Stern JB, Haupt HM. Pagetoid melanocytosis: tease or tocsin? Semin Diagn Pathol 1998;15:225-229.

119. Maize JC, Ackerman AB. Pigmented lesions of the skin. Clinicopathologic correlations. Philadelphia: Lea & Febiger; 1987.

120. Okun MR. Histological demarcation of lateral borders: an unsupportable criterion for distinguishing malignant melanoma from Spitz naevus and compound naevus. Histopathology 1998;33:158-162.

121. Hantschke M, Bastian BC, LeBoit PE. Consumption of the epidermis: a diagnostic criterion for the differential diagnosis of melanoma and Spitz nevus. Am J Surg Pathol 2004;28:1621-1625.

122. Braun-Falco M, Friedrichson E, Ring J. Subepidermal cleft formation as a diagnostic marker for cutaneous malignant melanoma. Hum Pathol 2005;36:412-415.

123. Clark WH Jr, Tucker MA, Goldstein AM. Parenchymal-stromal interactions in neoplasia: theoretical considerations and observations in melanocytic neoplasia. Acta Oncol 1995;34:749-757.

124. McGovern VJ. Spontaneous regression of melanoma. Pathology 1975;7:91-99.

125. Clark WH Jr, Tucker MA. Problems with lesions related to the development of malignant melanoma: common nevi, dysplastic nevi, malignant melanoma in situ, and radial growth phase malignant melanoma. Hum Pathol 1998;29:8-14.

126. Stretch JR, Denton KJ, Millard PR, Horak E. Paget's disease of the male breast clinically and histopathologically mimicking melanoma. Histopathology 1991;19:470-472.

127. Peison B, Benisch B. Paget's disease of the nipple simulating malignant melanoma in a black woman. Am J Dermatopathol 1985;7(Suppl):165-169.

128. Reed W, Oppedal BR, Eeg Larsen T. Immunohistology is valuable in distinguishing between Paget's disease, Bowen's disease and superficial spreading malignant melanoma. Histopathology 1990;16:583-588.

129. Gillett CE, Bobrow LG, Millis RR. S100 protein in human mammary tissue—immunoreactivity in breast carcinoma, including Paget's disease of the nipple, and value as a marker of myoepithelial cells. J Pathol 1990;160:19-24.

130. Rosen L, Amazon K, Frank B. Bowen's disease, Paget's disease, and malignant melanoma in situ. South Med J 1986;79:410-413.

131. Clemente C, Cochran A, Elder DE, et al. Histopathologic diagnosis of dysplastic nevi. Concordance among pathologists convened by the WHO melanoma programme. Hum Pathol 1991;22:313-319.

132. Steijlen PM, Bergman W, Hermans J, Scheffer E, van Vloten WA, Ruiter DJ. The efficacy of histopathological criteria required for diagnosing dysplastic naevi. Histopathology 1988;12:289-300.

133. Smoller BR, Egbert BM. Dysplastic nevi can be diagnosed and graded reproducibly: a longitudinal study. J Am Acad Dermatol 1992;27:399-402.

134. De Wit PE, van't Hof-Grootenboer B, Ruiter DJ, et al. Validity of the histopathological criteria used for diagnosing dysplastic naevi. An interobserver study by the pathology subgroup of the EORTC Malignant Melanoma Cooperative Group. Eur J Cancer 1993;29A:831-839.

135. Roush GC, Kirkwood JM, Ernstoff M, et al. Reproducibility and validity in the clinical diagnosis of the nonfamilial dysplastic nevus: work in progress. Recent Results Cancer Res 1986;102:154-158.

136. Weinstock MA. Dysplastic nevi revisited. J Am Acad Dermatol 1994;30:807-810.

137. Hastrup N, Clemmensen OJ, Spaun E, Sondergaard K. Dysplastic naevus: histological criteria and their inter-observer reproducibility. Histopathology 1994;24:503-509.

138. Piepkorn MW, Barnhill RL, Cannon-Albright LA, et al. A multiobserver, population-based analysis of histologic dysplasia in melanocytic nevi. J Am Acad Dermatol 1994;30:707-714.

139. McDermott NC, Hayes DP, al-Sader MH, et al. Identification of vertical growth phase in malignant melanoma. A study of interobserver agreement. Am J Clin Pathol 1998;110:753-757.

140. A nationwide survey of observer variation in the diagnosis of thin cutaneous malignant melanoma including the MIN terminology. J Clin Pathol 1997;50:202-205.

141. Liu W, Dowling JP, Murray WK, et al. Rate of growth in melanomas: characteristics and associations of rapidly growing melanomas. Arch Dermatol 2006;142:1551-1558.

142. Elder DE, Gimotty PA, Guerry D. Cutaneous melanoma: estimating survival and recurrence risk based on histopathologic features. Dermatol Ther 2005;18:369-385.

143. Nowell PC. The clonal evolution of tumor cell populations. Science 1976;194:23-28.

144. Oliveira Filho RS, Ferreira LM, Biasi LJ, Enokihara MM, Paiva GR, Wagner J. Vertical growth phase and positive sentinel node in thin melanoma. Braz J Med Biol Res 2003;36:347-350.

145. Bedrosian I, Faries MB, Guerry D 4th, et al. Incidence of sentinel node metastasis in patients with thin primary melanoma (< or = 1 mm) with vertical growth phase. Ann Surg Oncol 2000;7:262-267. Comment in Ann Surg Oncol 2000;7:251-252.

146. Kuehnl-Petzoldt C, Berger H, Wiebelt H. Verrucous-keratotic variants of malignant melanoma: a clinicopathologic study. Am J Dermatopathol 1982;4:403-410.

147. Smolle J, Hofmann-Wellenhof R, Kofler R, Cerroni L, Haas J, Kerl H. Computer simulations of histologic patterns in melanoma using a cellular automaton provide correlations with prognosis. J Invest Dermatol 1995;105:797-801.

148. Clark WH Jr, Mastrangelo MJ, Ainsworth AM, Berd D, Bellet RE, Bernardino EA. Current concepts of the biology of human cutaneous malignant melanoma. Adv Cancer Res 1977;24:267-338.

149. Paniago-Pereira C, Maize JC, Ackerman AB. Nevus of large spindle and/or epithelioid cells (Spitz's nevus). Arch Dermatol 1978;114:1811-1823.

150. Barr RJ, King DF. The significance of pseudoinclusions within the nuclei of melanocytes of certain neoplasms. In: Ackerman AB, ed. Pathology of malignant melanoma. New York: Masson; 1981:269-272.

151. Nakhleh RE, Wick MR, Rocamora A, Swanson PE, Dehner LP. Morphologic diversity in malignant melanomas. Am J Clin Pathol 1990;93:731-740.

152. Cachia AR, Kedziora AM. Subungual malignant melanoma with cartilaginous differentiation. Am J Dermatopathol 1999;21:165-169.

153. Sheibani K, Battifora H. Signet-ring cell melanoma: a rare morphologic variant of malignant melanoma. Am J Surg Pathol 1988;12:28-34.

154. Bastian BC, Kutzner H, Yen T, LeBoit PE. Signet-ring cell formation in cutaneous neoplasms. J Am Acad Dermatol 1999;41:606-613.

155. Livolsi VA, Brooks JJ, Soslow R, Johnson BL, Elder DE. Signet cell melanocytic lesions. Mod Pathol 1992;5:515-520.

156. Aloi FG, Coverlizza S, Pippione M. Balloon cell melanoma: a report of two cases. J Cutan Pathol 1988;15:230-233.

157. Abbott JJ, Amirkhan RH, Hoang MP. Malignant melanoma with a rhabdoid phenotype: histologic, immunohistochemical, and ultrastructural study of a case and review of the literature. Arch Pathol Lab Med 2004;128:686-688.

158. Borek BT, McKee PH, Freeman JA, Maguire B, Brander WL, Calonje E. Primary malignant melanoma with rhabdoid features: a histologic and immunocytochemical study of three cases. Am J Dermatopathol 1998;20:123-127.

159. Bhuta S, Mirra JM, Cochran AJ. Myxoid malignant melanoma. A previously undescribed histologic pattern noted in metastatic lesions and a report of four cases. Am J Surg Pathol 1986;10:203-211.

160. Olmstead PM, Lund HZ, Leonard DD. Monsel's solution: a histologic nuisance. J Am Acad Dermatol 1980;3:492-498.

161. Duray PH, Livolsi VA. Recurrent dysplastic nevus following shave excision. J Dermatol Surg Oncol 1984;10:811-815.

162. Jones RE. Questions to the editorial board and other authorities. What are your five most important histologic criteria for the diagnosis of malignant melanoma? Am J Dermatopathol 1984;6(Suppl 1):89-94.

163. Stolz W, Schmoeckel C, Welkovich B, Braun-Falco O. Semiquantitative analysis of histologic criteria in thin malignant melanomas. J Am Acad Dermatol 1989;20:1115-1120.

164. Kirkham N. Optimal handling and criteria for melanoma diagnosis. Histopathology 2000;37:467-469.

165. Slater DN. Doubt and uncertainty in the diagnosis of melanoma. Histopathology 2000;37:469-472.

166. Okun MR, Edelstein LM, Kasznica J, Kirkham N, Slater DN. What criteria reliably distinguish melanoma from benign melanocytic lesions? Histopathology 2000;37:464-472.

167. Barnhill RL. Childhood melanoma. Semin Diagn Pathol 1998;15:189-194.

168. Elder DE, Rodeck U, Thurin J, et al. Antigenic profile of tumor progression stages in human melanocytic nevi and melanomas. Cancer Res 1989;49:5091-5096.

169. Brocker EB, Suter L, Bruggen J, Ruiter DJ, Macher E, Sorg C. Phenotypic dynamics of tumor progression in human malignant melanoma. Int J Cancer 1985;36:29-35.

170. Kan Mitchell J, Imam A, Kempf RA, Taylor CR, Mitchell MS. Human monoclonal antibodies directed against melanoma tumor-associated antigens. Cancer Res 1986;46:2490-2496.

171. Brogelli L, Carli P, Reali UM, Pimpinelli N, Moretti S. Antigenic phenotype of radial growth phase melanomas with or without a vertical growth phase portion. Tumori 1988;74:157-162.

172. Herlyn M, Ross AH, Balaban G, et al. Cell biology of melanoma and nonmalignant melanocytic lesions. In: Elder DE, ed. Pathobiology of malignant melanoma. Basel: Karger; 1987:166-181.

173. Balaban GB, Herlyn M, Clark WH Jr, Nowell PC. Karyotypic evolution in human malignant melanoma. Cancer Genet Cytogenet 1986;19:113-122.

174. Frank NY, Margaryan A, Huang Y, et al. ABCB5-mediated doxorubicin transport and chemoresistance in human malignant melanoma. Cancer Res 2005;65:4320-4333.

175. Schatton T, Murphy GF, Frank NY, et al. Identification of cells initiating human melanomas. Nature 2008;451:345-349.

176. Cochran AJ, Wen DR, Herschman HR, Gaynor RB. Detection of S-100 protein as an aid to the identification of melanocytic tumors. Int J Cancer 1982;30:295-297.

177. Argenyi ZB, Cain C, Bromley C, et al. S-100 protein-negative malignant melanoma: fact or fiction? A light microscopic and immunohistochemical study. Am J Dermatopathol 1994;16:233-240.

178. Busam KJ, Chen YT, Old LJ, et al. Expression of melan-A (MART1) in benign melanocytic nevi and primary cutaneous malignant melanoma. Am J Surg Pathol 1998;22:976-982.

179. Clarkson KS, Sturdgess IC, Molyneux AJ. The usefulness of tyrosinase in the immunohistochemical assessment of melanocytic lesions: a comparison of the novel T311 antibody (anti-tyrosinase) with S-100, HMB45, and A103 (anti-melan-A). J Clin Pathol 2001;54:196-200.

180. De Vries TJ, Smeets M, de Graaf R, et al. Expression of gp100, MART-1, tyrosinase, and S100 in paraffin-embedded primary melanomas and locoregional, lymph node, and visceral metastases: implications for diagnosis and immunotherapy. A study conducted by the EORTC Melanoma Cooperative Group. J Pathol 2001;193:13-20.

181. Orchard GE. Comparison of immunohistochemical labelling of melanocyte differentiation antibodies melan-A, tyrosinase and HMB 45 with NKIC3 and S100 protein in the evaluation of benign naevi and malignant melanoma. Histochem J 2000;32:475-481.

182. Busam KJ, Jungbluth AA. Melan-A, a new melanocytic differentiation marker. Adv Anat Pathol 1999;6:12-18.

183. Fetsch PA, Marincola FM, Filie A, Hijazi YM, Kleiner DE, Abati A. Melanoma-associated antigen recognized by T cells (MART-1): the advent of a preferred immunocytochemical antibody for the diagnosis of metastatic malignant melanoma with fine-needle aspiration. Cancer 1999;87:37-42.

184. Jungbluth AA, Busam KJ, Gerald WL, et al. A103: an anti-Melan-a monoclonal antibody for the detection of malignant melanoma in paraffin-embedded tissues. Am J Surg Pathol 1998;22:595-602.

185. Miettinen M, Franssila K. Immunohistochemical spectrum of malignant melanoma. The common presence of keratins. Lab Invest 1989;61:623-628.

186. Ben-Izhak O, Stark P, Levy R, Bergman R, Lichtig C. Epithelial markers in malignant melanoma. A study of primary lesions and their metastases. Am J Dermatopathol 1994;16:241-246.

187. Boni R, Wellmann A, Man YG, Hofbauer G, Brinkmann U. Expression of the proliferation and apoptosis-associated CAS protein in benign and malignant cutaneous melanocytic lesions. Am J Dermatopathol 1999;21:125-128.

188. Björnhagen V, Bonfoco E, Brahme EM, Lindholm J, Auer G. Morphometric, DNA, and proliferating cell nuclear antigen measurements in benign melanocytic lesions and cutaneous malignant melanoma. Am J Dermatopathol 1994;16:615-623.

189. Barks JH, Thompson FH, Taetle R, et al. Increased chromosome 20 copy number detected by fluorescence in situ hybridization (FISH) in malignant melanoma. Genes Chromosomes Cancer 1997;19:278-285.

190. Wiltshire RN, Duray P, Bittner ML, et al. Direct visualization of the clonal progression of primary cutaneous melanoma: application of tissue microdissection and comparative genomic hybridization. Cancer Res 1995;55:3954-3957.

191. Bastian BC, Wesselmann U, Pinkel D, LeBoit PE. Molecular cytogenetic analysis of Spitz nevi shows clear differences to melanoma. J Invest Dermatol 1999;113:1065-1069.

192. Harvell JD, Kohler S, Zhu S, Hernandez-Boussard T, Pollack JR, Van de Rijn M. High-resolution array-based comparative genomic hybridization for distinguishing paraffin-embedded Spitz nevi and melanomas. Diagn Mol Pathol 2004;13:22-25.

193. Curtin JA, Fridlyand J, Kageshita T, et al. Distinct sets of genetic alterations in melanoma. N Engl J Med 2005;353:2135-2147.

194. Wang E, Marincola FM. cDNA arrays and the enigma of melanoma immune responsiveness. Cancer J 2001;7:16-24.

195. Bittner M, Meltzer P, Chen Y, et al. Molecular classification of cutaneous malignant melanoma by gene expression profiling. Nature 2000;406:536-540.

196. Su YA, Bittner ML, Chen Y, et al. Identification of tumor-suppressor genes using human melanoma cell lines UACC903, UACC903(+6), and SRS3 by comparison of expression profiles. Mol Carcinog 2000;28:119-127.

197. Jonsson G, Dahl C, Staaf J, et al. Genomic profiling of malignant melanoma using tiling-resolution array CGH. Oncogene 2007;26:4738-4748.

198. Alonso SR, Tracey L, Ortiz P, et al. A high-throughput study in melanoma identifies epithelial-mesenchymal transition as a major determinant of metastasis. Cancer Res 2007;67:3450-3460.

199. Jaeger J, Koczan D, Thiesen HJ, et al. Gene expression signatures for tumor progression, tumor subtype, and tumor thickness in laser-microdissected melanoma tissues. Clin Cancer Res 2007;13:806-815.

200. Winnepenninckx V, Lazar V, Michiels S, et al. Gene expression profiling of primary cutaneous melanoma and clinical outcome. J Natl Cancer Inst 2006;98:472-482.

201. Crowson AN, Magro CM, Mihm MC. Approach to the reporting of equivocal/border line nevomelanocytic lesions: the severely atypical dermoepidermal neromelanocytic proliferation as a transition step in lesions, a progression to malignant melanoma. In: Crowson AN, Magro CM, Mihm MC, eds. The melanocytic proliferations. A comprehensive textbook of pigmented lesions. New York: Wieley-Liss, 2001:477-500.

202. Elder DE, Xu X. The approach to the patient with a difficult melanocytic lesion. Pathology 2004;36:428-434.

203. McGinnis KS, Lessin SR, Elder DE, et al. Pathology review of cases presenting to a multidisciplinary pigmented lesion clinic. Arch Dermatol 2002;138:617-621.

9 HISTOGENETIC VARIANTS OF NONTUMORIGENIC MELANOMA (RADIAL GROWTH PHASE)

The variant patterns of radial growth phase lesions appear to have somewhat distinctive epidemiologic correlates, although they do not, in general, have prognostic significance (see Table 8-1). These variants can be regarded as clinicopathologic/epidemiologic syndromes of melanoma. The common superficial spreading melanoma, for example, occurs in young adults who indulge in recreational sun exposure, while the individual at greatest risk for lentigo maligna melanoma is a more elderly person with a history of lifelong outdoor work. All of the variants may present with or without an associated tumorigenic nodule within the radial growth phase. As has been discussed, some melanomas evolve directly to the vertical growth phase without an antecedent radial growth phase, resulting in a disparate appearance, termed nodular melanoma. Accurate diagnosis is greatly facilitated by an understanding of these morphologic variations. Interestingly, the clinicopathologic attributes that have been devised to separate these clinicopathologic entities over the years, such as nesting, scatter, chronic solar damage, patient age, circumscription, cell size, pigmentation, lesional location, cell and nuclear shape and size, and a thickened or hyperplastic epidermal contour, have recently been found to correlate with the fundamental genotype of the tumors (1), providing molecularly based support for the hypothesis that "all melanomas are not the same."

SUPERFICIAL ATYPICAL MELANOCYTIC PROLIFERATIONS OF UNCERTAIN SIGNIFICANCE (SAMPUS): UNCERTAINTY IN THE DIAGNOSIS OF NONTUMORIGENIC MELANOMA

As is also the case in tumorigenic melanomas, there are many superficial melanocytic proliferations in which criteria are conflicting. Depending on which criteria are emphasized by different observers, there will be disagreement among them as to the exact diagnosis, leading to uncertainty as to the biologic behavior of the lesion. It is our opinion that such uncertainty should be communicated clearly and directly to physicians and their patients, and that patients deserve to know and understand the differential diagnosis of their lesions and the potential consequences of each possible diagnosis. Only by such means can patients be offered appropriate management options with truly informed consent. It is helpful to divide these uncertain cases into two descriptive diagnostic categories, namely, superficial or nontumorigenic and deep or tumorigenic lesions.

The first or nontumorigenic category is that of superficial atypical melanocytic proliferation of uncertain significance (SAMPUS) (2). These are typically lesions in which the differential diagnosis lies between melanoma in situ or microinvasive radial growth phase melanoma and a benign simulant such as a junctional or superficial compound dysplastic nevus, a pigmented spindle cell nevus of Reed, a superficial Spitz nevus, or an atypical lentigo. In these cases, tumorigenic proliferation in the dermis is not present, and the prognosis is very good, with a very low probability of metastatic disease as long as local control can be achieved. If not excised, however, some such cases, at least as judged by anecdotal experience, persist at the local site and then have a propensity to regrow or recur, and perhaps in time to progress to a more fully malignant stage of melanocytic neoplasia. Until such progression (i.e., to vertical growth phase) occurs, these recurrences (or "persistences followed by regrowth") are not associated with competence for metastasis, and are amenable to local control by excision with clear margins (3). Many observers sign out these lesions as "atypical intraepidermal or superficial melanocytic proliferation," however, in our opinion, this term does not adequately convey the potential significance of a differential diagnosis that may include a melanoma.

In a relatively common scenario, such as that illustrated in figure 9-1, a few pagetoid melanocytes may be seen above the dermal-epidermal junction in an otherwise characteristic dysplastic nevus, or there may be an area suggestive of continuous or confluent proliferation between rete ridges (fig. 9-2). If there is no high-level and extensive (more than one high-power field or greater in width) pagetoid proliferation, no extensive continuous basal proliferation, no high-grade and uniform cytologic atypia, and no mitotic activity in these foci, we may interpret such lesions descriptively as, for example, "superficial atypical melanocytic proliferation of uncertain significance, see note." When a lesion is entirely in situ, the term "intraepidermal atypical melanocytic proliferation of uncertain significance" (IAMPUS) may be used (fig. 9-1). In a note we would add that "while we favor a diagnosis of a junctional nevus with moderate to focally severe melanocytic dysplasia, there are focal changes suggestive of evolving melanoma in situ, and this diagnosis cannot be ruled out." Sometimes this term may be appropriate to use for an inadequate biopsy, with a recommendation for complete excision to obtain additional diagnostic material (fig. 9-3). We believe that the presence of this uncertainty should be communicated to the patient and treatment options should be discussed and the differential diagnosis taken into consideration. For such SAMPUS lesions, we typically recommend consideration of a reexcision, aiming at a minimum for a clear margin of normal skin around the scar of the biopsy and any residual portion of the lesion.

Many clinicians may choose to apply minimal treatment for melanoma in situ, i.e., a clinical measured margin of 3 to 5 mm, with clear margins histologically (4,5). This approach should avoid the possibility of undertreatment of an in situ melanoma, which might then recur locally as in situ melanoma or as a more advanced lesion (figs. 9-4, 9-5). Although there are exceptional nevi in which epidermal or even dermal mitoses may be observed, this is rare and the diagnosis of a benign nevus should be made with extreme caution in the presence of any mitotic activity, especially if there is also cytologic atypia and if a diagnosis of a Spitz nevus cannot be established with certainty on other grounds. Also, the presence in the dermis of a tumorigenic proliferation of atypical melanocytes resembling those of an in situ melanoma in the overlying epidermis should lead to a diagnosis of melanoma.

SUPERFICIAL SPREADING MELANOMA (PAGETOID MELANOMA)

Definition. *Superficial spreading melanoma* is the common form of malignant melanoma. It is defined by the presence of a microinvasive or in situ radial growth phase that is composed of large epithelioid neoplastic melanocytes arranged in a pagetoid pattern within the epidermis. A vertical growth phase tumorigenic compartment may or may not be present as well (figs. 9-6, 9-7). This form of melanoma was termed *pagetoid melanoma* by McGovern (6), and this term aptly describes its most striking histologic characteristic.

Clinical Features. By definition, superficial spreading melanomas include a histologically nontumorigenic and microinvasive or in situ compartment, the radial growth phase. Clinically, this compartment appears as a plaque (if broad) or as a small papule when the lesion is small (less than 6 mm). These small papular lesions constitute a minority of cases but their incidence is increasing as more attention is paid to early diagnosis. The plaque exhibits the criteria discussed and summarized in chapter 7 under the "ABCDE" mnemonic (asymmetry, border irregularity, color variegation, diameter usually greater than 6 mm, elevation at least in microinvasive lesions) (figs. 9-6, 9-7). Most superficial spreading melanomas have discrete, well-defined although irregular borders, and the edge is usually palpable, in contrast to lentigo maligna melanoma and dysplastic nevi. A vertical growth phase tumorigenic nodule may be present within or at the edge of the radial growth phase. If so, its morphology and clinical significance are the same as a similar tumor nodule in other forms of melanoma, including melanomas of the nodular type.

Superficial spreading melanoma is the most common form of melanoma, accounting for about 80 percent of cases (7). Clinically and histologically, superficial spreading melanoma is more likely to be associated with a putative precursor nevus than other forms of melanoma (8), and attributes such as number and size of

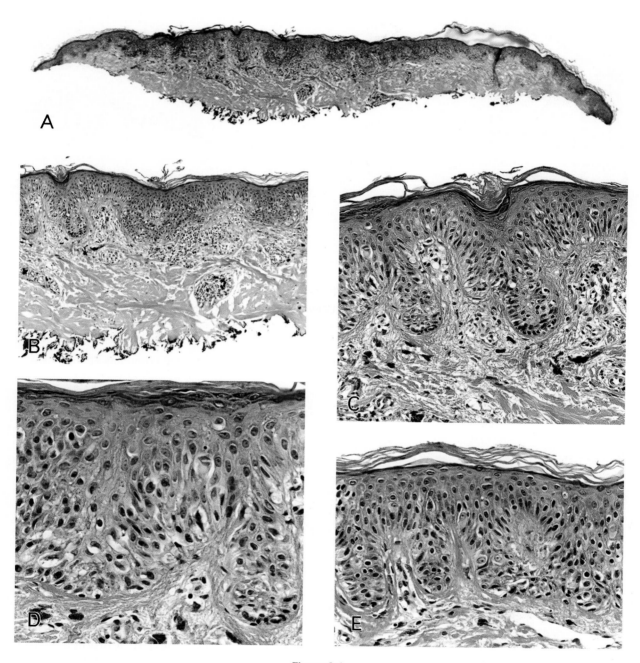

Figure 9-1

**SUPERFICIAL ATYPICAL MELANOCYTIC PROLIFERATION OF UNCERTAIN SIGNIFICANCE
(SAMPUS), EVOLVING MELANOMA IN SITU VERSUS SEVERE MELANOCYTIC DYSPLASIA**

A,B: A moderately cellular proliferation in the epidermis is associated with irregular thickening and thinning of the rete ridges and a patchy lymphocytic infiltrate in the dermis.

C: There is an increased number of nevoid to epithelioid melanocytes along the dermal-epidermal junction. Many are around the tips and sides of elongated rete ridges, but there is also proliferation between the rete.

D: In addition to the tendency to continuous proliferation between the rete ridges, there is focal pagetoid extension of single cells into the epidermis, generally not beyond the stratum spinosum.

E: The nuclei are somewhat enlarged, with open chromatin and small nucleoli. Criteria differentiating severe dysplasia and evolving melanoma in situ, with mixed lentiginous and pagetoid features, are conflicting.

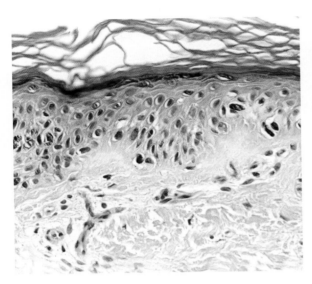 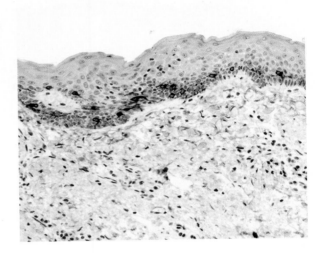

Figure 9-2

INTRAEPIDERMAL ATYPICAL MELANOCYTIC PROLIFERATION OF UNCERTAIN SIGNIFICANCE (IAMPUS)

Left: There is an increased number of single and nested melanocytes near the dermal-epidermal junction. Cytologic atypia is severe. There is no continuous basal or extensive pagetoid proliferation. The differential diagnosis is between severe melanocytic dysplasia and melanoma in situ.

Right: A Melan-A stain shows increased basal melanocytes, without clearly demonstrating a continuous proliferation.

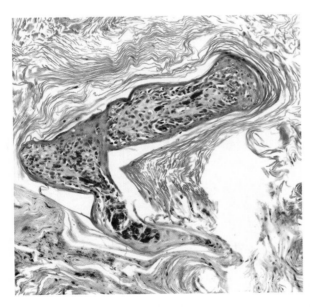

Figure 9-3

SUPERFICIAL ATYPICAL MELANOCYTIC PROLIFERATION OF UNCERTAIN SIGNIFICANCE (SAMPUS)

The uncertainty in this case arises from the submission of the specimen in the form of curettings, providing insufficient representation of the architecture. Cytologic atypia in this specimen is mild; however, the proliferation appears to be continuous, a potential indicator of melanoma in situ.

nevi are more strongly associated with risk for this form of melanoma than for other forms (7,9). Superficial spreading melanoma is the predominant form of melanoma that occurs in hereditary melanoma kindreds where dysplastic nevi are strong markers of melanoma risk (10), and is also the most common form of melanoma observed in association with dysplastic nevi in a nonhereditary setting (11). In addition, this is the form of melanoma that is increasing most rapidly in incidence (12).

Risk factors identified in epidemiologic studies that apply particularly to superficial spreading melanomas include the presence of dysplastic nevi, the total number of nevi, the number of large nevi, and the presence of irregular or variegated nevi. In addition to factors associated with nevi, behavioral characteristics, such as a history of episodic weekend or vacation exposure to the sun rather than chronic continuous occupational exposure, are also important risk factors for superficial spreading melanoma, unlike lentigo maligna melanoma, where the risk appears to be greatest on the chronically exposed skin of outdoor workers. In common with lentigo maligna melanoma, the risk of developing superficial spreading

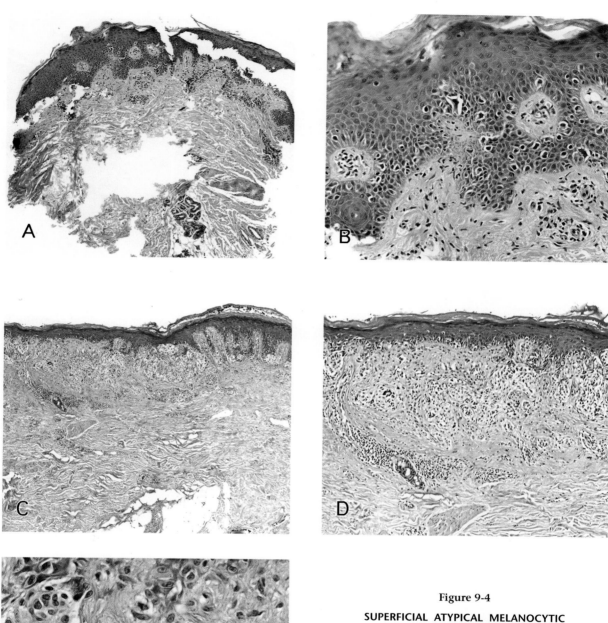

Figure 9-4

**SUPERFICIAL ATYPICAL MELANOCYTIC
PROLIFERATION OF UNCERTAIN
SIGNIFICANCE AND RECURRENT MELANOMA**

A,B: A fragmented biopsy from the thigh of a 44-year-woman contains an increased number of slightly enlarged melanocytes; however, there is no high-level pagetoid or continuous basal proliferation. This lesion was called a severely dysplastic nevus.

C–E: About 3 years later the lesion recurred as a melanoma of less than 1 mm in Breslow thickness, but with a tumorigenic vertical growth phase present, indicating potential competence for metastasis. A strong recommendation for complete excision is important in such a case.

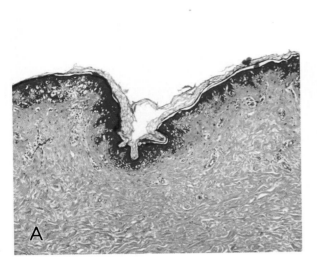

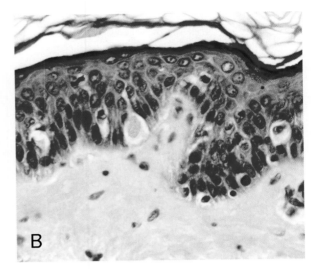

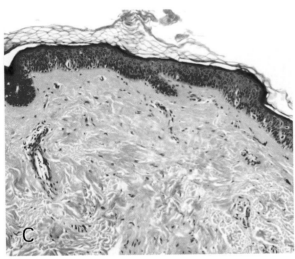

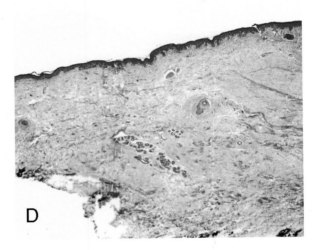

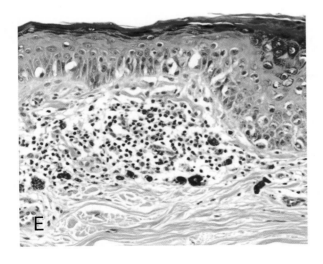

Figure 9-5

**MELANOMA IN SITU AND
RECURRENT INVASIVE MELANOMA**

A: A broad lesion is characterized by extensive proliferation of large epithelioid melanocytes, many of which are above the dermal-epidermal junction but mostly not beyond the mid-spinous layer. There is a tendency to continuous proliferation between irregularly elongated rete ridges.

B,C: Higher power demonstrates uniform, albeit mild to moderate, cytologic atypia. Subtle changes and increased atypical single cells in the epidermis extend close to a lateral specimen margin. Despite presenting sufficient criteria for diagnosis of melanoma in situ, this lesion was initially diagnosed as severe melanocytic dysplasia. A reexcision was not done. One year later, the recurrent lesion was excised.

D,E: This section shows a scar on the right, with an overlying and adjacent atypical intraepidermal proliferation.

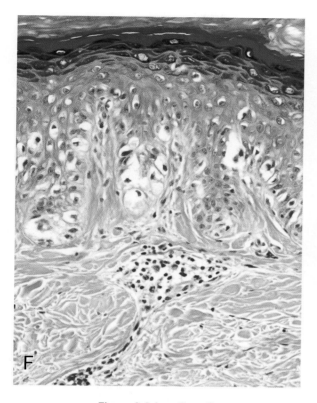

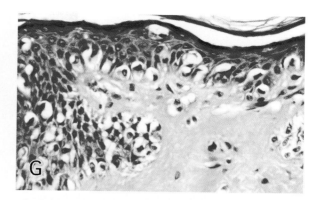

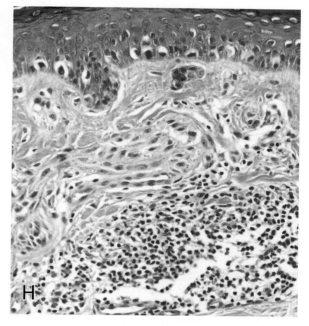

Figure 9-5 (continued)

F,G: Higher magnification demonstrates a continuous basal and pagetoid proliferation of uniformly atypical epithelioid melanocytes above the scar (F) and adjacent to it (G).

H: There is a focus of invasion in the form of a cluster of cells slightly larger than the largest intraepidermal cluster (minimal early tumorigenic and nonmitogenic vertical growth phase).

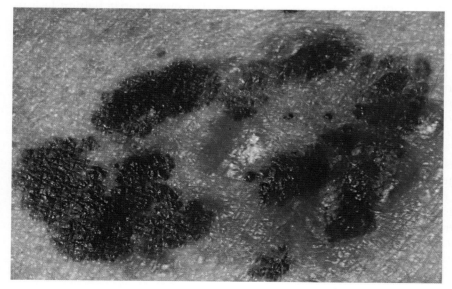

Figure 9-6

MALIGNANT MELANOMA, SUPERFICIAL SPREADING TYPE, RADIAL GROWTH PHASE WITH EXTENSIVE REGRESSION AND SMALL VERTICAL GROWTH PHASE PAPULES

The small papules are present within the geographic confines of the area of regression and within the pigmented residual radial growth phase component.

Figure 9-7

MALIGNANT MELANOMA, SUPERFICIAL SPREADING TYPE, WITH RADIAL GROWTH PHASE, EXTENSIVE REGRESSION, AND SEVERAL PAPULAR NODULAR FOCI OF VERTICAL GROWTH PHASE, ONE ULCERATED

Progression is occurring in the form of tumorigenic vertical growth phase within the geographic confines of the radial growth phase regression process.

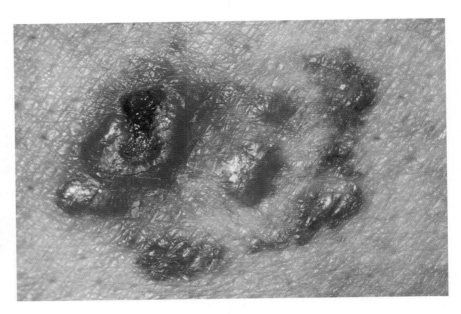

melanoma is greater in persons whose skin is more susceptible to sunburn (13).

Microscopic Findings. The two most important features that distinguish superficial spreading melanoma from the lentiginous forms of melanoma (lentigo maligna, acral- and mucosal-lentiginous melanomas) are the architectural pattern and the cell type in the radial growth phase compartment. This form of melanoma is associated with a prominent pagetoid pattern of proliferation of large epithelioid melanocytes in the epidermis (fig. 9-8). Perhaps because it is the most dramatic pattern observed in melanomas, this is also the best known, but it is neither present in all melanomas nor pathognomonic of melanoma, as discussed previously. A few pagetoid nests without many single cells above the junctional zone may be seen in benign lesions, especially in some Spitz or pigmented spindle cell nevi, and in acral nevi. In characteristic melanomas of the superficial spreading type, spread of single cells and nests is observed above the basement membrane zone (14). In some small lesions thought to be "early" in their evolution, the cells may be mainly basal, and single cells tend to predominate over nests (figs. 9-9, 9-10) (15). In other melanomas, nests may be more prominent (fig. 9-11). In a more prototypical superficial spreading melanoma, the pagetoid cells extend as far as the granular layer and usually into the stratum corneum (fig. 9-12), and it is the pigment in this location that accounts for

the black color of melanomas (pigment in the basement membrane zone appears brown and in the dermis it is blue). When a melanoma occurs in association with a preexisting dysplastic nevus, the two compartments are often readily distinguishable (fig. 9-13).

Cytologically, the lesional cells are characteristically large, with abundant cytoplasm and a low nuclear to cytoplasmic ratio. The cytoplasm contains finely divided ("dusty") melanin pigment granules, which ultrastructurally represent immature, partially melanized, often spherical and poorly formed melanosomes that are not organized into the larger, coarser compound melanosomes that characterize benign lesions and normal pigment in keratinocytes. A similar epithelioid cell type may be seen as a minority population in dysplastic nevi, but usually the cells in superficial spreading melanomas exhibit uniform cytologic atypia (nuclear changes that affect a majority of the lesional cells [fig. 9-9]). In other melanomas, pigment may be minimal or absent (fig. 9-8). The atypical nuclei are large compared to those of melanocytes or nevi (16), with irregular nuclear membranes and often with eosinophilic macronucleoli in a majority of the lesional cells. In some lesions, however, the atypia is surprisingly slight, and in one such variant the nuclei are small and darkly staining, indeed almost pyknotic in appearance. Mitotic figures are observed in the epidermis in only about one third of cases, but when present,

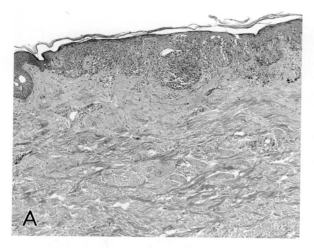

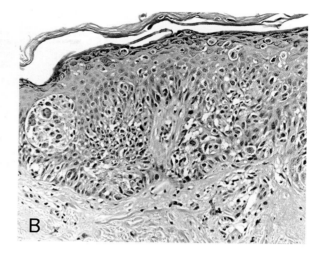

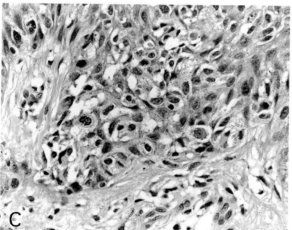

Figure 9-8

MALIGNANT MELANOMA, SUPERFICIAL SPREADING TYPE, CLASSIC PAGETOID PATTERN

A: Scanning magnification shows a broad, highly cellular melanocytic proliferation. The proliferation appears to be well circumscribed.

B: Higher magnification shows pagetoid extension of uniformly (albeit mildly to moderately) atypical melanocytes at all levels of the epidermis including the stratum corneum.

C: At high magnification, there is uniform cytologic atypia. A single mitosis is present.

constitute strong evidence in favor of melanoma over dysplasia.

When invasion occurs in an otherwise in situ melanoma, the cells in the dermis usually resemble those in the epidermis, failing to show the maturation typical of nevi (fig. 9-14). Invasive melanomas tend to have a brisker lymphocytic infiltrate and a denser, more diffuse fibroblastic stromal response that may obscure the invasive cells. When an associated nevus is present, the distinction between nevus and melanoma cells may be difficult. Continuity with the overlying in situ component may be a valuable clue that the entire lesion is melanoma. Conversely, cells, albeit atypical ones, that are in cytologic continuity with underlying definitive nevus cells are likely to be a component of the nevus. Some melanomas have a combination of both an underlying nevus and nevoid matura-

tion of the invasive component, an especially difficult combination to accurately interpret (fig. 9-15). Small or larger collections of dermal nevus cells are commonly seen beneath an in situ melanoma component, and these should not be misinterpreted as invasive melanoma (fig. 9-16).

Focally complete radial growth phase regression is commonly observed in superficial spreading and other histopathologic subtypes of melanoma. Occasionally, total or subtotal regression of the radial growth phase occurs (fig. 9-17). In this case, care must be taken to be sure that the regressed radial growth phase is completely excised in the definitive therapy specimen, as a few lesional cells may well be present at the periphery of an area of regression, as is evident from inspection of the clinical figures 9-6 and 9-7.

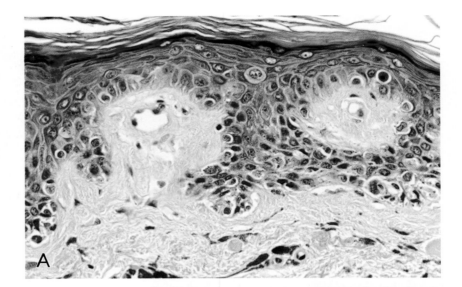

A

Figure 9-9

MELANOMA IN SITU, SUPERFICIAL SPREADING TYPE

A: Uniformly atypical melanocytes are present near the tips and sides of elongated rete ridges and extend up in a focal pagetoid pattern to the mid-spinous layer. This is not independently diagnostic of melanoma.

B: In another field, there is uniform atypia and a mid-epidermal pagetoid proliferation.

C: Another field shows uniform atypia and pagetoid extension down a skin appendage. Taken together, these appearances are diagnostic of melanoma in situ, primarily because of the severe uniform atypia. Architectural features, however, are incomplete, because there is no extensive or high-level pagetoid proliferation, and no extensive continuous basal proliferation.

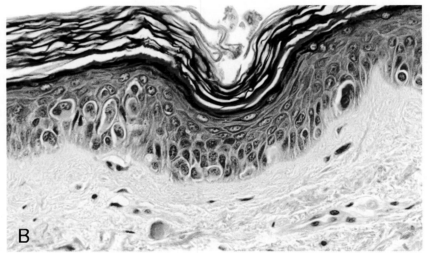

B

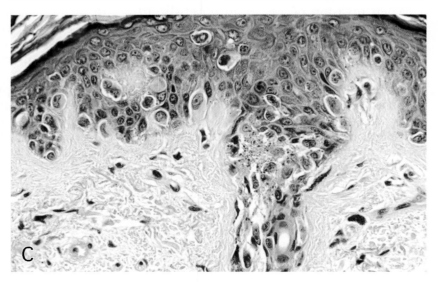

C

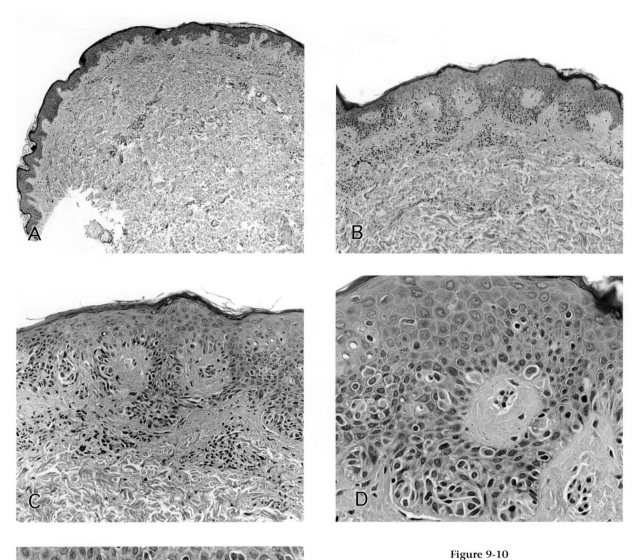

Figure 9-10

MELANOMA IN SITU, SUPERFICIAL SPREADING TYPE

This lesion occurred in a 49-year-old woman who is a member of a familial melanoma kindred, in which two siblings have had melanoma.

A: At scanning magnification, there is a fairly broad, moderately cellular melanocytic proliferation, with irregular thickening and thinning of the epidermis.

B: Higher magnification reveals nests bridging adjacent rete ridges. In addition, there is pagetoid extension of single cells into the epidermis.

C,D: Cytologically, there is uniform, generally moderate atypia in the form of nuclear enlargement and slight hyperchromatism. Focally, there is diffuse fibroplasia in the dermis and continuous proliferation in the epidermis. Although the pagetoid and continuous proliferation is not extensive, the combination of architectural and cytologic features minimally meets our criteria for melanoma in situ.

E: Only rare single cells, if any, are present in the dermis.

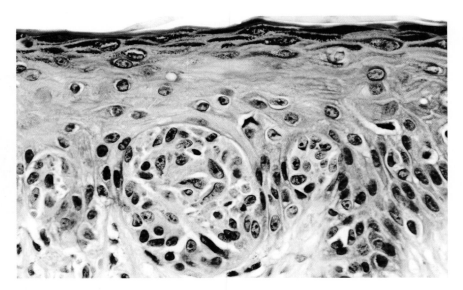

Figure 9-11

**MALIGNANT MELANOMA,
SUPERFICIAL
SPREADING TYPE**

There is a continuous basal proliferation with nest formation. Despite the absence of pagetoid proliferation in this field, the large epithelioid cell cytology is more consistent with superficial spreading melanoma than with lentigo maligna melanoma.

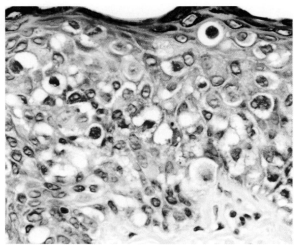

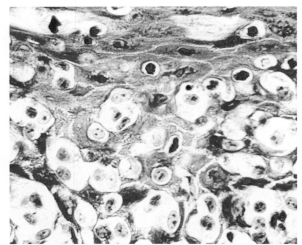

Figure 9-12

MELANOMA IN SITU, WITH PROMINENT PAGETOID PATTERN

In contrast to the "early" lesion in the previous two figures, here there is extensive high-level pagetoid proliferation coupled with cytologic atypia, which is moderate in the left figure and more severe on the right. The right figure shows extensive pagetoid proliferation of cells with clear cytoplasm and open chromatin. Immunohistochemical studies might be appropriate to confirm melanocytic differentiation in such a case.

Early Tumorigenic and/or Mitogenic Vertical Growth Phase. Mitotic figures may be observed in the dermis if there is a tumorigenic vertical growth phase compartment. In a nontumorigenic invasive melanoma, however, mitotic figures are not usually observed, and a mitotic figure in the dermis, even in a nontumorigenic melanoma, defines the presence of mitogenic vertical growth phase and competence for metastasis (fig. 9-18). The general characteristics of the tumorigenic vertical growth phase are similar among the various subtypes of melanoma (see Tumorigenic Melanoma, chapter 10). In a superficial spreading melanoma the tumorigenic compartment, if present, is likely to be composed of epithelioid cells arranged in nests larger than any junctional nests and generally more atypical and often less pigmented than those of the microinvasive or in situ radial growth phase compartment (figs. 9-19, 9-20).

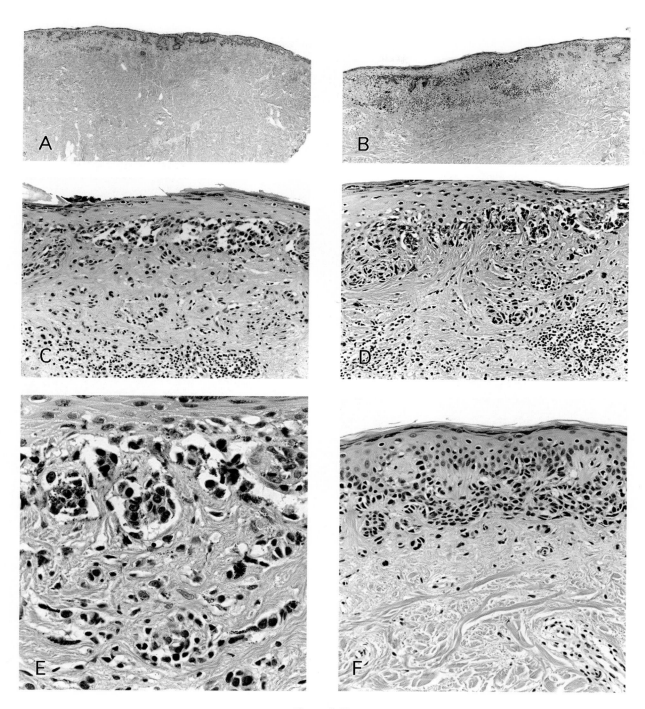

Figure 9-13

MALIGNANT MELANOMA, SUPERFICIAL SPREADING TYPE, INVASIVE BUT NONTUMORIGENIC

A: A broad superficial melanocytic proliferation arose in a dysplastic nevus, from the back of a 72-year-old man.

C–E: Cells in the papillary dermis resemble those in the epidermis. There is a continuous proliferation of uniformly atypical cells in this area (D), and a focal area of nontumorigenic and nonmitogenic invasion (E). This is a malignant melanoma, superficial spreading type.

F: Near the periphery of the lesion, mainly near the tips and sides of elongated rete ridges, the cells are smaller with lesser random atypia. Bridging occurs between adjacent rete ridges. This is a preexisting dysplastic nevus.

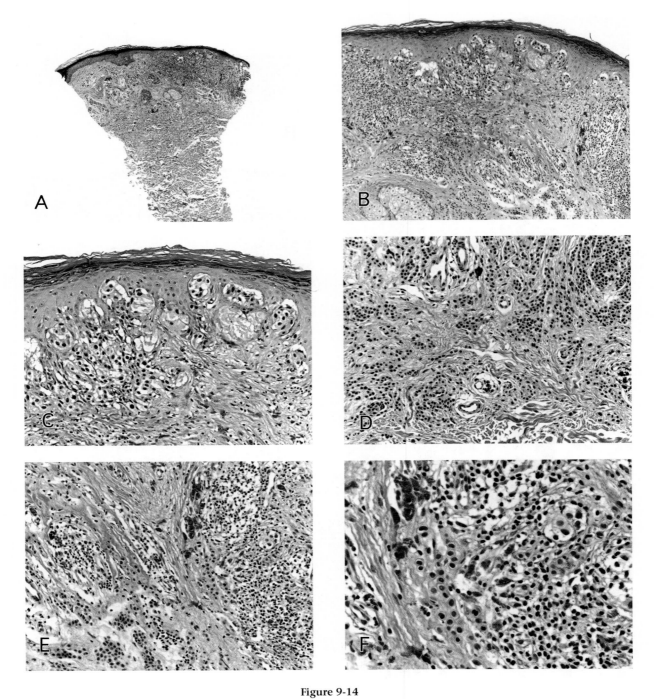

Figure 9-14

**MALIGNANT MELANOMA, SUPERFICIAL SPREADING TYPE,
NONTUMORIGENIC, CLARK LEVEL II, AND AN ASSOCIATED NEVUS**

A: The punch biopsy shows a complex lesion in the epidermis and dermis.
B: In the epidermis, there is extensive continuous and pagetoid proliferation of uniformly atypical cells.
C: Similar cells protrude into the dermis.
D: There is a population of much smaller cells at the base of the lesion with the characteristics of nevus cells.
E,F: There is no cytologic or architectural "blending" or "continuity" between the two cell types.

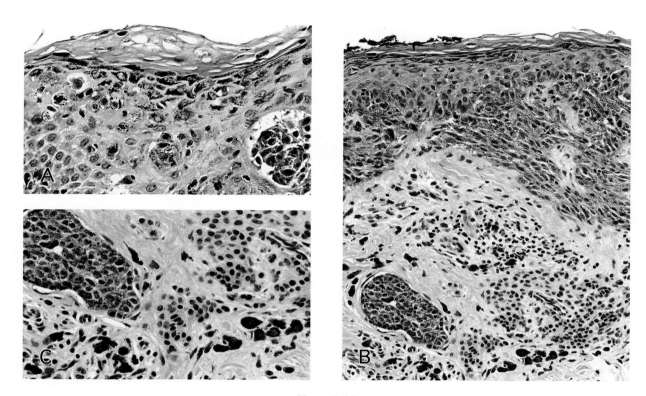

Figure 9-15

**MALIGNANT MELANOMA, SUPERFICIAL SPREADING TYPE, WITH A
SMALL NEVOID VERTICAL GROWTH PHASE AND ASSOCIATED NEVUS**

A: There is a confluent proliferation of uniformly atypical melanocytes at the dermal-epidermal junction, coupled with high-level and extensive pagetoid proliferation to all levels of the epidermis in the stratum corneum. In the dermis, there are small but atypical melanocytes in a cluster on the left, contrasted with authentic dermal nevus cells on the right.

B: The nevoid vertical growth phase on the left exhibits nuclear irregularity and hyperchromatism.

C: Nevus cells on the right exhibit more uniform nuclei and abundant cytoplasm.

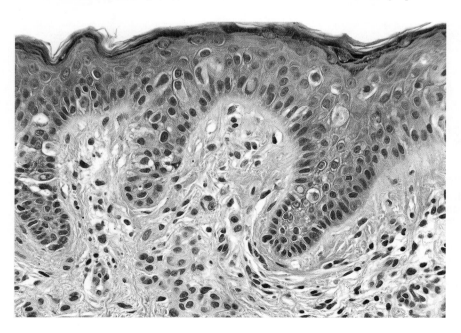

Figure 9-16

MELANOMA IN SITU, SUPERFICIAL SPREADING TYPE, WITH DERMAL NEVUS CELLS

Dermal nevus cells beneath an in situ melanoma component should not be overdiagnosed as invasive melanoma.

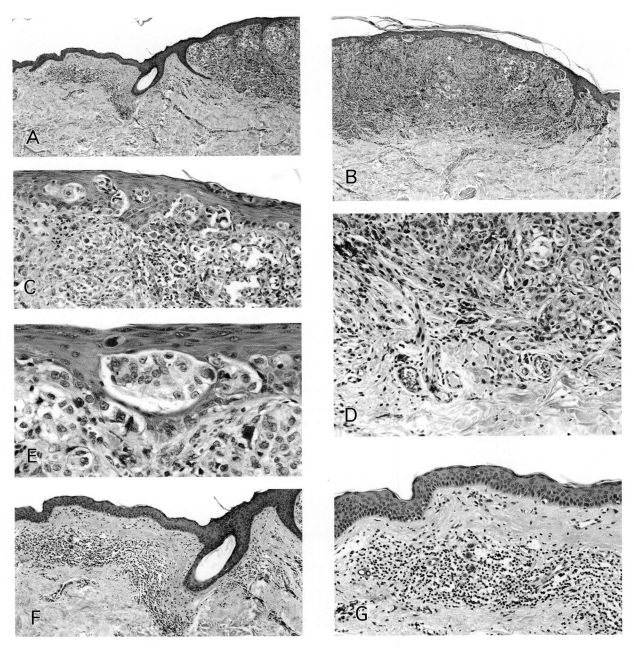

Figure 9-17

MALIGNANT MELANOMA WITH A TOTALLY REGRESSED RADIAL GROWTH PHASE

A: Malignant melanoma from the back of a 51-year-old man, Clark level IV, Breslow thickness 0.94 mm. At the left, the papillary dermis is widened with fibroplasia and a dense lymphocytic infiltrate. At the right, there is a tumorigenic dermal component.

B: The tumorigenic vertical growth phase expands the papillary dermis and infiltrates the upper reticular dermis (Clark level IV). There is pagetoid involvement of the epidermis above the vertical growth phase.

C: Small clusters of apoptotic cells resemble the Kamino bodies seen in Spitz nevi.

D: At the base, there is subtle infiltration of the upper reticular dermis.

E: Higher power shows uniformly severe cytologic atypia and pagetoid involvement of the epidermis.

F,G: In the area of regressed radial growth phase, the papillary dermis is widened with a band-like lymphocytic infiltrate. The histology of this type of melanoma should be recognized in a reexcision specimen, and should be reexcised if it extends to specimen margins. This patient was alive and well 14 years later.

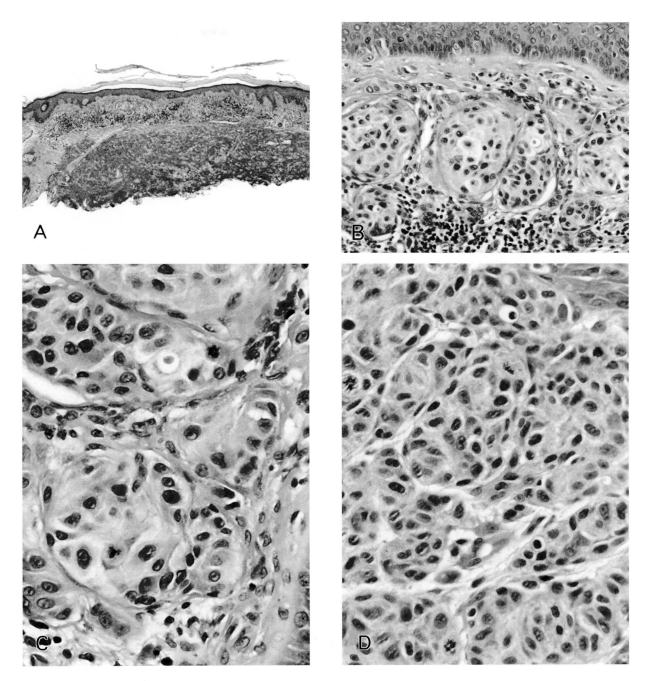

Figure 9-18

**MALIGNANT MELANOMA, SUPERFICIAL SPREADING TYPE,
WITH EARLY TUMORIGENIC AND MITOGENIC VERTICAL GROWTH PHASE**

A: This lesion, in a 32-year-old woman, shows a Breslow thickness of only 0.36 mm, yet has an early tumorigenic and mitogenic vertical growth phase invasive to Clark level III. This broad lesion is characterized by irregular thickening and thinning of the epidermis, a patchy to band-like lymphocytic infiltrate in the dermis, and extensive artifactual hemorrhage in the reticular dermis.

B: The cells in the dermis are arranged in clusters that vary in size and shape, and there is moderate uniform atypia.

C: Two mitoses are present in the dermal tumor in this field.

D: Five mitoses are seen in another field, some of them abnormal.

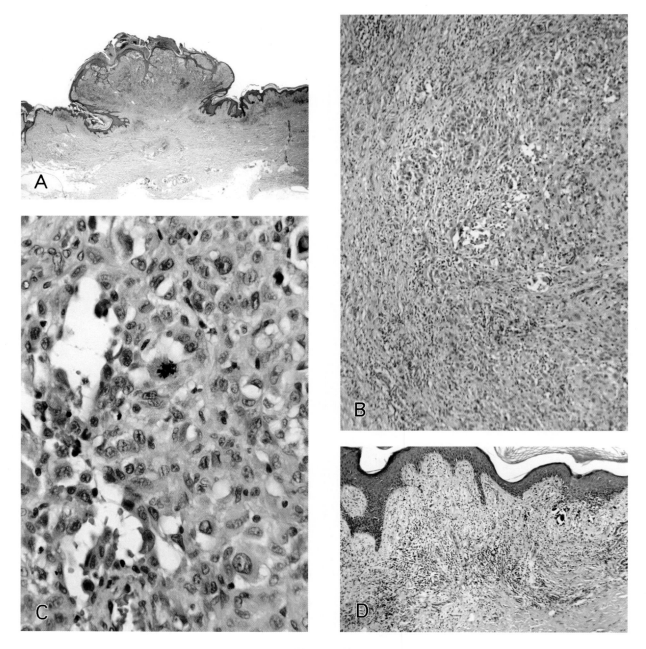

Figure 9-19

**MALIGNANT MELANOMA, SUPERFICIAL SPREADING TYPE,
TUMORIGENIC AND MITOGENIC VERTICAL GROWTH PHASE**

A: This lesion, from the leg of a 38-year-old man, has a Breslow thickness of 2.2 mm, mitotic rate of 2.7, and brisk tumor-infiltrating lymphocytes. There is a polypoid tumorigenic vertical growth phase component and adjacent alterations of the epidermis and papillary dermis.

B: High magnification at the base of the vertical growth phase shows "brisk" tumor-infiltrating lymphocytes present across the entire base of the tumor and among tumor cells.

C: In the tumorigenic vertical growth phase, mitotic figures, including an abnormal one, are readily detected. This patient was alive and well 9 years after diagnosis.

D: The adjacent papillary dermis shows the histologic features of regression: widened papillary dermis with diffuse fibroplasia, and lymphocytes and melanophages with absence of melanoma in the dermis and overlying epidermis.

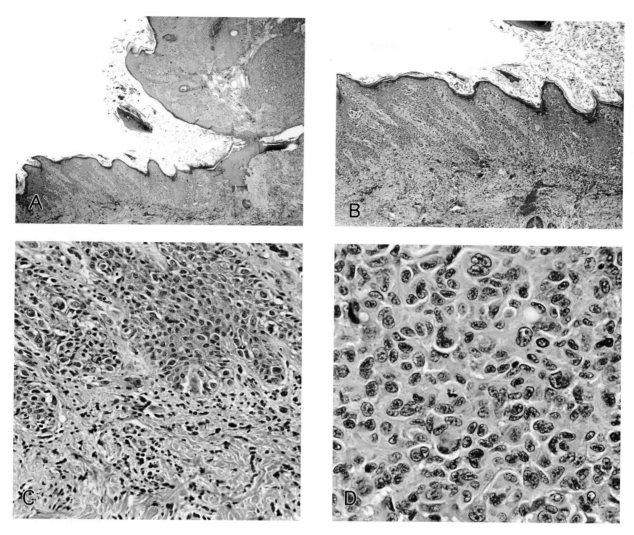

Figure 9-20

MALIGNANT MELANOMA, SUPERFICIAL SPREADING TYPE, TUMORIGENIC AND MITOGENIC, POLYPOID

A: This bulky tumorigenic melanoma occurred on the back of a 29-year-old woman. There is an adjacent radial or "horizontal" growth phase.

B: The radial growth phase is characterized by the continuous proliferation of uniformly atypical melanocytes along the dermal-epidermal junction and extensive pagetoid proliferation into the epidermis.

C: A few lesional cells of the radial growth phase protrude into the papillary dermis without tumorigenic proliferation.

D: In the tumorigenic vertical growth phase, there is severe uniform atypia, greater in degree than that in the radial growth phase, and mitotic activity. This woman died of her disease within 2 years.

Prominent spindle or dendritic cells, neurotropism, and desmoplasia are uncommon in the tumorigenic compartments of superficial spreading melanoma in contrast to the lentiginous forms of melanoma.

Differential Diagnosis. The differential diagnosis of superficial spreading melanoma includes the other forms of melanoma to be discussed in this section, and benign lesions, especially dysplastic nevi. This differential diagnosis has already been discussed (see Dysplastic Melanocytic Nevi, chapter 8) and is summarized in Table 9-1.

Conditions that may simulate superficial spreading melanoma because of the presence of a pagetoid pattern in the epidermis include

Table 9-1

FEATURES HELPFUL IN DIFFERENTIATING DYSPLASTIC NEVUS AND RADIAL GROWTH PHASE MELANOMA

Dysplastic Nevus	Radial Growth Phase Melanoma
May be less than 6 mm diameter, not often more than 10 mm	Usually greater than 6 mm, often much greater than 10 mm
Somewhat symmetrical	Often highly asymmetrical
Uniformly elongated, narrow, delicate rete ridges	Irregularly thickened epidermis, often with effaced rete ridges
No alteration of stratum corneum	May be hyperkeratotic
Nests predominate over single cells in the epidermis	Single cells predominate except in late lesions
Little or no pagetoid spread of lesional cells into epidermis	Usually obvious pagetoid spread into epidermis, extending to stratum corneum
Often symmetrically arranged about "shoulders" of a mature dermal nevus	If dermal nevus is present, it is likely to be asymmetrically placed
Patchy lymphocytic infiltrate in papillary dermis	Brisk band-like infiltrate
No regression	Regression common
No mitoses in epidermis or dermis	Intraepidermal mitoses in about one third of cases; no mitoses in dermis
Most cells are not atypical	Most cells are atypical
Scattered atypical epithelioid cells with dusty melanin pigment, nucleoli, anisokaryosis ("random atypia")	Epithelioid cells with dusty pigment, nucleoli, anisokaryosis predominate ("uniform atypia")
Cells in dermis, if any, are smaller than those in epidermis	Cells in dermis are similar to those in epidermis
Last lesional cells at lateral border are often in a nest	Last cells are often single and may be above the basal zone

mammary and extramammary Paget disease (17) and pagetoid squamous cell carcinoma (18). The differences between melanoma and Paget disease at scanning magnification include the generally larger size of the Paget cells with their more abundant cytoplasm, and the tendency of most of the Paget cells to be separated from the basal lamina by a layer of basal keratinocytes. Some lesions may form ill-defined glandular structures, and once the diagnosis is suspected, inspection at higher magnification may reveal mucin droplets that can be confirmed with a mucicarmine stain. Immunopathology for S-100 protein and HMB45 reactivity may be used to support the diagnosis of melanoma, while Paget disease is usually reactive with keratin, carcinoembryonic antigen (CEA) (19), and syndecan-1 (20).

Squamous cell carcinoma may present with a pagetoid pattern in which large, somewhat pale cells are scattered among a background population of benign cells. Usually, bridges (desmosomes) are recognized between the le-

sional cells at high power, and stains for low molecular weight keratin and syndecan-1 are positive (20). Pigment may be seen in the cells of Paget disease or in squamous carcinoma cells (transferred from benign melanocytes), and thus intracellular pigment alone is not pathognomonic of melanocytic differentiation. The differentiation of pagetoid intraepidermal proliferations is discussed at greater length with nontumorigenic melanomas.

The recurrent nevus phenomenon (discussed in chapter 2) may also show enlarged pigmented and apparently atypical melanocytic cells in a pagetoid array within the epidermal layer. While this pattern may initially mimic melanoma in situ of the superficial spreading type, the discrete localization of the recurrent nevus proliferation to a zone that overlies a superficial dermal scar should assist in its accurate recognition.

LENTIGO MALIGNA MELANOMA

Definition. *Lentigo maligna melanoma* constitutes about 10 percent of all melanomas, and typically presents as a large, flat, irregular, asymmetric and variably pigmented lesion of sun-exposed skin that is characterized histologically by an increased number of cytologically atypical melanocytes in the basal layers of the epidermis (21,22). Although most of the cells are single, some nests may be present, and in the center of the lesion there may be a tendency to intraepidermal pagetoid spread of lesional cells above the basal layer. Lentigo maligna melanoma may be in situ (termed lentigo maligna) or invasive, and the "invasive" cells may be tumorigenic or nontumorigenic as defined above. First described by Sir Jonathan Hutchinson in 1892 and named "lentigo melanosis" (23), lentigo maligna melanoma is also known today, especially in Australia where it is very prevalent, as *Hutchinson melanotic freckle* (24).

Although there is some controversy, most authors believe that lentigo maligna should be regarded as a form of in situ radial growth phase melanoma. In an alternative view, some of these lesions (such as those lacking confluent proliferation of uniformly atypical melanocytes) may be regarded as an atypical, potentially premalignant, proliferation (premalignant dysplasia) (25–27). In any event, the lesions are biologically benign when they are confined to the epidermis or when they are invasive but not tumorigenic, as previously discussed for all such in situ or microinvasive nontumorigenic lesions that are, with rare exceptions, incapable of metastasis (28).

It has recently been demonstrated that lentigo maligna melanomas are less likely to have the *BRAF* mutation that is common in superficial spreading melanomas. Because the latter are about four times as prevalent as lentigo maligna melanomas, the *BRAF* mutation is by far the most frequent in melanomas as a whole. In contrast, about 30 percent of melanomas on chronically sun-damaged skin (mostly lentigo maligna histogenetic type) but few if any melanomas on nonacral, nonchronically sun-exposed skin (mostly superficial spreading subtype) have an activating mutation in the oncogene *KIT* (29) that is also found in many mucosal melanomas (30). Clinical and histologic attributes in current use in making distinctions among the subtypes of melanoma have recently been shown to be highly predictive of these fundamental genetic differences (1), supporting the validity of these "clinicopathologic subtypes."

Clinical Features. Lentigo maligna melanoma occurs in Caucasians of fair complexion and is essentially never seen in dark-skinned subjects or races. Lesions occur on continuously sun-exposed areas of skin, most commonly on the face, but also on the forearms and backs of the hands, the ears in men, and the "V" of the neck (fig. 9-21) (9). The lesion occurs in a somewhat older population than does the more common superficial spreading melanoma, but may be seen occasionally in patients as young as the fourth decade of life (31,32). In a population-based study from Stockholm, the incidence of melanoma on the face was 3.4 times higher than on the skin outside the head-neck area and the lentigo maligna melanoma subtype was 74 times more common on the face (33). The mean age at diagnosis was significantly higher for patients with melanoma of the head and neck irrespective of histogenetic type.

Whatever their age, patients usually have evidence of severe chronic actinic skin damage not only at the lesional site, but also in other sun-exposed areas, and they typically have skin that burns on exposure to the sun and then tans lightly or not at all. Although lentigo maligna (melanoma in situ of the lentigo maligna type) probably begins as a small lesion, it usually cannot be reliably distinguished clinically from solar or actinic lentigo if it is less than 6 mm in diameter. Most lesions are larger than 10 mm, and neglected lesions of several centimeters in diameter are not rare (although most of these have foci of invasion).

A characteristic lentigo maligna is a broad, flat lesion that progressively enlarges and develops increasing irregularity of shape as well as increasing color variegation. As the lesion grows, the border becomes even more irregular, with an indefinite and impalpable edge, unlike most superficial spreading melanomas, where the border is usually discrete and palpable. As the lesion progresses, color variegation increases and the blue-black color so characteristic of melanoma appears. Often, a network of racemose interlacing lines of dark pigmentation appears in the tan background lesion. Blue-black or other dark colors in a pigmented lesion should prompt biopsy, as should areas of regression, conspicuous erythema

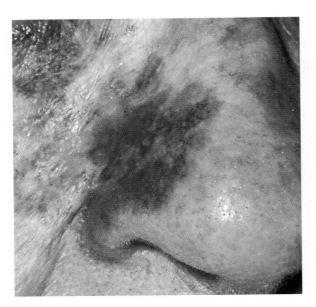 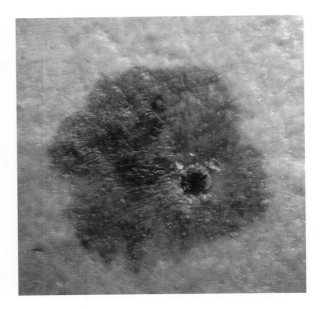

Figure 9-21

MALIGNANT MELANOMA, LENTIGO MALIGNA TYPE

Left: This large plaque of lentigo maligna melanoma displays the characteristic reticulated pattern in several areas. The areas of superficial regression centrally concealed a neurotropic vertical growth phase. (Fig. A from Plate VI, Fascicle 2, Third Series.)

Right: The lesion is broad, asymmetric, and irregularly colored tan-brown to dark brown. There is a tendency to a reticulated pattern and a fairly definite but nonpalpable border, all consistent with lentigo maligna or lentigo maligna melanoma. A punch biopsy site is seen.

or scale, large size, or a history of progressive growth. Some smaller lesions, which may be solar lentigines, can be followed photographically and left intact if they remain stable.

Lentigo maligna is difficult to recognize with specificity when small, so that the rate of progression of individual lesions to fully evolved melanoma is not known. Those lesions that are diagnosed clinically are usually completely excised for diagnosis and therapy, so that their natural history cannot be followed. Some incompletely excised (misdiagnosed or mistreated) lesions progress to frankly invasive and tumorigenic melanoma, often years later. Most observers believe that a significant number of lentigo maligna lesions (but not all and probably less than the majority) will progress inexorably but slowly over several years to microinvasion and later to the tumorigenic vertical growth phase (24). Vertical growth phase occasionally develops in small lesions, and sometimes it is of the desmoplastic and neurotropic type, with a very high chance for local recurrence if the lesion is not accurately diagnosed and adequately treated by complete local excision. Occasional

examples of amelanotic lentigo maligna melanoma have been described. These lesions may present as erythematous patches, and some of them have been mistaken clinically for inflammatory dermatoses, localized sclerosing disorders, or nonmelanoma skin cancers, sometimes with unfortunate results (34–36).

Although there has been some controversy about the matter (22), it seems likely that patients with lentigo maligna melanoma have no better prognosis than those with other forms of melanoma when other prognostic variables are controlled (37–39), except that there is a greater risk of local recurrence than with superficial spreading melanomas (40,41). There are, however, significant differences in the epidemiology and morphology compared with the more common superficial spreading melanoma. In a population-based study of melanomas in western Australia, the incidence of superficial spreading melanoma was 14.3 and of lentigo maligna melanoma 1.8/100,000 person-years. The incidence of lentigo maligna melanoma increases progressively with age, while superficial spreading melanoma is most common in middle

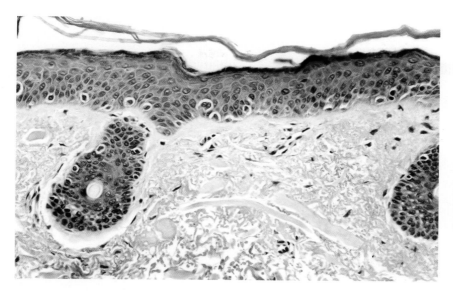

Figure 9-22

ATYPICAL INTRAEPIDERMAL MELANOCYTIC PROLIFERATION, CONSISTENT WITH EVOLVING LENTIGO MALIGNA

There is an increased number of single cells with mild atypia. Although the proliferation is not continuous, the appearance is highly suggestive of evolving lentigo maligna. Complete excision of this process is appropriate.

age. Lentigo maligna melanoma is much less likely to be associated with a precursor nevus (7,31). In a population-based study that included 13,000 melanomas, the different shapes of the age-incidence curves for lentigo maligna melanoma compared with other types suggested that different histologies reflect different responses to sunlight exposure as an etiologic factor. The findings were considered to strongly support the importance of considering the histologic subtype of cutaneous melanoma in future etiologic studies (42). These and other epidemiologic findings have suggested that lentigo maligna melanoma may be associated with chronic continuous occupational sun exposure, while superficial spreading melanoma is associated with intermittent, recreational sun exposure (43).

Microscopic Findings. Scanning magnification of lentigo maligna shows a broad and poorly circumscribed lesion situated in an atrophic epidermis, sometimes with a patchy lymphocytic infiltrate in the dermis. Severe dermal actinic elastosis is present in most cases. The atrophic epidermal pattern contrasts with the irregular thickening of the epidermis that occurs in superficial spreading melanomas, and also with the more uniform delicate rete ridge elongation of dysplastic nevi.

At higher magnification, lentigo maligna is characterized by an increased number of enlarged melanocytes in the basal epidermis (this "lentiginous" proliferation of melanocytes, unlike that in dysplastic nevi, is not associated

with keratinocytic proliferation and thus the rete ridges are not elongated). Early lesions, or the periphery of more centrally advanced lesions, may show a subtle increase in basal melanocytes in which cytologic atypia is not marked (figs. 9-22, 9-23). A Melan-A stain can be helpful in demonstrating the continuous proliferation along the dermal-epidermal junction (fig. 9-24). The lesional cells are sometimes heavily pigmented, and the pigment is often coarse, unlike the dusty pigment of superficial spreading melanomas. In addition to the single cells, nests are often present, which tend to "hang down" like raindrops from the interface (fig. 9-25). Occasionally, there are a few mitoses, but in lentigo maligna without associated invasion these are often absent and are hardly ever numerous.

The junctional melanocytes of lentigo maligna tend to be smaller than those of superficial spreading melanoma, with less cytoplasm and without the characteristic epithelioid shape. Because of their scant cytoplasm, these cells may appear to be fusiform to stellate in contour, with retraction spaces separating them from neighboring cells.

The nuclei of a few to a majority of the lesional cells are enlarged and may be hyperchromatic compared with normal melanocytes or nevus cells. More or less characteristic dendritic or "starburst" giant cells may be present, and multinucleated melanoma cells are helpful in distinguishing subtle lentigo maligna from

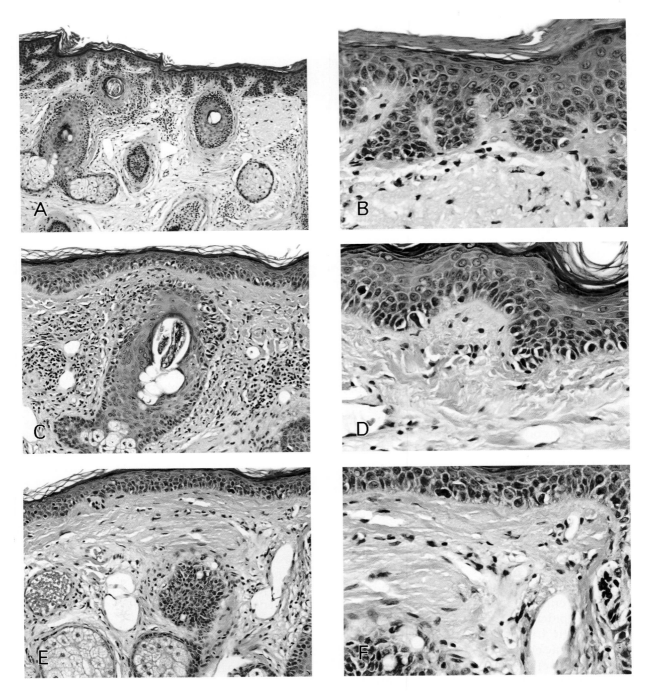

Figure 9-23

SUBTLE LENTIGO MALIGNA ADJACENT TO AN ACTINIC LENTIGO

A: Actinic lentigo, with a subtle increase of slightly atypical melanocytes, including involvement of hair follicles.

B: At higher magnification, rare, slightly atypical melanocytes are visualized, consistent with actinic lentigo.

C: Close to the previous field, epidermal atrophy and a suggestion of continuous basal proliferation of uniformly atypical nevoid epithelioid melanocytes are seen, with a similar proliferation involving a hair follicle.

D: Another field shows a subtle but focally continuous proliferation of uniformly atypical melanocytes.

E: There are a few nested and single cells in actinically damaged skin, with slight cytologic atypia.

F: High magnification demonstrates slight atypia.

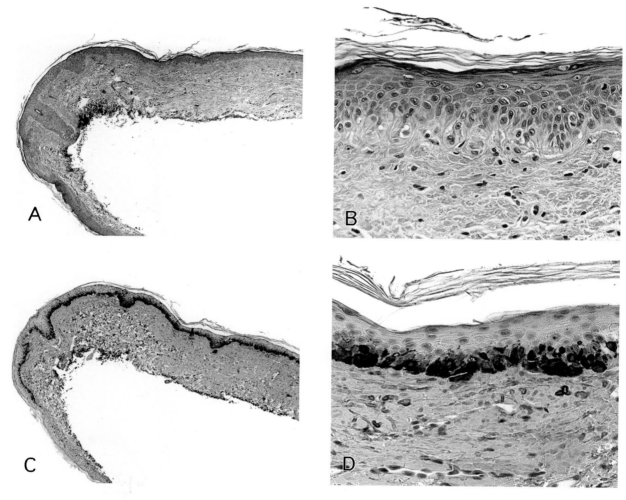

Figure 9-24

LENTIGO MALIGNA MELANOMA IN SITU

A: A shave biopsy of a subtle lesion in skin shows an atrophic epidermis.

B: Higher magnification shows uniformly atypical cells, which could potentially be confused with the keratinocytes of actinic keratosis.

C: Melan-A stain shows continuous proliferation along the dermal-epidermal junction.

D: High-power magnification demonstrates the continuous proliferation. The uniform atypia and the continuous proliferation together support the diagnosis of melanoma in situ, lentigo maligna type.

uninvolved sun-damaged skin (44). These features are often absent at the margin of the lesion; however, the margin may be quite subtle and is easily missed (fig. 9-26). Cytologic atypia with nuclear enlargement, irregularity, and hyperchromasia is variable and often slight, and nucleoli are occasionally, but not often, prominent.

It is characteristic for the cells of lentigo maligna to extend downward into the basal epithelium of hair follicles and sweat ducts, so that this intraepithelial lesion often involves

the deep margin of a shave biopsy specimen even when there is no invasion (fig. 9-27). In the center of the lesion, especially over areas of invasion, there may be cluster or nest formation, with some pagetoid spread of cells into the epidermis, but at the periphery of the lesion, the cells are single and basally located. In a region of pagetoid spread into the epidermis, there may be greater atypia of lesional cells, and the epidermis may be hyperplastic rather than atrophic. As with the clinical features, there is a range of severity

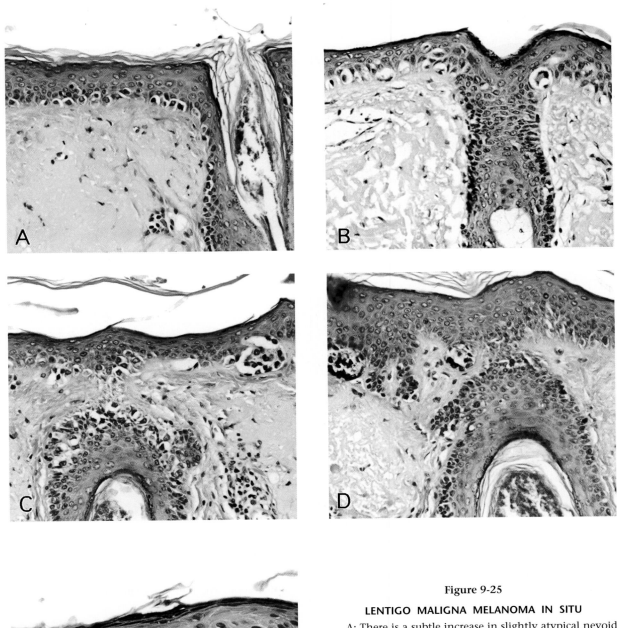

Figure 9-25

LENTIGO MALIGNA MELANOMA IN SITU

A: There is a subtle increase in slightly atypical nevoid melanocytes along the dermal-epidermal junction, without contiguous proliferation, highly suggestive but not diagnostic of evolving lentigo maligna.

B–D: Single cells demonstrate slight random atypia with hair follicle involvement, in chronically sun-damaged skin, consistent with lentigo maligna.

C–E: Nests of nevoid to epithelioid melanocytes with slight atypia "hanging down" from the epidermis in a characteristic "droplet" or "raindrop" pattern characteristic of lentigo maligna and lentigo maligna melanoma.

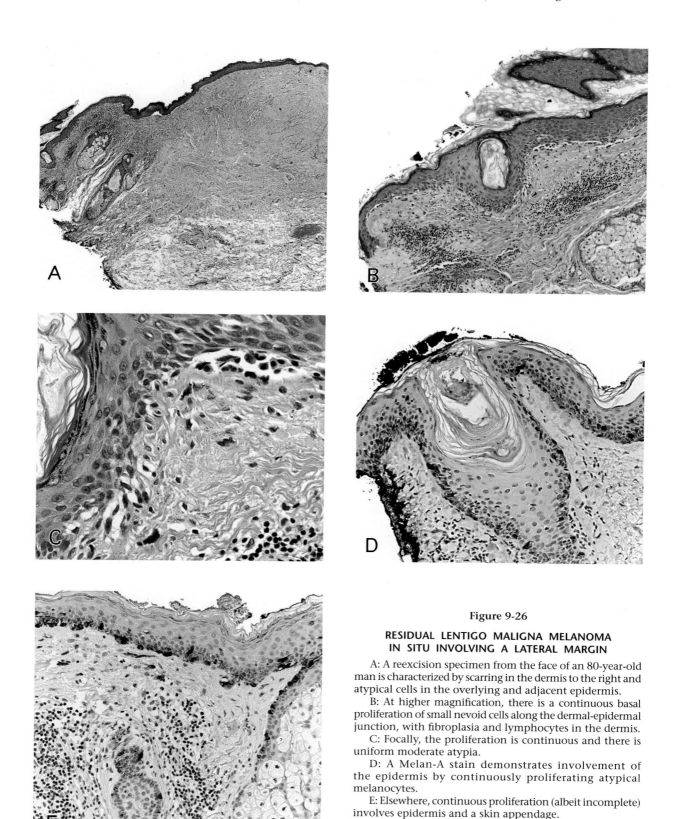

Figure 9-26

RESIDUAL LENTIGO MALIGNA MELANOMA IN SITU INVOLVING A LATERAL MARGIN

A: A reexcision specimen from the face of an 80-year-old man is characterized by scarring in the dermis to the right and atypical cells in the overlying and adjacent epidermis.

B: At higher magnification, there is a continuous basal proliferation of small nevoid cells along the dermal-epidermal junction, with fibroplasia and lymphocytes in the dermis.

C: Focally, the proliferation is continuous and there is uniform moderate atypia.

D: A Melan-A stain demonstrates involvement of the epidermis by continuously proliferating atypical melanocytes.

E: Elsewhere, continuous proliferation (albeit incomplete) involves epidermis and a skin appendage.

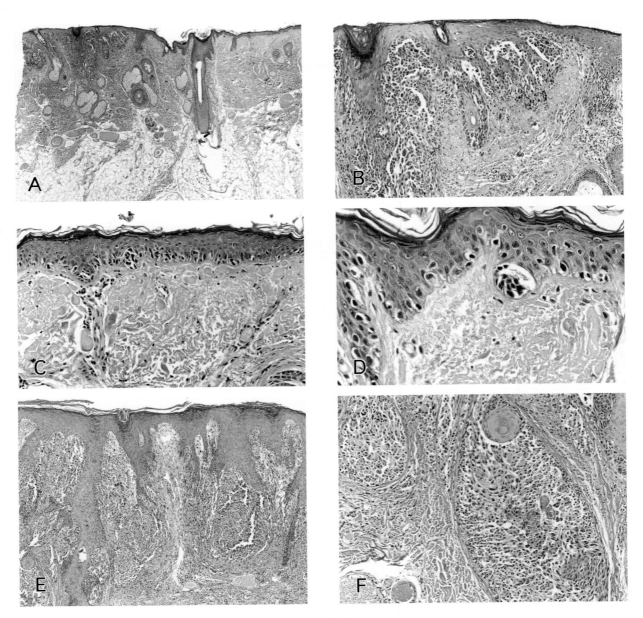

Figure 9-27

**MALIGNANT MELANOMA, LENTIGO MALIGNA TYPE, INVASIVE
BUT NOT TUMORIGENIC, WITH EXTENSIVE HAIR FOLLICLE INVOLVEMENT**

A: Scanning magnification shows a cellular proliferation, mainly intraepidermally on the left, with a more subtle intraepidermal proliferation on the right, all in sun-damaged skin. On the right, the epidermis is atrophic, while in the invasive area it is hyperplastic.

B: Higher magnification shows a cellular proliferation within the epidermis, extending down hair follicles. The cells are large and there is pagetoid extension into the epidermis. To the right of the lesion is a more subtle proliferation of smaller nevoid cells arranged as single cells and nests along the dermal-epidermal junction.

C: Although atypia is minimal, this appearance is consistent with melanoma in situ, lentigo maligna type. The presence of nests of atypical melanocytes above the elastosis in chronically sun-damaged skin is concerning for lentigo maligna, unless the lesion can be confidently diagnosed as a component of a junctional nevus.

D: The presence of atypical single cells is a clue to the correct diagnosis.

E: In the region of hair follicle invasion, the columns of cells extending down into the dermis are mostly in situ.

F: A few cells invade the papillary dermis and upper reticular dermis, in the region between the expanded hair follicles.

Table 9-2

FEATURES HELPFUL IN DIFFERENTIATING ACTINIC LENTIGO AND LENTIGO MALIGNA MELANOMA IN SITU

Feature	Actinic Lentigo	Atypical Actinic Lentigo	Lentigo Maligna (MIS LM Type)[a]
Rete pattern	Elongated	Partly effaced	Effaced
Basal melanocytic proliferation	Noncontiguous, noncontinuous	Noncontiguous, noncontinuous	Contiguous and continuous
Pagetoid melanocytic proliferation	Absent	Absent	Focally present usually
Cytologic atypia	Slight, random	Slight to moderate, random	Moderate to severe, uniform
Lesional cell nests	Absent	Absent	Focally present

[a]MIS LM = melanoma in situ, lentigo maligna.

of all of these signs, and in some lesions where the features are incompletely represented, especially when only a small biopsy is available for interpretation, a descriptive diagnosis may be the best that can be offered. Additional biopsies may be needed, either immediately or after a period of observation, during which time the features may become more evident clinically and histologically.

Some authors have considered lentigo maligna to be a form of premalignant dysplasia or atypical melanocytic proliferation, whereas others have considered it to be melanoma in situ. Flotte and Mihm (26) reviewed 50 cases of lentigo maligna, and identified two subsets of lesions. The first was characterized by atypical melanocytic hyperplasia (an increased number of single melanocytes), which they postulated to be correctly designated lentigo maligna. The second subset had the following features in addition to the melanocytic hyperplasia: individual and nests of cells at varying layers of the epidermis (pagetoid proliferation), confluence of melanocytes replacing the basilar region (contiguous and continuous proliferation), uniformity of cytologic atypia, and nesting of uniformly atypical melanocytes. These lesions were designated as malignant melanoma in situ, lentigo maligna type. The observations suggested that the lesions that have been termed lentigo maligna represent a spectrum of atypia, perhaps correlating with the clinical aggressiveness of the lesions. Lesions with the attributes of melanoma in situ within the epidermis were more likely to have a focus of dermal invasion elsewhere in the lesion (27).

Recently, another form of lentiginous melanoma that frequently affects the skin of older individuals has been described (45). Like melanoma in situ of the acral-lentiginous type, and in contrast to nevi, this variant shows contiguous and continuous replacement of the basal cell layer by atypical melanocytes, in addition to junctional nesting, which could lead to confusion with a lentiginous junctional nevus or a dysplastic nevus.

We tend to consider that any lesion meeting the criteria for lentigo maligna should be classified and managed as a melanoma in situ, with complete local excision and follow-up. Nevertheless, there is undoubted overlap between lesions of lentigo maligna and actinic lentigines, with some of the latter exhibiting atypical features (Table 9-2). There is overlap among all of the lesions, however, and in cases of uncertainty a descriptive diagnosis can be used, such as "superficial atypical melanocytic proliferation of uncertain significance (SAMPUS)," with a note describing the differential diagnosis and the reasons for the diagnostic dilemma (figs. 9-28, 9-29).

Tumorigenic and/or Mitogenic Vertical Growth Phase in Lentigo Maligna Melanoma. In a lentigo maligna (whether or not further qualified as in situ melanoma), there are no tumor cells in the dermis by definition. When lesional cells similar to those in the epidermis are present in the dermis, usually associated with some host reaction of fibroblasts and/or lymphocytes, the lesion is considered to be invasive. Once invasion is present, the later course and the pathology may be similar to other forms of melanoma (fig. 9-30), except that the tumorigenic vertical growth phase of lentigo maligna melanoma is more likely to be composed of spindle cells (sometimes with desmoplasia and/or neurotropism than is

Figure 9-28

SUPERFICIAL ATYPICAL MELANOCYTIC PROLIFERATION OF UNCERTAIN SIGNIFICANCE (SAMPUS): LENTIGO MALIGNA MELANOMA IN SITU VERSUS SEVERE MELANOCYTIC DYSPLASIA

A: Scanning magnification shows elongated rete ridges, with nests mainly at the tips.

B: At higher magnification, there are single cells between the rete ridges, but they are not continuous with one another. There is a small cluster of nevus cells in the dermis in the center of the field.

C: High magnification demonstrates generally mild but "random" atypia, involving a minority of the lesional cells.

D: Nests tend to become confluent; however, there is no continuous basal or pagetoid proliferation. Such lesions have been described as "nevoid lentigo maligna." They often occur on the torso of elderly individuals, and should be managed by complete excision and follow-up. This lesion was from the ear of a 62-year-old man, and in our opinion, should not be interpreted as an unequivocally benign nevus of special sites.

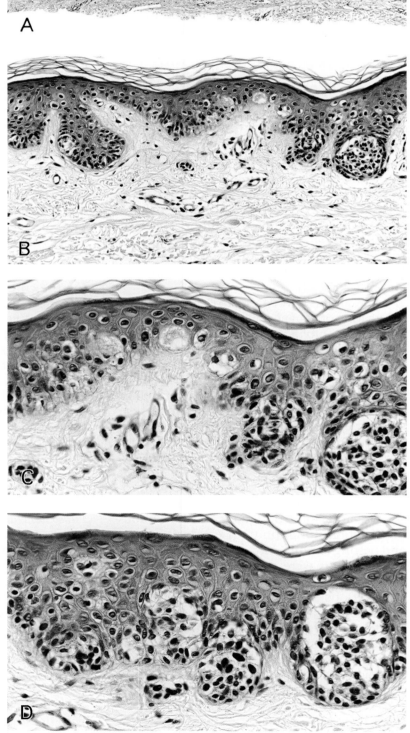

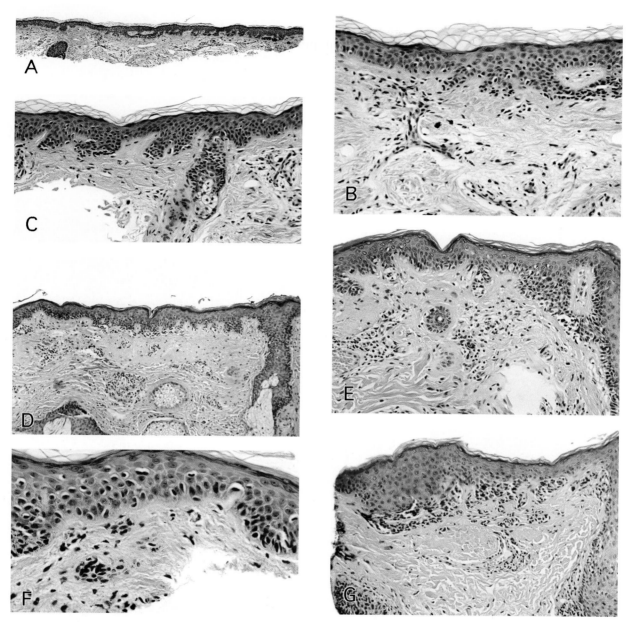

Figure 9-29

SUPERFICIAL ATYPICAL MELANOCYTIC PROLIFERATION OF UNCERTAIN SIGNIFICANCE (SAMPUS): SUBTLE LENTIGO MALIGNA VERSUS SEVERE MELANOCYTIC DYSPLASIA

A: The scanning magnification shows a shave biopsy of a lesion from the temple of a 50-year-old woman. It is characterized by elongated rete ridges, nests at the tips of the rete, and bridging nests.

B: In the dermis, there is diffuse fibroplasia.

C: Small nevoid melanocytes are present at the tips of rete ridges, an appearance that was considered most consistent with melanocytic dysplasia.

D: This lesion was not reexcised and recurred locally, and in the local recurrence, the cellularity is greater.

E–G: Single cells and nests hanging down from the epidermis in sun-damaged skin (E) are close to the new margins of the excision (F,G). This lesion fits into the category of "nevoid lentigo maligna" or a SAMPUS lesion, which should be treated by complete local excision and follow-up, especially if the patient has other clinically atypical nevi or a family or personal history of melanoma.

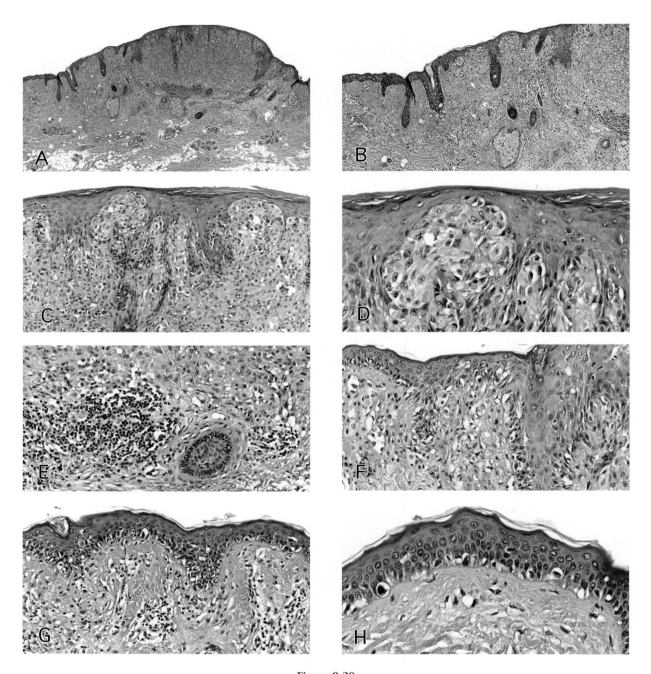

Figure 9-30

LENTIGO MALIGNA MELANOMA WITH VERTICAL GROWTH PHASE AND ADJACENT RADIAL GROWTH PHASE

A: Tumorigenic vertical growth phase is present to the right and predominantly in situ radial growth phase to the left of a lesion from the cheek of a 44-year-old.

B–F: The vertical growth phase is composed of epithelioid melanocytes showing little evidence of maturation from superficial to deep, with a predominantly noninfiltrative lymphocytic response at the base. Superficially, there is continuous proliferation of uniformly atypical melanocytes along the dermal-epidermal junction. The immediately adjacent in situ component is comprised of large cells with some tendency to pagetoid extension into the epidermis (F).

G: Further to the periphery, the proliferation is predominantly lentiginous (continuous, basal), with rare pagetoid melanocytes.

H: The far periphery of the lesion contains a few scattered atypical melanocytes at the dermal-epidermal junction.

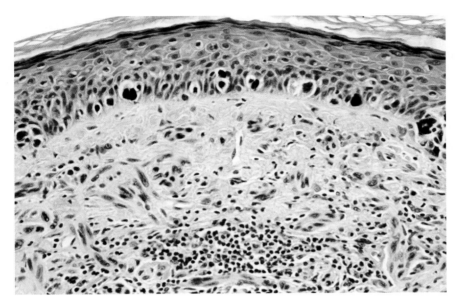

Figure 9-31

LENTIGO MALIGNA MELANOMA, WITH INVASIVE SPINDLE CELLS

An atypical intraepidermal melanocytic proliferation is consistent with lentigo maligna with uniform atypia (lentigo maligna melanoma in situ). An invasive spindle cell component with associated lymphocytes is seen in the dermis.

that of the more common form of superficial spreading melanoma (fig. 9-31).

Treatment and Prognosis. Since lentigo maligna melanomas commonly occur on cosmetically sensitive sites or adjacent to vital structures such as the eye, excisions are often planned with margins that are narrower than for other melanomas, and control of the margins may present histologic problems. In particular, it is important not to overinterpret minor degrees of hyperplasia and atypia of melanocytes in actinically damaged skin (fig. 9-32). These cells may show varying degrees of nuclear enlargement and hyperchromasia, but there is little or no proliferation, so that the atypical cells remain as solitary units separated by keratinocytes at the dermal-epidermal junction, and mitotic figures are not observed. Duve et al. (46) studied 722 reexcision scars of patients with benign and malignant nonmelanocytic lesions. Melanocytic hyperplasia was defined as variable numbers of increased melanocytes arranged as solitary units at the dermal-epidermal junction, and was present in 59 cases (8 percent), 56 from the sun-exposed skin of the face and neck and 3 from the trunk (p <0.00001). The most common sites were the nose and lower eyelids, but the forehead was also frequently involved.

Because of the poor circumscription and ill-defined borders of the in situ component of lentigo maligna melanoma, identification of the exact tumor border may be difficult,

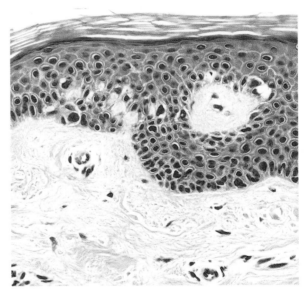

Figure 9-32

MELANOCYTIC ATYPIA IN CHRONICALLY SUN-DAMAGED SKIN

An isolated atypical melanocyte in chronically sun-damaged skin cannot be used as evidence of involvement by lentigo maligna.

especially in the presence of melanocytic hyperplasia, and this can complicate the evaluation of specimen margins. Weyers et al. (47) examined the epidermis adjacent to lesions of in situ melanoma in skin with elastosis as a marker for chronic sun-related injury, using

Table 9-3

FEATURES OF VALUE IN DISCRIMINATING MELANOCYTIC HYPERPLASIA FROM MELANOMA IN SITU IN CHRONICALLY SUN-DAMAGED SKIN

	Melanoma in Situ	Melanocytic Hyperplasia	Diagnostic Value[b]
Nests of melanocytes in epidermis	94%	4%	90
Melanocytes not equidistant from one another	100%	14%	86
Melanocytes present above junction	96%	12%	84
Melanocytes descend far down appendages	96%	12%	84
Lesion not uniformly pigmented	88%	4%	84
>15 melanocytes/0.5 mm in 2 adjacent fields	98%	14%	84
Pleomorphism of melanocytes	86%	8%	76
Enlarged melanocyte nuclei	80%	6%	74
Melanocytes touch one another	100%	30%	70

[a]Modified from Table 1 from Weyers W, Bonczkowitz M, Weyers I, Bittinger A, Schill WB. Melanoma in situ versus melanocytic hyperplasia in sun-damaged skin. Assessment of the significance of histopathologic criteria for differential diagnosis. Am J Dermatopathol 1996;18:560-566.

[b]Diagnostic value is the frequency of the feature in melanoma in situ minus the frequency in melanocytic hyperplasia.

skin with basal cell carcinomas as controls. The most valuable criteria for the diagnosis of melanoma, as opposed to melanocytic hyperplasia as may be seen in chronically sun-damaged skin, according to the authors are: presence of nests of melanocytes, irregular distribution of melanocytes, descent of melanocytes far down adnexal epithelial structures, irregular distribution of pigment, presence of melanocytes above the dermal-epidermal junction, a high number of melanocytes, pleomorphism of melanocytes, and atypical nuclei of melanocytes (Table 9-3). Other criteria, such as the collapse of cytoplasm around nuclei of melanocytes; flattening of rete ridges; differences in the area, shape, and contour of nuclei of melanocytes as assessed by nuclear morphometry; and presence of melanocytes stained by HMB45 and Ki-67/MIB-1 monoclonal antibodies, were considered in this study to be of little value.

Control of margins in reexcision specimens of lentigo maligna and lentigo maligna melanoma is complicated by the poor circumscription of the lesions, by the tendency to limit margin widths to preserve vital structures in the head and neck, or for cosmetic regions (fig. 9-26) (47). Perhaps, in part, as a consequence of these surgical limitations, and also no doubt because of the possible presence of "field cells" with precursor potential (48), local recurrence

is more common in lentiginous melanomas and in melanomas on sun-damaged and cosmetically sensitive skin than in other forms of melanoma (40,41). In a retrospective analysis of 1,996 patients followed by the Pigmented Lesion Group of the University of Pennsylvania (41,49), the incidence of locally recurrent melanoma was 2.2 percent, and lentigo maligna melanoma accounted for 37 percent of these local recurrences. Increased tumor thickness and microsatellites were associated with early local recurrence and decreased survival from time of recurrence. Nineteen percent of the local recurrences developed more than 5 years after the initial definitive treatment.

The preponderance of lentigo maligna melanoma among locally recurrent melanomas suggests a need for refinements in the techniques of margin identification and surgical excision of this melanoma type (41). Breuninger et al. (50) studied reexcision specimens by taking sections inward from a 10-mm initial margin, and found that 54 percent of lentigo maligna melanoma lesions had evidence of continuous subclinical spread more than 5 mm from the clinical border. As a result, they advocated the use of continuous vertical sections for the evaluation of these margins. Others have also advocated the use of similar micrographic techniques for mapping of the entire margin. Because of the difficulty of specifically recognizing subtle changes at the periphery of the lesions, most have recommended the use of paraffin rather than frozen sections, with delayed surgery for positive margins if necessary (51–56). This method also allows for the use of immunohistochemistry (54,55).

The presence of field cells, which are histologically unremarkable cells in the epidermis adjacent to a melanoma that carry some of the genetic abnormalities of the melanoma, has recently been described around acral melanomas (48); such cells are probably present in melanomas at other sites as well. It is likely that these cells, through continued progression, may account for local persistence, followed by recurrence, of some lesions. It may soon be possible to test for these cells by the use of fluorescent in situ hybridization (FISH) for increased copy number of chromosomes to identify genetically abnormal cells; the balance between excision of all of the abnormal cells, an acceptable cosmetic result, and an acceptable level of local recurrence needs to be determined through appropriately designed clinicopathologic studies.

"Recurrences" due to field cells represent persistence followed by regrowth, and clinical recurrence of in situ disease, although surgically troublesome because of functional and/or cosmetic issues, should be distinguished from the prognostically more significant local recurrence of tumorigenic melanoma. The latter is less common in our experience, and usually represents local metastasis (satellites and intransit metastases), rather than true local persistence and regrowth (57). Melanocytic hyperplasia and atypia may be seen in sun-damaged skin unrelated to the presence of a nearby melanoma. In a study of 180 specimens of melanoma and nonmelanoma skin cancers, contiguous melanocytes, atypical melanocytes, and follicular melanocytes were seen in sun-damaged skin surrounding both melanoma and nonmelanoma skin cancers, potentially mimicking melanoma in situ (58). These findings were more common in skin around melanomas. The authors urged caution when assessing the margins for melanoma in sun-damaged skin.

Although limited follow-up studies have demonstrated reasonable effectiveness for the micrographic technique with paraffin sections (56), there is no standard management for these lesions. In a survey of British dermatologists,

the preferred treatment option was dependent on the age of the patient. Dermatologists were far more likely to use surgery for patients under the age of 60 years and more likely to use cryotherapy/radiotherapy or merely to observe patients of increasing age. Where surgery was used, the excision margins chosen ranged from 0 to 10 mm (59).

As an alternative to the micrographically controlled method, Jeneby et al. (60) have recently described a method in use for some years at the University of Pennsylvania Pigmented Lesion Clinic. Using ultraviolet identification (Wood's lamp) to enhance recognition of the clinical margin, circumferentially arranged punch biopsy specimens were obtained and sent for formal pathologic review, including immunohistochemical staining. If the punch biopsies were positive for lentigo maligna or lentigo maligna melanoma, more peripheral punch biopsies were obtained. Once clear margins were obtained, definitive resection was performed. The specimen was then examined by routine histology. No patients required re-excision for positive surgical margins. Fourteen patients were cleared after their first series of biopsies, 3 patients required a second series of biopsies, 2 patients required a third session, and 1 patient required a fourth session. In a mean follow-up of 1 year, there was no evidence of recurrence. The procedure appeared to have reduced the need for repeat surgical excisions to obtain clear margins and may decrease the risk for recurrence by mapping accurately the true histologic margin (54). Caution is needed not only to reduce the incidence of recurrence but also to avoid excessive, potentially mutilating excisions (58).

ACRAL-LENTIGINOUS MELANOMA

Definition. *Acral-lentiginous melanoma* is defined by the presence of a microinvasive or in situ nontumorigenic radial growth phase compartment that is composed of uniformly atypical neoplastic melanocytes located mainly in and near the basal layer of an acral epidermis (a lentiginous pattern). A vertical growth phase compartment may or may not be present; the lesions are classified as acral-lentiginous on the basis of the morphology of the radial growth phase. This form of melanoma was first

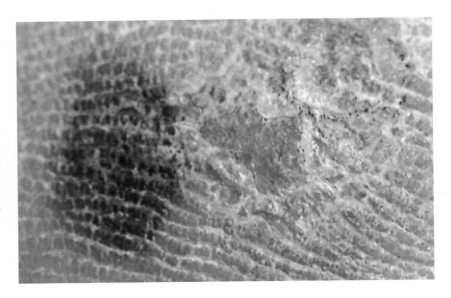

Figure 9-33

ACRAL-LENTIGINOUS MELANOMA

This small and flat lesion was nevertheless quite deeply invasive. Perhaps because of the tough stratum corneum in acral sites, these lesions tend to be endophytic rather than exophytic in their pattern of vertical growth. (Fig. F from Plate V, Fascicle 2, Third Series.)

described in 1977 (61), and there have been several subsequent reported series (62,63).

Clinical Features. Epidemiologically, acral-lentiginous melanomas are distinguished from all other cutaneous melanomas. They are similar to mucosal melanomas in that they occur with about equal frequency in people of all races, including those with cutaneous phenotypes other than the fair Caucasian complexion that is usual in other forms of cutaneous melanoma. In countries where non-Caucasians predominate, acral-lentiginous melanoma may be the most common form of the disease, although the total population-based incidence in these countries remains low (63,64). Compared with lentigo maligna melanoma, with which they share some lentiginous patterns of proliferation (see below), the lesions are not likely to be associated with chronic sun exposure in the dermis at the lesional site, nor are they especially prone to occur in individuals who are susceptible to sunburn or have a history of heavy recreational sun exposure. To the contrary, acral and mucosal lentiginous melanomas are about as common in dark-skinned races as in Caucasians. Unlike superficial spreading melanoma, this form of the disease is not commonly associated with nevi as either precursors or markers of increased risk, such as dysplastic nevi (7).

Acral-lentiginous melanomas most commonly occur on the volar skin of the soles of the feet (fig. 9-33), followed in frequency by the palmar skin of the hands, especially that of the

thumb. Subungual melanoma shares similar histologic characteristics (fig. 9-34). Clinically, the radial growth phase of acral-lentiginous melanoma is similar to that of other melanomas in most respects, but the border is more likely to be ill-defined and impalpable than that of superficial spreading melanoma. Indeed, even when invasive, the entire lesion may be impalpable at times, which is very unusual in invasive melanomas of other types. The cardinal clinical features of asymmetry, border irregularity, color variegation, and diameter greater than 6 mm (ABCD criteria [65]) are present in most examples of radial growth phase acral-lentiginous melanoma. Many of these lesions present as neglected primaries with a very large and dramatically atypical radial growth phase plaque within which there may be several large vertical growth phase tumor nodules, often with ulceration and secondary infection.

Subungual melanoma is a subset of acral-lentiginous melanoma, and these lesions are most common on the thumb and great toe (fig. 9-34). They present as patches of tan-brown to blue-black variegated pigmentation beneath the nail. In the beginning, the lesion is completely impalpable, and usually remains so until a bulky vertical growth phase appears to elevate the nail. In contrast to a subungual hematoma where the nail plate acts as a flap valve to keep the blood in the nail bed, the pigmentation of subungual melanoma extends in the nail epithelium into and beyond that of the contiguous nail cuticle

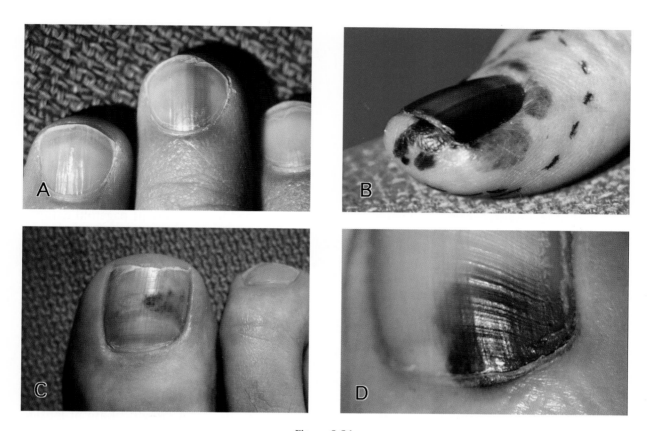

Figure 9-34

LONGITUDINAL MELANONYCHIA AND SUBUNGUAL MELANOMAS

A: This linear streak of brown is consistent with a junctional nevus of the nail matrix (longitudinal melanonychia).

B: Malignant melanoma of the acral-lentiginous type involves the nail cuticle and skin of the digit. Irregular pigmentation is seen in the nail. The neoplasm has spread within the epidermis to the skin of the digit proximally, laterally, and distally.

C: The variegated character of the pigment is concerning and should likely promote biopsy, or follow-up. Hutchinson sign, however, is negative.

D: A more subtle example of subungual acral-lentiginous melanoma, with early involvement of the nail cuticle (Hutchinson sign). Subungual hemorrhage or a benign nevus would remain confined to the nail bed and matrix, without "turning the corner" of the cuticle to involve the cuticle and skin, as here.

to involve the dorsal skin of the digit. This sign ("Hutchinson sign") was described in the 19th century by Sir Jonathan Hutchinson, who with Dubreuilh in France, is credited with having first described the radial growth phase of melanoma (66). Hutchinson sign in a subungual pigmented lesion should always prompt biopsy, which should include the full thickness of the nail and its bed (fig. 9-34).

The clinical signs of acral and subungual melanomas may be subtle. In a recent study of 53 cases with a final diagnosis of melanoma, Soon et al. (67) found that 18 were initially misdiagnosed. The list of misdiagnoses included wart, callus, fungal disorder, foreign body, crusty

lesion, sweat gland condition, blister, nonhealing wound, mole, keratoacanthoma, subungual hematoma, onychomycosis, ingrown toenail, and defective/infected toenail. Of the 18 misdiagnosed cases, 9 were clinically amelanotic.

In recent molecular studies, Bastian (48) demonstrated that chromosomal amplifications are frequent in melanomas on acral compared with nonacral sites, often associated with amplifications of cyclin D1 (68). These amplifications have allowed the detection of single basal melanocytes with gene amplifications in the histologically normal-appearing skin immediately adjacent to melanomas. These field cells may be considered to represent either subtle melanoma in situ or a precursor and are considered likely to represent minimal residual disease that could lead to local recurrence if not excised with safety margins (48). The incidence of local recurrence is higher in lentiginous melanomas, including lentigo maligna and acral lentiginous melanomas, than in the more common superficial spreading melanomas (48,69), perhaps due to a combination of site constraints on surgery and the field cells described by Bastian (48), which are histologically invisible. Such recurrences represent persistence followed by regrowth and clinical recurrence of in situ disease, and although surgically troublesome because of functional and/or cosmetic issues, they should be distinguished from prognostically more significant local recurrence of tumorigenic melanoma. It has also been demonstrated by the same group that *BRAF* mutations are uncommon in acral-lentiginous melanomas, while activating mutations of the oncogene *KIT* have been found in 36 percent of cases, a finding with obvious potential therapeutic consequences (29).

Since acral-lentiginous melanomas occur in areas of skin protected from direct sunlight by their location and by the thick keratin that covers these sites, it seems likely that etiologic agents other than ultraviolet light must play a role in their pathogenesis. Although the usual carcinogenic etiologic possibilities could be considered, namely chemical carcinogens, chronic trauma, and oncogenic viruses, there is little or no evidence other than anecdotes in favor of any of these agents.

Microscopic Findings. At scanning magnification, the epidermis is often uniformly thickened, without much accentuation of the rete ridge pattern (fig. 9-35). A thick keratin layer is physiologically present in these acral sites, but in acral-lentiginous melanomas this is often accentuated by pathologic hyperkeratosis. In an early lesion or at the periphery of a more advanced lesion, the cellularity may be low and the changes commensurately subtle, but toward the center of the lesion the cellularity typically becomes greater and there may be some tendency, occasionally marked, for pagetoid spread of lesional cells into the epidermis. There is often striking involvement of skin appendages (fig. 9-36).

In many lesions, there is a marked infiltrative lymphocytic host inflammatory response,

and when this response is particularly brisk, the major feature at scanning magnification may be a lichenoid pattern of lymphocytic infiltration at the dermal-epidermal junction. Among these lymphocytes, viable and degenerate neoplastic melanocytes can be discerned at higher magnification. Some of these neoplastic cells may be surrounded by rosetting lymphocytes, and the result of this inflammation may be the development of areas of apparently immunologic regression.

In contrast to the radial growth phase of superficial spreading melanoma, the lesional cells are not arranged in a prominent pagetoid pattern, except sometimes in the center of an advanced lesion. They are located mainly in the lower layers of the epidermis, especially at the periphery of the lesion where classification of the lesion is usually most straightforward. The cells essentially replace the majority of the basal keratinocytes and form a more or less continuous linear palisade of melanoma cells (contiguous and continuous basal melanocytic proliferation). This basal arrangement constitutes a lentiginous pattern, to some extent reminiscent of that seen in a lentigo simplex (see fig. 2-2).

As with the radial growth phase of lentigo maligna melanoma, atypical melanocytes may extend along adnexal structures, particularly within eccrine ducts and glands. Occasional superficial lesions show deep intraeccrine growth that involves coils within the deep dermis or subcutis, and this must be detected and considered when evaluating deep margins.

At higher magnification, there is an increased number of slightly to moderately enlarged melanocytes with moderately to severely (sometimes mildly) atypical nuclei. Eosinophilic or amphophilic nucleoli may be present; in some lesions these are not conspicuous and the majority of the cells have small, dark nuclei without an observable chromatin pattern. Mitoses are observed in about one third of radial growth phase cells. When present, they are of diagnostic assistance. In our experience, however, they are usually absent in a difficult lesion where the differential diagnosis may include a benign nevus.

A striking cytologic feature in some lesions is the presence of long dendrites that ramify among the benign keratinocytes. Such dendrites can only be seen in cells that are heavily pigmented or stained by immunohistochemistry (fig. 9-37). This

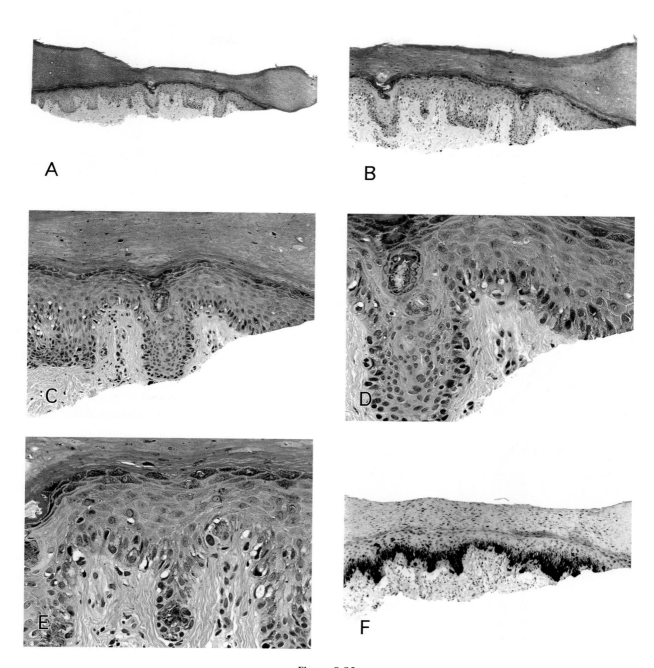

Figure 9-35

MELANOMA IN SITU, ACRAL-LENTIGINOUS TYPE

A: At scanning magnification, there is a moderately cellular proliferation, extending to a lateral margin on the right.

B: At higher magnification, there is continuous proliferation not only around the tips and sides, but also between the rete ridges.

C: The continuous proliferation extends to a lateral margin. There may be a small nest in the dermis. There is no tumorigenic proliferation.

D,E: Higher magnification shows uniform severe cytologic atypia.

F: A Melan-A stain shows continuous proliferation, more extensive than was apparent in the hematoxylin and eosin (H&E)-stained sections.

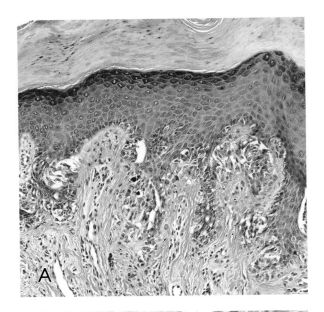

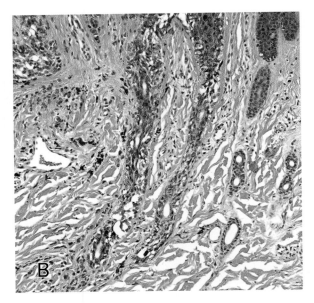

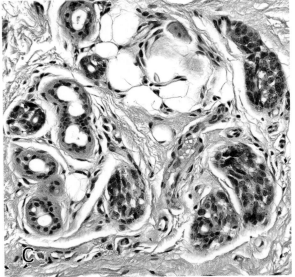

Figure 9-36

MALIGNANT MELANOMA, ACRAL-LENTIGINOUS TYPE

A: This melanoma has a predominantly nested and focal pagetoid proliferation.

B,C: Extensive involvement of skin appendages, such as these eccrine ducts, is characteristic in acral melanomas.

intracellular pigmentation seems to represent a form of pigmentary "constipation" or failure of the normal process of pigmentary transfer to keratinocytes. In some lesions, pigment is sparse or even absent in the radial growth phase, and in such cases dendrites are not visible. When pigment is absent, the lesions may clinically be mistaken for an inflammatory patch of some kind and the diagnosis may be delayed. At the histologic level, it is easy to miss a relatively subtle melanocytic proliferation among the cells of a dense lichenoid lymphocytic infiltrate if pigment is absent or sparse (fig. 9-38). The pigmentary changes are often focal in acral-lentiginous melanomas, so that amelanotic areas of radial growth phase melanoma may extend much further than the surgeon appreciates at the time of biopsy. Melanin pigment may be transmitted into the thickened stratum corneum, and unlike this phenomenon in acral nevi, which tend to produce discrete vertically aligned "smoke-stack" patterns, the intracorneal melanin in acral-lentiginous melanoma is often diffuse or irregularly distributed.

Tumorigenic and/or Mitogenic Vertical Growth Phase in Acral-Lentiginous Melanoma. The vertical

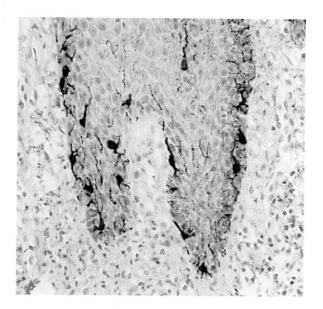

Figure 9-37

ACRAL-LENTIGINOUS MELANOMA

Increased dendritic melanocytes at the periphery of an acral-lentiginous melanoma are seen with the Melan-A stain.

growth phase compartment (if any) in an acral-lentiginous melanoma in some cases is composed of epithelioid cells, differing little or not at all from the vertical growth phase component of a superficial spreading melanoma. It is more likely, however, to be composed of plump atypical spindle cells, usually with enlarged nuclei, prominent nucleoli, and readily detectable mitoses (fig. 9-38). The spindle cells are often arranged in fascicles with a somewhat neuroid or schwannian pattern of differentiation, sometimes with desmoplasia. Frank neurotropism (invasion of the endoneurium or perineurium of cutaneous nerves) is common (discussed more fully with Desmoplastic Melanoma in chapter 10). We have observed neurotropism in as many as 7 percent of a series of acral-lentiginous lesions. Since neurotropic spread may extend beyond the apparent boundaries of the contiguous tumor, the margins of wide excision specimens should be carefully examined in such cases. It is helpful in neurotropic melanomas to advise the surgeon to identify the cutaneous nerves at the time of excision so that they can be examined specifically, and to ink the margins

of the specimen so that the true margin can be specifically identified.

Differential Diagnosis. The clinically trivial but epidemiologically significant distinction from superficial spreading melanoma involving acral skin may be difficult at times, and such cases may be signed out as unclassified melanomas indicating the presence or absence of radial, and especially, of vertical growth phase as appropriate. The value of the classification of acral melanoma lies not in any contribution to prognostication or therapy, but in the codification of diagnostic criteria that allow the accurate recognition of disparate morphologies, and in the insights that may result from the differing epidemiologic and molecular associations of acral-lentiginous and other forms of melanoma. Lentigo maligna melanoma does not occur on acral skin. Chronic sun exposure, a major epidemiologic association of lentigo maligna melanoma, does not affect acral skin because of the powerful light-scattering and -absorbing ability of the thick acral stratum corneum.

Lentiginous acral nevi constitute the other major potential differential diagnostic challenge. These benign lesions may be somewhat asymmetric in their scanning magnification appearance, raising a consideration of melanoma. There may also be slight to moderate nuclear atypia at higher magnification. Mitotic figures, however, are not observed, and there is no uniform, diffuse high-grade atypia of the type commonly seen in tumorigenic melanomas (fig. 9-39). Pagetoid spread of lesional cells into the epidermis, a subtle but diagnostically important finding that is often present focally in acral melanomas, may also occur in nevi in these sites; however, cytologic atypia is minimal or absent. The lichenoid lymphocytic infiltrate so characteristic of acral melanomas generally is not seen in the benign lesions, and there is no evidence of regression. Finally, the clusters of cells that may be present in the dermis are nevoid in configuration, lacking high-grade atypia and mitoses, and with evidence of maturation toward the base of the lesion. If there is extension into the reticular dermis, the pattern at the base of the lesion is the nevoid pattern of single cells or single files of cells predominating over fascicles, nests, or sheets of cells. Acral-lentiginous nevi are discussed in chapter 2.

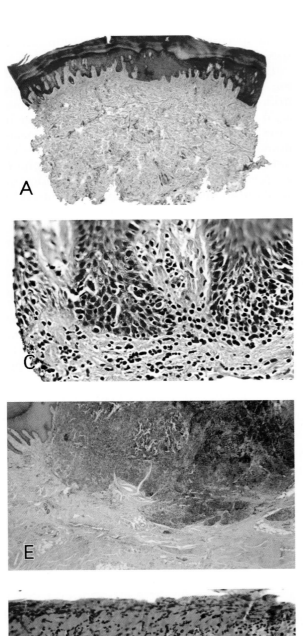

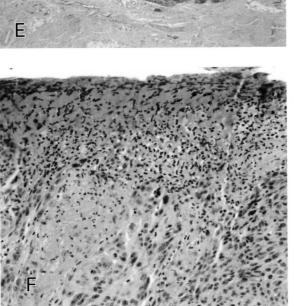

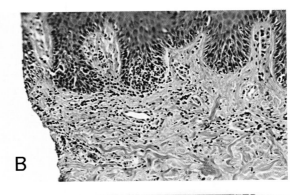

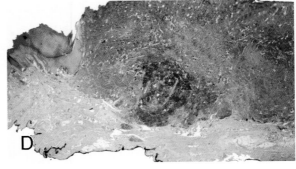

Figure 9-38

**MELANOMA IN SITU, ACRAL-LENTIGINOUS TYPE,
WITH TUMORIGENIC RECURRENCE**

A: This biopsy from a 38-year-old man shows irregular thickening and thinning of the epidermis at scanning magnification.

B,C: High magnification shows a subtle increase of atypical melanocytes along the dermal-epidermal junction, with a focally lichenoid lymphocytic infiltrate. This lesion was not reexcised.

D: Three years later, the lesion recurred as a bulky tumorigenic melanoma with an adjacent acral-lentiginous radial growth phase (at the left).

E: The tumorigenic melanoma extended deep into the reticular dermis, and measured 5.1 mm in Breslow thickness.

F: Superficially, the lesion is ulcerated, with invasive tumorigenic spindle cells.

G: Cytologically, there are frequent mitoses and uniform atypia with nuclear enlargement and prominent nucleoli.

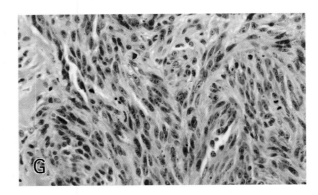

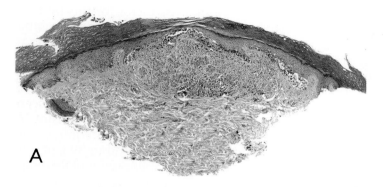

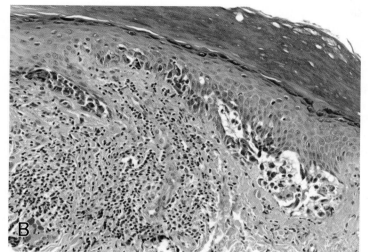

Figure 9-39

ACRAL MELANOMA, WITH SMALL TUMORIGENIC VERTICAL GROWTH PHASE

A: Scanning magnification shows a tumorigenic component, Clark level III, Breslow thickness 0.44 mm.

B: High magnification shows an adjacent in situ component composed of confluent, uniformly atypical epithelioid melanocytes along the dermal-epidermal junction.

C: Lesional cells in the tumorigenic vertical growth phase show severe uniform atypia with mitotic activity (tumorigenic and mitogenic [arrow] malignant melanoma).

MUCOSAL-LENTIGINOUS MELANOMA (NONTUMORIGENIC COMPARTMENT)

Definition. Although many mucosal melanomas are entirely in the vertical growth phase at presentation and should thus be termed nodular melanomas, many exhibit a radial growth phase nontumorigenic compartment, usually with a lentiginous architecture and often with a dendritic cytology similar to acral-lentiginous melanomas, and are termed *mucosal-lentiginous melanomas.*

Clinical Features. Clinically, the plaques of radial growth phase mucosal-lentiginous melanomas exhibit the cardinal features of any melanoma in this phase of tumor progression. The borders are ill-defined and impalpable, and we have seen examples of lesions where extensive areas of the radial growth phase were amelanotic. Such lesions may simulate an inflammatory patch or may even be difficult to distinguish from normal mucosa, resulting sometimes in the unexpected histologic involvement of resection margins that seemed to be widely clear clinically and grossly. A tumorigenic vertical growth phase nodule, if present, is a more or less spheroid mass that may itself be largely amelanotic and commonly is ulcerated at presentation.

In a population-based study, mucosal melanomas accounted for less than 5 percent of the total number of melanoma cases (70). The vulva and to a much lesser extent the vagina (71,72), oral cavity (73,74), and nasopharynx and sinuses (75, 76) are the most common sites. A few cases occur in the anal area (77) and in the distal urethra (78, 79). All other sites, including deep viscera such as the esophagus (80,81), gallbladder (82), urinary bladder (83–85), bowel (86), trachea (87), bronchial tree (88), and lung (87,89) are anecdotal or the subject of a few case reports only.

These lesions need to be distinguished from metastases, which are in general more common at some of these sites. Criteria for this distinction include the presence of an overlying, and especially, adjacent in situ component, and exclusion of a primary elsewhere. Even so, some of these lesions may represent metastatic melanoma from an unknown primary site, and if this is this case, the clinical course is likely to reveal the true diagnosis as time passes. Lesions of the lip may represent bona fide mucosal melanomas in some instances, but those lip lesions that predominantly involve the lower lip of chronically sun-exposed individuals are more likely to represent actinically induced lentigo maligna melanomas. As for the other mucosal melanomas, it seems clear that the local effect of sunlight does not play a role in their pathogenesis. Further, the occurrence of mucosal melanomas in persons of all races and geographic locations (like their acral counterparts) would suggest that skin susceptibility to the effects of sunlight is not a risk factor for this form of melanoma; however, the lesions are sufficiently rare as to have precluded effective population-based epidemiologic analysis to date.

In studies of malignant mucosal melanomas of the vulva, vagina, and head and neck, the common mutation in the *BRAF* gene has been rarely detected, unlike in melanomas arising in sun-exposed sites. In contrast, mutations of the oncogene *KIT* have been found in 39 percent, often associated with amplifications of this gene (29). These findings again support the view that the various subtypes of melanoma are not equivalent and that distinct genetic alterations may underlie the well-recognized differences in risk factors and behavioral patterns discussed in previous sections (90,91). It has been concluded from these data that patients with melanomas should not be collectively regarded as a uniform group as new strategies are developed that target specific genetic alterations (90).

Microscopic Findings. The histologic features are similar to those observed in acral-lentiginous melanoma (fig. 9-40). There are increased numbers of uniformly atypical melanocytes, often with prominent dendrites, arranged in a lentiginous pattern in the basal layer of the epithelium. An associated lichenoid lymphocytic infiltrate with admixed plasma cells is often observed. There may be areas of regression, characterized by the absence of melanoma cells and by the presence of fibrosis in the superficial lamina propria, with a scattering of lymphocytes and melanophages. Characteristic pagetoid superficial spreading melanoma patterns are rarely seen as a predominant pattern in mucosal melanomas, but usually at least a few cells are observed above the basal lamina, a finding that may be of diagnostic assistance. Like acral melanomas, mucosal melanomas often present with a spindle cell type in the vertical growth phase, and desmoplastic (92–94) as well as neurotropic (95) features are common (fig. 9-40). In one instance of a neurotropic but not desmoplastic mucosal melanoma of the lip, we have seen extension of tumor as far as the mandibular nerve at the angle of the jaw, but more often, nerve involvement is confined to the immediate vicinity of the tumor.

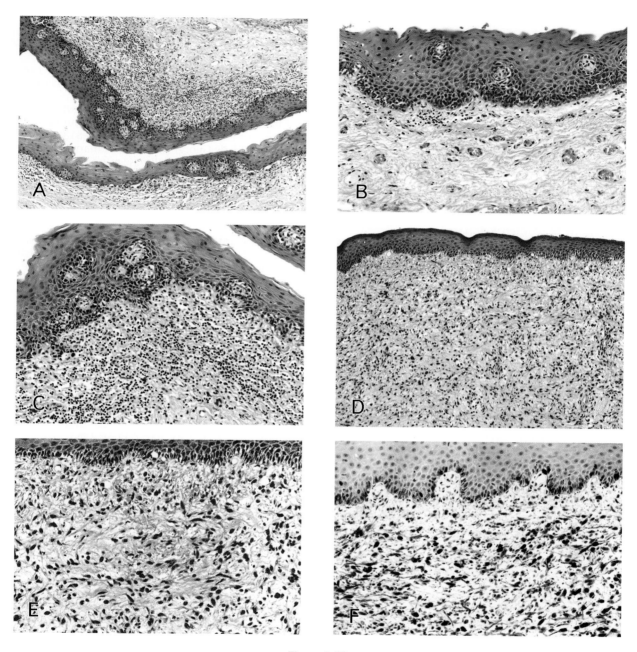

Figure 9-40

MUCOSAL-LENTIGINOUS MELANOMA OF THE VULVA

A: This portion of an extensive biopsy from a 78-year-old woman shows a lichenoid lymphocytic infiltrate almost obscuring an atypical melanocytic proliferation.

B: In another area, there are a few atypical melanocytes, with associated hyperpigmentation of basal keratinocytes.

C: Lichenoid lymphocytic inflammation partly obscures continuous proliferation of atypical melanocytes along the dermal-epidermal junction.

D: A tumorigenic component consists of invasive spindle cells separated by collagen fiber bundles (desmoplastic tumorigenic vertical growth phase).

E: Bland tumor cells are separated by newly synthesized collagen fibers.

F: S-100 protein stains strongly and diffusely. Note the subtle proliferation of atypical melanocytes in the overlying epidermis.

REFERENCES

1. Viros A, Fridyland J, Bauer J, Curtin J, Pinkel D, Bastian BC. Histomorphological signature of mutation status in melanoma. 2007. In: American Association for Cancer Research Annual Meeting: Proceedings; 2007 Apr 14-18; Los Angeles, CA. Philadelphia: AACR; 2007. Abstract nr {154}.

2. Elder DE, Xu X. The approach to the patient with a difficult melanocytic lesion. Pathology 2004; 36:428-434.

3. Yu LL, Heenan PJ. The morphological features of locally recurrent melanoma and cutaneous metastases of melanoma. Hum Pathol 1999;30:551-555.

4. Thorn M, Ponten F, Johansson AM, Bergstrom R. Rapid increase in diagnosis of cutaneous melanoma in situ in Sweden, 1968-1992. Cancer Detect Prev 1998;22:430-437.

5. National Institutes of Health Consensus Development Conference Statement on Diagnosis and Treatment of Early Melanoma, January 27-29, 1992. Am J Dermatopathol 1993;15:34-43.

6. McGovern VJ. The classification of melanoma and its relationship with prognosis. Pathology 1970;2:85-98.

7. Clark WH Jr, Elder DE, Van Horn M. The biologic forms of malignant melanoma. Hum Pathol 1986;5:443-450.

8. Bevona C, Goggins W, Quinn T, Fullerton J, Tsao H. Cutaneous melanomas associated with nevi. Arch Dermatol 2003;139:1620-1624.

9. Holman CD, Armstrong BK. Cutaneous malignant melanoma and indicators of total accumulated exposure to the sun: an analysis separating histogenetic types. J Natl Cancer Inst 1984;73:75-82.

10. Greene M, Clark WH Jr, Tucker MA, Kraemer KH, Elder DE, Fraser MC. High risk of malignant melanoma in melanoma-prone families with dysplastic nevi. Ann Intern Med 1985;102:458-465.

11. Holly EA, Kelly JW, Shpall SN, Chiu SH. Number of melanocytic nevi as a major risk factor for malignant melanoma. J Am Acad Dermatol 1987;17:459-468.

12. Crocetti E, Carli P. Only superficial spreading melanoma is causing the melanoma epidemics? Eur J Epidemiol 2004;19:91-92.

13. Rhodes AR, Weinstock MA, Fitzpatrick TB, Mihm MC Jr, Sober AJ. Risk factors for cutaneous melanoma. A practical method for recognizing predisposed individuals. JAMA 1987;258:3146-3154.

14. Stolz W, Schmoeckel C, Welkovich B, Braun-Falco O. Semiquantitative analysis of histologic criteria in thin malignant melanomas. J Am Acad Dermatol 1989;20:115-1120.

15. Maize JC, Ackerman AB. Pigmented lesions of the skin: clinicopathologic correlations. Philadelphia: Lea & Febiger; 1987.

16. Sorensen FB. Objective histopathologic grading of cutaneous malignant melanomas by stereologic estimation of nuclear volume: prediction of survival and disease-free period. Cancer 1989;63:1784-1798.

17. Pizzichetta MA, Canzonieri V, Massarut S, et al. Pigmented mammary Paget's disease mimicking melanoma. Melanoma Res 2004;14:S13-S15.

18. Stante M, de Georgi V, Massi D, Chiarugi A, Carli P. Pigmented Bowen's disease mimicking cutaneous melanoma: clinical and dermoscopic aspects. Dermatol Surg 2004;30:541-544.

19. Kohler S, Rouse RV, Smoller BR. The differential diagnosis of pagetoid cells in the epidermis. Mod Pathol 1998;11:79-92.

20. Bayer-Garner IB, Reed JA. Immunolabeling pattern of syndecan-1 expression may distinguish pagetoid Bowen's disease, extramammary Paget's disease, and pagetoid malignant melanoma in situ. J Cutan Pathol 2004;31:169-173.

21. Clark WH Jr, Mihm MC Jr. Lentigo maligna and lentigo-maligna melanoma. Am J Pathol 1969;55:39-67.

22. McGovern VJ, Shaw HM, Milton GW, Farago GA. Is malignant melanoma arising in a Hutchinson's melanotic freckle a separate disease entity. Histopathology 1980;4:235-242.

23. Hutchinson J. Senile freckles. Arch Surg (London) 1892;3:319.

24. McGovern VJ. Melanoma. Histologic diagnosis and prognosis. New York: Raven Press; 1983:3-24.

25. Reed RJ. A classification of melanocytic dysplasias and malignant melanomas. Am J Dermatopathol 1984;6:195-206.

26. Flotte TJ, Mihm MC Jr. Lentigo maligna and malignant melanoma in situ, lentigo maligna type. Hum Pathol 1999;30:533-536.

27. Tannous ZS, Lerner LH, Duncan LM, Mihm MC Jr, Flotte TJ. Progression to invasive melanoma from malignant melanoma in situ, lentigo maligna type. Hum Pathol 2000;31:705-708.

28. Elder DE, Guerry D 4th, Epstein MN, et al. Invasive malignant melanomas lacking competence for metastasis. Am J Dermatopathol 1984;6:55-62.

29. Curtin JA, Busam K, Pinkel D, Bastian BC. Somatic activation of KIT in distinct subtypes of melanoma. J Clin Oncol 2006;24:4340-4346.

30. Rivera RS, Nagatsuka H, Gunduz M, et al. C-kit protein expression correlated with activating mutations in KIT gene in oral mucosal melanoma. Virchows Arch 2008;452:27-32.

31. English DR, Heenan PJ, Holman CD, et al. Melanoma in Western Australia in 1980-81: incidence and characteristics of histological types. Pathology 1987;19:383-392.

32. Durnick A, Stolz W, Landthaler M, Vogt T. Lentigo maligna and lentigo maligna melanoma in young adults. Dermatol Surg 2004;30:813-816.

33. Gillgren P, Mansson-Brahme E, Frisell J, Johansson H, Larsson O, Ringborg U. Epidemiological characteristics of cutaneous malignant melanoma of the head and neck—a population-based study. Acta Oncol 1999;38:1069-1074.

34. McKenna DB, Cooper EJ, Kavanagh GM, Davie RM, McLaren KM, Tidman MJ. Amelanotic malignant melanoma following cryosurgery for atypical lentigo maligna. Clin Exp Dermatol 2000;25:600-604.

35. Conrad N, Jackson B, Goldberg L. Amelanotic lentigo maligna melanoma: a unique case presentation. Dermatol Surg 1999;25:408-411.

36. Rahbari H, Nabai H, Mehregan AH, Mehregan DA, Mehregan DR, Lipinski J. Amelanotic lentigo maligna melanoma: a diagnostic conundrum—presentation of four new cases. Cancer 1996;77:2052-2057.

37. Clark WH Jr, Elder DE, Guerry D 4th, et al. Model predicting survival in stage I melanoma based on tumor progression. J Natl Cancer Inst 1989;81:1893-1904.

38. Cox NH, Aitchison TC, Sirel JM, MacKie RM. Comparison between lentigo maligna melanoma and other histogenetic types of malignant melanoma of the head and neck. Br J Cancer 1996;73:940-944.

39. Koh HK, Michalik E, Sober AJ, et al. Lentigo maligna melanoma has no better prognosis than other types of melanoma. J Clin Oncol 1984;2:994-1001.

40. Schmid-Wendtner MH, Baumert J, Eberle J, Plewig G, Volkenandt M, Sander CA. Disease progression in patients with thin cutaneous melanomas (tumour thickness < or = 0.75 mm): clinical and epidemiological data from the Tumour Center Munich 1977-98. Br J Dermatol 2003;149:788-793.

41. Wildemore JK 4th, Schuchter L, Mick R, et al. Locally recurrent malignant melanoma characteristics and outcomes: a single-institution study. Ann Plast Surg 2001;46:488-494.

42. Newell GR, Sider JG, Bergfelt L, Kripke ML. Incidence of cutaneous melanoma in the United States by histology with special reference to the face. Cancer Res 1988;48:5036-5041.

43. Holman CD, Armstrong BK. Cutaneous malignant melanoma and indicators of total accumulated exposure to the sun: an analysis separating histogenic types. J Natl Cancer Inst 1984;73:75-82.

44. Cohen LM. The starburst giant cell is useful for distinguishing lentigo maligna from photodamaged skin. J Am Acad Dermatol 1996;35:962-968

45. King R, Page RN, Googe PB, Mihm MC. Lentiginous melanoma: a histologic pattern of melanoma to be distinguished from lentiginous nevus. Mod Pathol 2005;18:1397-1401.

46. Duve S, Schmoeckel C, Burgdorf WH. Melanocytic hyperplasia in scars. A histopathological investigation of 722 cases. Am J Dermatopathol 1996;18:236-240.

47. Weyers W, Bonczkowitz M, Weyers I, Bittinger A, Schill WB. Melanoma in situ versus melanocytic hyperplasia in sun-damaged skin. Assessment of the significance of histopathologic criteria for differential diagnosis. Am J Dermatopathol 1996;18:560-566.

48. Bastian BC. Understanding the progression of melanocytic neoplasia using genomic analysis: from fields to cancer. Oncogene 2003;22:3081-3086.

49. Papadopoulos T, Rasiah K, Thompson JF, Quinn MJ, Crotty KA. Melanoma of the nose. Br J Surg 1997;84:986-989.

50. Breuninger H, Schlagenhauff B, Stroebel W, Schaumburg-Lever G, Rassner G. Patterns of local horizontal spread of melanomas: consequences for surgery and histopathologic investigation. Am J Surg Pathol 1999;23:1493-1498.

51. Anderson KW, Baker SR, Lowe L, Su L, Johnson TM. Treatment of head and neck melanoma, lentigo maligna subtype: a practical surgical technique. Arch Facial Plast Surg 2001;3:202-206.

52. Hill DC, Gramp AA. Surgical treatment of lentigo maligna and lentigo maligna melanoma. Australas J Dermatol 1999;40:25-30.

53. Johnson TM, Headington JT, Baker SR, Lowe L. Usefulness of the staged excision for lentigo maligna and lentigo maligna melanoma: the "square" procedure. J Am Acad Dermatol 1997;37:758-764.

54. Robinson JK. Margin control for lentigo maligna. J Am Acad Dermatol 1994;31:79-85.

55. Stonecipher MR, Leshin B, Patrick J, White WL. Management of lentigo maligna and lentigo maligna melanoma with paraffin-embedded tangential sections: utility of immunoperoxidase staining and supplemental vertical sections. J Am Acad Dermatol 1993;29:589-594.

56. Clayton BD, Leshin B, Hitchcock MG, Marks M, White WL. Utility of rush paraffin-embedded tangential sections in the management of cutaneous neoplasms. Dermatol Surg 2000;26:671-678.

57. Heenan PJ, Ghaznawie M. The pathogenesis of local recurrence of melanoma at the primary excision site. Br J Plast Surg 1999;52:209-213.

58. Barlow JO, Maize J Sr, Lang PG. The density and distribution of melanocytes adjacent to melanoma and nonmelanoma skin cancers. Dermatol Surg 2007;33:199-207.

59. Mahendran RM, Newton-Bishop JA. Survey of U.K. current practice in the treatment of lentigo maligna. Br J Dermatol 2001;144:71-76.

60. Jeneby TT, Chang B, Bucky LP. Ultraviolet-assisted punch biopsy mapping for lentigo maligna melanoma. Ann Plast Surg 2001;46:495-499.

61. Arrington JH 3rd, Reed RJ, Ichinose H, Krementz ET. Plantar lentiginous melanoma: a distinctive variant of human cutaneous malignant melanoma. Am J Surg Pathol 1977;1:131-143.

62. Coleman WP 3rd, Loria PR, Reed RJ, Krementz ET. Acral lentiginous melanoma. Arch Dermatol 1980;116:773-776.

63. Kukita A, Ishihara K. Clinical features and distribution of malignant melanoma and pigmented nevi on the soles of the feet in Japan. J Invest Dermatol 1989;92(Suppl):210S-213S.

64. Elwood JM. Epidemiology and control of melanoma in white populations and in Japan. J Invest Dermatol 1989;92(Suppl):214S-221S.

65. Friedman RJ, Rigel DS, Kopf AW. Early detection of malignant melanoma: the role of physician examination and self-examination of the skin. CA Cancer J Clin 1985;35:130-151.

66. Hutchinson J. Melanosis often not black: melanotic whitlow. Br Med J 1886;1:491.

67. Soon SL, Solomon AR Jr, Papadopoulos D, Murray DR, McAlpine B, Washington CV. Acral lentiginous melanoma mimicking benign disease: the Emory experience. J Am Acad Dermatol 2003;48:183-188.

68. Sauter ER, Yeo UC, von Stemm A, et al. Cyclin d1 is a candidate oncogene in cutaneous melanoma. Cancer Res 2002;62:3200-3206.

69. Rokuhara S, Saida T, Oguchi M, Matsumoto K, Murase S, Oguchi S. Number of acquired melanocytic nevi in patients with melanoma and control subjects in Japan: Nevus count is a significant risk factor for nonacral melanoma but not for acral melanoma. J Am Acad Dermatol 2004;50:695-700.

70. Iversen K, Robins RE. Mucosal malignant melanomas. Am J Surg 1980;139:660-664.

71. Ariel IM. Malignant melanoma of the female genital system: a report of 48 patients and review of the literature. J Surg Oncol 1981;16:371-383.

72. Wechter ME, Gruber SB, Haefner HK, et al. Vulvar melanoma: a report of 20 cases and review of the literature. J Am Acad Dermatol 2004;50:554-562.

73. Rapini RP, Golitz LE, Greer RO Jr, Krekorian EA, Poulson T. Primary malignant melanoma of the oral cavity. A review of 177 cases. Cancer 1985;55:1543-1551.

74. Garzino-Demo P, Fasolis M, Maggiore GM, Pagano M, Berrone S. Oral mucosal melanoma: a series of case reports. J Craniomaxillofac Surg 2004;32:251-257.

75. Mesara BW, Burton WD. Primary malignant melanoma of the upper respiratory tract. Clinicopathologic study. Cancer 1968;21:217-225.

76. Lengyel E, Gilde K, Remenar E, Esik O. Malignant mucosal melanoma of the head and neck. Pathol Oncol Res 2003;9:7-12.

77. Werdin C, Limas C, Knodell RG. Primary malignant melanoma of the rectum. Evidence for origin from rectal mucosal melanocytes. Cancer 1988;61:1364-1370.

78. Weiss J, Elder D, Hamilton R. Melanoma of the male urethra: surgical approach and pathological analysis. J Urol 1982;128:382-385.

79. Oliva E, Quinn TR, Amin MB, et al. Primary malignant melanoma of the urethra: a clinicopathologic analysis of 15 cases. Am J Surg Pathol 2000;24:785-796.

80. Gollub MJ, Prowda JC. Primary melanoma of the esophagus: radiologic and clinical findings in six patients. Radiology 1999;213:97-100.

81. Symmans WF, Grimes MM. Malignant melanoma of the esophagus: histologic variants and immunohistochemical findings in four cases. Surg Pathol 1991;4:222-234.

82. Heath DI, Womack C. Primary malignant melanoma of the gallbladder. J Clin Pathol 1988;41:1073-1077.

83. Kojima T, Tanaka T, Yoshimi N, Mori H. Primary malignant melanoma of the urinary bladder. Arch Pathol Lab Med 1992;116:1213-1216.

84. Lund L, Storgard L, Noer H. Primary malignant melanoma of the urinary bladder. Scand J Urol Nephrol 1992;26:205-206.

85. Ainsworth AM, Clark WH Jr, Mastrangelo M, Conger KB. Primary malignant melanoma of the urinary bladder. Cancer 1976;37:1928-1936.

86. Elsayed AM, Albahra M, Nzeako UC, Sobin LH. Malignant melanomas in the small intestine: a study of 103 patients. Am J Gastroenterol 1996;91:1001-1006.

87. Dountsis A, Zisis C, Karagianni E, Dahabreh J. Primary malignant melanoma of the lung: a case report. World J Surg Oncol 2003;1:26

88. Pasquini E, Rastelli E, Muretto P, et al. Primary bronchial malignant melanoma. A case report. Pathologica 1994;86:546-548.

89. Wilson RW, Moran CA. Primary melanoma of the lung: a clinicopathologic and immunohistochemical study of eight cases. Am J Surg Pathol 1997;21:1196-1202.

90. Cohen Y, Rosenbaum E, Begum S, et al. Exon 15 BRAF mutations are uncommon in melanomas arising in nonsun-exposed sites. Clin Cancer Res 2004;10:3444-3447.

91. Edwards RH, Ward MR, Wu H, et al. Absence of BRAF mutations in UV-protected mucosal melanomas. J Med Genet 2004;41:270-272.

92. Prasad ML, Patel SG, Busam KJ. Primary mucosal desmoplastic melanoma of the head and neck. Head Neck 2004;26:373-377.

93. Kavanagh BD, Campbell RL, Patterson JW, O'Neill RL, Cardinale RM, Kaugars GE. Desmoplastic malignant melanoma of the palatal alveolar mucosa: sustained disease-free survival after surgery and postoperative radiotherapy. Oral Surg Oral Med Oral Pathol Oral Radiol Endod 2000;89:465-470.

94. Mulvany NJ, Sykes P. Desmoplastic melanoma of the vulva. Pathology 1997;29:241-245.

95. Chang PC, Fischbein NJ, McCalmont TH, et al. Perineural spread of malignant melanoma of the head and neck: clinical and imaging features. AJNR Am J Neuroradiol 2004;25:5-11.

10 HISTOGENETIC VARIANTS OF TUMORIGENIC MELANOMA (VERTICAL GROWTH PHASE)

Just as there is variation among the different types of radial growth phase melanomas, so there is important variation in the tumorigenic vertical growth phase compartments of melanomas (see Table 8-1). These may have nosologic and diagnostic as well as prognostic and management significance, as discussed in the sections following.

NODULAR MELANOMA

Definition. *Nodular melanoma* is a malignant tumor of epidermal melanocytes that evolves apparently de novo out of clinically normal skin (see fig. 8-5G). By definition, there is no clinical or histologic evidence of a preexisting

nontumorigenic radial growth phase compartment, although there may be a preexisting nevus or in situ growth directly above the tumor nodule. Occasionally, there is extension of a junctional component slightly beyond the most lateral dermal nest; by convention, if this component does not extend more than three rete ridges, the lesion is placed in the nodular category (fig. 10-1).

Nodular melanoma is perhaps the "default" or prototypic tumorigenic melanoma. The morphology of a nodular melanoma does not differ from that of a melanoma with an adjacent nontumorigenic compartment, except for the lack of the latter. It is likely that nodular melanomas evolve

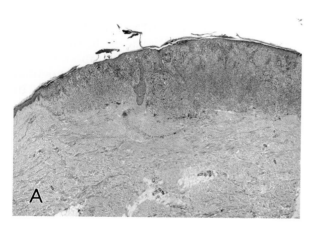
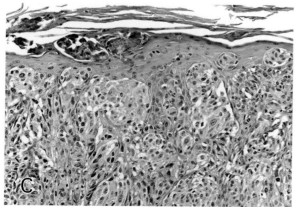
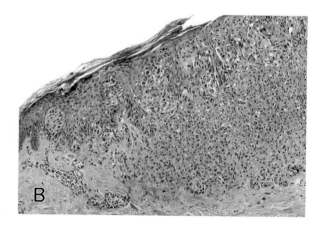

Figure 10-1

TUMORIGENIC MELANOMA, NODULAR TYPE

A,B: A junctional component extends not more than three rete ridges from the lateral border of the dermal component, qualifying the lesion as the nodular subtype.

C: The cells in the junctional component resemble those in the dermal component, suggesting that they are part of the same clonal process rather than remnants of an antecedent phase of progression.

from a "telescoped" or overgrown radial growth phase of one of the defined types—superficial spreading lentigo maligna, acral-lentiginous, or mucosal-lentiginous melanoma (see Table 8-1) (1). Because superficial spreading melanoma is the most common type of radial growth phase melanoma, nodular melanoma in general tends to share the epidemiology of this subtype.

Despite these considerations, a recent study (2) found differential expression between nodular and superficial spreading melanomas for human pituitary tumor-transforming gene 1 (*hPTTG1*), which is a protooncogene that codes for securin, a protein involved in sister chromatid separation. In this series of 29 nodular and 29 superficial spreading melanomas, matched for all histologic prognostic parameters, securin expression significantly correlated with the nodular subtype and was not related to thickness. The data suggest that *hPTTG1* may act as an oncogene in the vertical growth phase, and that there may be a real biologic difference between the vertical growth phases of nodular and superficial melanomas.

Clinical Features. It is important to be aware that the ABCD clinical criteria for the diagnosis of melanoma do not apply to most nodular melanomas. Nodular melanomas may be quite symmetric, are commonly poorly pigmented or even amelanotic, although there are usually at least a few flecks of visible pigment (see fig. 8-5G), and the border of the lesion may be smooth and well defined. In contrast to that of radial growth phase melanomas, the surface of the nodule is often shiny and smooth with a loss of skin-marking patterns. In other lesions, hyperkeratosis may result in a rough, verrucous surface texture. Since these lesions grow much more rapidly than do indolent radial phase plaques, there is usually a history of growth and change, and this evidence of change is often the main presenting symptom. Unfortunately, these melanomas are difficult to recognize clinically (3), and often grow rapidly, presenting with aggressive histologic features despite relatively short clinical histories (4). Therefore, patients often present with "late" symptoms such as bleeding or oozing or even with satellites or nodal metastases, even when the clinical course has been relatively short (5). In Australia, nodular melanomas comprise less than 15 percent of

all melanomas but account for up to 70 percent of those thicker than 3 mm (6,7).

The prognostic significance of the vertical growth phase of a nodular melanoma is similar to that of a melanoma with a tumorigenic vertical growth phase that has an adjacent radial growth phase plaque, if the thickness and other microstaging characteristics of the two tumors are similar (8). The prognosis of patients with nodular melanoma is, however, on average, worse than that of other melanomas because they are all, by definition, in the vertical growth phase. By contrast, 40 to 50 percent of superficial spreading melanomas are entirely in the radial growth phase, during which the survival rate is close to 100 percent (9,10). Since all nodular melanomas are in the vertical growth phase, they are all capable of metastasis, and the risk of metastasis is related to the thickness of the tumor as well as other microstaging characteristics (discussed in a later section) (8).

Microscopic Findings. The microscopic features of nodular melanoma are those of vertical growth phase melanoma. Since nodular melanomas do not arise in a recognizable radial growth phase, there is no surrounding in situ or microinvasive compartment adjacent to the dermal tumor (figs. 10-2–10-4). The epidermis is usually involved by cells similar to those in the dermal tumor, and these cells usually extend upward in a typical pagetoid pattern. A few cells may be observed in the epidermis a short distance from the tumor; by definition, this involvement does not extend more than three rete ridges lateral to the vertical growth phase in nodular melanoma. This criterion is of necessity arbitrary, and it is possible, indeed likely, that nodular melanomas arise in the epidermis in a stepwise tumor progression sequence similar to that proposed for melanomas with a radial growth phase. Thus, it is possible that all or some nodular melanomas are preceded by a short-lived intraepidermal phase analogous to a radial growth phase. Some nodular melanomas indeed present with an adjacent putative precursor dysplastic nevus, and in some of the lesions, remnants of the dermal component of some form of benign nevus are seen deep to the vertical growth phase tumor. These associations suggest that nodular melanomas may evolve in a stepwise manner similar to other melanomas, but the pace of evolution of

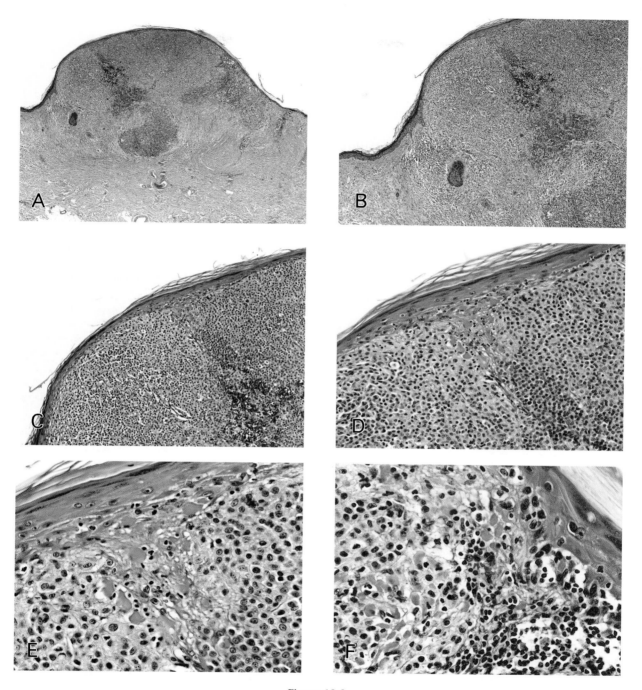

Figure 10-2

TUMORIGENIC MELANOMA, NODULAR TYPE, WITH KAMINO BODIES

A: The bulky tumor nodule from a locally recurrent lesion in a 63-year-old woman has an overall symmetric profile but with asymmetrically distributed cytologic variants and host responding elements.

B: There is no adjacent radial growth phase.

C: Lesional cells exhibit uniform cytologic atypia, and mitoses are present.

D,E: Globoid eosinophilic Kamino bodies are present. Although these are more characteristic of Spitz nevi, they may be seen in melanomas.

F: There is a moderate to brisk tumor-infiltrating lymphocyte response, with associated apoptotic lesional cells.

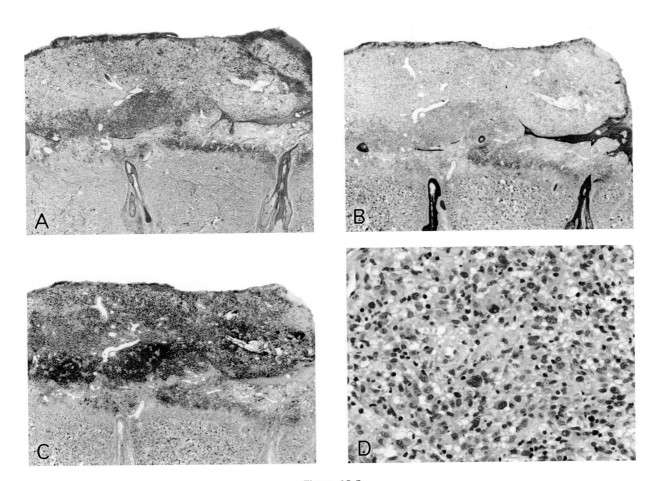

Figure 10-3

MALIGNANT MELANOMA, TUMORIGENIC, NODULAR TYPE, POLYPOID

A: The bulky, polypoid tumor has a collaret of hyperplastic epidermis and an extensive overlying ulcer.

B: Keratin stains the collaret.

C: S-100 protein stain highlights the dermal tumor.

D: Routine staining demonstrates severe cytologic atypia, not as uniform in this example as in most cases, with an associated infiltrative lymphocytic response.

the vertical growth phase from its antecedent steps is sufficiently rapid that the radial growth phase is obliterated, and this results in a lesion that is sufficiently different in its behavior and general appearance as to warrant separate description and classification.

Since there is no radial growth phase in a nodular melanoma, the criteria for diagnosis must be based on the morphology of the vertical growth phase alone. Since many of the criteria for the diagnosis of melanoma are characteristics of the radial growth phase, there may, as a result, be some difficulty in diagnosing nodular melanomas. This is especially true when the lesional

cells exhibit some tendency toward differentiation along nevoid lines, as in nevoid melanomas (fig. 10-4), and in so-called minimal deviation melanoma, which was originally described as a variant of nodular melanoma (melanomas with radial growth phase, irrespective of the morphology of the vertical growth phase, do not qualify as "minimal deviation" by definition) (11–13). Most nodular melanomas present with readily evident cytologic features of malignancy, including nuclear hyperchromatism, irregularity of the nuclear membranes, large eosinophilic nucleoli, and easily detectable mitotic figures. Although the lesions are often symmetric at scanning

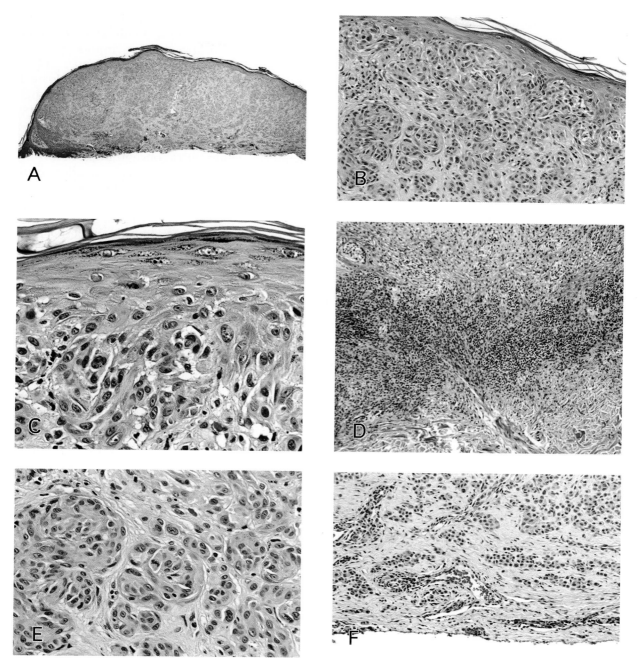

Figure 10-4

TUMORIGENIC MELANOMA, NODULAR TYPE, WITH NEVOID VERTICAL GROWTH PHASE

A: A shave biopsy of a nodular tumor shows no adjacent intraepidermal component.

B,C: The tumor is composed, superficially, of uniformly atypical epithelioid melanocytes arranged mainly in nests that vary in size and shape. Confluent nests are in the overlying epidermis, and mitotic activity is seen.

D: Toward the base, the cells are smaller, indicative of a tendency to maturation. The cells at the base, however, are cytologically "continuous" with those above, indicating that they represent nevoid differentiation of melanoma cells.

E: The more superficially located cells are uniformly atypical and have mitotic activity.

F: Although the cells at the base are smaller than those at the top, they remain relatively large compared to authentic nevus cells, and they do not disperse well as single cells into the reticular dermis collagen.

magnification (unlike radial growth phase melanomas), the cytologic features tend to be pleomorphic, varying from one part of the lesion to another, especially with respect to pigment synthesis and cytoplasmic configuration.

The most common cell type is the large epithelioid cell, which is either amelanotic or has finely divided "dusty" melanin pigment in its cytoplasm. This cell is indistinguishable from the predominant cell of the vertical growth phase of superficial spreading melanoma. Some nodular melanomas, especially those that arise on severely sun-damaged skin, are composed predominantly of spindle cells, similar to those that may be seen in the vertical growth phase of some lentigo maligna melanomas, and in these cells the pigment, if any, is apt to be coarser.

Differential Diagnosis. The differential diagnosis of nodular melanoma is different from that of radial growth phase melanoma, which is a plaque lesion with dysplastic nevus as the major differential consideration. Nodular melanoma must be differentiated from other cutaneous lesions that present with a nodular configuration.

Globoid dermal and compound nevi are usually not difficult to distinguish from nodular melanomas because of their characteristic patterns at scanning magnification, and the lack of high-grade nuclear atypia and mitoses in their lesional cells. In occasional longstanding dermal nevi, enlarged hyperchromatic nuclei may be seen, usually superficially, in a pattern that has been likened to the benign, presumably degenerative phenomenon of "ancient change" in schwannomas. These nevi, however, like almost all benign acquired dermal nevi (non-Spitz nevi), have no mitotic figures in the dermis, and few mitoses, if any, in their epidermal component. The exceptions to this in our experience are a few lesions of children or young adolescents that had rare mitoses, and in the setting of pregnancy. The reticulin pattern of nevi, in which single cells at the base of the lesion are surrounded by reticulin fibers, tends to differ from that of melanomas, in which reticulin tends to outline groups of cells (14). This stromal pattern is also reflected in the tendency for the clustered, nested, or expansile and coalescent growth of melanoma cells that is seen at the base of lesions in routine sections.

Banal acquired nevi typically elicit no lymphocytic host response, while most nodular melanomas have at least a few lymphocytes, and occasionally, a brisk response that may call to mind a halo nevus. Indeed, since some halo nevi contain relatively large cells with somewhat atypical nuclei, this differential diagnosis can be difficult. The absence of mitoses within melanocytic cells and the typical clinical setting of a small, symmetric lesion with a concentric halo occurring often as one of several lesions in an adolescent are reassuring in these circumstances.

Nevoid melanomas present special difficulties and are discussed later in the chapter.

Spindle and epithelioid cell nevi, especially Spitz nevi, often present as nodular lesions, and some are very difficult to distinguish from nodular melanoma. Generally, Spitz nevi are more symmetric but nodular melanomas may be symmetric, unlike superficial spreading melanomas, which have an asymmetric radial growth phase. The symmetry is usually imperfect in nodular melanoma, however, especially at the cytologic level. This implies that cell size, cell shape, or melanin production may vary abruptly within the melanoma, especially from side to side. Although Spitz nevi typically contain spindle as well as epithelioid cells, there are continuous transitional forms between these two types, and the nuclei are characteristically monomorphous throughout the lesions, suggesting that the two cell types are really a single dimorphic cell type. The cells of some nodular melanomas may exhibit a similar variation in shape, but many melanomas clearly have more than a single cell type, as judged by the existence of populations with disparate nuclear and cytoplasmic morphologies, and the absence of transitional forms.

The epidermal component of Spitz nevi tends to be composed of nests predominating over single cells (15), and to be discontinuous. McGovern (14) emphasized that continuous proliferation of atypical melanocytes in the junction region for the entire extent of the lesion, with absence of a clustered (nested) pattern, indicates that an invasive lesion may be melanoma. In most Spitz nevi, the cells are similar to one another from side to side throughout the lesion, while tending to mature (i.e., become smaller) as they descend to the base of the lesion. Almost all Spitz nevi that are thicker than 0.5

mm involve the reticular as well as the papillary dermis, and the pattern of involvement of the reticular dermis is that of single cells or single files of cells predominating over fascicles and nests at the base of the lesion, a pattern that is seen in banal nevi also. In melanomas that invade the reticular dermis, the infiltrating cells are arranged in clusters, pointed at the infiltrating front like the blade of a spear, with little tendency for separation into single cells (except in desmoplastic melanoma).

The distinction of nodular melanoma and Spitz nevus can be one of the most difficult diagnostic dilemmas that pathologists face. As McGovern pointed out (14), equivocal lesions usually behave in a benign manner; however, when there is continued uncertainty, these lesions, in our opinion, should be signed out descriptively (melanocytic tumors of uncertain malignant potential [MELTUMP]), and managed with therapy that considers the "worst-case scenario." Such management should include a discussion of the diagnostic uncertainty with the patient, and consideration of reexcision and periodic follow-up, with a consideration of sentinel lymph node sampling if appropriate to the differential diagnosis.

Epithelioid cell histiocytoma is another lesion composed of large cuboidal cells that can simulate a nodular melanoma. These lesions usually form superficial tumors, often with a collaret. They lack an in situ melanoma component, and do not demonstrate significant cytologic atypia. The lesional cells are negative for S-100 protein, HMB45, and Melan-A, and positive for CD68. The rare deep type could simulate metastatic melanoma in the dermis (16–18).

In nodular tumors composed mainly of spindle cells, a classic differential diagnosis includes spindle cell nodular melanoma, spindle cell squamous carcinoma, atypical fibroxanthoma, and occasionally, other spindle cell neoplasms including leiomyosarcoma and neurothekeoma. Most of these tumors, other than leiomyosarcoma, tend to occur in sun-damaged skin. Features suggestive or diagnostic of melanoma include a continuous/contiguous lentiginous or pagetoid pattern in the epidermis (as long as pagetoid squamous cell carcinoma can be ruled out), and finely divided, dusty melanin pigment in the lesional cells. Occasional pig-

mented nonmelanoma tumors are observed in the skin, however, including basal cell carcinoma, squamous cell carcinoma in situ (Bowen disease), invasive squamous cell carcinoma, and metastatic carcinoma. In these circumstances, the tumor cells have taken up melanin that has been synthesized by reactive proliferating benign melanocytes. Usually, this melanin occurs in the form of large, coarsely granular, compound melanosomes, rather than the finely divided dusty premelanosomes that are seen in most melanomas. Some melanomas have coarse pigment, however. Squamous cell carcinoma, like melanoma, originates from the epidermis. This diagnosis is suggested by the presence of desmosomal bridges between atypical cells or by evidence of keratinization. Atypical fibroxanthoma may show a Grenz, or clear, zone between the tumor cells in the papillary dermis and the epidermis, and the diagnosis is suggested by the presence of histiocytic and giant cells in addition to spindle cells. The marked bizarre nuclear pleomorphism and hyperchromatism with atypical mitoses that characterize these lesions are paradoxically more pronounced than in most melanomas, despite the better prognosis of patients with atypical fibroxanthoma. Reticulin stains may show a "mesenchymal" pattern of reticulin fibers about individual cells, in contrast to the "epithelial" pattern of clusters of cells surrounded by reticulin that is more characteristic of melanoma.

Neurothekeoma is a benign cutaneous lesion of probable nerve sheath origin, and is divided into two histologically defined subtypes: myxoid and cellular. Either type may contain mitoses. The myxoid type is distinguished from rare myxoid examples of cutaneous melanoma by its dermal location, lobular pattern, bland cytology, and myxoid stroma. The cellular variant sometimes resembles melanoma because of its content of large epithelioid cells with abundant eosinophilic to amphophilic cytoplasm. Although the nuclei are usually not atypical, there may be overlap, presenting a difficult diagnostic problem. Only the myxoid variants of neurothekeoma stain for S-100 protein. Husain et al. (19) concluded that when the histologic differential diagnosis is between cellular neurothekeoma and melanoma, an S-100 protein–positive lesion should be regarded as a melanoma. Antibodies to S-100A6 protein (20), microphthalmia transcription factor (MITF), and NKI/C3 (21) have all been proposed recently as helpful diagnostic markers for cellular neurothekeoma.

In many histologically malignant spindle cell tumors, the cell of origin cannot be reliably determined in routine sections, and in these circumstances, immunopathology is valuable. Reactivity with S-100 protein antigen is diagnostic of melanoma in a lesion of the type under consideration here if keratin stains are negative. HMB45 and Melan-A/MART reactivities are highly specific for melanocytic differentiation, although less sensitive than S-100 protein, especially in spindle cell lesions (22,23). In the interpretation of S-100 protein reactions, it must be remembered that many cutaneous neoplasms may become populated by benign dendritic S-100 protein–positive Langerhans cells. These cells should not be misinterpreted as melanoma cells, an error that can usually be avoided by comparing the nuclei of the S-100 protein–reactive cells to those of neoplastic cells elsewhere in the tumor. The finding of dendritic cells is quite common, for example, in atypical fibrous histiocytomas and in some poorly differentiated squamous cell carcinomas. An analogous phenomenon, mentioned above, is the presence of a population of benign melanocytes or Langerhans cells in nonmelanocytic tumors. This finding is commonplace in pigmented seborrheic keratoses and basal cell carcinomas, and is occasionally observed in poorly differentiated metastatic carcinomas that may be mistaken for melanomas.

Many nodular melanomas have little pigment, and any pigment that is present is most likely to be superficially located, as also is the case in pigmented benign nevi. The presence of pigment deep in a bulky tumor argues against a banal or Spitz nevus, especially if there is less pigment or no pigment superficially, or if pigment is haphazardly scattered throughout the neoplasm. Heavily pigmented nodular melanomas must be differentiated from blue nevi and their variants. Common blue nevi are distinguished by their low cellularity and the absence of atypia or mitoses. Cellular blue nevi are perhaps more likely to be misinterpreted as melanomas than most benign nevi because of their relative unfamiliarity, coupled with their

cellularity, the typical presence of plump spindle and epithelioid and/or nevoid cells, and their heavy pigmentation which extends into the lower third of the lesion, characteristically into the deep reticular dermis or panniculus. The presence of an associated common blue nevus component and the characteristic "dumbbell" architecture should lead to their consideration at scanning magnification as forms of blue nevi. Criteria for malignancy should then be sought at higher power, including high-grade nuclear atypia, mitoses, and necrosis. If any of these features are present in more than a subtle degree, the lesion may be malignant.

Lesions meeting these criteria are extraordinarily rare in our experience; more often than not, the criteria are equivocal. For example, there may be a few mitoses or subtle focal necrosis, or the nuclei may appear atypical with prominent nucleoli, but the other criteria are lacking. In such cases, a diagnosis of "atypical cellular blue nevus" may be appropriate, and some authorities consider that such lesions also meet the criteria for a form of so-called minimal deviation melanoma.

There are examples of atypical dermal pigment-synthesizing melanocytic tumors that do not fit readily into any category, and in these cases we use the descriptive term, melanocytic tumor of uncertain malignant potential (MELTUMP). We endeavor to avoid arbitrarily categorizing these equivocal lesions into a diagnostic category of nodular melanoma with its connotations of a highly aggressive neoplasm. The descriptive diagnosis reflects uncertainty, and implies a probabilistic statement as to the likely behavior of the lesion, which can be amplified and clarified in descriptive notes attached to the diagnosis. Although this is probably a heterogeneous group of cases, our experience suggests that most of these lesions will have a benign course, although some recur locally if not completely excised, and occasional examples metastasize, sometimes to the regional lymph nodes only.

DESMOPLASTIC MELANOMA

Definition. *Desmoplastic melanoma* is a variant pattern of the tumorigenic or vertical growth phase component of melanoma that is characterized by a spindle cell pattern and associated with collagen

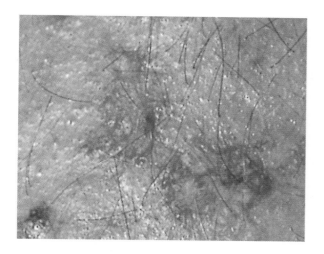 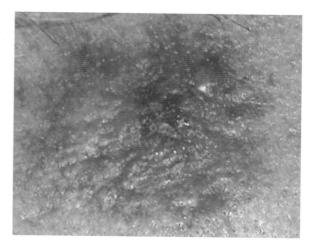

Figure 10-5

DESMOPLASTIC MELANOMA

This diagnosis may be challenging clinically as well as histologically, as these lesions may lack most of the characteristics of classic melanomas. In other cases, the desmoplastic vertical growth phase arises in a more characteristic radial growth phase, usually one of the lentiginous types. (Figures C and D from Plate VI, Fascicle 2, Third Series.)

production and with patterns suggestive of neuro-fibromatous or schwannian differentiation. Nerve invasion is a common feature of desmoplastic melanoma, but neurotropism occurs in some spindle cell melanomas that lack the desmoplastic pattern, so that neurotropic melanoma is considered in the next section as a separate entity.

Clinical Features. Desmoplastic melanoma, first described by Conley, Lattes, and Orr in 1971 (24), is a vertical growth phase variant that may or may not be associated with a detectable radial growth phase component at the time of histologic examination. If a radial growth phase is present, it is usually one of the lentiginous variants, namely, lentigo maligna, acral-lentiginous, or mucosal-lentiginous melanoma. The demography of desmoplastic melanoma is that of these variants, so that desmoplastic melanomas are most common on the exposed skin of middle-aged to elderly fair-skinned sun-sensitive Caucasians in association with lentigo maligna, but they may also be seen on acral (25) and mucosal (26,27) sites. Acral and mucosal melanomas are about as frequent in fair- as in dark-skinned people, and desmoplastic melanoma is seen in all races with equal frequency in these sites.

Since the diagnosis of a desmoplastic melanoma is not usually made until a lesion has been excised and examined histologically, few details are available about the clinical morphology. If a

radial growth phase is present, it has the characteristics already described of breadth, border irregularity, poor circumscription, and pigmentary variegation that characterize these lesions. The radial growth phase of many desmoplastic melanomas is almost completely amelanotic, however, and this lack of pigment can contribute to delay in diagnosis (fig. 10-5) (28,29). All desmoplastic melanomas, by definition, have a tumorigenic vertical growth phase, which sometimes presents as an indurated nodule but is sometimes flat, especially in acral sites (28). The desmoplastic vertical growth phase is almost always amelanotic or very sparsely pigmented, and it is usually not ulcerated so that, again, clinical signs may be very subtle (29), or the lesion may deceptively present as a nonmelanocytic tumor or reactive/reparative process (30). Even when neural invasion is demonstrated histologically, pain is not a common clinical complaint. In a review of 25 patients and 83 cases from the literature since the first description in 1971, the average age was 61.2 years, the sex distribution was about equal, 21 cases occurred on the head and neck, and all but one case were associated with lentigo maligna or an atypical junctional melanocytic proliferation (31).

Microscopic Findings. Although desmoplastic melanoma is defined in terms of its dermal tumorigenic vertical growth phase component,

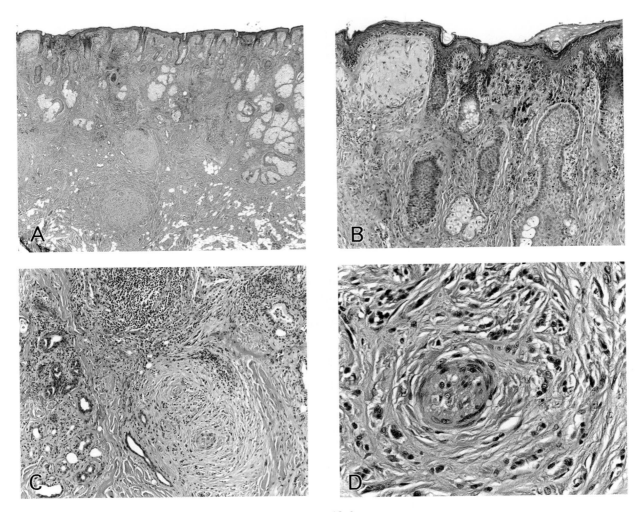

Figure 10-6

MALIGNANT MELANOMA, DESMOPLASTIC AND NEUROTROPIC

A: Scanning magnification shows extensive involvement of the dermis by a tumor composed of epithelioid to spindle cells, which tend to be clustered in some areas and diffuse in others. Nodular clusters of lymphocytes are also visible at this magnification.

B: Superficially, there is an atypical intraepidermal melanocytic proliferation, focally consistent with melanoma in situ, lentigo maligna type.

C: In the dermis, lesional cells tend to cluster around small cutaneous nerves.

D: The tumor surrounds nerves (perineural invasion), and is within the endoneurium (endoneurial invasion).

most examples have an epidermal and/or micro-invasive radial growth phase component as well (fig. 10-6) (28,31). There is considerable variation in the cellularity and degree of cytologic atypia exhibited by the lesional cells in the epidermis and papillary dermis. The most common pattern is a lentiginous (contiguous and continuous predominantly basal) proliferation of moderately to severely atypical melanocytes arranged mostly as single cells in the basal layer

of an atrophic epidermis, associated with actinic elastosis in the dermis, and meeting the criteria for lentigo maligna melanoma. A desmoplastic vertical growth phase may also be observed in association with acral-lentiginous and mucosal-lentiginous radial growth phase proliferations, although this is less common. Another group of cases is associated with miscellaneous atypical intraepidermal proliferations of variable but usually low cellularity and nuclear grade

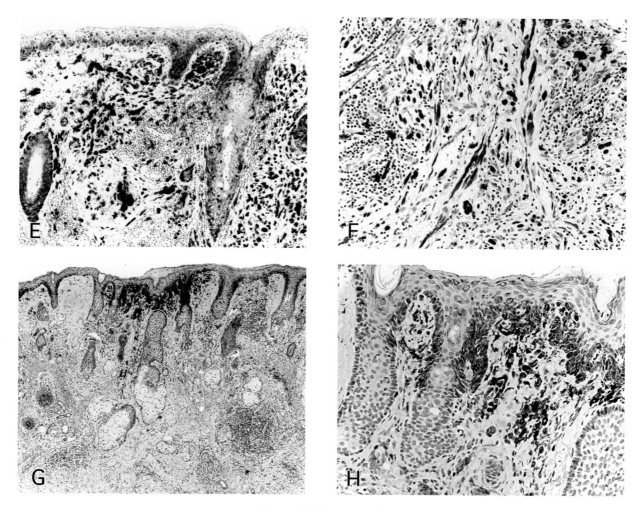

Figure 10-6 (continued)
E: S-100 protein strongly and diffusely stains the lesional cells throughout the dermis and epidermis.
F: Fascicles of tumor cells infiltrate the reticular dermis (S-100 protein stain).
G: A Melan-A preparation stains cells superficially; the spindle cells at the base of the lesion do not stain.
H: Melan-A stains the superficial cells in the dermis and epidermis, which tend, in this superficial part of the tumor, to be epithelioid rather than spindled in configuration.

that may not meet formal criteria for in situ or microinvasive melanoma (32), but presumably represent precursors of the desmoplastic tumorigenic component of the lesion. Such lesions can present difficulties in diagnosis, especially when shave biopsies are submitted, leading to delay in diagnosis (fig. 10-7). Finally, some desmoplastic melanomas ("de novo" lesions) have no discernable intraepithelial component (see Neurotropic Melanoma).

At scanning magnification, the two main components of a characteristic desmoplastic melanoma are usually evident, one a junctional lentiginous and/or focally pagetoid proliferation of epithelioid or cuboidal melanocytes in the superficial epidermis and/or papillary dermis, and the other a tumorigenic proliferation of spindle cells extending from the papillary dermis into the reticular dermis (fig. 10-6). A few lesions have no evident epidermal component, but the tumorigenic dermal component, which defines the lesion, is always present, usually extending into the reticular dermis to a thickness of 1.5 mm or greater. This dermal component is subtle in some lesions due to low cellularity and low nuclear grade; in other lesions the appearance

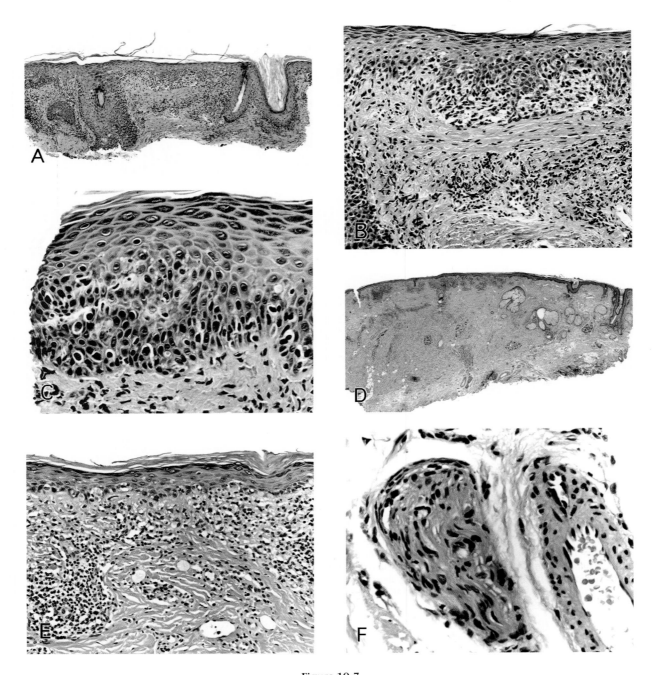

Figure 10-7

MALIGNANT MELANOMA, DESMOPLASTIC AND NEUROTROPIC

A: A biopsy of a lesion in a 58-year-old man shows lentiginous basal and pagetoid proliferation of atypical melanocytes in the epidermis extending to the margins.

B: Higher magnification shows confluent nests and pagetoid extension of single cells into the epidermis.

C: Lesional cells extend to a lateral margin.

D: This lesion was not definitively treated and later recurred as a bulky dermal tumor beneath a dermal scar with an atypical proliferation in the overlying epidermis.

E: The epidermis has a lentiginous proliferation of uniformly atypical melanocytes. The dermis has a band-like lymphocytic infiltrate with fibrosis.

F: There is perineural and endoneurial invasion of small cutaneous nerves.

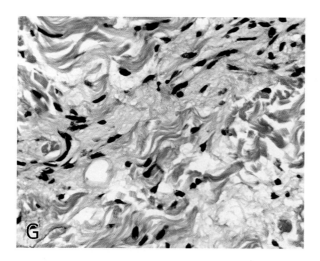
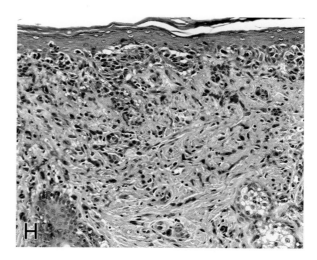

Fig. 10-7 (continued)
G: In the dermis, spindle cells in a delicate desmoplastic matrix infiltrate preexisting collagen fibers.
H: An S-100 protein stain with red chromogen highlights spindle cells infiltrating from the junction into the dermis.

suggests a high-grade neural sarcoma, and in other lesions, the dermal component may mimic and be mistaken for a scar or an inflammatory process (fig. 10-8), especially in a reexcision specimen where a pathologist knows that an earlier biopsy was done. These problems frequently result in underdiagnosis: the lesion is not recognized as melanoma or its true extent is not recognized. This error may result in inadequate therapy and later in local recurrences at the biopsy site if the desmoplastic tumor extends to a margin or if there is neurotropic spread to the margin.

In a characteristic desmoplastic melanoma, however, the dermal tumor is readily evident as a region in the reticular dermis where the normal collagen bundle pattern is replaced by a cellular proliferation of spindle cells separated by delicate collagen bundles (figs. 10-7, 10-8). Sometimes this collagen production is so conspicuous as to suggest fibromatosis. Within this collagenous or "desmoplastic" tumor, often concentrated where the tumor interfaces with the adjacent reticular dermis, there is usually a highly characteristic host response consisting of nodular clusters of mature small lymphocytes, sometimes with a few plasma cells. Combined with the atypical or frankly malignant melanocytic proliferation in the epidermis and papillary dermis, a diagnosis of desmoplastic melanoma is often suggested at scanning mag-

nification. Other histologic features of desmoplastic melanoma include multinucleate cells, myxoid areas, storiform patterns reminiscent of malignant fibrous histiocytoma, and areas with a smooth muscle-like appearance (28).

At higher magnification, the dermal tumor is composed of narrow, elongated spindle cells whose long axes are considerably greater than their diameters. Often, these cells are disposed in bundles or fascicles. The bundles as well as the lesional cell nuclei are often "wavy" or S-shaped in their conformation, like those of a neurofibroma or schwannoma (15). Upon close inspection, these cells, at least focally, contain nuclei with angulated contours and condensed heterochromatin, in contradistinction to activated fibroblasts within a scar that contain nuclei with evenly contoured nuclear membranes and delicately distributed chromatin. The spindle cell nuclei and their inconspicuous cell bodies are separated by delicate collagen fibers.

Trichrome and reticulin stains reveal a delicate network of reticulin fibers that surrounds each cell in the fasciculated spindle cell areas of the lesion, although there may be areas where epithelioid cells are arranged in sheets and nests, with an "epithelial" pattern of reticulin that surrounds groups or clusters of cells (fig. 10-6H). If there is pigment, it is likely to be in these epithelioid cells. The cells of a desmoplastic melanoma

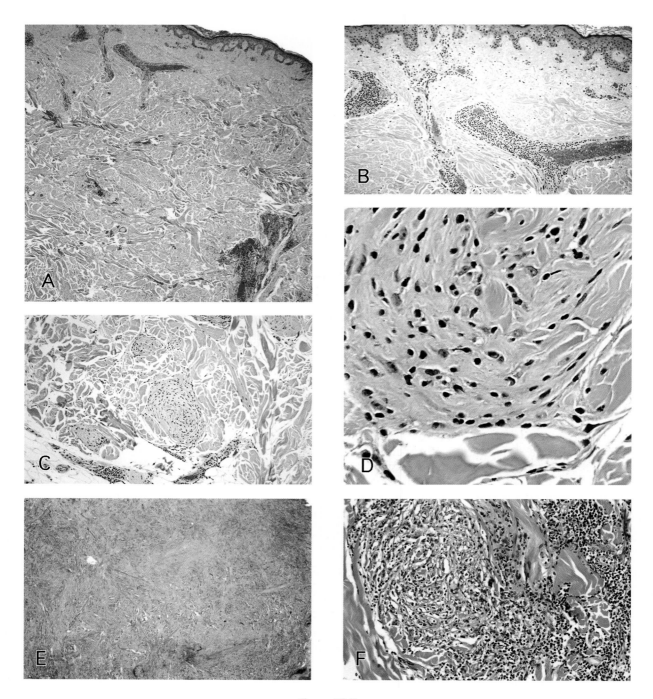

Figure 10-8

DESMOPLASTIC MELANOMA, WITH AN INFLAMMATORY PATTERN

A: At scanning power, an increased number of cells are in a perivascular position.
B: Higher magnification demonstrates perivascular lymphocytes predominating.
C: There is a subtle proliferation of spindle cells arranged in clusters and forming a delicate desmoplastic stroma.
D: These cells have minimal cytologic atypia.
E: This lesion was interpreted as an inflammatory condition and some years later recurred as this bulky tumor.
F: The recurrence consisted of spindle to epithelioid melanocytes with a brisk infiltrative lymphocytic response.

may thus exhibit not only melanocytic but also fibroblastic and schwannian characteristics at the light microscopic level.

Ultrastructurally, the cells have been shown to contain newly synthesized collagen fibers as may be seen in fibroblasts, to synthesize incomplete basement membranes as is more characteristic of melanocytic and Schwann cell lesions (33,34), and in some cases, to contain melanosomes as evidence of melanocytic differentiation (34).

Melanosomes have been found in most published ultrastructural studies of desmoplastic melanoma, but macroscopic and light microscopic evidence of melanin synthesis may be difficult to find in the dermal tumors. If an epidermal component is present, pigment is most likely to be observed in large cuboidal or epithelioid cells in the epidermis or in the superficial dermis. This finding, together with patterns of a nested or pagetoid intraepidermal proliferation characteristic of melanoma, may offer convincing evidence of melanocytic differentiation and thus indicate that a difficult spindle cell proliferation in the dermis is desmoplastic melanoma. The spindle cells themselves, however, are likely to be amelanotic, and while they may react with S-100 protein (28), they are typically negative with HMB45 and most other melanoma markers in our experience.

For those uncommon lesions with no intraepidermal component, the diagnosis of desmoplastic melanoma rests on the identification of pigment in the dermis, and this pigment, if present, is most likely to be found in the superficial nested epithelioid cell population. Sometimes these epithelioid cells appear to blend with the spindle cells as they extend from the papillary dermis into the upper reticular dermis, suggesting that the epithelioid cells with "melanocytic" differentiation are capable of differentiating into cells with fibroblastic as well as schwannian characteristics. Lesions that occupy the papillary dermis and upper reticular dermis should probably be termed desmoplastic melanoma even if there is no obvious epidermal component and especially if there is melanin pigment, prominent clusters of nevoid epithelioid cells, or any evidence of a regressed radial growth phase. Otherwise, similar lesions that are confined to the lower half of the reticular

dermis or panniculus may be termed malignant schwannoma or malignant peripheral nerve sheath tumor, especially when pigment is lacking (15). If there is strong and diffuse S-100 protein staining, the current convention is to favor the diagnosis of desmoplastic melanoma. The prognosis of patients with these deep-seated, "nerve-centered" tumors is very poor, with a marked propensity for neurotropic local recurrence (28).

Most desmoplastic melanomas are recognized as melanoma, and thus as frank malignancies, by the intraepidermal pattern of growth and the presence of clusters of atypical, epithelioid and nucleolated cells with mitoses in the upper dermis. Since these cells seem to differentiate into the spindle cell type at the base of the lesion, the spindle cells are also recognized as malignant cells, and indeed, the spindle cells often exhibit recognizable nuclear atypia with occasional mitoses. Further, the pattern of growth in the dermis is infiltrative and destructive (35,36), and there is often a history of expansile growth. Many lesions exhibit nerve invasion (neurotropic desmoplastic melanoma, see next section). Although mitoses are usually demonstrable in desmoplastic melanomas, the mitotic rate is often very low, and the prognosis, in our experience, may be surprisingly good (considering the thickness of many of these lesions), as long as local control can be achieved.

Busam (35,36) has emphasized that there is variation among lesions classified as desmoplastic melanoma. The desmoplasia may be prominent throughout the entire tumor, in which case the lesion is termed "pure" desmoplastic melanoma or may represent a portion of an otherwise nondesmoplastic melanoma, termed "combined" desmoplastic melanoma. Evidence is also emerging that for patients with thick melanomas, the presence of a predominantly paucicellular fibrosing tumor histology (pure desmoplastic melanoma) is a favorable prognostic factor for survival.

Differential Diagnosis. Desmoplastic melanoma may be confused with a number of different lesions, including a variety of melanocytic and nonmelanocytic lesions that may be associated with spindle cells in the dermis. There is morphologic overlap with malignant epithelioid schwannoma if pigment is absent or with malignant melanocytic schwannoma if there is pigment. We favor the diagnosis of desmoplastic or neurotropic melanoma in a desmoplastic spindle cell tumor that involves the papillary dermis or epidermis unless there is convincing evidence of origin from a cutaneous nerve and epidermal origin can be ruled out or appears unlikely. Lesions of the deep dermis, panniculus, or deep soft tissues are more likely to be of schwannian origin; however, a tumor of the dermis and perhaps involving the panniculus is probably best called a desmoplastic melanoma if there is strong and diffuse S-100 protein positivity.

In lesions where there is little or no nuclear atypia and mitotic figures are absent, there is morphologic overlap with benign desmoplastic Spitz nevi. Lesions that show only one or two mitoses in a number of section planes may represent low-grade malignancies that could be regarded as a form of minimal deviation melanoma, and some of these lesions can only be signed out descriptively as MELTUMPS. Clinically, we have seen recurrent desmoplastic melanomas mistaken for keloids, but the eosinophilic bands of collagen that define the latter are not seen commonly in desmoplastic melanoma.

Desmoplastic melanoma may be mistaken for an inflammatory process or a cellular or hyperplastic scar (fig. 10-8). This is a fairly common error that can be avoided by a high index of suspicion and a careful evaluation of reexcision scars and recurrent lesions for evidence of melanocytic differentiation and cellular atypia, especially in lesions of the head and neck and in acral and mucosal lentiginous melanomas. A curious "angiomatoid" variant of desmoplastic melanoma has also been described as a pattern that could mimic a vascular neoplasm or a scar (fig. 10-9) (37). Although S-100 protein staining is helpful in the evaluation of scars, it must be recognized that indeterminate spindle cells and dermal Langerhans cells, small cutaneous nerve twigs, and dendritic cells may all react with this antibody in scars. If possible, the primary tumor should be examined when a reexcision specimen is to be signed out. In this manner, we have discovered more than once that a primary lesion was desmoplastic or neurotropic (unannounced as such in the surgical history). This finding should lead to a careful examination of the reexcision specimen, including any areas of apparent scarring as well as the specimen margins, including small cutaneous nerves.

Evidence of melanocytic differentiation also helps to distinguish desmoplastic melanomas from fibromatoses, a differential diagnosis that may be suggested by patterns seen at least focally in some desmoplastic melanomas. The cellular and storiform pattern of dermatofibrosarcoma protruberans (DFSP) is not seen in desmoplastic melanoma, although occasional lesions produce a DFSP-like "honeycomb" architecture upon infiltration of the subcutis. Atypical fibroxanthoma is much more cellular than desmoplastic melanoma, with a more prominent epithelioid cell component, much greater cellularity, and bizarre nuclear atypia. Although the distinction is of lesser significance clinically, we do not believe that melanomas composed mainly of spindle cells should be termed desmoplastic melanomas unless the pattern of individual neoplastic spindle cells surrounded by reticulin and delicate collagen fibers is seen in the tumorigenic component of the lesion. This distinction may be biologically important as well, as many reports of more aggressive and metastasizing variants of desmoplastic melanoma may actually include lesions better classified as spindle cell melanomas.

Table 10-1 summarizes features that may be of assistance in the accurate diagnosis of a desmoplastic melanoma.

Immunopathology in the Differential Diagnosis. Desmoplastic melanomas usually express S-100 protein strongly and diffusely, in contrast to malignant peripheral nerve sheath tumors. This is a relatively nonspecific marker that is also expressed by important differential diagnostic conditions including benign nevi, neurofibromas, and other benign and malignant neoplastic and non-neoplastic conditions. It has been recently demonstrated that nondescript spindle cells thought to represent Schwann cells, with a minority of Langerhans cells and cells of uncertain lineage in actively healing scars in excisions of nonmelanocytic lesions, may express S-100 protein antigen, suggesting that this marker should be used with caution in the interpretation of possible residual tumor in scars (38). With due attention to other morphologic considerations, such as the density of a positive cellular infiltrate (e.g., cells in small aggregates

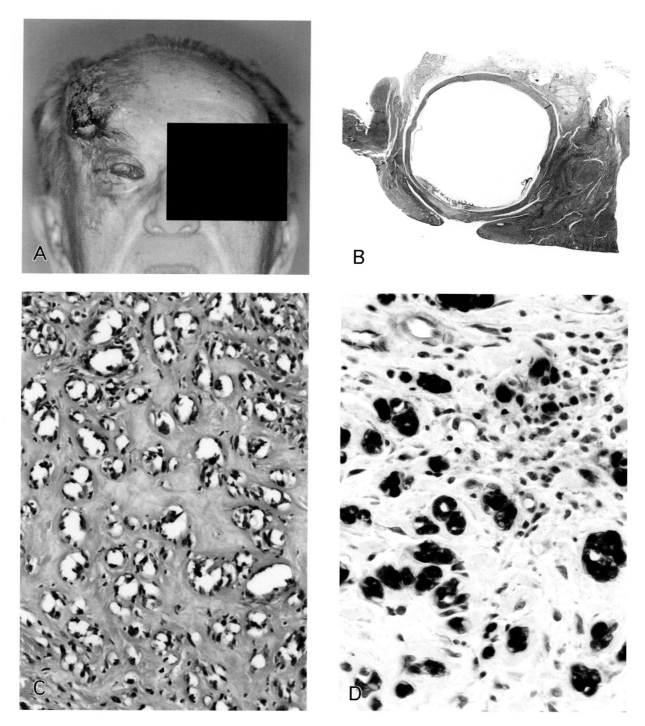

Figure 10-9

LENTIGO MALIGNA MELANOMA, DESMOPLASTIC ANGIOMATOID PATTERN

A: This bulky tumor involves the right frontal and eyebrow region, has infiltrated the orbit, and is destroying the globe.
B: A whole mount section shows tumor in the orbit surrounding the globe.
C: Histologically, this is a peculiar tumorigenic melanoma with a prominent angiomatoid stromal component.
D: S-100 protein stains clusters of neoplastic cells in the angiomatoid stroma.

and fascicles versus single interstitial cells), cytologic atypia, or continuity with more readily evident areas of the tumor, S-100 protein can be valuable in more accurately delineating the extent of a desmoplastic melanoma (fig. 10-6), especially in a biopsy specimen where false-positive reactivity in a scar is not an issue (39).

More specific markers of melanocytic differentiation and more useful if positive, include HMB45, Melan-A, and tyrosinase. Their sensitivity in desmoplastic melanoma is lower than for conventional melanomas, especially in the spindle cell component (40–42). Additionally, the transcription factor MITF may have some utility especially if convincingly positive, but its sensitivity and specificity are insufficient for use as a reliable diagnostic test for desmoplastic melanoma (42–48). This marker stains fibroblasts and macrophages, so its use cannot be recommended for the detection of subtle residual melanoma in a scar (40). In a study of desmoplastic/spindle cell melanoma versus scar, neurofibroma, malignant peripheral nerve sheath tumor, and atypical fibroxanthoma, the sensitivity and specificity of the adhesion molecule Mel-CAM were high (47); however, this marker is also expressed in a variety of mesenchymal tumors and carcinomas. In a study of eight HMB45-negative desmoplastic malignant melanomas with multiple markers including MITF, tyrosinase, Melan-A, and MAGE-1, MAGE-1 was positive in three, and the other markers were negative (23). In a recent study, strong expression of the adhesion molecule N-cadherin was found in 10 of 21 desmoplastic melanomas, and its expression correlated with poor prognosis (49). Another study demonstrated expression of clusterin in a minority of desmoplastic melanomas (50). Nerve growth factor receptor (NGFR) has also recently been described as a useful marker, including in atypical cases where S-100 protein staining is weak (51).

A reasonable approach to the histologic confirmation of desmoplastic melanoma would include the initial use of S-100 protein with one or more of the more specific markers, Melan-A, HMB45, tyrosinase, Mel-CAM, or possibly MITF, N-cadherin, or NGFR, with careful attention to the possibility of false-positive reactivity in scars. If the initial more specific markers are negative, then the remainder of the available panel may

Table 10-1

FEATURES OF DESMOPLASTIC MALIGNANT MELANOMA

Spindle cell vertical growth phase present by definition

Individual spindle cells separated by thin collagen fibers

Epithelioid cells often present superficially, blend with spindle cells in lower two thirds of lesion

Lentiginous radial growth phase often present adjacent to desmoplastic tumor (lentigo maligna, acral-lentiginous melanoma)

Nodular clusters of lymphocytes in dermal tumor

Scant pigment, slight atypia, rare mitoses in dermal spindle cells, more obvious in epithelioid cells (dermis and epidermal)

Spindle cells in wavy bundles, with S-shaped nuclei, invade endoneurium of cutaneous nerves in neurotropic cases

be used. If only S-100 protein is positive, the diagnosis of desmoplastic melanoma may still be appropriate if the morphologic findings are consistent. If pigment is present, or if silver stains for melanin are positive, the diagnosis of a melanocytic as opposed to another type of spindle cell lesion gains support. None of the markers mentioned above, of course, is effective in distinguishing between benign and malignant melanocytic lesions, including neurotized nevi, blue nevi, and cellular blue nevi, except that strong staining for HMB45 perhaps can be taken as evidence against a desmoplastic melanoma and in favor of a sclerotic spindle cell nevus (52,53).

Prognosis. Because most desmoplastic melanomas involve the reticular dermis, they are all tumorigenic, usually at Clark level IV or V, and usually their Breslow thickness is well over 1.5 mm (and often several millimeters) at presentation. Thus, as discussed in the section on prognosis in melanoma, they have potential competence for metastasis. Perhaps because of other microstaging characteristics that tend to be favorable, such as mitotic rate and the presence of tumor-infiltrating lymphocytes, the prognosis for patients with these lesions is considerably better than might be expected from the thickness of the lesion alone, as long as the lesions have been prospectively recognized and definitively treated in a manner sufficient to prevent local recurrence.

Local recurrence is common in desmoplastic melanomas for at least three reasons. First, the lesions may be subtle, especially at their borders, both clinically and histologically, so that margin involvement may be missed, leading almost inevitably to recurrence. Second, because of the location of these lesions close to vital structures such as the eye, surgical management is sometimes constrained, leading to inadequate margins. Finally, the presence of neurotropism, which is common in desmoplastic melanoma, may increase the likelihood of an undetected positive margin and result in recurrence. Local recurrence may follow persistence and regrowth of either the nontumorigenic or the tumorigenic component. In the former case, the prognosis is good. In contrast, in the case of recurrent tumorigenic desmoplastic melanoma, the recurrent tumor is typically more cellular than the primary, mitoses are more frequent, surgical resection is often more difficult or impossible, and the prognosis is typically poor. Therefore, local eradication of the neoplasm at the time of first presentation is critical. The possibility of a neurotropic component should be carefully sought in biopsies and excision specimens, with special attention to the deep and lateral specimen margins.

In desmoplastic melanomas that have been completely resected with definitive margins, local recurrence is uncommon and appears to be related mainly to the presence of neurotropism. In a study in which the clinical presentation and follow-up of patients with melanomas with desmoplasia and/or neurotropism were compared with those of other types of cutaneous stage I melanomas, all followed for a minimum of 8 years, the overall survival was 80 percent or better in both groups and desmoplasia was not associated with a statistically significant worse prognosis, even after adjustment for other prognostic factors (54). It was considered that the more clinically aggressive behavior of desmoplastic melanomas observed in previous studies was secondary to initial misdiagnosis or inadequate margin assessment of these lesions. Neurotropism was associated with a statistically significant decrease in survival in patients with desmoplastic melanoma, and was also related to an increase in the frequency of local recurrence of melanoma. In the largest study of 280 cases (29),

the 5-year survival rate was 75 percent although the median tumor thickness was 2.5 mm and all of the desmoplastic melanomas exceeded 1.5 mm in thickness and were graded as Clark level IV or V. Significant predictors of overall survival were a high mitotic rate and tumor thickness. There was a significant increase in local recurrence when neurotropism was present (29,54).

Busam et al. (55) have recently emphasized (as mentioned above) that desmoplasia may be prominent throughout the entire tumor (pure desmoplastic melanoma, with a better prognosis) or represent a portion of an otherwise nondesmoplastic melanoma (combined desmoplastic melanoma). In a multivariate analysis considering Clark level (IV versus V), desmoplastic melanoma subtype (pure versus combined), tumor mitotic rate, and tumor thickness, only histologic subtype (P = 0.02) and Clark level (P = 0.05) were independently significant by Cox regression analysis. Therefore, distinguishing pure from combined or mixed forms of desmoplastic melanoma is clinically relevant for prognosis, in that pure forms are associated with a longer disease-specific survival period. In addition, despite their often having thick primary tumors, patients with pure desmoplastic melanoma have a lower incidence of positive sentinel nodes compared with patients with mixed or with nondesmoplastic melanomas, suggesting that sentinel node biopsy may not be warranted in these patients (50,56). Nevertheless, in another recent series, nodal recurrence was seen in 16 percent of patients with desmoplastic melanoma, although these had not been separated into pure or mixed forms (57).

NEUROTROPIC MELANOMA AND NEUROTROPISM

Definition. *Neurotropic melanoma* is a malignant melanoma that invades and extends along nerves, either in the perineural space or in the endoneurium. Many examples exhibit a desmoplastic vertical growth phase, and most are composed mainly of spindle cells (fig. 10-6). Accordingly, neurotropic melanoma may in many instances represent an aggressive variant of spindle cell/desmoplastic melanoma.

Clinical Features. The age of onset and characteristic anatomic locations are similar to those of desmoplastic melanoma. In the original report of Reed and Leonard (32), the median age was 62 years. The youngest patient was 28, and 4 of the 22 patients were under 40. Most of the lesions were on the head and neck, and 4 were on the lip, apparently a site of predilection since it is common in our experience also.

There are usually no specific clinical characteristics indicative of neurotropism in a melanoma, which, however, can be potentially imaged by magnetic resonance imaging (MRI) if clinically suspected (58). In particular, there are only a few reported cases of sensory changes in these lesions (28). Neurotropism is most often seen histologically in the vertical growth phase compartment of one of the lentiginous forms of melanoma: lentigo maligna melanoma, acral-lentiginous melanoma, or mucosal-lentiginous melanoma (32,59).

The prognosis of patients with neurotropic melanoma is considered to be poor, although there are no multivariate analyses of large series of this rare lesion. Most neurotropic melanomas are thick, bulky vertical growth phase melanomas, so that a poor survival would, in general, be expected. In the original series (32), more than 50 percent of the patients with a follow-up of 2 to 9 years died of their disease. Neurotropic melanoma is associated with a striking propensity for local recurrence even after formal wide local excision, and the prognosis after local recurrence is very poor (28,29,60).

Microscopic Findings. In an excision biopsy or reexcision specimen from any melanoma, the tissue surrounding the borders of the contiguous tumor should be carefully scrutinized for the possibility of spread, whether in the form of neurotropism, satellitosis, or lymphatic invasion. Neural involvement may be seen within the confines of the tumor itself (contiguous neurotropism), but noncontiguous spread beyond the borders of the tumor is more significant because it may extend to and beyond the margins of the specimen. In such cases, local recurrence is a possibility if the nerve involvement at the margin is not recognized and dealt with by extending the resection. In our experience, neurotropism and microscopic satellites are the most frequent causes of the uncommon phenomenon of local recurrence following definitive wide local excision of a primary cutaneous melanoma (figs. 10-10, 10-11). When

we observe neurotropism in a biopsy specimen, we alert the surgeon that a wide excision with ample margins (e.g., the traditional 3 to 5 cm margins) should be considered. We also request that the grossly apparent cutaneous nerves at the margins be identified with sutures, so that they can be isolated and examined histologically. It is important in these cases to ink the margins and examine them carefully with multiple perpendicular block sections.

The nerve involvement in some lesions is subtle at a histopathologic level. Sometimes, clusters of lymphocytes around and within the nerves draw attention to the neoplastic cells within the nerves, but in other cases, the invasion must be searched for at higher magnification. Such a search should be done in all lentiginous melanomas with vertical growth phase, especially those with spindle cell or desmoplastic features. Neurotropism may take the form of extensive invasion of the perineurium (perineural invasion) or as subtle hypercellularity of neural bundles owing to intraneural infiltration by malignant cells (endoneurial invasion) (fig. 10-11). A survey of lentiginous melanomas done by the authors revealed nerve involvement in about 20 percent of the cases, so the phenomenon is not as rare as is supposed. Most of these cases were instances of contiguous neurotropism, where the involved nerves were within the tumor and widely clear of the margins. In the less common cases of noncontiguous neurotropism, the neoplastic cells extended a considerable distance from the primary tumor. We have observed intraneural spread of tumor from a neurotropic melanoma of the lip to the mandibular nerve, extending as far as the angle of the jaw. Although neurotropism is commonly associated with a lentiginous nontumorigenic component, giving rise to a spindle cell tumorigenic component, we have observed this phenomenon in superficial spreading melanomas in association with epithelioid cell differentiation in the tumorigenic component (fig. 10-12).

As in desmoplastic melanoma, the neoplastic cells in most cases of neurotropic melanoma are reactive with S-100 protein, but the sensitivity of this antigen in the diagnosis appears to be less than in common epithelioid cell melanomas, and a negative result does not exclude melanoma (61). Similarly, the sensitivity of HMB45,

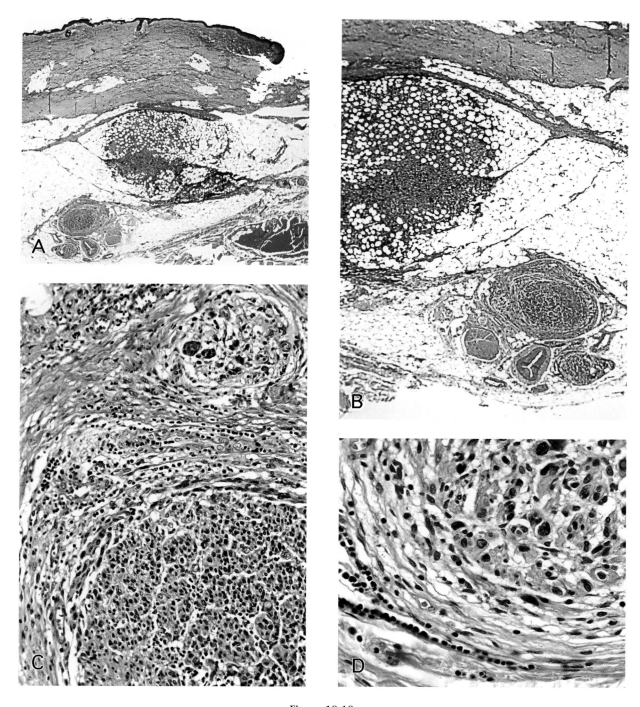

Figure 10-10

NEUROTROPIC MELANOMA, LOCALLY RECURRENT

A: Scanning magnification shows a tumor, mainly in the subcutis, with expanded and hypercellular nerves at the bottom center.

B: The tumor cells are honeycombing the subcutaneous fat and expanding nerves at the base of the image.

C: An expanded peripheral nerve is extensively involved by tumor cells, mostly epithelioid cells in this instance, with a sprinkling of lymphocytes.

D: Atypical epithelioid cells are within the endoneurium of the nerve.

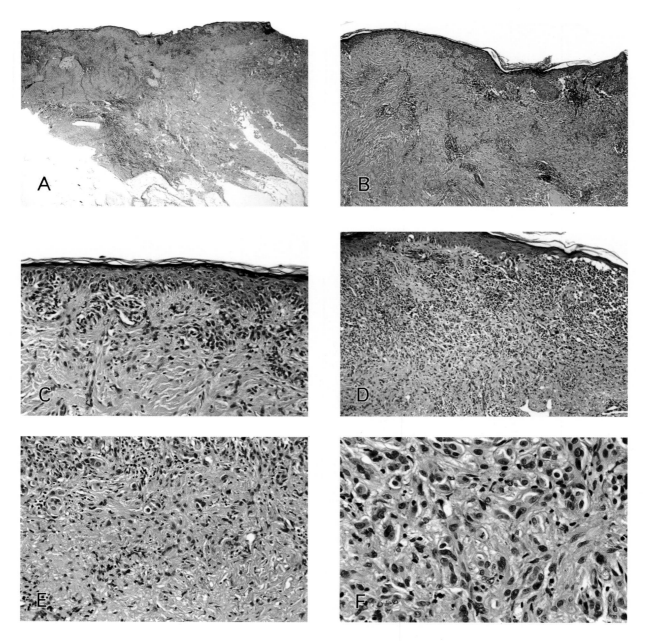

Figure 10-11

DESMOPLASTIC AND NEUROTROPIC MELANOMA AND LOCAL RECURRENCE

A: The architecture of the reticular dermis is altered by extensive involvement by a desmoplastic tumor, most prominently seen at the upper left. More superficially, there are nodular clusters of lymphocytes and extension of the papillary dermis, with hyperplasia of the epidermis (top right).

B: There is an increased number of melanocytes, mainly along the dermal-epidermal junction (top right). The architecture of the papillary and upper reticular dermis is altered by fibroplasia, with a cellular infiltrate and nodular clusters of lymphocytes.

C: Higher magnification shows atypical spindle cells separating from nested, more epithelioid cells and infiltrating the dermis.

D: The spindle cells are admixed in some areas with prominent tumor-infiltrating lymphocytes.

E: Spindle cells infiltrate elastotic dermal fibers.

F: More superficially, an epithelioid cell component shows prominent mitotic activity.

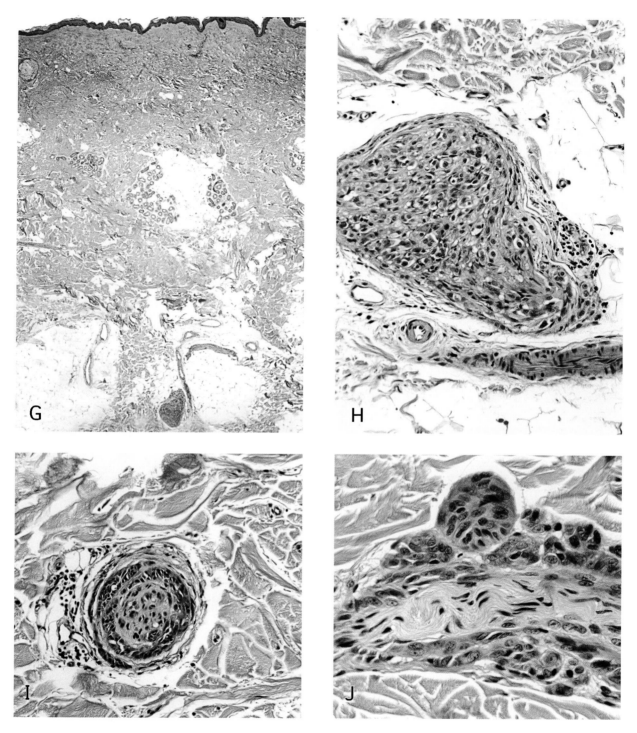

Figure 10-11 (continued)

G: This lesion recurred locally, in the form of nerve involvement (bottom).

H: A nerve is expanded and largely replaced by uniformly atypical epithelioid melanocytes.

I: This nerve is surrounded by spindle to epithelioid melanocytes.

J: An epithelioid cell tumor surrounds a peripheral nerve in the recurrence. Recurrences of desmoplastic melanomas are commonly neurotropic and often have a more epithelioid character than the primary tumor.

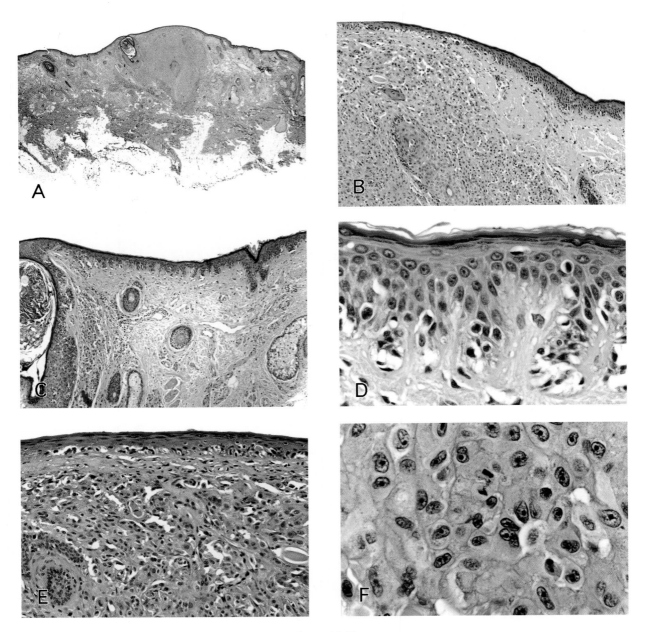

Figure 10-12

**MALIGNANT MELANOMA, LENTIGO MALIGNA TYPE, WITH
EPITHELIOID TUMORIGENIC VERTICAL GROWTH PHASE AND NEUROTROPISM**

A: Scanning magnification shows a bulky tumor from a 62-year-old. In the adjacent epidermis are more subtle alterations. The epidermis over the tumor and adjacent to it contains a slightly increased number of nevoid to epithelioid melanocytes arranged along the dermal-epidermal junction.

B: The tumor cells infiltrate elastotic fibers of the dermis and collagen fibers of the reticular dermis.

C: Lentiginous proliferation of slightly atypical melanocytes constitutes lentigo maligna melanoma in situ, with involvement of a hair follicle.

D: Uniform, albeit moderate, atypia of lesional cells, which are arranged in nests that tend to hang down from the epidermis. There is somewhat more elongation of rete ridge in this case than in most examples of lentigo maligna.

E: Cells of the tumorigenic vertical growth phase are epithelioid, with uniformly atypical nuclei and prominent nucleoli. Frequent mitotic figures are present.

F: Nuclear membranes are irregular and chromatin is irregularly clumped.

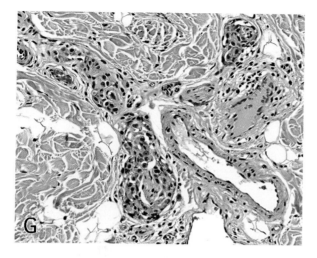

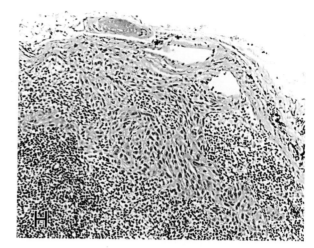

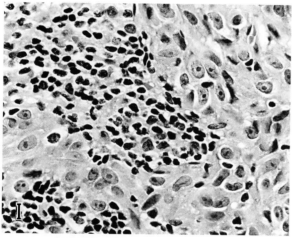

Figure 10-12 (continued)

G: Epithelioid cells surround nerves in the reticular dermis.

H: This lesion was associated with a positive sentinel node.

I: Uniformly atypical epithelioid cells with prominent nucleoli are in the stroma of the lymph node.

Melan-A, and other markers (reviewed above) in the diagnosis of desmoplastic and neurotropic melanomas has been disappointing.

Differential Diagnosis. As originally described, the concept of neurotropic melanoma included a description of neural (or schwannian) patterns of growth in the vertical growth phase. Although most examples of neurotropic melanoma have such patterns of differentiation, this, in our view, is an association primarily of desmoplastic melanoma and need not be a requirement for the diagnosis of neurotropic melanoma. Desmoplastic and neurotropic melanoma are closely associated but not synonymous entities. Most desmoplastic melanomas, in our experience, are also neurotropic, but some pure spindle cell neurotropic melanomas and most of the few epithelioid cell melanomas that we have seen with definite neurotropism do not exhibit the desmoplastic

collagen pattern, and may not exhibit convincing schwannian differentiation either.

Neurotropic melanoma also overlaps with primary dermal tumors, some of which may be regarded as superficial malignant epithelioid schwannomas, which have been termed *nerve-centered desmoplastic melanomas* by Jain and Allen (fig. 10-13) (28). These lesions are usually amelanotic but may focally express the occasional capacity of Schwann cells for melanogenesis (15,28), and exemplify the close inter-relationships that can be discerned among the neoplastic proliferations derived from cutaneous neural crest derivatives.

At a clinical level, the precise classification of individual cases into these various closely related diagnostic categories is less important than the recognition of the nerve involvement, which is associated with an increased propensity for local

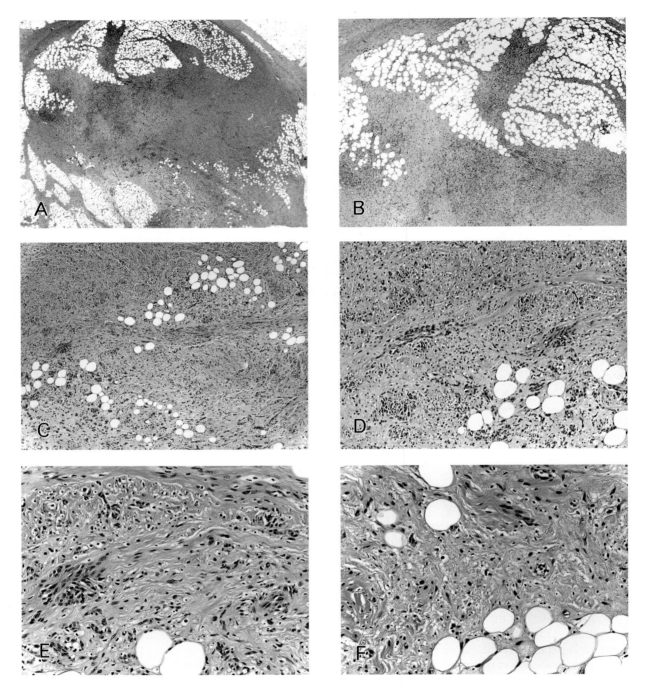

Figure 10-13

NERVE-CENTERED SUBCUTANEOUS DESMOPLASTIC AND NEUROTROPIC MALIGNANT MELANOMA

A: The tumor, from the back of a 78-year-old man, infiltrates the subcutaneous tissue. It is associated with desmoplasia.
B: The tumor infiltrates and honeycombs the fat.
C: The tumor is composed predominantly of spindle cells separated from one another by a desmoplastic stroma.
D: The cells are arranged in wavy fiber bundles and involve apparent preexisting nerves (upper center).
E: Wavy fiber bundles infiltrate the desmoplastic stroma.
F: Atypical spindle cells and smaller hyperchromatic cells are present in a delicate desmoplastic stroma.

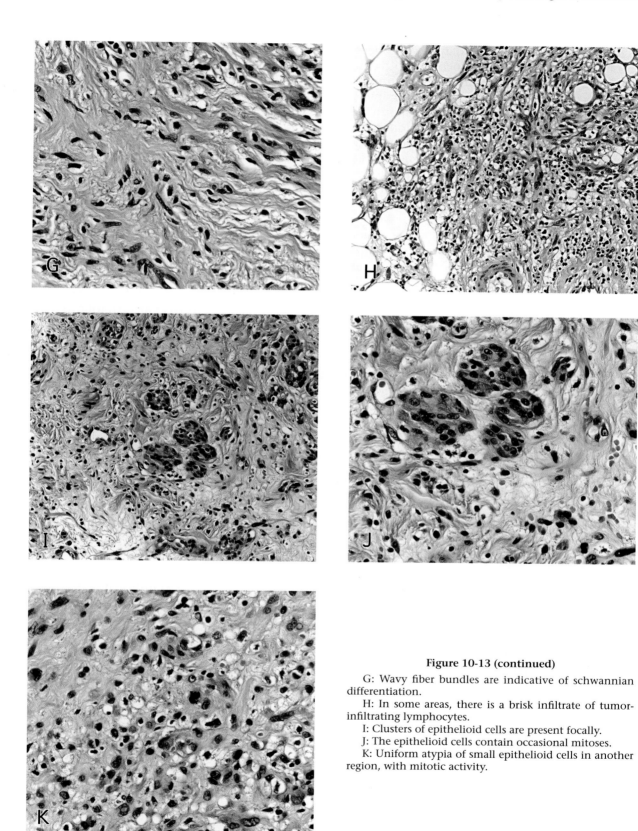

Figure 10-13 (continued)

G: Wavy fiber bundles are indicative of schwannian differentiation.

H: In some areas, there is a brisk infiltrate of tumor-infiltrating lymphocytes.

I: Clusters of epithelioid cells are present focally.

J: The epithelioid cells contain occasional mitoses.

K: Uniform atypia of small epithelioid cells in another region, with mitotic activity.

recurrence. The neurotropism may be prominent or subtle, and may occur in association with desmoplastic, acral-lentiginous, mucosal-lentiginous, or lentigo maligna melanoma, or as a prominent feature in a pigment-synthesizing superficial cutaneous spindle cell malignancy that does not completely fulfill the characteristics of these other forms of melanoma. It is these latter lesions that we categorize as neurotropic melanomas.

Cellular neurothekeoma, considered to be a benign tumor of nerve sheath origin, tends to present in children or young adults, often in the head and neck area, as a relatively large dermal tumor composed of fascicles of polygonal and spindle cells with eosinophilic or pale-staining cytoplasm, and with neuroid characteristics (structures resembling nerve trunks) (61–63). Low-grade cellular atypia and rare mitotic activity are commonly present, and multinucleate giant cells are often observed. Necrosis is absent. Because of the abundant cytoplasm, the nested pattern of the lesional cells, the cellular atypia, and the neuroid differentiation, the differential diagnosis may include neurotropic melanoma, but there is no radial growth phase proliferation in the epidermis and no melanin pigment. The lesions are negative with routine antibodies to S-100 protein, while tending to react with antibodies to the S-100A6 protein, MITF, and NKI/C3 antigens (20,21). Reexcision with clear margins is recommended as definitive treatment for cellular neurothekeoma, whose course is typically benign (64).

MALIGNANT MELANOMAS IN CONGENITAL MELANOCYTIC NEVI

Nodular tumors of melanocytes often arise in the dermal component of giant congenital nevi, and exhibit histologic indicators of malignancy including frequent mitoses, areas of necrosis, high-grade nuclear atypia with macronucleoli, and destructive patterns of growth without maturation (65,66). Despite these characteristics of malignancy, the behavior of these lesions is unpredictable, and in some cases, an unexpectedly benign course is documented. Similarly, melanomas may arise in small or giant congenital melanocytic nevi either by the pathway of an antecedent radial growth phase (figs. 10-14, 10-15), or, rarely, as a dermal tumor nodule unconnected with the epidermis. Most examples of the latter phenomenon, in our opinion, are cases

of proliferative nodules occurring in congenital nevi, which typically have a benign course.

Clinical Features. The incidence of malignancy in congenital melanocytic nevi has been discussed in some detail in previous sections. Although the incidence is clearly increased, these are uncommon neoplasms and there are few published descriptions of the lesions (67). In their review of seven cases and of the literature, Hendrickson and Ross (65) concluded that the "usual" origin of melanoma from a radial growth phase component in the epidermis and papillary dermis was the exception rather than the rule for melanomas that arose in giant congenital nevi. The lifetime incidence of melanoma in giant congenital nevi is 4 to 6 percent based on population studies (68,69). In a prospective single-center study, Gari et al. (70) followed 47 individuals with large (over 20 cm) congenital nevi for a mean of 53 months. A single primary central nervous system (CNS) melanoma developed in a 2-month-old child who died of her disease at the age of 21 months.

The incidence of melanoma in small congenital nevi is controversial. Although there is no doubt that the phenomenon occurs, its clinical and especially its epidemiologic significance can be questioned (71–73). In an interesting study, the prevalence of small congenital nevi was higher in melanoma cases versus controls, and it was determined that the relative risk of developing melanoma was increased approximately four-fold in individuals having these nevi on their skin (73).

Most of the lesions described have presented as dermal tumors or swellings, not necessarily associated with conspicuous pigmentary changes. When the lesions are deep-seated, surface ulceration is usually absent. Superficially located malignant melanomas also occur in giant congenital nevi and these lesions may arise in the epidermal component, may be associated with pigmentary changes, may ulcerate, and may metastasize, just like melanomas arising in skin not involved by a congenital nevus.

Microscopic Findings. As noted by Hendrickson and Ross (65), the literature presents a bewildering variety of patterns that have been noted in lesions that occur in giant congenital nevi. Most of these lesions present as cellular

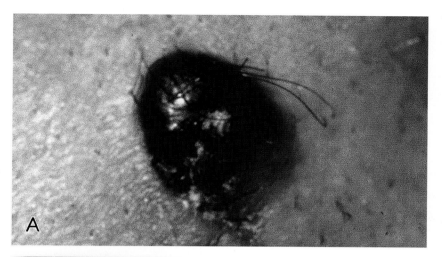

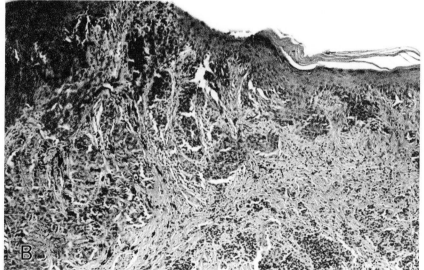

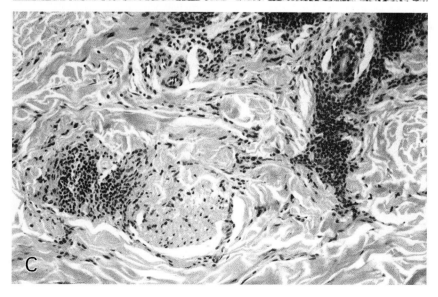

Figure 10-14

**MALIGNANT MELANOMA
ARISING IN A
CONGENITAL NEVUS**

A: A bulky black tumor nodule
arises in a blue-black plaque, which
in turn has arisen in a brown papule
(right periphery of the lesion).
On the left are large pigmented,
uniformly atypical cells forming a
tumor that infiltrates the reticular
dermis. On the right are small cells in
the dermis consistent with the cells
of a congenital melanocytic nevus.

B: There is a confluent and
continuous proliferation of uniformly atypical cells in the overlying
epidermis, consistent with a radial
growth phase component.

C: At the base of the lesion,
nevus cells are present among
reticular dermis collagen bundles,
within arrector pili muscle and
around a sweat duct.

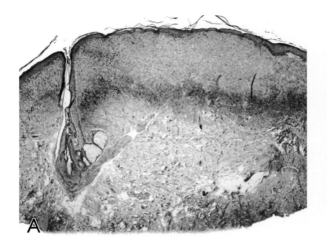

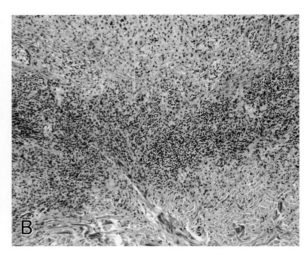

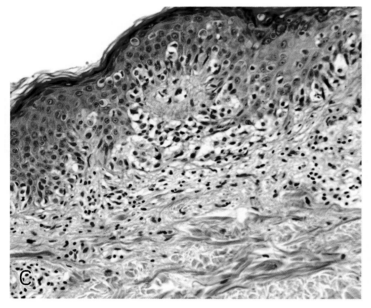

Figure 10-15

MALIGNANT MELANOMA ARISING IN A SMALL CONGENITAL NEVUS

A: Superficial large cells with abundant cytoplasm create a pale-staining tumor. At the base are smaller cells with less cytoplasm forming a blue lesion, which represents a residual congenital pattern dermal nevoid component.

B: At the base of the tumor, lymphocytes are admixed with small nevoid cells that extend into the upper reticular dermis.

C: In the adjacent epidermis, a pagetoid proliferation of uniformly atypical epithelioid cells is consistent with an in situ component of superficial spreading melanoma.

D: Just beneath the epidermis, the cells are larger, with frequent mitoses.

E: At the base of the lesion, in a different area from the subjacent nevus, there is infiltration of the reticular dermis by melanoma cells smaller than those near the epidermis, indicative of nevoid maturation within the lesion.

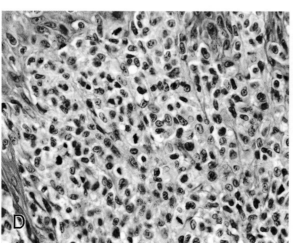

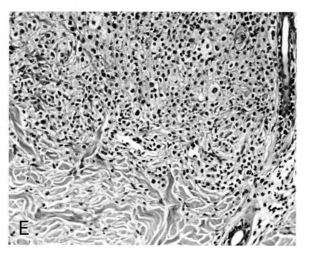

and atypical dermal nodules, often having no connection with the epidermis. These authors described several different cellular variations. Small round cells, reminiscent of the cells of neuroblastoma or lymphoma, and also described in the early report of Reed et al. (74), appear to be the single most common cell type to be found in these rare cancers. Mitoses may be frequent, and scanty melanin pigment may be demonstrable with difficulty.

Spindle cell components containing melanin are cytologically benign or malignant, and recall the differentiation of common or cellular blue nevi. The cytologically benign forms are seen in the areas of "neurotization" that are common in giant congenital nevi. More cellular and atypical spindle cell nodules, especially when associated with necrosis, have been described as "malignant blue nevi" but perhaps more appropriately should be termed "spindle cell melanomas occurring in giant congenital nevi." Some of these lesions have recurred locally and later metastasized (65). Spindle cell components with neural-supportive differentiation include cytologically benign areas that morphologically resemble or are indistinguishable from cutaneous neurofibromas and areas with prominent and fascinating formation of pseudo-Meissnerian corpuscles. Lamellar structures are reminiscent of Meissnerian corpuscles, the latter occurring in some primitive spindle cell neoplasms that have been seen in giant congenital nevi.

Epithelioid cell elements, with or without melanin, are most often seen as components of tumors that appear to have arisen in the dermal component of the giant nevi; only occasionally are they seen in contact with the epidermis in a pattern similar to that of common melanomas.

Components with specific mesenchymal ("ectomesenchymal") differentiation that have been reported in giant congenital nevi include rhabdomyoblasts, lipoblasts, and ganglion cells. All have been described as components of complex neoplastic nodules; islands of benign cartilage have been described in the background nevi (65).

It must be emphasized, however, that the patterns described above are not in themselves diagnostic of malignancy, even when seen as components of cellular nodules in congenital nevi. The features that we use to suggest the possibility of malignant behavior include, in particular, sharp demarcation of the tumor nodule from the surrounding nevus with compression of adjacent structures, ulceration or spontaneous necrosis at the architectural level, cytologic atypia, and mitotic activity. Cytologically, high cellularity with a high nuclear to cytoplasmic ratio and high-grade nuclear atypia with macronucleoli and frequent mitoses are very disturbing features (66). Some nodular tumors that lack necrosis and frequent mitoses, and that blend with the surrounding nevus cells rather than compressing them, are best classified descriptively ("congenital nevus with atypical proliferative nodule"). More atypical lesions may be provisionally classified as melanomas, especially in patients beyond the first 6 months of life, but with the caveat that the behavior may be better than expected if evaluated by conventional prognostic attributes for adults.

Biologic Behavior and Differential Diagnosis. In their review, Hendrickson and Ross (65) provide a number of useful generalizations regarding the management of patients with giant congenital nevi. First, a biopsy of the changing areas in the giant nevus is mandatory, and close clinical observation of individuals whose nevi cannot be excised is important because of the significant incidence of melanoma. Second, the possibility of leptomeningeal melanosis should be considered in patients with midline or scalp nevi, because such patients have developed meningeal melanomas (70,74). This possibility can be evaluated with MRI scanning (75). Histologically, peculiar differentiation is expected in neoplasms arising in giant congenital nevi, often without evidence of an epidermal origin, and these findings do not suggest a metastasis from another site. These neoplasms may be multiple and occur synchronously or metachronously, and their morphology may vary widely in multiple lesions from the same patient. Some alarmingly cellular neoplasms may not behave aggressively, and most of these cellular and atypical but biologically benign neoplasms have low mitotic rates. Conversely, cellular spindle cell lesions resembling cellular blue nevi that exhibit necrosis, mitoses, and high-grade nuclear atypia should be labeled malignant because they have a demonstrable capacity for metastasis.

MALIGNANT BLUE NEVUS

Definition. *Malignant blue nevus* is a malignant dermal tumor composed of neoplastic, spindle-shaped and occasionally epithelioid, pigment-synthesizing cells that form a bulky cutaneous tumor that extends through the dermis without conspicuously involving the epidermis. It is classically associated with elements resembling a residual or associated benign or cellular blue nevus, but in addition, has areas of increased cellularity, cellular atypia, necrosis, and mitotic activity. The term has been applied in three ways (76–78). Most commonly, malignant blue nevus is a melanoma that arises in association with a cellular blue nevus (also referred to as a *malignant cellular blue nevus*). Others use the term to refer to melanomas arising in association with a blue nevus, while in a less restrictive usage, the term may be applied to melanomas that mimic cellular blue nevi, lack a benign component, and appear to arise de novo. In a recent study of 10 cases of malignant blue nevi, 6 proved to be de novo melanomas mimicking cellular blue nevus, but lacking a clearcut benign component (76); 2 melanomas arose in association with a common blue nevus and 2 with a cellular blue nevus.

Clinical Features. Malignant blue nevi are extraordinarily rare. Most studies have focused on their microscopic morphology, so that clinical information is scant. Combining two series of 21 "fully documented" cases from the literature with the 10 cases of Granter et al. (76), the average age at diagnosis was 40 to 48 years (range, 10 to 80 years), and the sex ratio was about equal. Eleven of the 21 cases occurred on the scalp, and 3 on the foot. Nine cases occurred on the posterior trunk, at least 5 near the sacrococcygeal area, which is a common location for cellular blue nevus (78). The lesional size ranged from 0.5 cm to greater than 3.0 cm in diameter, and some were multi-nodular. Most were blue or blue-black, and there was commonly a history of progressive enlargement.

In another study of seven cases, the most frequent location of malignant blue nevus was the scalp (79). Clinically, the tumor generally consisted of a blue nodule, about 2.5 cm in diameter. In some cases, there had been a history of a longstanding, apparently stable lesion that began to change progressively. In cases that metastasized, the average duration of disease from initial recognition of a pigmented lesion to metastasis was 16 years in one review of 11 cases, indicating to these observers that this may be an indolent disease (77). Metastases have been documented in at least 15 cases, however, and at least 10 of these have been responsible for the death of the patient. In a more recent study of seven cases with follow-up, three local recurrences occurred within 2 years, and visceral metastases, which were all followed by death from disease, occurred within 4 years in three cases (76).

Microscopic Findings. As seen in a generous biopsy or an excision specimen, a malignant blue nevus is a bulky dermal tumor composed of heavily pigmented spindle cells (fig. 10-16). In a recent abstract of 12 cases, the diagnosis was based on "the presence of cytologically malignant melanocytes, usually forming nodules, in a blue nevus background" (80). Granter et al. (76) similarly emphasized the focal or complete loss of the characteristic cellular architecture of benign common blue or cellular blue nevi and the development of a sheet-like pattern, often composed of epithelioid cells, with necrosis, nuclear hyperchromasia, pleomorphism, prominent nucleoli, excessive mitotic activity, and an infiltrative border. The epithelioid cells were present in about half of their cases, and exhibited the characteristic melanoma morphology, including large nuclei and prominent nucleoli, with fine melanin dispersed in the cytoplasm.

Malignant blue nevus frequently extends through the reticular dermis to involve the fat, in some instances with a "dumbbell" pattern similar to that seen in many cellular blue nevi. The tumor thickness ranges from 4 to 20 mm or more (76). Features of benign blue nevus or cellular blue nevus may be seen in samples from different areas of these neoplasms, suggesting that malignant blue nevus may evolve, at least in some instances, from a preexisting "precursor" cellular blue nevus. In the study of Granter et al. (76), the malignant and benign components were easily distinguished in the four cases that arose in association with a common or cellular blue nevus. Abrupt transition between a benign blue nevus and melanoma was readily recognized at scanning magnification as distinctive nodules of epithelioid to spindled cells with a

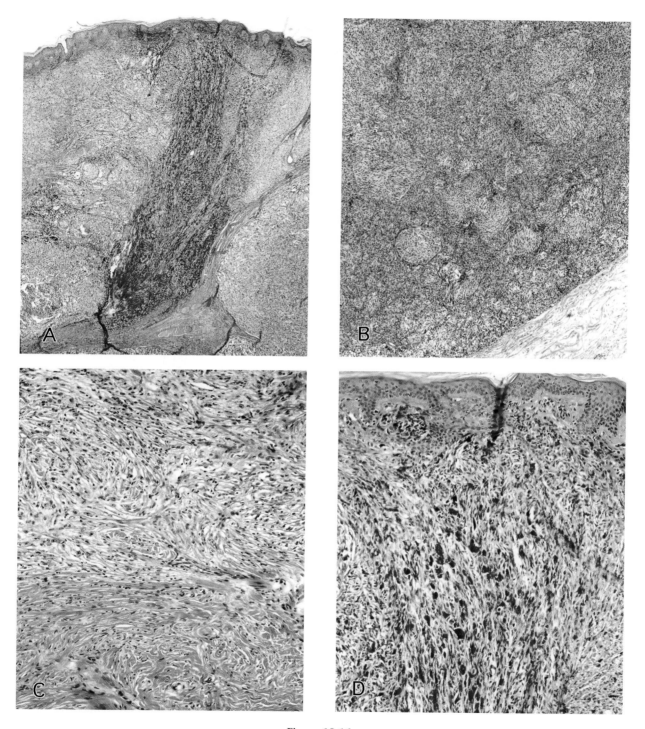

Figure 10-16

MALIGNANT BLUE NEVUS

A: A bulky tumor spans the dermis and enters the subcutis.
B: A mixed-biphasic pattern of cellular blue nevus is seen in some areas.
C: A banal blue nevus-like pattern is seen in other areas.
D,E: Elsewhere, there are sheets of uniform epithelioid cells with high-grade atypia and mitotic activity.

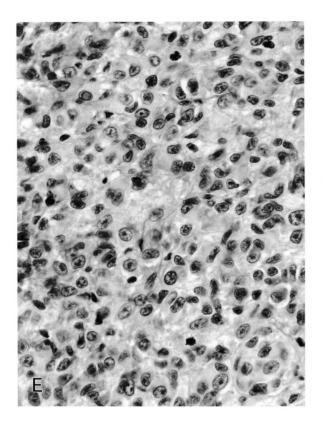
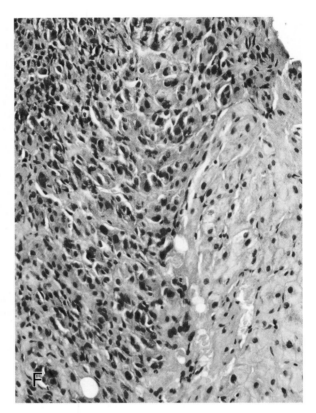

Figure 10-16 (continued)

F: This tumor metastasized to the liver.

sheet-like growth pattern. These considerations suggest that any neoplasm found to exhibit features of a cellular blue nevus on incisional biopsy should be completely excised and examined histologically to rule out malignancy.

The features that suggest malignancy at scanning magnification in a lesion of this type include large size (many malignant blue nevi are larger than 3 cm; most cellular blue nevi are smaller than 2 cm), high cellularity, cytologic atypia, and necrosis. The biphasic pattern of clear nested and pigmented fascicular cells seen in cellular blue nevus is less evident or absent in malignant blue nevus. At higher power, nuclear atypia, pleomorphism, hyperchromasia, and prominent nucleoli are usually evident, and mitoses have been described in most if not all of the metastasizing lesions. Necrosis has not been observed in all malignant blue nevi, including some fatal lesions, and the mitotic rate is often not greater than 2 to 3 per 10 high-power fields (76,80). Thus, the absence of necrosis or of fre-

quent mitoses does not rule out malignancy. Conversely, since mitoses may be present in cellular blue nevi, the use of a few mitoses as a sole or even major criterion is not advised (76).

The reliability of adjunct diagnostic methods, such as cell cycle marker antigens, remains uncertain, especially in borderline cases (76). In a recent study of seven cases by image analysis, there was no single histopathologic criterion for the diagnosis of malignant blue nevus (79). In this series, the AgNOR measurement was significantly higher in malignant blue nevus than in common blue nevus or cellular blue nevus. This parameter may have some validity if it is confirmed in other series; however, the accurate counting of AgNORs is difficult to accomplish in routine practice. In another study of comparative genomic hybridization of cellular blue nevi and related lesions, chromosomal aberrations were present in the majority of the lesions that showed moderate to severe cytologic atypia and a high mitotic rate, and every lesion with necrosis demonstrated genomic abnormalities, suggesting that this type of analysis may have diagnostic utility in difficult cases (81).

Although some of the reported lesions considered to represent malignant blue nevus have metastasized only to regional lymph nodes or skin, visceral metastases have occurred in other cases, and these patients have all died of their disease (77). As discussed in the section on cellular blue nevus in chapter 4, benign "metastases" may be seen in lymph nodes draining cellular blue nevi. These, however, tend to be small and peripheral, and the lymph node architecture is not extensively replaced. Authentic metastases from a malignant blue nevus, in contrast, are larger, destructive, and associated with necrosis. The metastatic cells show high-grade nuclear atypia and frequent mitoses, and the cytology may appear similar to that in the primary lesion, with heavily pigmented spindle cells predominating (77).

Differential Diagnosis. Although this lesion is extremely rare as judged by the paucity of convincing case reports (and no large series), lesions are encountered that meet some but not all of the criteria. These may be divided into two groups. First, there is a group of lesions with some or all of the features of a cellular blue nevus and with some atypical features, including perhaps a mitosis or two, but where the criteria for malignancy are not convincing. We have classified some such lesions descriptively as MELTUMPs while others may be classified as "atypical cellular blue nevi," especially when the features just mentioned are subtly expressed. Although these lesions usually do not metastasize, local recurrence is possible if they are not completely excised, and such recurrence or persistence may be followed by progression to a more cellular, anaplastic and aggressive neoplasm. In addition, fully malignant behavior cannot entirely be ruled out in a cellular blue nevus-like lesion, especially when there is cytologic atypia, even in the absence of the other members of the "triad" of atypia, mitotic activity, and necrosis (76).

In other cases, an obviously malignant spindle cell melanocytic tumor may lead to a consideration of malignant blue nevus. If there are no associated features of benign or cellular blue nevus in such a tumor and especially if there is a junctional component present we, like Maize and Ackerman (15), consider the neoplasm to be a form of common malignant melanoma, which may be classified as a nodular melanoma if there is no radial growth phase. The presence of a radial growth phase in association with a pigmented, spindle cell vertical growth phase similarly rules out the diagnosis of a malignant blue nevus. Such lesions should be diagnosed as malignant melanomas, and classified according to the morphology of the radial growth phase compartment. Most of these heavily pigmented vertical growth phase nodules occur in relation to a lentiginous radial growth phase variant, such as lentigo maligna, acral-lentiginous, or mucosal-lentiginous melanoma. When these heavily pigmented, spindle cell vertical growth phase nodules of nodular or lentiginous melanoma are distinguished from malignant blue nevi, the diagnosis of the latter becomes very rare in our experience.

There also exists a small group of cases which lack a benign component but closely mimic a benign cellular blue nevus. Some of these have the dumbbell pattern of extension into the subcutis, and some have the mixed-biphasic or alveolar architecture characteristic of cellular blue nevi. Diagnosis in these cases is based on nuclear enlargement, increased nuclear to cytoplasmic ratio, prominent nucleoli, and increased mitotic rate (76). These lesions are difficult to distinguish from benign cellular blue nevi, and some may be best interpreted prospectively as MELTUMPs.

In clear cell sarcoma (melanoma of soft parts), the diagnosis of malignancy is usually not in question, but the tumor may be confused with either primary or metastatic melanoma and heavily pigmented examples may raise the question of a malignant blue nevus. Clear cell sarcomas lack the benign blue nevus component that may be seen in cellular, atypical and malignant blue nevi. In doubtful cases, a reticulin stain demonstrating an "epithelial" pattern outlining cell groups rather than single cells helps distinguish sarcoma. In addition, genetic testing for the characteristic chromosomal t(12;22)(q13;q12) translocation which results in a fusion between the Ewing sarcoma gene (*EWSR1*) and activating transcription factor 1 (ATF1) may be definitive if needed (82). MITF is frequently positive in these lesions, although this is not necessarily helpful in separating them from malignant blue nevi and melanoma variants. In a recent study, immunoreactivity in a nuclear pattern for MITF was present in 26 of 32 tumors (78 percent), S-100 protein expression was seen in all cases, HMB45 staining in 96 percent, and focal Melan-A positivity was seen in 69 percent (83). Cellular neurothekeoma has been discussed in the section on neurotropic melanoma, with which it is more likely to be confused (61). Deep penetrating nevi, including those with atypical features, may overlap with cellular and malignant blue nevi and are discussed in chapter 2.

NEVOID AND MINIMAL DEVIATION MELANOMAS

Definition. Although no doubt closely related to minimal deviation melanoma, *nevoid melanoma* is potentially different biologically. *Nevoid melanoma* is a lesion that, to a greater or lesser extent, mimics a benign nevus histologically, especially with regard to architectural features. Usually, the resemblance is most apparent at scanning magnification, which can lead to a missed diagnosis if sufficient attention is not paid to cytologic and more subtle architectural features (fig. 10-17).

The term *minimal deviation melanoma* is applied to a diagnostically difficult and heterogeneous group of melanocytic tumors that are considered to be malignant melanomas of indeterminate risk. The lesions are architecturally atypical expansile tumors (hence not nevoid), meeting the criteria for vertical growth phase disease, but the degree of cytologic atypia in the vertical growth phase is less than that observed in common forms of melanoma. Most examples of minimal deviation melanoma simulate, in terms of their aggregate architectural characteristics, to a greater or lesser degree, some variant form of benign melanocytic lesion (e.g., congenital pattern nevi, spindle and epithelioid cell nevi, halo nevi).

Clinical Features. Nevoid melanoma has been defined as "a rare variant of melanoma characterized by deceptive morphologic features reminiscent of a benign melanocytic nevus" (84). The term is attributed to Levene, who described a case of "verrucous and nevoid melanoma" in 1980 (85,86). Schmoeckel et al. (87) in 1985 described 33 patients with nevoid melanoma followed for at least 5 years; 15 developed metastases and 8

died of disseminated melanoma. In a study of 20 cases, 4 tumors recurred and 3 metastasized, with subsequent death of the patients (84). It was concluded that nevoid melanoma can be distinguished from a benign nevus by a high index of suspicion, a careful analysis of the architecture, and attention to the cytologic features, and that the data do not support the notion that patients with nevoid melanoma have a better prognosis than do those with ordinary melanoma. The few such studies that have been conducted may preferentially include those lesions that were originally regarded as nevi but that have declared themselves biologically as malignant as a result of metastatic spread. Accordingly, those lesions that were considered to be nevi but with histologic characteristics of nevoid melanoma that failed to metastasize may per force be excluded from such studies, potentially skewing results.

In a clinicopathologic study of 21 cases of so-called minimal deviation melanoma, some of the lesions presented as nonpigmented, pink or flesh-colored nodules and were interpreted as Spitz nevi or as hemangiomas clinically, while other lesions that were pigmented were recognized as melanomas (11). The lesions occurred on all regions of the skin. The age range was from 5 to 73 years and the sex ratio was about equal. Some of the lesions arose within preexisting nevi, including congenital nevi.

Microscopic Findings. In a study of seven cases, Wong et al. (88) defined nevoid melanomas as being characterized by a "deceptively benign histological appearance with an architecture resembling that of benign melanocytic nevi on scanning magnification." They described two architectural patterns, namely, a dome-shaped pattern in two of their cases and a verrucoid pattern in five. The dome-shaped lesions were characterized by a smooth epidermal surface and a proliferation of epithelioid melanoma cells with an inconspicuous intraepidermal component resembling Spitz nevi. There was some evidence of maturation in the form of gradual diminution in the size of the dermal nests toward the bases of the lesions. However, the pattern of dermal organization in cords and strands of melanoma cells and the persistence of cellular atypia extending to the bases of the tumors were considered important in recognizing the lesions as malignant melanomas. The

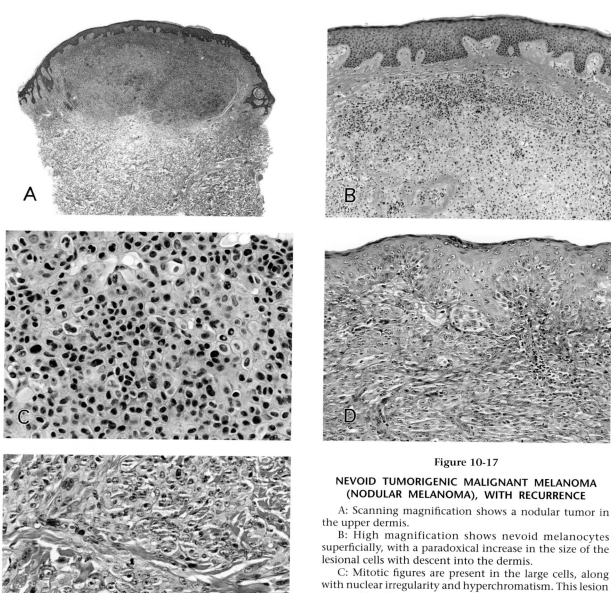

Figure 10-17

NEVOID TUMORIGENIC MALIGNANT MELANOMA (NODULAR MELANOMA), WITH RECURRENCE

A: Scanning magnification shows a nodular tumor in the upper dermis.

B: High magnification shows nevoid melanocytes superficially, with a paradoxical increase in the size of the lesional cells with descent into the dermis.

C: Mitotic figures are present in the large cells, along with nuclear irregularity and hyperchromatism. This lesion recurred locally (D and E).

D: There is confluent proliferation of uniformly atypical spindle to epithelioid cells, with a few nests in the overlying epidermis.

E: Mitotic activity was present in the tumorigenic dermal recurrence.

verrucoid lesions were broad, exophytic tumors with a verrucous epidermal surface resembling that of papillomatous dermal nevi. Distinguishing features were continuous proliferation of melanocytes along the dermal-epidermal junction and confluent sheets of melanoma cells in the dermis without evidence of true maturation (88). McNutt

(89,90) has also emphasized this "sheet-like" pattern of growth in the dermis, with filling and expansion of the verrucous papillae in the verrucous variant, rather than looser, nested pattern of proliferation of benign dermal nevus cells. In addition, in our opinion like that of others, the presence of mitotic figures is almost an absolute

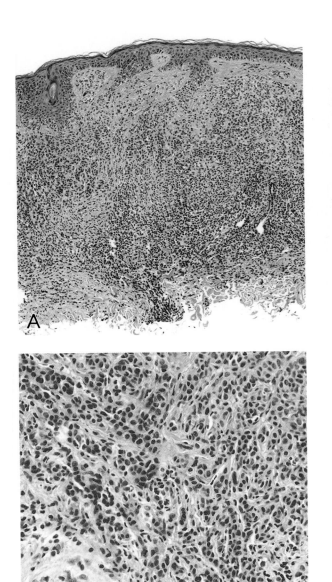

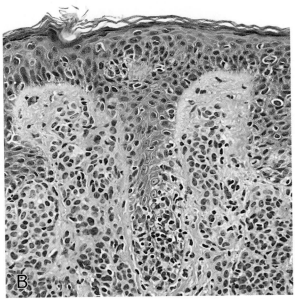

Figure 10-18

NEVOID MELANOMA WITH HALO REACTION

A: Scanning magnification shows a tumor with a brisk infiltrative lymphocytic response.

B: Higher power shows nevoid melanocytes and ill-defined nests and sheets in the upper dermis. Only a few atypical melanocytes are in the overlying epidermis.

C: Toward the base of the lesion, there is some evidence of maturation to a smaller cell type.

requirement for an unqualified diagnosis of a nevoid melanoma (84).

Schmoeckel et al. (87) described the microscopic features of his series of nevoid melanomas as follows: "some of the following histologic characteristics were always observed: cellular atypia, mitoses, infiltration of adnexa, and in the deeper dermis, infiltrative growth, pigmented tumor cells, sharply demarcated tu-

mor nests, and the absence of maturation" (figs. 10-17–10-21). In the recent study by Zembowicz et al. (84) of 20 cases, 13 of which had a nodular and 7 a verrucous architecture, the features were suggestive of a nevus at scanning magnification; however, more careful inspection demonstrated subtle pleomorphism and impaired maturation with depth, invariably accompanied by multiple dermal mitoses.

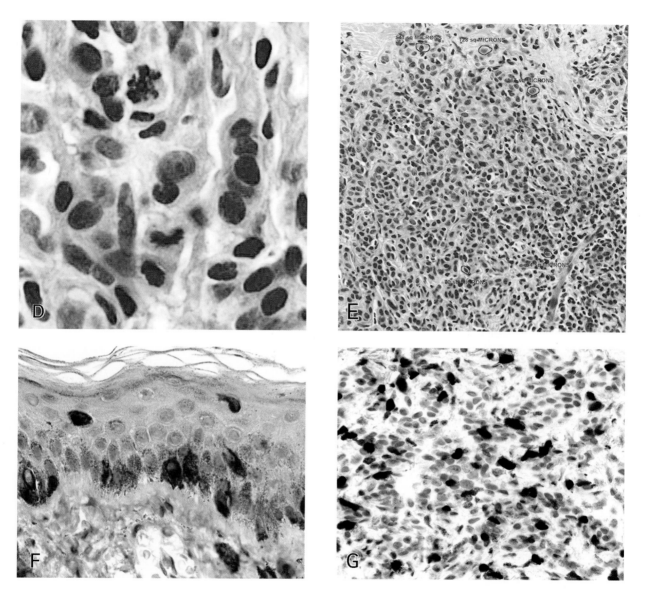

Figure 10-18 (continued)

D: Two mitotic figures are present in a high-power field within this smaller cell type.

E: Lesional cells mature from a larger cell superficially to a smaller cell toward the base of the specimen.

F: A Melan-A stain reveals increased, somewhat enlarged, epithelioid melanocytes in the epidermis; some are present in a suprabasal position.

G: A Ki-67 study demonstrates numerous reactive cells; many of these, however, are lymphocytes or other infiltrating cells.

McNutt et al. (89,90) have emphasized that nevoid melanomas mimic ordinary compound or dermal nevi when the melanoma cells are small, or Spitz nevi when the cells are large. In comparison with ordinary melanomas and nevi, the pattern of HMB45 staining was strong in the dermal component of the nevoid melanomas, while in nevi, the upper dermal component stained less than the junctional component, and the deepest components were negative. Spitz nevi and cellular blue nevi also had positive dermal cells, limiting the specificity of this finding for melanoma. In staining for a proliferation marker, such as Ki-67, the melanomas

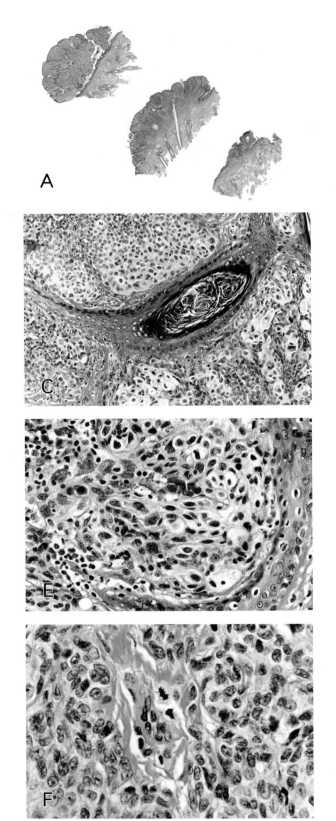

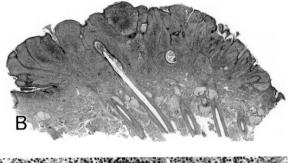

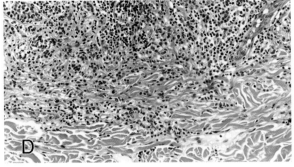

Figure 10-19

NEVOID AND VERRUCOUS MELANOMA

A: Scanning magnification shows a verrucous lesion from the scalp of a 34-year-old man characterized by expansile groups of cells at the tips of greatly expanded dermal papillae. There is confluent growth of similar cells in the papillary and upper reticular dermis.

B: Expansion of the papillae by the nevoid melanoma cells in the dermis is a clue to the diagnosis.

C: At higher magnification, there is cytologic atypia, which is moderate to severe in some foci and uniform; however, there is blending with adjacent less atypical cells.

D: At the base of the lesion is a lymphocytic infiltrate. Lesional cells extend into the reticular dermis without dispersing as single cells. There is clear evidence, however, of nevoid maturation.

E: Uniformly atypical cells are near the surface of the lesion.

F: Occasional mitotic figures are detected within the lesion.

G: A Ki-67 study shows a focally elevated proliferation rate, although not more than 10 percent.

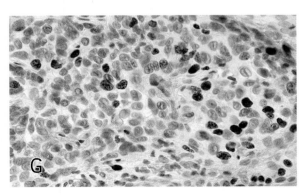

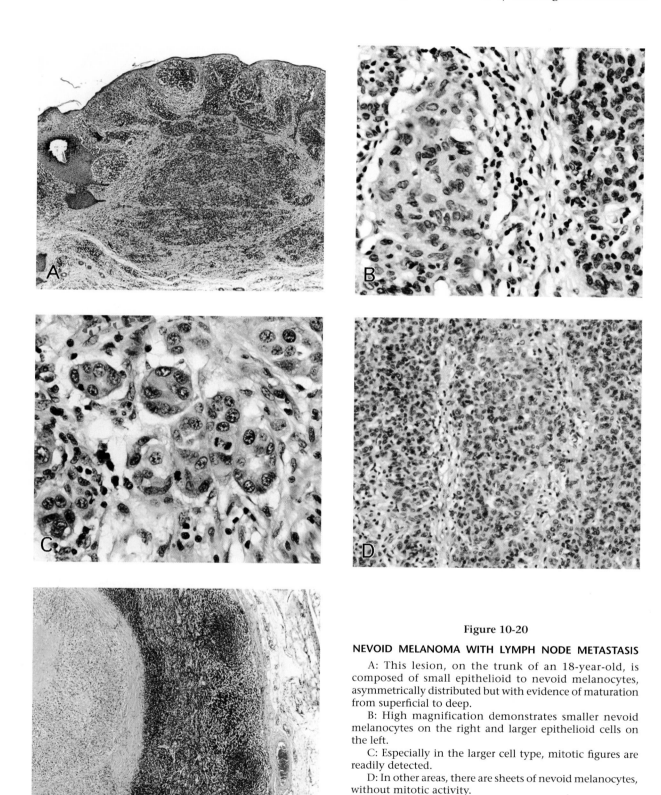

Figure 10-20

NEVOID MELANOMA WITH LYMPH NODE METASTASIS

A: This lesion, on the trunk of an 18-year-old, is composed of small epithelioid to nevoid melanocytes, asymmetrically distributed but with evidence of maturation from superficial to deep.

B: High magnification demonstrates smaller nevoid melanocytes on the right and larger epithelioid cells on the left.

C: Especially in the larger cell type, mitotic figures are readily detected.

D: In other areas, there are sheets of nevoid melanocytes, without mitotic activity.

E: This lesion metastasized to a regional lymph node.

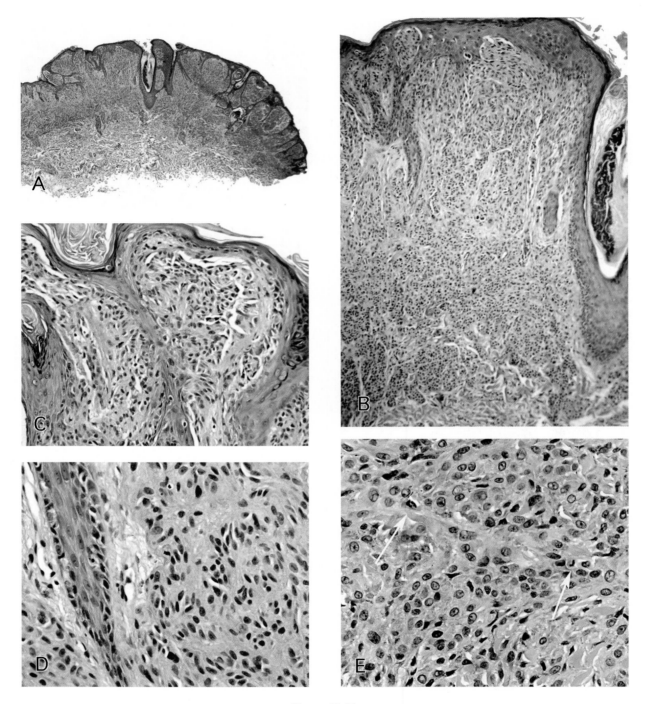

Figure 10-21

NEVOID MELANOMA WITH LYMPH NODE METASTASIS

A: Scanning magnification shows a lesion resembling a small congenital pattern nevus.

B: There is evidence of maturation from superficial to deep; however, the lesional cells fail to disperse as single cells into the reticular dermis at the base.

C: At the surface, the lesional cells tend to be large spindle and/or epithelioid cells, reminiscent of a Spitz nevus, with clefting artifact.

D–F: Mitotic figures are present in these superficial cells and there is an admixture of smaller cells, unlike Spitz nevus.

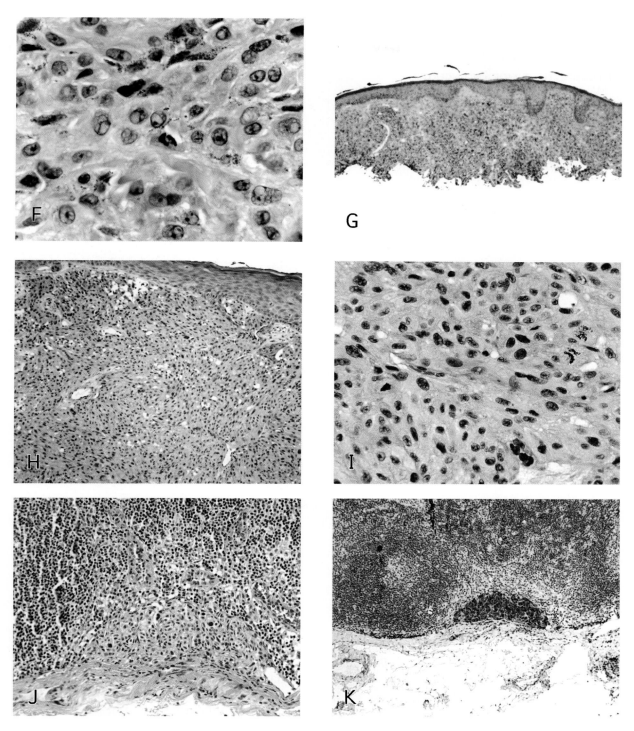

Figure 10-21 (continued)
G: The lesion recurred as this cellular tumor.
H: The recurrence consists of monotonously atypical spindle cells arranged in sheets with an ill-defined nested pattern.
I: Frequent abnormal mitotic figures are present. The lesion was also associated with a small lymph node metastasis (J and K).
J: Nevoid melanocytes are present beneath the capsule, indicative of a metastasis rather than a capsular nevus.
K: The lesion is strongly S-100 protein positive.

Figure 10-22

MELANOCYTIC TUMOR OF UNCERTAIN MALIGNANT POTENTIAL (MELTUMP): NEVUS VERSUS NEVOID MELANOMA

A: At scanning magnification, the lesion from a 42-year-old woman resembles a small congenital pattern nevus.

B,C: There is evidence of maturation of the dermal component from larger cells superficially (B) to smaller cells at the base (C).

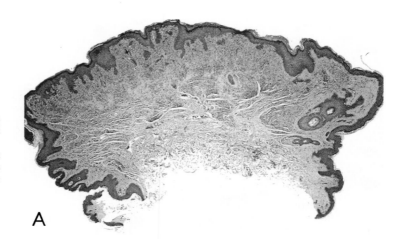

A

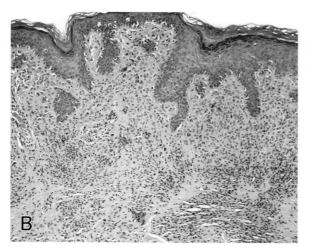

B

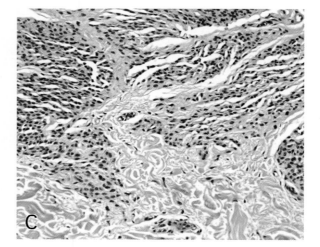

C

had strong nuclear staining throughout the lesion, while the Spitz nevi had more staining at the top of the lesion than at the bottom. The patterns of HMB45 and MIB-1 staining, interpreted with caution, could be used along with standard histologic criteria for the diagnosis of nevoid melanoma. Some differentiated or "nevoid" metastatic melanomas are difficult to distinguish from benign nevi (fig. 10-22) or from primary nevoid melanoma, and clinicopathologic correlation may be required to make this distinction.

As defined by Reed and colleagues (91), minimal deviation melanoma presents as an expansile, tumorigenic vertical growth phase lesion typically nodular in configuration, with no radial growth phase compartment or with an ill-defined intraepidermal component. The most important aspect of the lesion that differentiates it from a common form of malignant melanoma is the lesser degree of atypia of the cells in the vertical growth phase nodule. At the same time, the lesion exhibits features that preclude a diagnosis of one of the common forms of benign nevus, such as a common acquired nevus, spindle and epithelioid cell nevus, or blue nevus. The cells of the nodule are characteristically monomorphous, in contrast to many advanced melanomas in which there may be multiple cell types suggestive of multiple subclones. Categories of minimal deviation melanoma based on the predominant cell type in the vertical growth phase include a spindle cell type (pigmented and nonpigmented), a mixed spindle-epithelioid cell type (in which a single cell type exists in configurations ranging from plump and elongated to round), and a small epithelioid or nevoid cell type (13).

On a clinicopathologic basis, six classes of minimal deviation melanoma have been

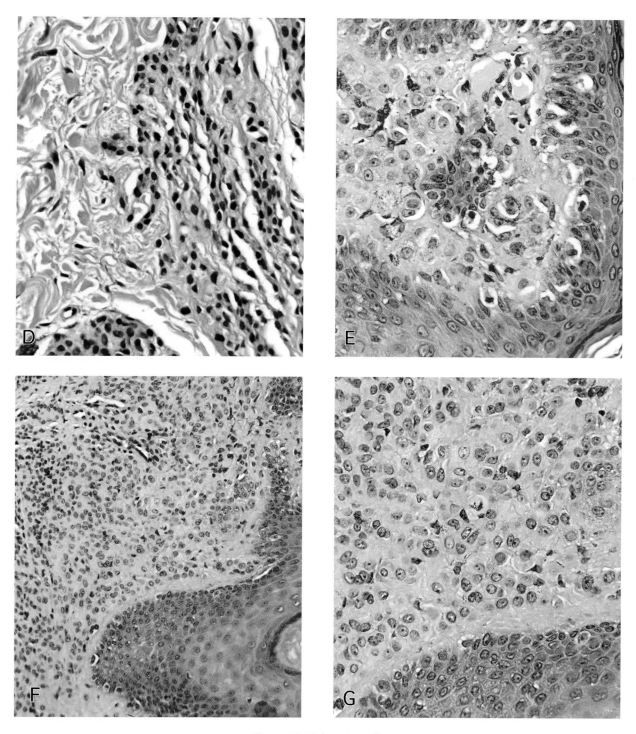

Figure 10-22 (continued)

D: The small cells disperse among reticular dermis collagen bundles at the base (left of image).

E: Superficially, there are atypical epithelioid melanocytes in the dermis and overlying epidermis (on the right).

F: There is cellular sheet-like growth in some areas of the lesion.

G: A rare lesional cell mitosis is present. This lesion is either a nevus with mitoses or a nevoid melanoma; the cellularity and atypia suggest that the latter diagnosis is more likely.

categorized (13,66). These include: 1) small nodules of melanocytes usually less than 0.76 mm thick, showing moderate nuclear atypism and expansile growth, discussed in chapter 8 as "probable early vertical growth phase"; 2) melanomas that share some features with a Spitz nevus, discussed in chapter 3; 3) a "halo nevus" variant, characterized by aggregated nests of cells constituting an expansile mass and suffused by lymphocytes in a manner reminiscent of a halo nevus. These lesions do not necessarily express a histologic halo and do not evolve from a characteristic benign halo nevus; 4) miscellaneous proliferations occurring in congenital melanocytic nevi; 5) melanomas occurring in the dermal component of a nevus (rare except in the context of congenital nevi) (see chapter 5); and 6) pigmented spindle cell lesions, most examples of which are tumors that share some attributes with benign pigmented spindle cell nevi but exhibit more marked atypia and, especially, tend to involve the reticular dermis in a pattern of invasive fascicular growth (see chapter 3). Other categories of spindle cell lesions that may have some attributes of minimal deviation melanoma are discussed elsewhere in this Fascicle, and include desmoplastic and neurotropic melanomas, and atypical and malignant blue nevi. Many of these lesions fall into the category of MELTUMP.

The *minimal deviation melanoma, Spitz variant*, is characterized by an expansile nodule of atypical spindle cells in association with a remnant of a common or atypical Spitz nevus (13). The lesions are larger than most common Spitz nevi, and measure one to several centimeters in diameter. The pattern of involvement of the reticular dermis is different than in the typical Spitz nevus. The delicate infiltrative pattern of small nevoid cells between the reticular dermis collagen fibers that characterizes Spitz nevus is not seen. Instead, there is either expansile growth of the nodule with compression of surrounding structures or infiltration of reticular dermis collagen by broad tongues and fascicles of cells that show little or no tendency to maturation. Within the nodule, the fascicles of tumor cells tend to be closely aggregated and tortuous, and there is a delicate tumor stroma, in contrast to most Spitz nevi, where the lesional cells permeate among largely unaltered

preexisting collagen fibers. Lesions like this are commonly diagnosed today as malignant melanomas with nevoid and "spitzoid" features (88). In our experience, some of these tumors metastasize to regional lymph nodes, but have not subsequently disseminated or caused the death of the patient (66).

The *pigmented spindle cell variant of minimal deviation melanoma* has been described as a solid, expansile nodule in the dermis, with at least moderate cytologic atypia, dense irregular nuclear membranes, mitoses, and overall asymmetry (13). A lymphocytic host response and neurotropism with invasion of the endoneurial space of adjacent nerves are additional signs of possible malignancy in such a lesion. Neurotropism alone may be seen in benign blue nevi, congenital nevi, and Spitz nevi, and is not diagnostic of malignancy as a single finding. These lesions usually differ substantially from the common benign pigmented spindle cell nevus, which is typically a superficial lesion confined to the papillary dermis. Involvement of the reticular dermis in such a lesion is a suspicious finding, especially if an expansile nodule is formed, mitoses or necrosis is observed, and the lesional cells do not mature to a small nevoid cell type.

The original concept of minimal deviation melanoma included that of borderline melanoma, separating those lesions that qualified architecturally as level III lesions (borderline) from those termed minimal deviation that involved the reticular dermis (level IV). While the concept of borderline and minimal deviation melanoma was forward-thinking in that it recognized rare "gray-zone" lesions with histopathologic characteristics intermediate between those of fully benign nevi and overt melanoma variants, it also produced considerable confusion. Nonetheless, recognition of this important concept spawned new and important studies, such as those outlined above that have delineated distinctive clinicopathologic melanoma variants, such as nevoid melanoma. While in this section we have endeavored to extensively review the concept of minimal deviation melanoma, we seldom if ever make this diagnosis; rather, the vast majority of such lesions are considered in the MELTUMP category. This permits the option of therapeutic intervention based on the worst scenario, while at the same time recognizing that such lesions are as yet incompletely studied and characterized in terms of their biologic potential and clinical outcome.

Prognosis. In the only follow-up study of patients with lesions designated as minimal deviation melanoma, 21 patients were followed for an average of 57 months, and only 2 died of metastatic melanoma (11). These data were considered to support the suspicion that minimal deviation lesions do not behave in the same aggressive fashion as do common varieties of melanoma, but it was correctly noted that comparisons need to be done with a large series of patients matched for lesion thickness and other prognostic variables. Until this has been done, we consider that the concept of minimal deviation melanoma has theoretical and descriptive value, but is of uncertain predictive or prognostic importance. The concept of minimal deviation melanoma represents an ambitious attempt to categorize heterogeneities among vertical growth phase melanomas, and emphasizes that there are examples of melanocytic lesions that are difficult to characterize either as unequivocally benign or malignant. In these circumstances, and also as emphasized above, it is usually our own preference to express uncertainty unambiguously, signing such cases out descriptively as MELTUMP (see next section).

The concept of minimal deviation melanoma also emphasizes that there are examples of thick melanomas where the prognosis is unexpectedly good, and links this improved prognosis to characteristics associated with "differentiation" of the lesional cells. This prognostic advantage may be identified in other ways, for example, by models that are more complex and more powerful than a simple thickness evaluation. The examples of minimal deviation melanoma that we have studied have typically been very thick lesions but have been associated with highly favorable predicted survival rates in a six-variable prognostic model for vertical growth phase melanoma, primarily because of their low mitotic rates.

There is increasing awareness that rare gray-zone melanocytic lesions exist: those with architectural features that show some overlap with melanoma but with less malignant cytology (minimal deviation melanoma) and those with architectural features that show some overlap with nevi but with more malignant cytology (nevoid melanoma) may be biologically distinctive entities. On the other hand, there are many reports of recurrence, metastasis, and death associated with nevoid melanoma (84,86–88,92), and we agree with the conclusion of Schmoeckel et al. (87) that "such cases do not appear to have a lower degree of malignancy and should be treated as normal malignant melanomas."

PIGMENTED EPITHELIOID MELANOCYTIC TUMORS (PIGMENTED EPITHELIOID MELANOCYTOMA)

Rarely, melanocytic tumors are composed of epithelioid and dendritic melanocytes containing abundant quantities of coarsely divided pigment that may obscure nuclear detail (93). Occasionally, these cells are difficult to differentiate from melanophages. Some of these lesions show prominent epidermal involvement by heavily pigmented epithelioid melanocytes distributed in a pagetoid pattern, and a deeper dermal component that is broader in the papillary dermis than in the reticular dermis. Despite their unusual pigmented cytology, these lesions may have an architectural pattern that is characteristic of nodular melanoma (figs. 10-23–10-26). Melanin bleach stains reveal prominent nucleoli and mitoses. A few tumors metastasize. The "melanophagic" differentiation has been likened to the heavily pigmented cells that characterize some melanomas that occur spontaneously or experimentally in animals (e.g., in horses or Sinclair swine [94–96]). Such lesions are provisionally categorized in our files as *malignant melanomas, nodular type, melanophagic variant* (or, with reference to their morphologic counterpart in vertebrate animals, *animal type melanoma*). They are also referred to as *melanoma with prominent pigment*.

Zembowicz et al. (97) recently described 41 lesions observed in the course of a study of borderline melanocytic tumors, characterized by features similar to those previously described as animal type melanoma and also to the epithelioid blue nevus of Carney complex (myxomas [especially cardiac], spotty skin pigmentation, endocrine overactivity, and schwannomas) (97–99). These lesions were considered to be histologically indistinguishable, and were

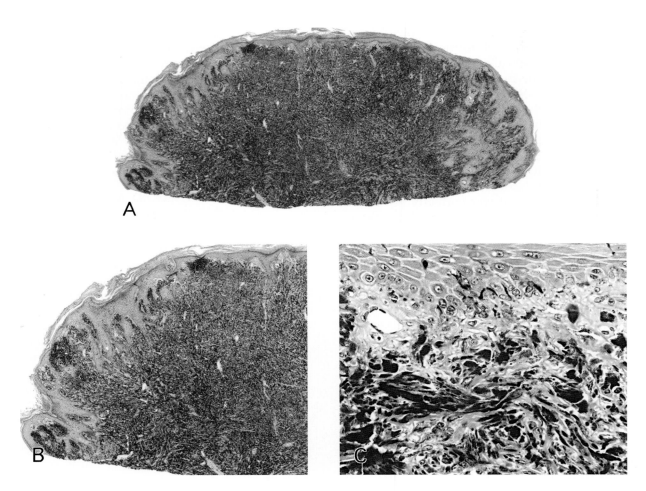

Figure 10-23

PIGMENTED EPITHELIOID MELANOCYTOMA

A: This heavily pigmented lesion, from the scalp of a 34-year-old African-American woman, is composed of heavily pigmented cells with associated irregular epidermal hyperplasia.

B: The tumor extends through the papillary dermis without filling or greatly expanding it, and infiltrates the reticular dermis. It is transected at the base.

C: The tumor is comprised of heavily pigmented spindle to epithelioid cells with coarsely divided melanin pigment. In the overlying epidermis, there are a few heavily pigmented dendritic melanocytes.

grouped together under the designation of *pigmented epithelioid melanocytoma* (PEM). The lesions occurred in both sexes of diverse ethnic backgrounds and ages (range, 0.6 to 78 years). The tumors had a wide distribution, with the extremities being the most common site. They were characterized by a deep proliferation of heavily pigmented epithelioid and/or spindled melanocytes that extended into the deep dermis, to a mean thickness of 3.3 mm. Maturation was generally absent. Five lesions were part of a combined nevus. Ulceration was present in 7 cases, and tumor necrosis in 1 case.

The regional lymph nodes were sampled in 24 cases, and in 11 of these (46 percent), none of which was associated with the Carney complex, the lymph nodes contained metastases. Liver metastases occurred in 1 case. Although none of the patients died of the disease, clinical follow-up was short (mean, 32 months; range, up to 67 months). There were no histologic criteria separating PEMs with nodal involvement from those without nodal involvement, and the only feature more common in PEM in patients without the Carney complex than in epithelioid blue nevi of Carney complex was ulceration. From

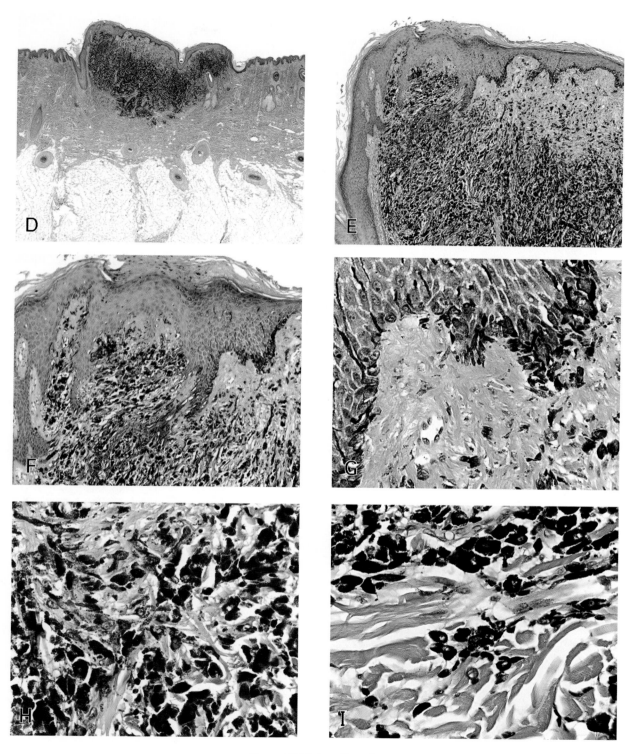

Figure 10-23 (continued)

D–I: This tumor was reexcised (D–I). In the reexcision specimen, there is superficial scarring with prominent dendritic melanocytes in the overlying epidermis, reminiscent of the recurrent ("persistent") nevus phenomenon (E–G). At the base, the heavily pigmented lesional cells infiltrate the dermal collagen (H,I).

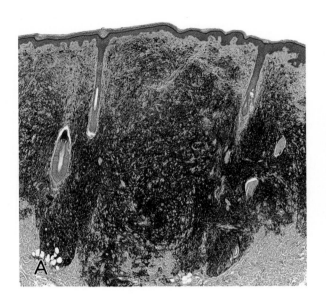

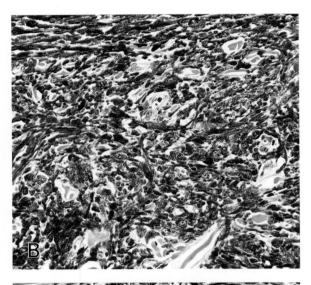

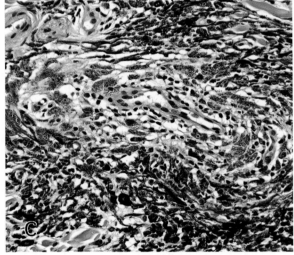

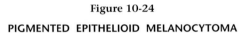

Figure 10-24

PIGMENTED EPITHELIOID MELANOCYTOMA

A: This tumor extensively involves the reticular dermis. Heavily pigmented epithelioid to spindle to dendritic cells are arranged in an ill-defined fascicular pattern. There is a sprinkling of perivascular lymphocytes and macrophages associated with the lesion.

B,C: Pigmented macrophages (in a perivascular position here) are distinguished with some difficulty from the pigmented epithelioid cells of the melanocytoma.

D,E: A melanin bleach stain demonstrates rather uniform nuclei without marked cytologic atypia. An occasional mitotic figure is observed.

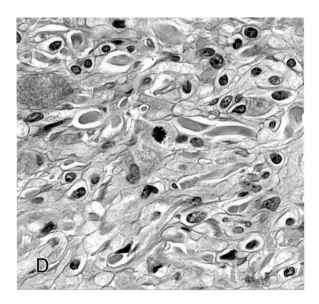

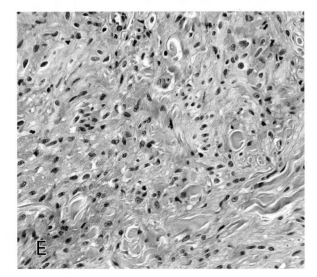

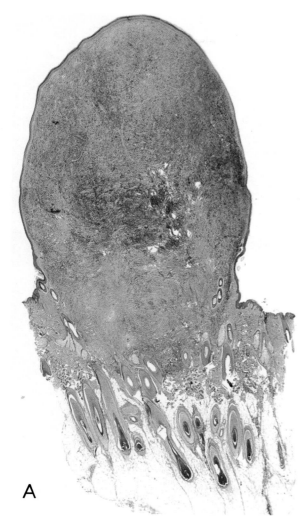

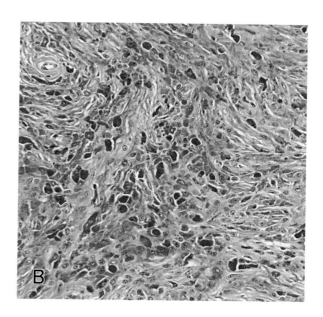

Figure 10-25

PIGMENTED EPITHELIOID MELANOCYTOMA

A: This polypoid lesion greatly expands the reticular dermis in an upward direction.

B: Spindle to epithelioid cells are arranged in a fascicular pattern. Most contain abundant melanin pigment.

C: There are some more epithelioid/nevoid areas.

D: In another area, the proliferation is predominantly spindle cell and fascicular. Lesions of this type were often formerly called cellular blue nevi, monophasic spindle cell type.

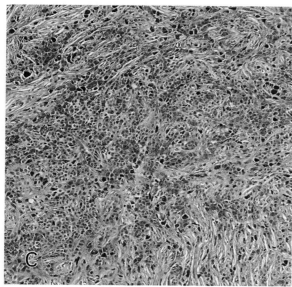

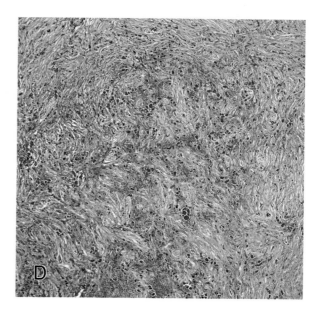

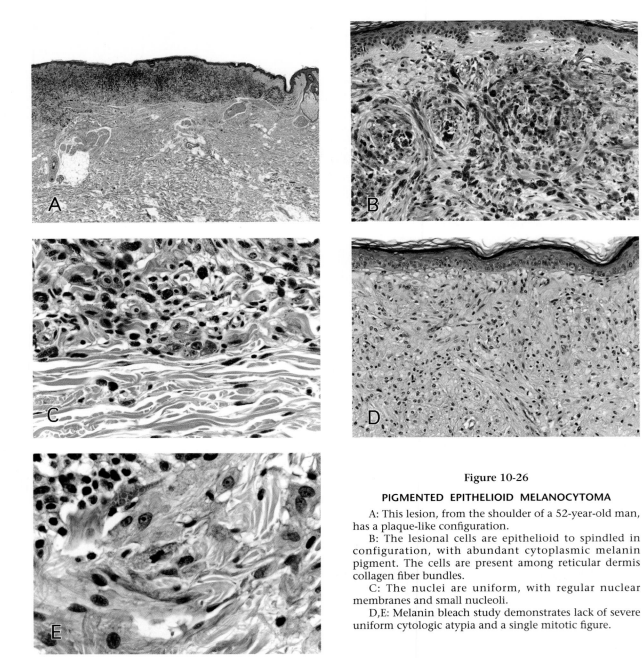

Figure 10-26

PIGMENTED EPITHELIOID MELANOCYTOMA

A: This lesion, from the shoulder of a 52-year-old man, has a plaque-like configuration.

B: The lesional cells are epithelioid to spindled in configuration, with abundant cytoplasmic melanin pigment. The cells are present among reticular dermis collagen fiber bundles.

C: The nuclei are uniform, with regular nuclear membranes and small nucleoli.

D,E: Melanin bleach study demonstrates lack of severe uniform cytologic atypia and a single mitotic figure.

these observations, it was suggested that PEM is a unique low-grade variant of melanoma with frequent lymph node metastases but an indolent clinical course, and it was recommended that PEM should be considered as a provisional histologic entity encompassing both animal type melanoma and epithelioid blue nevus.

These lesions should also be distinguished from unusually heavily pigmented examples of banal (spindle cell) blue nevi (fig. 10-27). In a recent study, mutations of the protein kinase A regulatory subunit type, 1alpha (R1alpha), coded by the *PRKAR1A* gene, which is found in more than half of Carney complex patients, is also found in most PEMs but not in equine melanomas, nevi including deep penetrating and cellular blue nevi, or human melanomas (99). The study supports the concept that PEM

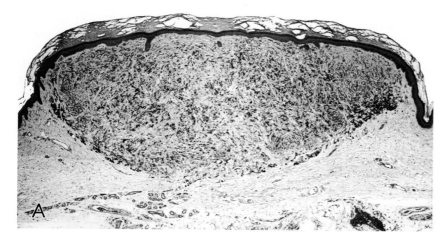

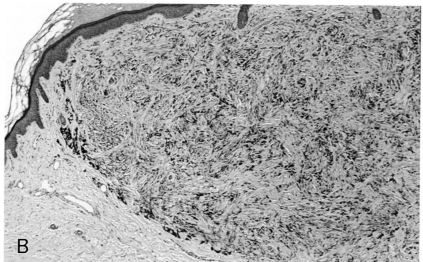

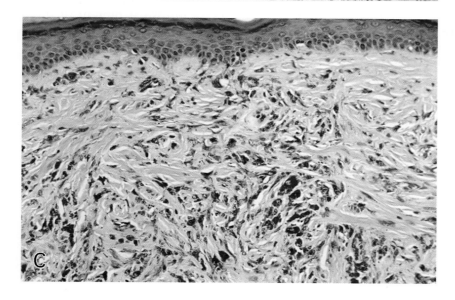

Figure 10-27

BLUE NEVUS VERSUS PIGMENTED EPITHELIOID MELANOCYTOMA

A: This large dome-shaped tumor involves the bulk of the reticular dermis.

B: Spindle cells are placed among reticular dermis collagen fiber bundles.

C: The lesional cells are elongated spindle cells, more consistent with a blue nevus than with pigmented epithelioid melanocytoma, in our opinion.

is a distinct melanocytic tumor occurring in a sporadic setting and in the context of Carney complex. In addition, loss of expression of R1alpha offers a useful diagnostic test that could help to distinguish this tumor from lesions that may mimic it histologically.

While the concept of PEM is an ambitious attempt to synthesize several seemingly separate entities under a common nomenclature, there remain several concerns with this notion and related terminology. One is the conceptual reclassification of a lesion formerly regarded as a benign epithelioid blue nevus as a melanoma, albeit low-grade. Conversely, the concept that a lesion with a 46 percent incidence of associated lymph node involvement is "low-grade" in the face of limited follow-up may be questioned. In addition, the possibility exists that some authentic heavily pigmented melanomas may be regarded as nonmalignant due to the misinterpretation of the term "melanocytoma." Perhaps the most salient concern is that PEMs appear to represent a heterogeneous group of lesions with potentially distinctive clinicopathologic and biologic characteristics. Hence, premature clustering under the category of melanoma could result in overly aggressive therapy for some, or conversely, under the moniker of melanocytoma, undertreatment for others. An alternative approach pending further evaluation of such lesions is to consider three main subtypes of PEM tumors as follows.

True Epithelioid Blue Nevus

In the initial reports of epithelioid blue nevus by Carney and Ferreiro (98,100), the lesions were described as heavily pigmented, poorly circumscribed dermal tumors containing two types of cells: one intensely pigmented, globular, and fusiform; the other lightly pigmented, polygonal, and spindled. The cells were situated among collagen bundles singly, in short rows and small groups, and occasionally in fascicles. The nuclei were vesicular, with pale chromatin and a single prominent nucleolus. If mitoses were detected, they were few (1 to 2 per section of the entire lesion). The 21 tumors were described in 11 patients, all of whom had the Carney complex. With follow-up of 1 to 27 years (mean, 11), none recurred locally or metastasized. The importance of detection of such lesions was emphasized in

terms of alerting the clinician to the possibility of Carney complex and potentially fatal left atrial myxomas, necessitating consideration of cardiac ultrasound to screen for the latter.

Subsequently, it was recognized that epithelioid blue nevi are not invariably associated with the Carney complex (101,102). Additionally, variant forms were recognized, including epithelioid blue nevi of the classic or Carney type, and of the combined type (with either hybrid features of epithelioid blue nevus and deep penetrating nevus or of epithelioid blue nevus and dermal Spitz nevus). In a study by Groben et al. (103) of 33 cases, rare mitoses were present in occasional lesions. However, follow-up of 6 to 162 months (average, 31 months) showed no evidence of metastases or local recurrence after excision. Similarly, Izquierdo et al. (104) have described a variant of epithelioid blue nevus involving either the mucosa of the glans penis or the labium minoris. These lesions appear to be benign. We have recently encountered one such lesion in consultation on the vulva of a young woman for which aggressive surgery had been planned based on an initial diagnosis of PEM/low-grade melanoma. Like benign epithelioid blue nevi of other sites, mitoses in such lesions are absent and high-grade cellular atypia is lacking. HMB45 may be positive in epithelioid blue nevi, and should not influence a decision toward malignancy. We generally recommend conservative excision for such lesions. Because of the difficulty in distinguishing between epithelioid blue nevi and the lesions formerly termed animal type melanomas, if even a rare mitosis is present or there is atypia, a lesion of this type, in our opinion, should be placed in the category to be discussed in the section following, a pigmented epithelioid melanocytoma (or melanocytic tumor) of uncertain malignant potential.

Pigmented Epithelioid Melanocytoma of Uncertain Malignant Potential

In the series of Zembowicz et al. (97), as discussed above, comparison of cases previously categorized as animal type melanomas with Carney complex–associated epithelioid blue nevus revealed no consistent distinguishing characteristics. There was a 41 percent incidence of sentinel lymph node involvement; however, none of these cases were associated with the complex. We consider that the unqualified term PEM for non-Carney–associated lesions may lead to undertreatment in some cases, and we therefore suggest adding the qualifier "of uncertain malignant potential" (PEMUMP) to this diagnosis in order to more explicitly describe the biologic potential of such tumors. This category includes those lesions that superficially resemble epithelioid blue nevus, but upon closer inspection (often facilitated by a melanin bleach) show foci of significant cytologic atypia and a few (or more) mitotic figures (fig. 10-24). Such lesions tend to include those previously designated as melanophagic and animal type melanomas.

In a recent publication, Antony et al. (105) suggested the use of the term *pigment synthesizing melanoma* (PSM) for the lesion also known as animal type melanoma, arguing that this term was expressive of the biologic potential of the lesions and likely to be more acceptable to patients and their physicians. The histologic diagnosis of PSM in 14 cases described by these authors was based on the finding of an "asymmetrical, predominantly intradermal tumor formed of deeply pigmented, round or short, spindle-shaped dendritic melanocytes with some degree of hyperchromatism and a single nucleolus." Numerous melanophages were invariably present. Cytologic atypia although always present was not pronounced, while the mitotic rate was usually low (mean, 2 per 10 high-power fields). The Breslow thickness ranged from 1.1 to 7.5 mm (mean, 3.3 mm). Perineural and lymphovascular invasion were not seen. In a median follow-up period of 5 years, six patients had no evidence of disease, three had local recurrence in the form of satellite nodules adjacent to the scar, four had spread to regional lymph nodes, and one patient had distant metastases to the liver. There were no deaths. It was concluded that PSM is a distinctive, possibly low-grade variant of melanoma usually lacking the histologic features (other than thickness) predictive of aggressive behavior seen in ordinary melanoma, and that these lesions should be managed "in the same way as other melanomas with wide local excision."

While the behavior of lesions in this general category is potentially malignant, we, like others, have seen several patients with long disease-free survival periods, despite the often relatively advanced microstage (characterized by high Breslow thickness and Clark level, although ulceration, high mitotic rate, and lymphovascular invasion are usually absent). Although these lesions show atypia, they sometimes do not meet the criteria for fully evolved melanocytic malignancy. For this reason, as well as in view of the limited outcome data, we prefer to classify these tumors in the uncertain malignant potential category. While therapeutic recommendations for such tumors have not been completely formulated, some clinicians and oncologists excise these lesions with margins used for ordinary melanomas of similar depth, as well as consider sentinel lymph node sampling for purposes of staging.

Tumoral Melanosis Mimicking Pigmented Epithelioid Melanoma

This last category includes lesions that present as nodular clusters of authentic melanophages. Such lesions may be examples of complete regression of a pigmented vertical growth phase nodule of melanoma, a rare phenomenon that differs from the partial regression that is often observed in the radial growth phase component of common melanomas. Similar cases of nodular or "tumoral" melanosis may result from the regression of nonmelanocytic neoplasms, such as certain basal cell carcinomas that become heavily pigmented due to an embedded population of hyperplastic benign melanocytes (106,107). Melanin bleach stains help exclude cytologic atypia when nuclear detail is obscured. Immunohistochemistry for melanocytic and histiocytic markers (MART-1 and CD68, respectively) using a red chromogen distinct from the brown melanin pigment may also exclude a persistent or predominant melanocytic component in such lesions. A Giemsa counterstain, which renders melanin a green color that is more readily distinguished from other chromogens, may also be helpful in evaluating these neoplasms (108). Patients with tumoral melanosis should be carefully evaluated and followed since a preceding completely regressed melanoma cannot be excluded.

We occasionally have observed expansile zones of melanophages resembling tumoral melanosis in sentinel lymph nodes. As with primary cutaneous sites, such foci must be regarded as suspicious for zones of regression of metastatic melanoma and are reported as such.

MALIGNANT MELANOCYTIC SCHWANNOMA

Definition. *Malignant melanocytic schwannoma* is a malignant neoplasm derived from Schwann cells, typically originating in a large peripheral nerve, and composed focally of epithelioid pigment-synthesizing cells.

Clinical Features. The lesions usually present as deep-seated bulky neoplasms, only occasionally involving the dermis or subcutaneous tissues (109). Sometimes there is a history of a longstanding tumor followed by the recent onset of more rapid growth. In a review of 34 cases (110), the spinal nerve roots were the single most common site of presentation; tumors in this site commonly present with spinal cord compression.

Gross Findings. On gross examination, the lesions are usually several centimeters in diameter, and often appear circumscribed or partially encapsulated. The spinal root lesions may show the dumbbell configuration typical of schwannomas in that area. Pigment is usually appreciable on gross sectioning, and sometimes the lesions are jet black throughout. Carney (111) initially described 40 cases of a related lesion termed "psammomatous melanotic schwannoma," which is familial (autosomal dominant) in about 50 percent of the cases, and which presented mostly in visceral organs. These tumors are often associated with a complex of myxomas in heart, skin, and breast; spotty pigmentation described as lentigines and blue nevi; and endocrine overactivity variously presenting as Cushing syndrome, sexual precocity, or acromegaly.

Microscopic Findings. At scanning magnification, malignant melanocytic schwannomas are often circumscribed but not well encapsulated, and their borders may be frankly infiltrative and destructive. Most, if not all, dermal lesions involve nerves, and this neurotropism is similar in morphology and clinical significance to that of neurotropic melanoma. Indeed, there is complete overlap between the dermal component of neurotropic melanoma and dermal malignant melanocytic schwannoma, so much so that many consultants prefer to classify these tumors as *"nerve-centered" desmoplastic (and/or*

neurotropic) malignant melanomas (fig. 10-13) (28). This distinction is to some extent arbitrary and may have little clinical significance. In our own practice, we use the term melanoma for lesions that involve the epidermis or at least the papillary dermis, and for malignant lesions that show strong and diffuse S-100 protein reactivity (112). Compared to ordinary desmoplastic melanomas, these "nerve-centered" lesions tend to occur in a younger age group (mean, 53 years), with a marked male preponderance. Most of the lesions occur on the head and neck (28).

Cytologically, there is a variable pattern from region to region, with spindle cells predominating throughout the tumor but with considerable variation in cellularity. Focal areas of epithelioid or round/cuboidal differentiation often present as islands within the spindle cell background. In areas of lower cellularity, the cells are arranged in fascicles of spindle cells with wavy cytoplasm and S-shaped nuclei. In these areas, there is abundant intercellular eosinophilic collagenous and basement membrane-like material, as can be demonstrated with a reticulin stain. In areas of higher cellularity, the cells may be plumper, with more cytoplasm but less intercellular material. It is in these areas of plump spindle or epithelioid cells that pigment is most likely to be seen. The pigment is often arranged in coarse granules as well as the fine granules more characteristic of common melanomas, and sometimes a dendritic cytoplasmic configuration is outlined by the pigment. Mitoses are not necessarily frequent, but are always detectable given sufficient sampling. The presence of even a single mitosis in a neural tumor should lead to a very careful consideration of malignancy, as should melanocytic differentiation and pigment synthesis, which are rare in benign schwannomas, if they occur at all. Most of these tumors do not show extensive necrosis, but if present, this is also an important sign of malignancy. In Carney's series of psammomatous melanocytic schwannomas (111), the natural history was indolent, and most of the cases were cured by excision. Four incompletely excised tumors recurred, however, and 4 of the 31 patients eventually died of metastatic disease, indicating the malignant potential of these lesions. The metastasizing tumors exhibited necrosis, large nucleolated cells, and/or mitoses.

The few examples of this tumor that have been studied immunohistochemically have commonly reacted with S-100 protein and with HMB45, a reaction pattern similar to that of melanomas. The pattern is somewhat different from that of benign schwannomas, which are usually unreactive with HMB45.

Differential Diagnosis. When pigment is prominent, the lesions are often initially misinterpreted as metastatic melanoma. This distinction is important, as the prognosis for a patient with primary malignant schwannoma is likely to be much better than that for metastatic melanoma. The plump spindle or epithelioid and pigmented cells may be indistinguishable from those of a metastatic melanoma in particular areas of these tumors, and the diagnosis must be made by recognizing the more characteristic neural tumor patterns in other regions of the neoplasm. It is possible that some examples of so-called metastatic melanoma presenting in soft tissue with no known primary site might represent primary pigment-synthesizing neoplasms of peripheral nerve tissue that lack evident neural differentiation, but this phenomenon is not likely to explain the more common node-based malignant melanomas that appear to be metastases from an unknown primary site (113).

Primary desmoplastic and neurotropic malignant melanomas overlap morphologically with malignant epithelioid schwannomas. If there are characteristic patterns of melanoma in the epidermis, these lesions are readily recognized, but we have seen tumors that lack epidermal involvement while exhibiting both melanocytic and neural differentiation, and we prefer to categorize these tumors as malignant melanocytic schwannomas rather than melanomas. This distinction, however, unlike that between the primary and metastatic tumors discussed above, may have little or no prognostic or therapeutic importance.

CLEAR CELL SARCOMA

Definition. *Clear cell sarcoma* is a soft tissue neoplasm originally described by Enzinger (114) that is composed of rounded or spindle cells, usually with pale-staining cytoplasm, often arranged in nests and fascicles that are separated by delicate fibrous septa (115). As a result of these growth patterns, the tumors resemble melanoma, and indeed, about half of them contain melanin

pigment and melanosomes. Immunohistochemical reactivity is similar to that of melanoma, so that these lesions are synonymously known as *malignant melanoma of soft parts.*

The lesions are characterized by a t(12;22) chromosome translocation in which there is fusion of the Ewing sarcoma gene *EWS* with the transcriptional factor gene *ATF1* (116). The *EWS* gene, which encodes an RNA binding protein, is also involved in Ewing sarcoma, certain primitive neuroectodermal tumors, and desmoplastic small round cell tumors. It has been demonstrated that the *EWS-ATF1* fusion gene product functions as an efficient constitutive transcriptional activator, unlike the normal ATF1 which needs to be activated (117). This or a related fusion gene is present in 90 percent of cases and can be useful in establishing the diagnosis (118–120).

Clinical Features. The lesions typically arise in association with tendons and aponeuroses, especially in the extremities, and in particular, in the foot and ankle region, where 43 percent of 141 cases described by Enzinger and Weiss occurred (114). The lesions present as a slowly enlarging mass, often of considerable duration (average, 2 years), associated with pain in about half of the cases. Even after appropriate management by radical excision or, if necessary, by amputation, the ultimate prognosis is poor, although perhaps somewhat better than would be the case for common cutaneous melanomas of similar large size. Only 34 of Enzinger and Weiss' patients were free of disease, with an average time to recurrence of 2.6 years. In other studies, the median survival has been approximately 4 years, with 5-year survival rates of about 50 percent and a 10-year survival of 36 percent (116,121–123). For patients who present with localized disease, the 5-year disease-free survival rate in one study was 65 percent (122). Some patients exhibit a prolonged course punctuated by multiple recurrences and ultimately terminated by disseminated disease.

Prognosis is related to tumor size: the prognosis of patients with tumors larger than 5 cm is very poor (121). Patients with a tumor 2 cm or smaller may have better survival rate than patients with a larger but still-localized tumor. Adjuvant radiotherapy to the primary tumor site may have a beneficial effect on survival. In a recent study that included 52 patients who presented with localized disease, significant prognostic factors included sex, tumor size, tumor depth, TNM stage, and chemotherapy (123). Most patients with a local recurrence or regional lymph node metastasis develop distant metastasis, and most of these die of their tumor. It has been emphasized that early diagnosis and initial radical surgery are essential for a favorable outcome, and that once regional lymph node metastasis or hematogenous dissemination has occurred, the prognosis is dismal (122).

Gross Findings. The resected lesions are circumscribed but not usually encapsulated, and usually in the 2- to 6-cm size range (and thus considerably larger than most common cutaneous melanomas). The cut surface is gray-white and sometimes lobulated. Occasional cases exhibit focal brown melanin pigmentation, and there may be foci of hemorrhage and spontaneous necrosis. The lesions are attached to tendons or aponeuroses in most instances, and there is no connection with the overlying epidermis, although large lesions may secondarily involve the dermis from below.

Microscopic Findings. At scanning magnification, the pattern is that of nests and fascicles of clear cells with rounded polygonal or plump fusiform cytoplasm, separated by collagenous septa (fig. 10-28). This "packeted" appearance is also seen in some melanomas, but not often in such a well-developed form as is usual in clear cell sarcoma and therefore is a helpful diagnostic clue. Foci of necrosis or hemorrhage may be apparent at low power, especially in larger lesions. The border of the tumor is histologically infiltrative and destructive of surrounding tissues, despite the circumscription that may be apparent at gross examination. Pigment is not often prominent at low power, but may be appreciated at higher magnification. The lesional cells are fairly uniform, with round-oval vesicular nuclei and prominent basophilic nucleoli, similar to melanoma cells. The cytoplasm is usually clear, but may, in some cells and in some lesions, be predominantly eosinophilic, more like that seen in melanomas. Tumor giant cells are a characteristic feature, having multiple nuclei but otherwise similar to the mononuclear tumor cells. Mitotic figures are readily detectable, but the mitotic rate is often low compared to melanomas of comparable size.

Necrosis is common, especially in large tumors. The stroma is occasionally mucinous, as is also true of occasional melanomas, and as in melanoma, the nests of cells are outlined by reticulin fibers as revealed by reticulin stains. Melanin is detected with silver stains like Fontana preparations in 50 percent of cases; the Warthin-Starry stain at pH 3.2 is even more sensitive.

Ultrastructurally, the nuclear features are as described at the light microscopic level. The cytoplasm contains prominent swollen mitochondria, membrane-bounded vesicles, variable ribosomes, and glycogen granules. Melanosomes are present in some tumors, their incidence no doubt depending on the assiduous searching of multiple sections.

The immunohistochemistry of clear cell sarcoma is similar to that of malignant melanoma. In an early study of six cases with a panel of antibodies, four were reactive for S-100 protein antigen, and five with HMB45 (124). All six lesions contained vimentin, while five cases expressed neuron-specific enolase and four expressed the class II histocompatibility antigen LN3. Cytokeratin, epithelial membrane antigen, carcinoembryonic antigen, desmin, muscle-specific actin, and leukocyte common antigen were absent. Clear cell sarcoma is positive for CD117 (c-kit) in about 50 percent of cases (125). The tumors are usually positive for MITF, and the EGF receptor variant ERBB3 has recently been shown to be overexpressed (82,126).

Differential Diagnosis. The differential diagnosis of clear cell sarcoma includes other epithelioid and clear cell sarcomas and metastatic melanoma. Distinguishing metastatic melanoma is very important, both with respect to prognosis and treatment. Synovial sarcoma can be distinguished by its lack of S-100 protein and HMB45 reactivity and by its biphasic epithelial and spindle cell patterns with cytokeratin and epithelial membrane antigen reactivity. The immunohistochemical profile of epithelioid sarcoma is similar to that of synovial sarcoma. Epithelioid leiomyosarcoma is distinguished by its desmin and muscle-specific reactivity. Clear cell metastatic carcinomas, including renal carcinoma, are distinguished by keratin reactivity. Malignant epithelioid or melanocytic schwannomas may be a consideration, but clear cell sarcoma is not associated with a large peripheral nerve

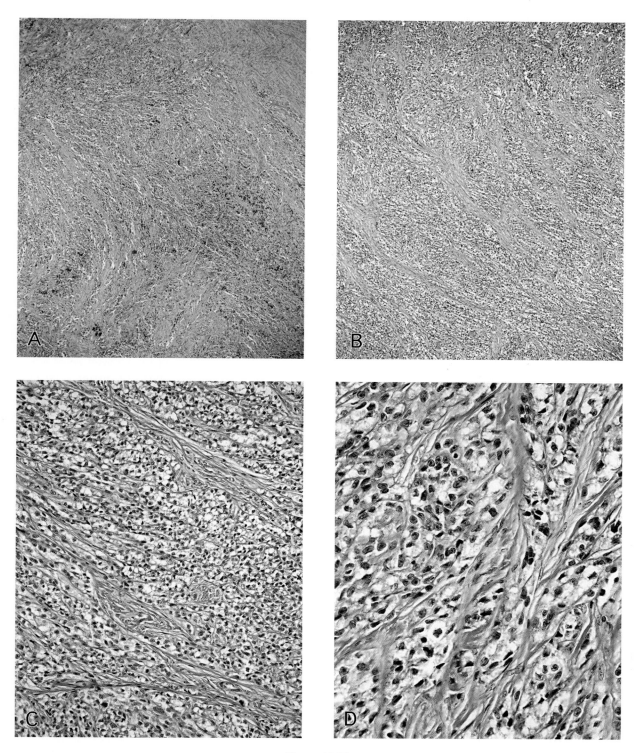

Figure 10-28

CLEAR CELL SARCOMA

A bulky subcutaneous tumor is composed of large cells with clear cytoplasm and prominent nucleoli embedded in a dense fibrous stroma.

and has not been reported in association with neurofibromatosis. Furthermore, neural sarcomas do not typically react with HMB45, which is regarded as highly specific for melanoma, but also reacts with most clear cell sarcomas. Cellular and malignant blue nevi are usually much more heavily pigmented, and there is an associated blue nevus component of small spindle cells among the collagen bundles.

Although clear cell sarcoma cannot reliably be distinguished from melanoma and is regarded as a primary malignant melanoma of soft tissue, it is important to distinguish it from metastatic melanoma. Histologically, the cells of metastases from a cutaneous primary are usually more epithelioid or rounded, with eosinophilic cytoplasm. The metastatic tumors rarely exhibit such a prominent packeted appearance, and mitoses are usually more frequent. Subcutaneous metastatic melanoma is rare in the absence of a known primary or of widespread metastatic disease elsewhere.

DERMAL MELANOCYTIC TUMORS OF UNCERTAIN MALIGNANT POTENTIAL (MELTUMP)

Definition. *Dermal melanocytic tumors of uncertain malignant potential* (MELTUMP) is a descriptive term for an ill-defined group of dermal melanocytic tumors that are often quite bulky and frequently exophytic, and exhibit one or several features indicative of possible malignancy, such as nuclear atypia, macronucleoli, mitotic activity, necrosis, or ulceration, but exhibit these features in number or degree insufficient to justify a malignant diagnosis. This is clearly a heterogeneous group of cases that may be related to cellular and atypical blue nevi, minimal deviation melanomas, and atypical Spitz tumors, and also perhaps to some benign lesions including combined nevi and deep penetrating nevi. Some lesions, such as pigmented epithelioid melanocytoma, carry an intrinsic connotation of uncertain malignant potential (97). Potentially tumorigenic lesions that may generate uncertainty because of atypical features are listed in Table 10-2.

Clinical Features. There are few clinical data for this heterogeneous group of tumors. Most of these lesions have been seen in consultation, often with a history of slow growth of

Table 10-2

EXAMPLES OF LESIONS THAT MAY SIMULATE MELANOMA AND GENERATE UNCERTAINTY

Compound nevocellular nevi with dermal mitoses and atypia

Spitz nevi with atypical features (atypical Spitz tumors)

Pigmented spindle cell nevi with dermal atypia

Dysplastic nevi with dermal atypia

Halo and inflamed nevi with atypia

Desmoplastic nevi with unusual features

Cellular blue nevi with atypia

Some deep penetrating nevi

Pigmented epithelioid melanocytoma

Any Spitz nevus in older individuals

Nevi lacking maturation

a blue-black pigmented nodule. The clearest example of an uncertain diagnosis is a lesion that has been reviewed by a panel of experts, with equal numbers favoring either a benign or a malignant diagnosis. For such a difficult or impossible diagnostic problem, the descriptive diagnosis of "uncertain" is clearly the only correct interpretation.

Cerroni and Kerl (127) published an important study in which six experts reviewed 71 cases of mostly "difficult" melanocytic tumors, many of which were thick, tumorigenic lesions. These cases were discussed at the International Society of Dermatopathology meeting in Graz, Austria, in 2001. Although the overall agreement for these difficult cases was about 80 percent, there was substantial disagreement. The diagnostic disagreement was concentrated in particular areas. Benign nevi in general, and in particular, Spitz nevus variants in adults and nevoid/spitzoid melanomas, accounted for the majority of the disagreement. Ironically, although there was almost perfect agreement for childhood Spitz nevi, one of these later metastasized and caused the death of the patient. The existence in this series of cases that elicit "perfect disagreement" (i.e., three observers for a malignant and three for a benign diagnosis) clearly indicates that the state of the art in histologic diagnosis still leaves room for uncertainty in diagnosis; in such a case, the only correct diagnosis is a descriptive diagnosis of MELTUMP.

Microscopic Findings. The tumors that we have placed in this descriptive category have tended to be bulky neoplasms, several millimeters in diameter and thickness. They are composed of pigmented, often spindle shaped cells that have abundant cytoplasm and contain finely divided but sometimes coarse melanin pigment (figs. 10-29–10-33). The cells may be arranged in nested clusters, and the overall cellularity is relatively low compared to fully malignant melanomas. There may be features of schwannian differentiation, such as spindle cells surrounding clusters of plumper, more epithelioid cells in a pattern reminiscent of neurosustentacular cells, or wavy spindle cell fiber bundles similar to those observed in neurofibromas (fig. 10-29). Cells may be seen in peripheral nerves, a finding that may also be seen in benign blue nevi and Spitz nevi and is not automatically indicative of malignancy. The nuclei are often large and may contain eosinophilic or amphophilic nucleoli. There may be occasional mitoses, but not more than one or a few per section plane. If the mitotic rate is greater than 2/mm^2, the diagnosis is usually melanoma. Abnormal mitoses are not typically observed (if so, the lesion would likely be termed malignant melanoma). Focal areas of individual cell necrosis may be present, but there are no areas of confluent geographic necrosis, and the lesions do not spontaneously ulcerate. Most of these lesions have only a few scattered stromal lymphocytes, but a few have a more prominent lymphocytic response and melanophages may be fairly numerous. There may be a few enlarged melanocytes in the epidermis but, importantly, there is no atypical intraepidermal component that can be construed as the radial growth phase of a malignant melanoma of any of the common types.

Another category of a MELTUMP lesion is characterized by atypia of the epidermal component, which may fall short or minimally meet the criteria for melanoma in situ. Clusters of cells in the dermis also exhibit atypia, generally without mitotic activity, and are larger than the largest intraepidermal clusters or nests, raising suspicion of a tumorigenic lesion. These lesions, in contrast to the bulky tumors discussed above, are likely to be thin, low-stage lesions, with a

good prognosis. Nevertheless, the presence of a possible tumorigenic component suggests a lesion with some, albeit low, competence for metastasis (fig. 10-34).

Ancillary diagnostic techniques, such as the use of the proliferation marker Ki-67 (128–131), mutational analysis (132), morphometric techniques including DNA microdensitometry, karyometry, argyrophilic staining of nucleolar organizer regions (131), and chromosomal analysis by comparative genomic hybridization (133,134), are beginning to be used to provide additional diagnostic information, but in the present state of knowledge, are rarely definitive. These techniques have been discussed more fully in the sections that deal with specific entities in the differential diagnosis of MELTUMP.

Differential Diagnosis. This descriptive diagnosis is one of exclusion, and the differential diagnosis includes specific neoplasms that are described elsewhere in this Fascicle. Deep penetrating nevi give some cause for concern because of cellular atypia, but atypia alone in the absence of mitoses or necrosis should not lead to a diagnosis of malignancy. Cellular neurothekeoma, discussed in the section on neurotropic melanoma, is a benign dermal nerve sheath tumor that may mimic a low-grade melanocytic tumor. In these lesions, pigment and necrosis are absent, and mitotic activity is low (61).

Common blue nevi are not usually suspected of malignancy because of their low cellularity and lack of significant atypia. Cellular blue nevi that exhibit a characteristic dumbbell configuration at scanning magnification and an alveolar cytoarchitectural pattern are easily recognized with specificity. Lesions that lack these features yet present as a bulky neoplasm of dermal pigment-synthesizing melanocytes are difficult to place into any nosologic category. When a few mitoses are present or there is subtle focal necrosis, the term "atypical cellular blue nevus" is often used, and this diagnosis is considered to be predictive of benign behavior. We have seen a few such lesions, however, that have recurred after incomplete therapy and progressed to a more cellular, high-grade neoplasm, and we prefer to express our uncertainty about the biologic potential and histogenesis of such lesions directly. If a recognizable radial growth phase of melanoma is observed adjacent to a nodule of

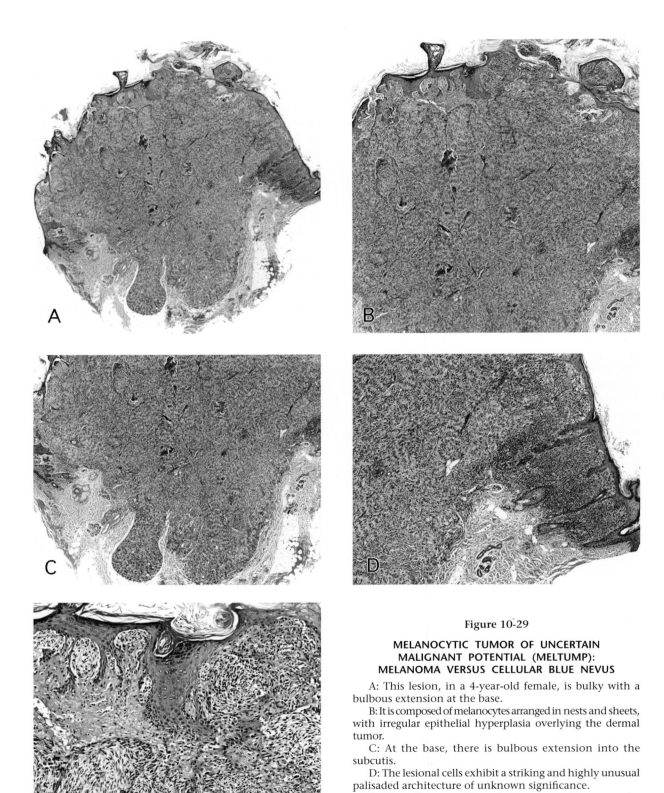

Figure 10-29

MELANOCYTIC TUMOR OF UNCERTAIN MALIGNANT POTENTIAL (MELTUMP): MELANOMA VERSUS CELLULAR BLUE NEVUS

A: This lesion, in a 4-year-old female, is bulky with a bulbous extension at the base.

B: It is composed of melanocytes arranged in nests and sheets, with irregular epithelial hyperplasia overlying the dermal tumor.

C: At the base, there is bulbous extension into the subcutis.

D: The lesional cells exhibit a striking and highly unusual palisaded architecture of unknown significance.

E: The cells are uniform from side to side across the lesion.

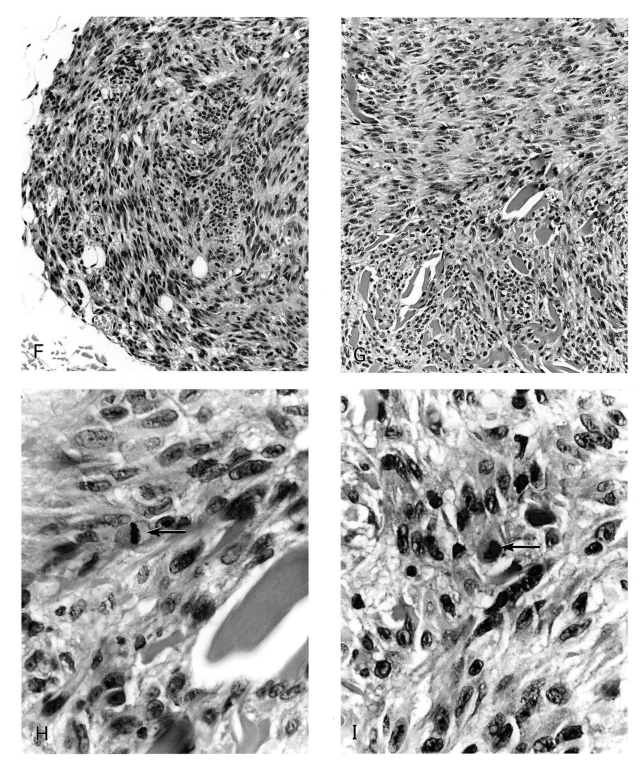

Figure 10-29 (continued)

F,G: There is little or no evidence of maturation from superficial to deep.
H,I: Only a rare mitotic figure (arrows) is observed.

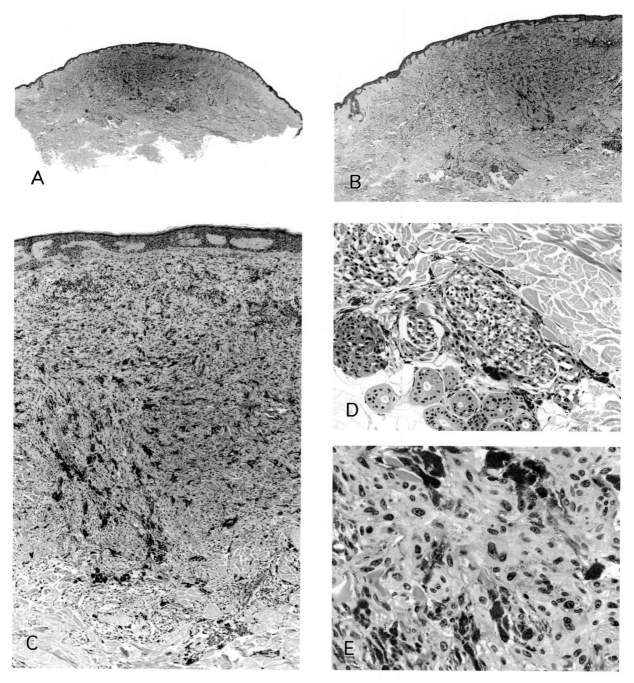

Figure 10-30

MELANOCYTIC TUMOR OF UNCERTAIN MALIGNANT POTENTIAL (MELTUMP): CELLULAR NODULE VERSUS MALIGNANT MELANOMA

A,B: This lesion has two major components: a congenital pattern nevus evident at the upper right and left, and a more cellular asymmetric proliferation of pigmented cells extending into the reticular dermis.

C–E: The cellular proliferation is highly infiltrative, with irregular and jagged borders. The nodule tends to blend with the more nevoid cells superficially (D). Large cells at the base of the tumor have finely divided cytoplasmic melanin pigment and associated melanophages (D,E).

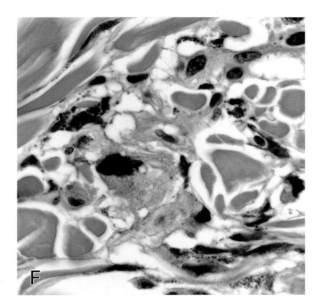

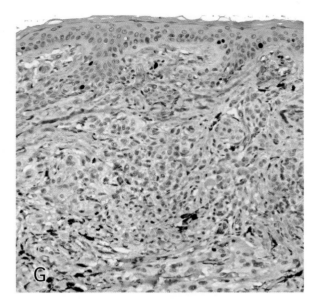

Figure 10-30 (continued)

D–F: Moderate to severe cytologic atypia is present in the form of nuclear enlargement and irregularity, and nucleoli. Rare mitotic figures were seen, including this abnormal one (F).

G: The Ki-67 proliferation rate was minimal.

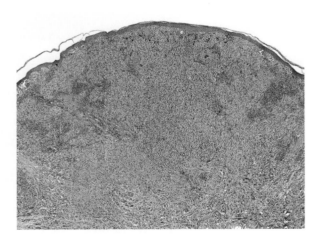

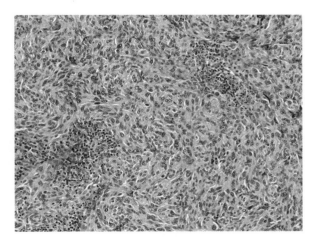

Figure 10-31

MELANOCYTIC TUMOR OF UNCERTAIN MALIGNANT POTENTIAL (MELTUMP): ATYPICAL SPITZ NEVUS VERSUS SPITZOID MELANOMA

Left: This bulky tumor deeply invades the reticular dermis. Lesional cells are large spindle to epithelioid cells.

Right: The pattern of growth in sheets is unusual for Spitz nevus. We would interpret this lesion as a MELTUMP if mitotic activity was low or as a melanoma if activity was greater than 2/mm².

this type, or if there are changes of melanoma in the epidermis above the nodule, the lesion is appropriately classified as a vertical growth phase tumor of malignant melanoma. Usually, the radial growth phase in these circumstances is one of the lentiginous variants: lentigo maligna, acral-lentiginous, or mucosal-lentiginous melanoma. These lentiginous melanomas are more likely than superficial spreading melanomas to be associated with well-differentiated spindle cells in their associated tumorigenic vertical growth phase compartments.

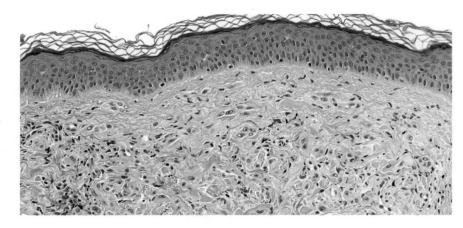

Figure 10-32

ATYPICAL DERMAL SPITZOID MELANOCYTIC PROLIFERATION

We would likely interpret this lesion as a dermal Spitz nevus if the mitotic rate was zero or very low or as a MELTUMP if mitoses were present, especially in a patient older than 30 years.

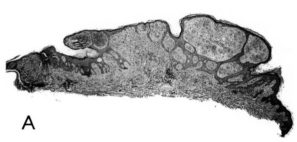

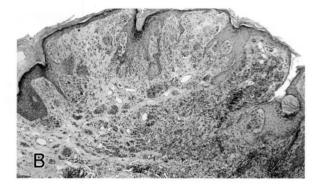

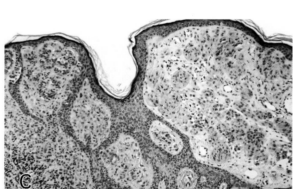

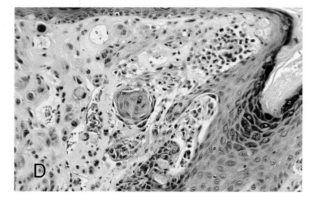

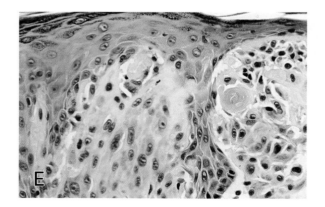

Figure 10-33

MELANOCYTIC TUMOR OF UNCERTAIN MALIGNANT POTENTIAL (MELTUMP): ATYPICAL SPITZ NEVUS VERSUS SPITZOID MELANOMA

A,B: This asymmetric lesion has a heterogeneous population of cells ranging from small to large which are not uniform from side to side across the lesion.

C: The mixture of small and larger cells argues against a diagnosis of Spitz nevus.

D: Epithelioid cells are superficial, with a few eosinophilic Kamino bodies at the junction.

E: Uniformly atypical large epithelioid cells with globoid eosinophilic Kamino bodies at the dermal-epidermal junction.

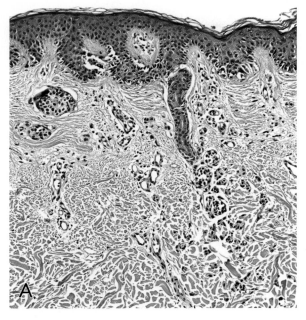

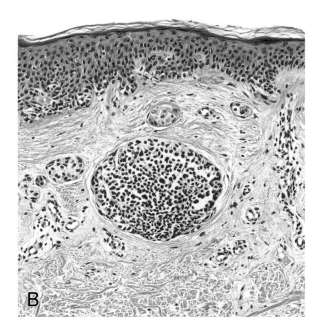

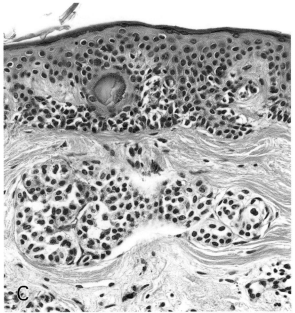

Figure 10-34

MELANOCYTIC TUMOR OF UNCERTAIN MALIGNANT POTENTIAL (MELTUMP): SEVERE DERMAL AND EPIDERMAL DYSPLASIA VERSUS EARLY TUMORIGENIC MALIGNANT MELANOMA

A: At low-power magnification, there is a nested and lentiginous proliferation mainly near the tips and sides of elongated rete ridges, with bridging nests. In the dermis, there is lamellar fibroplasia as well as clusters of nevoid melanocytes.

B,C: Two clusters of cells in the dermis are considerably larger than the largest intraepidermal clusters; however, there is nevoid maturation and there are no dermal mitoses. In our opinion, these changes are most consistent with severe dermal and epidermal melanocytic dysplasia.

Possibly related lesions include the ill-defined lesions characterized by dendritic cells stuffed with abundant and coarsely divided pigment that obscures the nucleus. Sometimes these cells are difficult to distinguish from melanophages, and the initial differential may therefore include tumoral melanosis. Some of these lesions, despite their unusual cytology, have features suggestive or diagnostic of nodular malignant melanoma, and a few have metastasized. Some related lesions, where criteria for malignancy are not deemed to have been fully met, are placed in the descriptive category of "uncertain malignant potential." These lesions overlap with the tumors discussed earlier in the chapter as "pigmented epithelioid melanocytoma" (97) or "pigment synthesizing melanoma" (105).

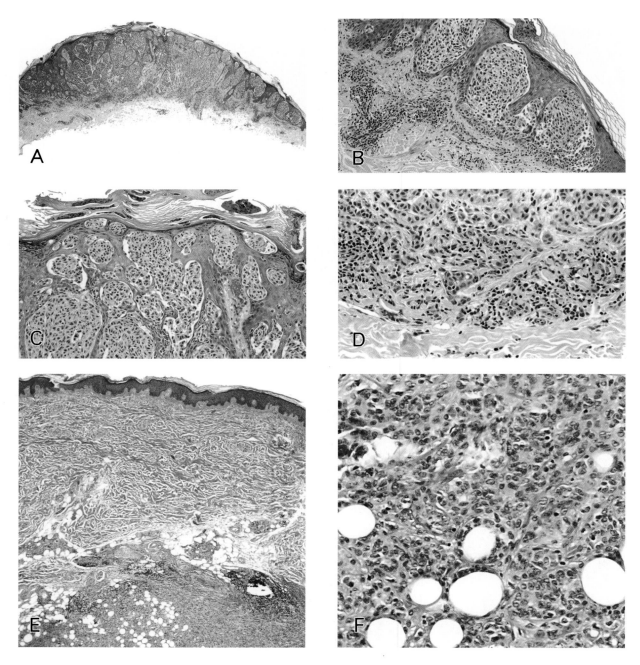

Figure 10-35

**MALIGNANT MELANOMA, TUMORIGENIC (SPITZOID) WITH
LARGE SPINDLE AND EPITHELIOID CELLS, AND LOCAL METASTASIS**

A: Scanning magnification shows a lesion characterized by large spindle and epithelioid cells arranged in nests with clefting artifact, reminiscent of a Spitz nevus.

B: There are large nests of cells with clefting artifact; however, the cells are not uniformly large spindle and/or epithelioid cells.

C: There is pagetoid extension of single cells as well as cells in nests to the stratum corneum.

D: There was little or no evidence of maturation from superficial to deep and the cells do not disperse as single cells into the reticular dermis.

E: Two years after excision and definitive therapy of the above described lesion, a dermal metastasis presented.

F: The metastasis consists of uniformly atypical, small epithelioid cells.

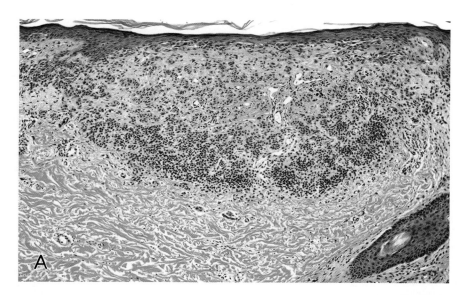

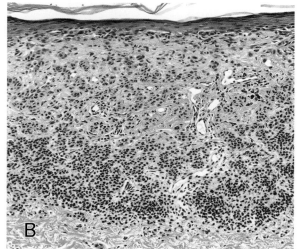
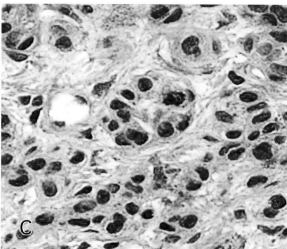

Figure 10-36

**MELANOCYTIC TUMOR OF UNCERTAIN
MALIGNANT POTENTIAL (MELTUMP): NEVOID
MELANOMA VERSUS NEVUS WITH MITOSIS**

A: There is a continuous proliferation of uniformly atypical cells along the dermal-epidermal junction superficially. Large cells in the upper papillary dermis mature to a smaller nevoid cell type at the base of the lesion and disperse into the reticular dermis.

B: Nevoid maturation occurs from superficial to deep, with dispersed single cells at the base.

C: A single mitotic figure is observed in the superficial epithelioid cell population.

The concept of MELTUMP allows for patient safety because the recommended therapy is to apply the minimal treatment for melanoma, based on the putative microstage of the tumor (i.e., the microstaging attributes that would have been applied if the lesion had been interpreted as a melanoma). The differential diagnosis, of course, includes malignant melanomas that mimic benign lesions. Figures 10-35–10-39 are examples of lesions that could be considered "uncertain," but which, in our opinion, are more appropriately classified directly as malignant melanomas. Use of the term MELTUMP for lesions with such hybrid features should segregate such borderline

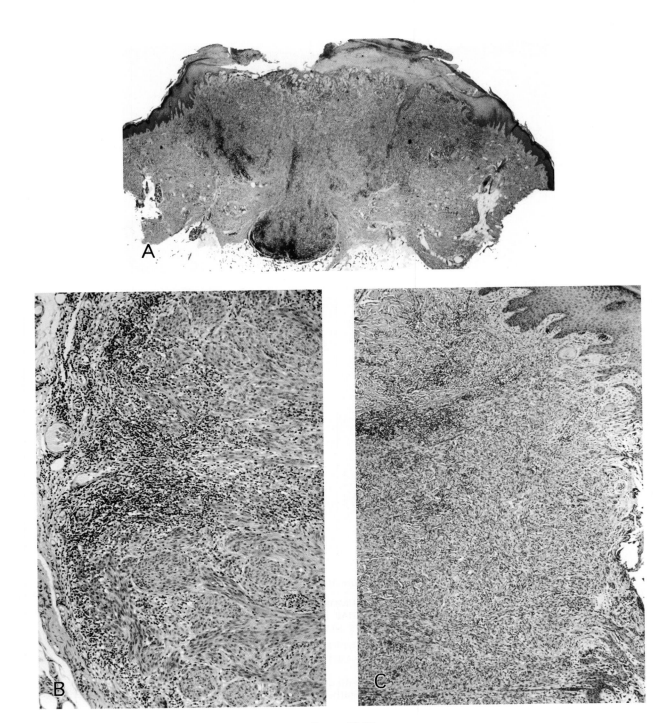

Figure 10-37

MELANOCYTIC TUMOR OF UNCERTAIN MALIGNANT POTENTIAL (MELTUMP): MELANOMA VERSUS SPITZ NEVUS

A: This bulky tumor, in a 10-year-old patient, is covered by a scaley crust and has a bulbous extension into the dermis and subcutis at the base.

B: At the base, the lesional cells remain cohesive rather than separating into the reticular dermis and there is a brisk tumor-infiltrating lymphocytic response.

C: Superficially, there is an ill-defined nested pattern and there are sheets of uniformly atypical spindle to epithelioid melanocytes.

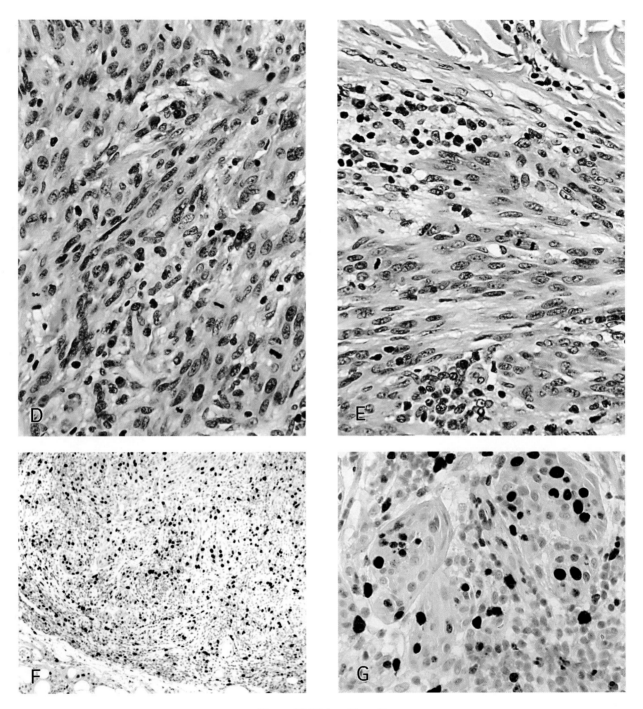

Figure 10-37 (continued)

D,E: Frequent mitotic figures are present. This degree of mitotic activity is not consistent with an unqualified diagnosis of a Spitz nevus.

F,G: The Ki-67 activity in this lesion was relatively high. Despite the age of the patient and the spitzoid appearance of the lesion in some respects, we favor a diagnosis of malignant melanoma in this case and would recommend definitive management based on that diagnosis.

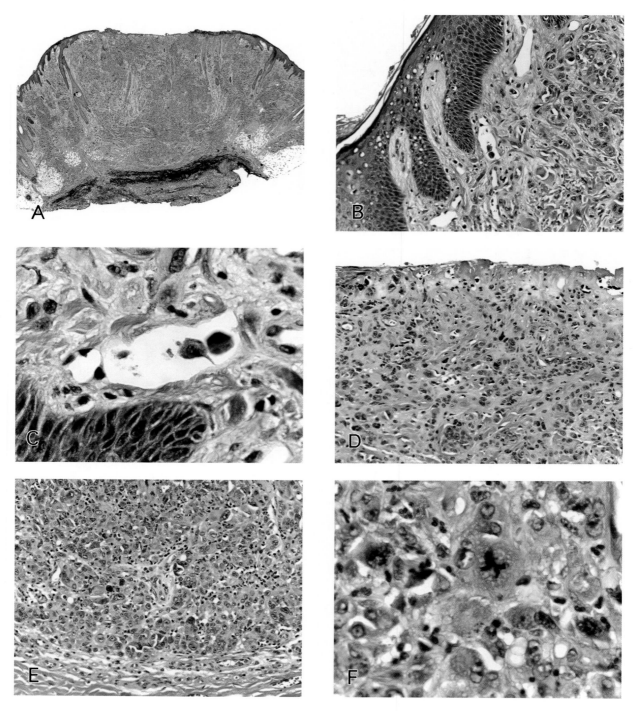

Figure 10-38

MALIGNANT MELANOMA, WITH SPITZOID FEATURES

A,B: This lesion from the scalp of a 2-year-old child presents as a bulky tumor spanning the reticular dermis. The lesional cells are uniformly large and epithelioid.

C: Tumor cells are seen in a lymphatic channel.

D,E: The surface is ulcerated. There is no evidence of maturation from superficial to deep.

F: Abnormal mitotic figures are observed and the overall mitotic rate is 5/mm^2.

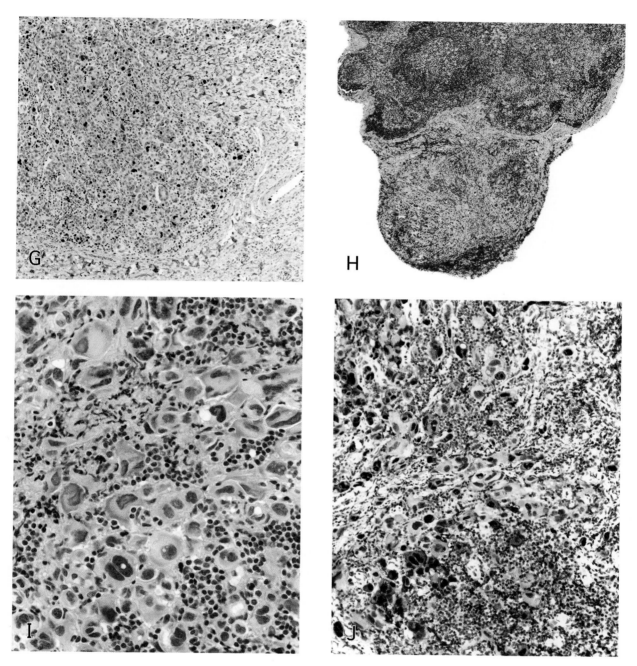

Figure 10-38 (continued)

G: The Ki-67 proliferation rate was low to moderate.

H: A reexcision was done and a sentinel lymph node sampling procedure was performed. This was positive for metastatic melanoma.

I: Higher magnification shows uniformly atypical epithelioid melanocytes infiltrating the node.

J: S-100 protein is positive in the lymph node.

tumors for 1) consideration for therapy along the lines of the worst-case scenario (equivalently microstaged melanoma), 2) further study in order to better define clinicopathological characteristics of members of this group, and 3) appreciation by patients, clinicians, and litigators

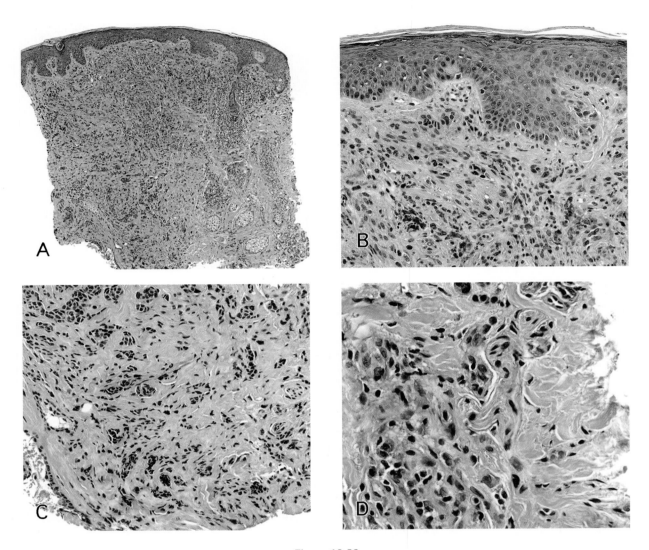

Figure 10-39

**MELANOCYTIC TUMOR OF UNCERTAIN MALIGNANT POTENTIAL (MELTUMP): DEEP PENETRATING
NEVUS VERSUS CONGENITAL NEVUS, CELLULAR BLUE NEVUS, AND MELANOMA**

A: This lesion, from the nose of a 19-year-old patient, shows an infiltrative melanocytic neoplasm extending into the reticular dermis and to both margins of the punch biopsy specimen. The lesion is composed of uniform epithelioid melanocytes with scant, finely divided melanin pigment and interstitial melanophages and lymphocytes.

B: There is no in situ component of a melanoma.

C: There is some evidence of maturation from superficial to deep.

D: Tumor cells are present around a small cutaneous nerve near the margin. The diagnostic features of this lesion are conflicting. For example, there is uniform atypia and a highly infiltrative pattern; yet there is evidence of maturation, and mitotic figures were rare or absent. It was recommended that this lesion be completely excised in the hope of obtaining a more precise diagnosis. Follow-up material is not available. The diagnosis remains uncertain.

that such a category separate from atypical nevi exists in terms of our present limitations in predicting outcome.

Some lesions cannot be classified descriptively because the submitted specimen does not provide sufficient information for a more specific classification (see fig. 9-3). In such a case, we recommend complete excision in order to obtain more diagnostic material.

REFERENCES

1. Heenan PJ, Holman CD. Nodular malignant melanoma: a distinct entity or a common end stage? Am J Dermatopathol 1982;4:477-478.

2. Winnepenninckx V, Biec-Rychter M, Belien JA, et al. Expression and possible role of hPTTG1/securin in cutaneous malignant melanoma. Mod Pathol 2006;19:1170-1180.

3. Chamberlain AJ, Fritschi L, Kelly JW. Nodular melanoma: patients' perceptions of presenting features and implications for earlier detection. J Am Acad Dermatol 2003;48:694-701.

4. Liu W, Dowling JP, Murray WK, et al. Rate of growth in melanomas: characteristics and associations of rapidly growing melanomas. Arch Dermatol 2006;142:1551-1558.

5. Demirci H, Shields CL, Shields JA, Eagle RC, Honavar SG. Bilateral breast metastases from choroidal melanoma. Am J Ophthalmol 2001;131:521-523.

6. Kelly JW, Chamberlain AJ, Staples MP, McAvoy B. Nodular melanoma. No longer as simple as ABC. Aust Fam Physician 2003;32:706-709.

7. Chamberlain AJ, Fritschi L, Giles GG, Dowling JP, Kelly JW. Nodular type and older age as the most significant associations of thick melanoma in Victoria, Australia. Arch Dermatol 2002;138:609-614.

8. Clark WH Jr, Elder DE, Guerry D 4th, et al. Model predicting survival in stage I melanoma based on tumor progression. JNCI 1989;81:1893-1904.

9. Elder DE, Guerry D 4th, Epstein MN, et al. Invasive malignant melanomas lacking competence for metastasis. Am J Dermatopathol 1984;6:55-61.

10. Clark WH Jr, Elder DE, Van Horn M. The biologic forms of malignant melanoma. Hum Pathol 1986;5:443-450.

11. Phillips ME, Margolis RJ, Merot Y, et al. The spectrum of minimal deviation melanoma: a clinicopathologic study of 21 cases. Hum Pathol 1986;17:796-806.

12. Muhlbauer JE, Margolis RJ, Mihm MC Jr, Reed RJ. Minimal deviation melanoma: a histologic variant of cutaneous malignant melanoma in its vertical growth phase. J Invest Dermatol 1983;80(Suppl):63s-65s.

13. Reed RJ. Minimal deviation melanoma. In: Mihm MC Jr, Murphy GF, Kaufman N, eds. Pathobiology and recognition of malignant melanoma. Baltimore: Williams & Wilkins; 1988:110-152.

14. McGovern VJ. Melanoma, histological diagnosis and prognosis. New York: Raven Press; 1983:3-24.

15. Maize JC, Ackerman AB. Pigmented lesions of the skin: clinicopathologic correlations. Philadelphia: Lea & Febiger; 1987.

16. Busam KJ, Granter SR, Iversen K, Jungbluth AA. Immunohistochemical distinction of epithelioid histiocytic proliferations from epithelioid melanocytic nevi. Am J Dermatopathol 2000;22:237-241.

17. Jones EW, Cerio R, Smith NP. Epithelioid cell histiocytoma: a new entity. Br J Dermatol 1989;120:185-195.

18. Glusac EJ, McNiff JM. Epithelioid cell histiocytoma: a simulant of vascular and melanocytic neoplasms. Am J Dermatopathol 1999;21:1-7.

19. Husain S, Silvers DN, Halperin AJ, McNutt NS. Histologic spectrum of neurothekeoma and the value of immunoperoxidase staining for S-100 protein in distinguishing it from melanoma. Am J Dermatopathol 1994;16:496-503.

20. Fullen DR, Lowe L, Su LD. Antibody to S100a6 protein is a sensitive immunohistochemical marker for neurothekeoma. J Cutan Pathol 2003;30:118-122.

21. Page RN, King R, Mihm MC, Googe PB. Microphthalmia transcription factor and NKI/C3 expression in cellular neurothekeoma. Mod Pathol 2004;17:230-234.

22. Kocan P, Jurkovic I, Boor A, et al. Immunohistochemical study of melanocytic differentiation antigens in cutaneous malignant melanoma. A comparison of six commercial antibodies and one non-commercial antibody in nodular melanoma, superficially spreading melanoma and lentigo maligna melanoma. Cesk Patol 2004;40:50-56.

23. Xu X, Chu AY, Pasha TL, Elder DE, Zhang PJ. Immunoprofile of MITF, tyrosinase, melan-A, and MAGE-1 in HMB45-negative melanomas. Am J Surg Pathol 2002;26:82-87.

24. Conley J, Lattes R, Orr W. Desmoplastic malignant melanoma (a rare variant of spindle cell melanoma). Cancer 1971;28:914-936.

25. Paladugu RR, Winberg CD, Yonemoto RH. Acral lentiginous melanoma. A clinicopathologic study of 36 patients. Cancer 1983;52:161-168.

26. Prasad ML, Patel SG, Busam KJ. Primary mucosal desmoplastic melanoma of the head and neck. Head Neck 2004;26:373-377.

27. Benda JA, Platz CE, Anderson B. Malignant melanoma of the vulva: a clinical-pathologic review of 16 cases. Int J Gynecol Pathol 1986;5:202-216.

28. Jain S, Allen PW. Desmoplastic malignant melanoma and its variants. A study of 45 cases. Am J Surg Pathol 1989;13:358-373.

29. Quinn MJ, Crotty KA, Thompson JF, Coates AS, O'Brien CJ, McCarthy WH. Desmoplastic and desmoplastic neurotropic melanoma: experience with 280 patients [see comments]. Cancer 1998;83:1128-1135.

30. Krenek G, Orengo IF, Baer S, Byrd D. Desmoplastic malignant melanoma presenting as an erythematous nodule tumor. Cutis 1998;61:275-276.

31. Egbert B, Kempson R, Sagebiel RW. Desmoplastic malignant melanoma. A clinicohistopathologic study of 25 cases. Cancer 1988;62:2033-2041.

32. Reed RJ, Leonard DD. Neurotropic melanoma. A variant of desmoplastic melanoma. Am J Surg Pathol 1979;3:301-311.

33. DiMaiao SM, Mackay B, Smith JL, Dickersin GR. Neurosarcomatous transformation in malignant melanoma: an ultrastructural study. Cancer 1982;50:2345-2354.

34. From L, Hanna W, Kahn HJ, Gruss J, Marks A, Baumal R. Origin of the desmoplasia in desmoplastic malignant melanoma. Hum Pathol 1983;14:1072-1080.

35. Busam KJ, Zhao H, Coit DG, et al. Distinction of desmoplastic melanoma from non-desmoplastic melanoma by gene expression profiling. J Invest Dermatol 2005;124:412-418.

36. Busam KJ. Cutaneous desmoplastic melanoma. Adv Anat Pathol 2005;12:92-102.

37. Baron JA, Monzon F, Galaria N, Murphy GF. Angiomatoid melanoma: a novel pattern of differentiation in invasive periocular desmoplastic malignant melanoma. Hum Pathol 2000;31:1520-1522.

38. Robson A, Allen P, Hollowood K. S100 expression in cutaneous scars: a potential diagnostic pitfall in the diagnosis of desmoplastic melanoma. Histopathology 2001;38:135-140.

39. Eng W and Tschen JA. Comparison of S-100 versus hematoxylin and eosin staining for evaluating dermal invasion and peripheral margins by desmoplastic malignant melanoma. Am J Dermatopathol 2000;22:26-29.

40. Busam KJ, Iversen K, Coplan KC, Jungbluth AA. Analysis of microphthalmia transcription factor expression in normal tissues and tumors, and comparison of its expression with S-100 protein, gp100, and tyrosinase in desmoplastic malignant melanoma. Am J Surg Pathol 2001;25:197-204.

41. Clarkson KS, Sturdgess IC, Molyneux AJ. The usefulness of tyrosinase in the immunohistochemical assessment of melanocytic lesions: a comparison of the novel T311 antibody (anti-tyrosinase) with S-100, HMB45, and A103 (anti-melan-A). J Clin Pathol 201;54:196-200.

42. Granter SR, Weilbaecher KN, Quigley C, Fletcher CD, Fisher DE. Microphthalmia transcription factor: not a sensitive or specific marker for the diagnosis of desmoplastic melanoma and spindle cell (non-desmoplastic) melanoma. Am J Dermatopathol 2001;23:185-189.

43. Busam KJ, Chen YT, Old LJ, et al. Expression of melan-A (MART1) in benign melanocytic nevi and primary cutaneous malignant melanoma. Am J Surg Pathol 1998;22:976-982.

44. Jungbluth AA, Busam KJ, Gerald WL, et al. A103: an anti-Melan-a monoclonal antibody for the detection of malignant melanoma in paraffin-embedded tissues. Am J Surg Pathol 1998;22:595-602.

45. King R, Googe PB, Weilbaecher KN, Mihm MC, Fisher DE. Microphthalmia transcription factor expression in cutaneous benign, malignant melanocytic, and nonmelanocytic tumors. Am J Surg Pathol 2001;25:51-57.

46. Orchard GE. Comparison of immunohistochemical labelling of melanocyte differentiation antibodies melan-A, tyrosinase and HMB 45 with NKIC3 and S100 protein in the evaluation of benign naevi and malignant melanoma. Histochem J 2000;32:475-481.

47. Koch MB, Shih IM, Weiss SW, Folpe AL. Microphthalmia transcription factor and melanoma cell adhesion molecule expression distinguish desmoplastic/spindle cell melanoma from morphologic mimics. Am J Surg Pathol 2001;25:58-64.

48. Miettinen M, Fernandez M, Franssila K, Gatalica Z, Lasota J, Sarlomo-Rikala M. Microphthalmia transcription factor in the immunohistochemical diagnosis of metastatic melanoma: comparison with four other melanoma markers. Am J Surg Pathol 2001;25:205-211.

49. Attis MG, Burchette JL, Selim MA, Pham T, Soler AP. Differential expression of N-cadherin distinguishes a subset of metastasizing desmoplastic melanomas. Hum Pathol 2006;37:899-905.

50. Busam KJ, Kucukgol D, Eastlake-Wade S, Frosina D, Delgado R, Jungbluth AA. Clusterin expression in primary and metastatic melanoma. J Cutan Pathol 2006;33:619-623.

51. Radfar A, Stefanato CM, Ghosn S, Bhawan J. NGFR-positive desmoplastic melanomas with focal or absent S-100 staining: further evidence supporting the use of both NGFR and S-100 as a primary immunohistochemical panel for the diagnosis of desmoplastic melanomas. Am J Dermatopathol 2006;28:162-167.

52. Kucher C, Zhang PJ, Pasha T, et al. Melan-A and Ki67 as useful markers to discriminate desmoplastic melanoma from sclerotic nevi. USCAP Abstracts 2004.

53. Xu X, Elder DE. A practical approach to selected problematic melanocytic lesions. Am J Clin Pathol 2004;121(Suppl.):S3-32.

54. Baer SC, Schultz D, Synnestvedt M, Elder DE. Desmoplasia and neurotropism. Prognostic variables in patients with stage I melanoma. Cancer 1995;76:2242-2247.

55. Busam KJ, Mujumdar U, Hummer AJ, et al. Cutaneous desmoplastic melanoma: reappraisal of morphologic heterogeneity and prognostic factors. Am J Surg Pathol 2004;28:1518-1525.

56. Pawlik TM, Ross MI, Prieto VG, et al. Assessment of the role of sentinel lymph node biopsy for primary cutaneous desmoplastic melanoma. Cancer 2006;106:900-906.

57. Posther KE, Selim MA, Mosca PJ, et al. Histopathologic characteristics, recurrence patterns, and survival of 129 patients with desmoplastic melanoma. Ann Surg Oncol 2006;13:728-739.

58. Chang PC, Fischbein JN, McCalmont TH, et al. Perineural spread of malignant melanoma of the head and neck: clinical and imaging features. AJNR Am J Neuroradiol 2004;25:5-11.

59. Kossard S, Doherty E, Murray E. Neurotropic melanoma: a variant of desmoplastic melanoma. Arch Dermatol 1987;123:907-912.

60. Shields JA, Elder D, Arbizo V, Hedges T, Augsburger JJ. Orbital involvement with desmoplastic melanoma. Br J Ophthalmol 1987;71:279-284.

61. Barnhill RL, Mihm MC Jr. Cellular neurothekeoma. A distinctive variant of neurothekeoma mimicking nevomelanocytic tumors. Am J Surg Pathol 1990;14:113-120.

62. Rosati LA, Fratamico FC, Eusebi V. Cellular neurothekeoma. Appl Pathol 1986;4:186-191.

63. Garcia RI, Szabo G. Melanosomes in dermal Schwann cells of human and rodent skin. Arch Dermatol Res 1979;264:83-87.

64. Busam KJ, Mentzel T, Colpaert C, Barnhill RL, Fletcher CD. Atypical or worrisome features in cellular neurothekeoma: a study of 10 cases. Am J Surg Pathol 1998;22:1067-1072.

65. Hendrickson MR, Ross JC. Neoplasms arising in congenital giant nevi: morphologic study of seven cases and a review of the literature. Am J Surg Pathol 1981;5:109-135.

66. Clark WH Jr, Elder DE, Guerry D 4th. Dysplastic nevi and malignant melanoma. In: Farmer ER, Hood AF, eds. Pathology of the skin. Norwalk, CD: Appleton & Lange; 1990.

67. Watt AJ, Kotsis SV, Chung KC. Risk of melanoma arising in large congenital melanocytic nevi: a systematic review. Plast Reconstr Surg 2004;113:1968-1974.

68. Lorentzen M, Pers M, Bretteville-Jensen G. The incidence of malignant transformation in giant pigmented nevi. Scand J Plast Reconstr Surg 1977;71:163-167.

69. Rhodes AR. Pigmented birthmarks and precursor melanocytic lesions of cutaneous melanoma identifiable in childhood. Pediatr Clin North Am 1983;30:435-463.

70. Gari LM, Rivers JK, Kopf AW. Melanomas arising in large congenital nevocytic nevi: a prospective study. Pediatr Dermatol 1988;5:151-158.

71. Illig L, Weidner F, Hundeiker M, et al. Congenital nevi less than or equal to 10 cm as precursors to melanoma. 52 cases, a review, and a new conception. Arch Dermatol 1985;121:1274-1281.

72. Rhodes AR, Melski JW. Small congenital nevocellular nevi and the risk of cutaneous melanoma. J Pediatr 1982;100:219-224.

73. Kopf AW, Levine LJ, Rigel DS, Friedman RJ, Levenstein M. Congenital-nevus-like nevi, nevi spili, and cafe-au-lait spots in patients with malignant melanoma. J Dermatol Surg Oncol 1985;11:275-280.

74. Reed WB, Becker SW, Becker SW Jr, Nickel WR. Giant pigmented nevi, melanoma, and leptomeningeal melanosis. Arch Dermatol 1965;91:100-119.

75. Foster RD, Williams ML, Barkovich AJ, Hoffman WY, Mathes SJ, Frieden IJ. Giant congenital melanocytic nevi: the significance of neurocutaneous melanosis in neurologically asymptomatic children. Plast Reconstr Surg 2001;107:933-941.

76. Granter SR, McKee PH, Calonje E, Mihm MC Jr, Busam K. Melanoma associated with blue nevus and melanoma mimicking cellular blue nevus: a clinicopathologic study of 10 cases on the spectrum of so-called 'malignant blue nevus'. Am J Surg Pathol 2001;25:316-323.

77. Goldenhersh MA, Savin RC, Barnhill RL, Stenn KS. Malignant blue nevus. Case report and literature review. J Am Acad Dermatol 1988;19:712-722

78. Rodriguez HA, Ackerman LV. Cellular blue nevus. Cancer 1968;21:393-405.

79. Gayraud A, Lorenzato M, Sartelet H, et al. [Malignant blue nevus: clinicopathologic study with AgNOR measurement. Seven cases]. Ann Dermatol Venereol 2002;129:1359-1364. [French]

80. Connelly J, Smith L. Malignant blue nevus. Lab Invest 1990;62:21A.

81. Maize JC Jr, McCalmont TH, Carlson JA, Busam KJ, Kutzner H, Bastian BC. Genomic analysis of blue nevi and related dermal melanocytic proliferations. Am J Surg Pathol 2005;29:1214-1220.

82. Schaefer KL, Brachwitz K, Wai DH, et al. Expression profiling of t(12;22) positive clear cell sarcoma of soft tissue cell lines reveals characteristic up-regulation of potential new marker genes including ERBB3. Cancer Res 2004;64:3395-3405.

83. Hisaoka M, Ishida T, Kuo TT, et al. Clear cell sarcoma of soft tissue: a clincopathologic, immunohistochemical, and molecular analysis of 33 cases. Am J Surg Pathol 2008;32:452-460.

84. Zembowicz A, McCusker M, Chiarelli C, et al. Morphological analysis of nevoid melanoma: a study of 20 cases with a review of the literature. Am J Dermatopathol 2001;23:167-175.

85. Levene A. On the histological diagnosis and prognosis of malignant melanoma. J Clin Pathol 1980;33:101-124.

86. Suster S, Ronnen M, Bubis JJ. Verrucous pseudonevoid melanoma. J Surg Oncol 1987;36:134-137.

87. Schmoeckel C, Castro CE, Braun-Falco O. Nevoid malignant melanoma. Arch Dermatol Res 1985;277:362-369.

88. Wong TY, Suster S, Duncan LM, Mihm MC Jr. Nevoid melanoma: a clinicopathological study of seven cases of malignant melanoma mimicking spindle and epithelioid cell nevus and verrucous dermal nevus. Hum Pathol 1995;26:171-179.

89. McNutt NS. "Triggered trap": nevoid malignant melanoma. Semin Diagn Pathol 1998;15:203-209.

90. McNutt NS, Urmacher C, Hakimian J, Hoss DM, Lugo J. Nevoid malignant melanoma: morphologic patterns and immunohistochemical reactivity. J Cutan Pathol 1995;22:502-517.

91. Reed RJ, Ichinose H, Clark WH Jr, Mihm MC Jr. Common and uncommon melanocytic nevi and borderline melanomas. Semin Oncol 1975;2:119-147.

92. Cassarino DS, Fullen DR, Sondak VK, Duray PH. Metastatic nevoid melanoma in a 4 1/2-year-old child. J Cutan Pathol 2003;30:647-651.

93. Crowson AN, Magro CM, Mihm MC. Malignant melanoma with prominent pigment synthesis: "animal type" melanoma—a clinical and histological study of six cases with a consideration of other melanocytic neoplasms with prominent pigment synthesis. Hum Pathol 1999;30:543-550.

94. Levene A. Equine melanotic disease. Tumori 1971;57:133-168.

95. Clark WH Jr, Min BH, Kligman LH. The developmental biology of induced malignant melanoma in guinea pigs and a comparison with other neoplastic systems. Cancer Res 1976;36:4079-4091.

96. Oxenhandler RW, Adelstein EH, Haigh JP, Hook RR Jr, Clark WH Jr. Malignant melanoma in the Sinclair miniature swine: an autopsy study of 60 cases. Am J Pathol 1979;96:707-720.

97. Zembowicz A, Carney JA, Mihm MC. Pigmented epithelioid melanocytoma: a low-grade melanocytic tumor with metastatic potential indistinguishable from animal-type melanoma and epithelioid blue nevus. Am J Surg Pathol 2004;28:31-40.

98. Carney JA, Ferreiro JA. The epithelioid blue nevus. A multicentric familial tumor with important associations, including cardiac myxoma and psammomatous melanotic schwannoma. Am J Surg Pathol 1996;20:259-272.

99. Zembowicz A, Knoepp SM, Bei T, et al. Loss of expression of protein kinase, a regulatory subunit 1alpha in pigmented epithelioid melanocytoma but not in melanoma or other melanocytic lesions. Am J Surg Pathol 2007;31:1764-1775.

100. Carney JA, Gordon H, Carpenter PC, Shenoy BV, Go VL. The complex of myxomas, spotty pigmentation, and endocrine overactivity. Medicine (Baltimore) 1985;64:270-283.

101. O'Grady TC, Barr RJ, Billman G, Cunningham BB. Epithelioid blue nevus occurring in children with no evidence of Carney complex. Am J Dermatopathol 1999;21:483-486.

102. Moreno C, Requena L, Kutzner H, de la CA, Jaqueti G, Yus ES. Epithelioid blue nevus: a rare variant of blue nevus not always associated with the Carney complex. J Cutan Pathol 2000;27:218-223.

103. Groben PA, Harvell JD, White WL. Epithelioid blue nevus: neoplasm Sui generis or variation on a theme? Am J Dermatopathol 2000;22:473-488.

104. Izquierdo MJ, Pastor MA, Carrasco L, et al. Epithelioid blue naevus of the genital mucosa: report of four cases. Br J Dermatol 2001;145:496-501.

105. Antony FC, Sanclemente G, Shaikh H, Trelles AS, Calonje E. Pigment synthesizing melanoma (so-called animal type melanoma): a clinicopathological study of 14 cases of a poorly known distinctive variant of melanoma. Histopathology 2006;48:754-762.

106. Maloney ME, Jones DB, Sexton FM. Pigmented basal cell carcinoma: Investigation of 70 cases. J Am Acad Dermatol 1992;27:74-78.

107. Szpak CA, Shelburne J, Linder J, Klintworth GK. The presence of stage II melanosomes (premelanosomes) in neoplasms other than melanomas. Mod Pathol 1988;1:35-43.

108. Kamino H, Tam ST. Immunoperoxidase technique modified by counterstain with azure B as a diagnostic aid in evaluating heavily pigmented melanocytic neoplasms. J Cutan Pathol 1991;18:436-439.

109. Harkin JC, Reed RJ. Tumors of the peripheral nervous system. Atlas of Tumor Pathology, 2nd Series, Fascicle 3. Washington, DC: Armed Forces Institute of Pathology; 1969.

110. Killeen RM, Davy CL, Bauserman SC. Melanocytic schwannoma. Cancer 1988;62:174-183.

111. Carney JA. Psammomatous melanotic schwannoma. A distinctive, heritable tumor with special associations, including cardiac myxoma and the Cushing syndrome. Am J Surg Pathol 1990;14:206-222.

112. Cruz J, Reis-Filho JS, Lopes JM. Malignant peripheral nerve sheath tumour-like primary cutaneous malignant melanoma. J Clin Pathol 2004;57:218-220.

113. Reintgen DS, McCarty KS, Woodard B, Cox E, Seigler HF. Metastatic malignant melanoma with an unknown primary. Surg Gynecol Obstet 1983;156:335-340.

114. Enzinger FM, Weiss SW. Soft tissue tumors. St Louis: CV Mosby; 1983:615-617.

115. Meis-Kindblom JM. Clear cell sarcoma of tendons and aponeuroses: a historical perspective and tribute to the man behind the entity. Adv Anat Pathol 2006;13:286-292.

116. Dim DC, Cooley LD, Miranda RN. Clear cell sarcoma of tendons and aponeuroses: a review. Arch Pathol Lab Med 2007;131:152-156.

117. Fujimura Y, Ohno T, Siddique H, Lee L, Rao VN, Reddy ES. The EWS-ATF-1 gene involved in malignant melanoma of soft parts with t(12;22) chromosome translocation, encodes a constitutive transcriptional activator. Oncogene 1996;12:159-167.

118. Antonescu CR, Tschernyavsky SJ, Woodruff JM, Jungbluth AA, Brennan MF, Ladanyi M. Molecular diagnosis of clear cell sarcoma: detection of EWS-ATF1 and MITF-M transcripts and histopathological and ultrastructural analysis of 12 cases. J Mol Diagn 2002;4:44-52.

119. Antonescu CR, Nafa K, Segal NH, Dal CP, Ladanyi M. EWS-CREB1: a recurrent variant fusion in clear cell sarcoma—association with gastrointestinal location and absence of melanocytic differentiation. Clin Cancer Res 2006;12:5356-5362.

120. Coindre JM, Hostein I, Terrier P, et al. Diagnosis of clear cell sarcoma by real-time reverse transcriptase-polymerase chain reaction analysis of paraffin embedded tissues: clinicopathologic and molecular analysis of 44 patients from the French sarcoma group. Cancer 2006;107:1055-1064.

121. Sara AS, Evans HL, Benjamin RS. Malignant melanoma of soft parts (clear cell sarcoma): a study of 17 cases, with emphasis on prognostic factors. Cancer 1990;65:367-374.

122. Deenik W, Mooi WJ, Rutgers EJ, Peterse JL, Hart AA, Kroon BB. Clear cell sarcoma (malignant melanoma) of soft parts: a clinicopathologic study of 30 cases. Cancer 1999;86:969-975.

123. Kawai A, Hosono A, Nakayama R, et al. Clear cell sarcoma of tendons and aponeuroses: a study of 75 patients. Cancer 2007;109:109-116.

124. Swanson PE, Wick MR. Clear cell sarcoma. An immunohistochemical analysis of six cases and comparison with other epithelioid neoplasms of soft tissue. Arch Pathol Lab Med 1989;113:55-60.

125. Sarlomo-Rikala M, Kovatich AJ, Barusevicius A, Miettinen M. CD117: a sensitive marker for gastrointestinal stromal tumors that is more specific than CD34. Mod Pathol 1998;11:728-734.

126. Li KK, Goodall J, Goding CR, et al. The melanocyte inducing factor MITF is stably expressed in cell lines from human clear cell sarcoma. Br J Cancer 2003;89:1072-1078.

127. Cerroni L, Kerl H. Tutorial on melanocytic lesions. Am J Dermatopathol 2001;23:237-241.

128. Gimotty PA, Van Belle P, Elder DE, et al. Biologic and prognostic significance of dermal Ki67 expression, mitoses, and tumorigenicity in thin invasive cutaneous melanoma. J Clin Oncol 2005;23:8048-8056.

129. Kucher C, Zhang PJ, Pasha T, et al. Expression of Melan-A and Ki-67 in desmoplastic melanoma and desmoplastic nevi. Am J Dermatopathol 2004;26:452-457.

130. Vollmer RT. Use of Bayes rule and MIB-1 proliferation index to discriminate Spitz nevus from malignant melanoma. Am J Clin Pathol 2004;122:499-505.

131. Li LX, Crotty KA, Scolyer RA, et al. Use of multiple cytometric markers improves discrimination between benign and malignant melanocytic lesions: a study of DNA microdensitometry, karyometry, argyrophilic staining of nucleolar organizer regions and MIB1-Ki67 immunoreactivity. Melanoma Res 2003;13:581-586.

132. van Dijk MC, Bernsen MR, Ruiter DJ. Analysis of mutations in B-RAF, N-RAS, and H-RAS genes in the differential diagnosis of Spitz nevus and spitzoid melanoma. Am J Surg Pathol 2005;29:1145-1151.

133. Harvell JD, Kohler S, Zhu S, Hernandez-Boussard T, Pollack JR, Van de Rijn M. High-resolution array-based comparative genomic hybridization for distinguishing paraffin-embedded Spitz nevi and melanomas. Diagn Mol Pathol 2004;13:22-25.

134. Bauer J, Bastian BC. Distinguishing melanocytic nevi from melanoma by DNA copy number changes: comparative genomic hybridization as a research and diagnostic tool. Dermatol Ther 2006;19:40-49.

11 METASTATIC MALIGNANT MELANOMA

GENERAL FEATURES

Although it is a truism, it is worth stating that metastasis, usually to a vital organ such as the brain (fig. 11-1), is the central problem posed by malignant melanoma, since there are very few deaths attributable to local disease alone. The diagnosis of metastatic melanoma is usually fairly straightforward histologically. Most metastases, whether in the skin or elsewhere, are relatively easy to recognize as malignancies because of the presence of high-grade nuclear atypia, frequent mitoses, infiltrative patterns of growth, and often, extensive areas of necrosis. If there are problems in diagnosis, these likely relate to the recognition of a particular malignant tumor as a metastatic rather than a primary neoplasm, and as a melanoma rather than some other form of malignancy. Another problem is identifying a locally recurrent tumor following complete excision of the primary melanoma as a metastatic event, rather than a consequence of inadequate or incomplete excision of the primary tumor, which is rare (1).

Features that suggest the diagnosis of metastatic malignant melanoma are listed in Table 11-1. Melanin pigment may be obvious, subtle (oligomelanotic melanoma), or absent (amelanotic melanoma). If pigment is present in an oligomelanotic melanoma, it is most likely seen around areas of necrosis, suggesting that ischemia can induce this form of differentiation in these injured cells. Less specific but suggestive features that may be seen at scanning magnification in an amelanotic lesion include a tendency to a nested or packeted pattern of growth and the presence of epithelioid and spindle cells in a single lesion, a finding unusual in other epithelial tumors. Other features, such as an infiltrative border, a destructive pattern of growth in the tissues, a sparse lymphocytic response, and necrosis are those of metastatic and malignant tumors in general, and are not specific for melanoma.

Cutaneous metastatic melanoma may be defined as "local" (closely related to the excision site), "regional" (between the site and/or in the

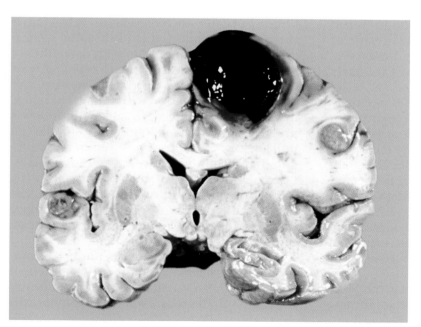

Figure 11-1

METASTATIC MALIGNANT MELANOMA

This bulky tumor has undergone hemorrhage, resulting in raised intracranial pressure and herniation. Other amelanotic metastases are also present (left and right hemispheres).

Table 11-1

HISTOLOGIC FEATURES OF METASTATIC MELANOMA

Configuration	Nodule, circumscribed or infiltrative, necrosis common
Growth Pattern	Nests (characteristic) or sheets, delicate stroma usually
Differentiation	Epithelioid, spindle, blastic, rarely nevoid (mixed differentiation characteristic)
Cytology	Cytoplasmic pigment common, usually "dusty," nuclear "pseudoinclusions," large eosinophilic or amphophilic nucleoli, dendritic cells often (especially using silver stains)
Host Response	Sparse lymphocytes often, rarely brisk, sparse plasma cells common, occasionally fibrosis

regional nodes), or "distant" (nonregional). Precise definitions have varied among studies, making comparisons difficult. Often, lesions within 5 cm of the local site, described as "satellites," are included in the local recurrence category. Yu and Heenan (605), however, have argued that when the primary tumor has been completely excised, these lesions represent local metastases rather than persistence followed by local recurrence of the primary tumor. Lesions beyond 5 cm, described as "in-transit metastases," are indistinguishable from satellites, which are also metastases. While satellites and in-transit metastases may represent either lymphatic or hematogenous spread from the primary site, distant and nonregional metastases are likely to be hematogenous.

The incidence of local metastases is closely related to tumor thickness, and the prognosis for patients with local metastases is poor. In a follow-up study, the incidence of locally metastatic tumors rose from 2 percent for tumors less than 0.99 mm, to 14 percent for tumors between 5 and 6 mm in thickness. Over a median postoperative follow-up period of 11 years, 67 percent of patients with locally metastatic disease died of disseminated malignant melanoma, compared with a 31 percent mortality for those without local disease metastasis (2).

Metastatic melanoma may present in the papillary dermis, the reticular dermis, or the subcutis, and often in more than one of these sites. The usual lesion is a more or less spherical mass composed of epithelioid and/or spindle cells. The presence of both spindle and epithelioid cell types in an unknown lesion is a clue to melanoma compared with another type of tumor.

At the cytologic level, a nuclear feature common to many metastatic melanomas, especially those of the common epithelioid type, is the presence of large, amphophilic or eosinophilic nucleoli. The presence of round intranuclear "pseudoinclusions" may be a striking feature. Pseudoinclusions are composed of material that resembles the cytoplasm of the tumor cell, and electron micrographs confirm that the "inclusions" are invaginations of the cytoplasm into the nucleus. They are suggestive of melanoma in an appropriate cellular environment, but not specific, since they may be seen in a variety of neoplasms, including leukemia and lymphoma, leiomyosarcoma, meningioma, glioma, granular cell tumors, liposarcoma, hepatoma, and benign hepatocytes, as well as in benign melanocytic lesions (see fig. 2-8D) (3). Some melanoma cell nuclei, although not often in metastases, exhibit a "bubbly" nuclear pattern similar to that seen in some schwannomas.

Three general types of tumor cells, epithelioid, spindle, and small "blastic" cell types, are distinguished in metastatic melanomas. The cytologic phenotype of the metastatic cells may reproduce that of the cells of the primary tumor, but often such correlation is lacking. If there is a correlation, it is likely to be seen in the epithelioid and spindle cell types, either of which may metastasize "true to type," at least for a period, although with a tendency to lesser degrees of pigmentation with time. If a change in cell type is observed, it is likely to follow a progression from a predominantly spindle cell morphology in the primary tumor, to a predominantly epithelioid cell type in the metastasis, and then often to small blastic cells as the tumor disseminates throughout the viscera. The blastic cell type is most often seen in autopsy material, apparently representing the end-stage of the dedifferentiation phenomenon.

The epithelioid cell type is the most common in metastases. Predominantly epithelioid metastases, however, may also show a minority of plump spindle cells, even when spindle cells were not prominent in the primary tumor, and such a dichotomous cellular phenotype should suggest the diagnosis of melanoma. Purely or predominantly spindle cell metastases, especially when heavily pigmented, may resemble blue nevi. Features aiding in the distinction include the presence of epithelioid cells, mitoses, and inflammation in the melanomas, although these features are subtle in some instances (4). Spindle cell metastatic melanomas may also have alternating hypercellular and hypocellular areas, numerous mitoses, and foci of necrosis, simulating a malignant peripheral nerve sheath tumor (MPNST). Tumors with a microscopic appearance compatible with an MPNST but showing strong diffuse S-100 protein staining and featuring remnants of lymph node may represent metastatic malignant melanoma and should elicit a search for a primary melanoma (5).

Unusual and variant forms of metastatic melanoma have been described. *Myxoid metastatic melanoma* may mimic various epithelial and soft tissue lesions (6). *Angiotropic metastatic melanoma* is a rare pattern of metastasis of melanoma, in the form of a malignant spindle-cell neoplasm invading the wall of a deep cutaneous blood vessel. Immunohistochemistry confirms the diagnosis of angiotropic metastatic melanoma and rules out primary leiomyosarcoma (7). *Angiomatoid metastatic melanoma* mimicking a vascular malignancy has been described (8). Heavily pigmented metastatic melanomas with a spindle cell component can be mistaken for a primary benign or malignant blue nevus (4).

The occurrence of metastatic melanoma is often considered an indicator of fatal outcome, but especially in the case of regionally metastatic melanoma, where the metastasis is initially at least confined to the regional lymph nodes, there is a substantial incidence of long-term survival, which also depends on the characteristics of the primary tumor, the characteristics of the metastases, and host factors (9). In a multivariable analysis of 1,273 stage III melanomas from a single institution, favorable prognostic factors included involvement of a single node, age less than 50 years, a primary tumor on the extremity, a disease-free interval greater than 6 months, a thickness less than 1.5 mm, and female sex (10). The most favorable risk group constituted 18 percent of a population of stage III cases, and

had actuarial 5- and 10-year survival rates of 58 percent and 49 percent, respectively.

EPIDERMOTROPIC METASTATIC MELANOMA

Definition. *Epidermotropic metastatic melanoma* is a metastasis of melanoma to the papillary dermis that secondarily involves the epidermis, resulting in an appearance that may simulate a primary melanoma or, in differentiated lesions, a benign nevus.

Clinical Features. Epidermotropic metastatic melanoma, in our experience, often presents as multiple lesions occurring in crops over prolonged periods of time. In most cases, the lesions occur in a limb proximal to a primary melanoma. Some patients present with distant metastatic disease after several years, during which time dozens of cutaneous metastases are excised; others remain free of detectable disease. The unusual differentiated metastases may represent examples of local spread of cells from the primary tumor that have tropism for the papillary dermis but are not (at least initially) competent to establish themselves as a metastatic deposit at a distant site.

Microscopic Findings. Atypical melanocytes are in the epidermis and upper dermis (papillary dermis), much as in primary melanomas (fig. 11-2) (11). Thus, epidermal involvement is not a sine qua non for a primary lesion. Since there is rarely any significant spread beyond the dermal tumor, a true radial growth phase of melanoma is not usually well simulated, and unlike most nodular melanomas (which, by definition, have no radial growth phase), the lesion is more or less confined to the superficial dermis. There have been cases of epidermotropic metastases in which there was prominent lateral spread (12). An occasional helpful finding is the presence of tumor cells in endothelium-lined channels (11); this finding is consistent with lymphatic invasion, which is rarely demonstrable in primary melanomas, and is certainly very rare in the small primaries that might simulate a nevus.

A characteristic that causes diagnostic difficulty in some cases is a tendency for the lesional cells to show marked nevoid differentiation, so that they simulate a benign compound nevus. The lesions can usually be distinguished from nevi by the presence of a large epithelioid cell

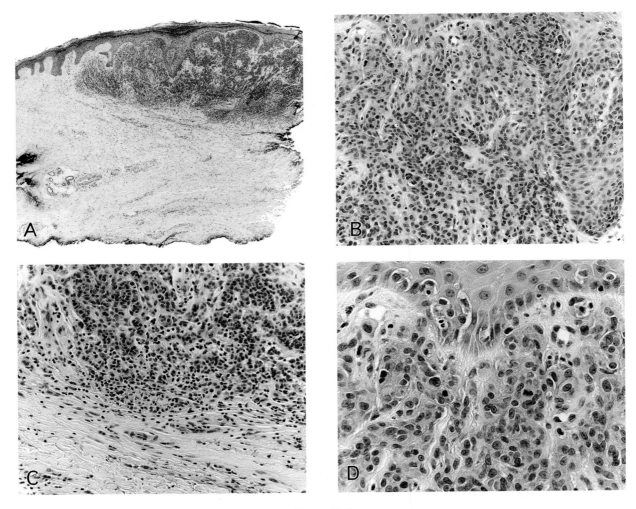

Figure 11-2

EPIDERMOTROPIC NEVOID METASTATIC MELANOMA

A: Symmetric neoplasm in the upper dermis, closely applied to the epidermis.

B: Higher magnification shows epithelioid nevoid melanocytes, with nests in the epidermis and evidence of maturation from superficial to deep.

C: Lesional cells at the base are smaller than those superficially and there is a sprinkling of lymphocytes.

D: Mitotic figures are present in the dermal component and there is uniform, albeit moderate, atypia. Easily detectable lymphatic invasion, not seen in this case, is often a clue to the diagnosis of epidermotropic nevoid metastatic melanoma.

type at the surface (although often with differentiation to small cells at the base), of nuclear atypia often with macronucleoli, and of a few mitoses (which are sometimes found only by careful searching) (fig. 11-3). Often, a patchy lymphocytic infiltrate is present, a finding that is rare in banal nevi. Clinically, these lesions present as crops of pink papules in the region of a treated melanoma, often in a limb. In a few difficult cases that we have observed, the distinction between metastatic melanoma and benign disease has been almost impossible to make histologically, until the occurrence of crops of the lesions in a drainage area of a prior melanoma leads to reconsideration of an initial benign diagnosis.

SATELLITES AND IN-TRANSIT METASTASES

Satellites of primary melanomas are, by definition, cutaneous metastases (discontinuous foci of tumor) that are located in the dermis or subcutaneous tissue within 5 cm of the primary

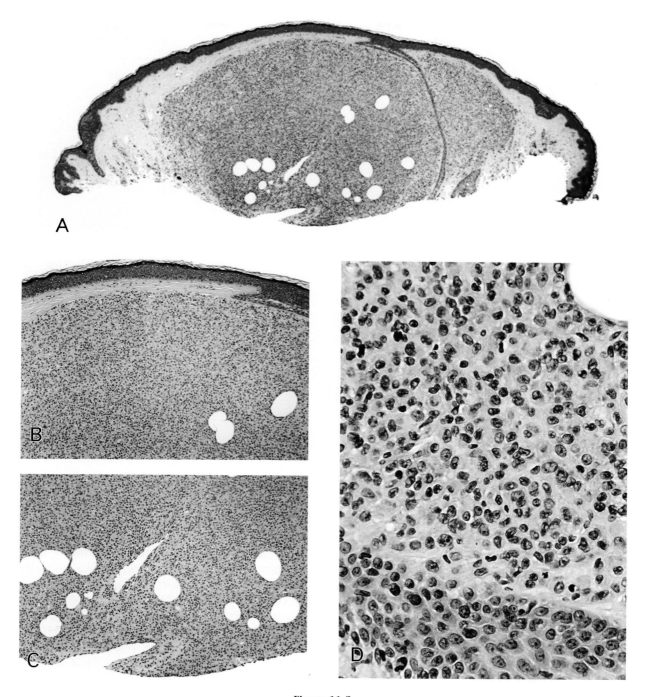

Figure 11-3

NEVOID METASTATIC MELANOMA

A: The tumor, in the upper dermis, has a striking epidermal collaret. Lesional cells are small nevoid to epithelioid melanocytes. There is no pigment.

B: Immunohistochemical studies are necessary to define melanocytic differentiation.

C: The tumor infiltrates the reticular dermis and subcutaneous fat.

D: Mitotic figures are usually detectable, sometimes with difficulty in these lesions.

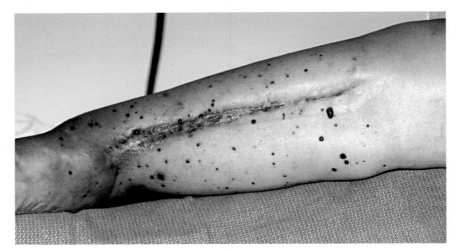

Figure 11-4

SATELLITES AND IN-TRANSIT METASTASES

Top: Satellites and in-transit metastases around a primary melanoma excision site.

Bottom: Amelanotic deposits of metastatic melanoma in skin.

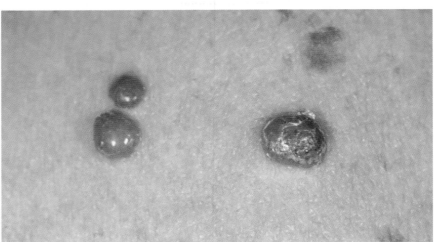

melanoma (fig. 11-4) (13,14). This definition arbitrarily distinguishes them from *in-transit metastases*, which are located beyond 5 cm but are still regional (in the same node drainage area).

Satellites may be located in the papillary or reticular dermis, or in the subcutaneous fat. They may be found deep to the primary tumor, when they are likely to be seen in the primary excisional or incisional biopsy, or they may be found adjacent to the primary tumor, often in the definitive wide excision specimen. Satellites may be clinically visible or they may be inapparent at the time of initial presentation. Their possible presence in the skin adjacent to a primary melanoma is a justification for the procedure of wide local excision of melanomas, since clinically inapparent foci of tumor in the region of the primary might serve as loci for continued growth of tumor and later presentation as a lo-

cal recurrence. Grossly visible satellites formed an important part of the clinical descriptions of melanomas in the first half of this century, but with earlier diagnosis of melanoma today, they are now rarely seen. Apparently isolated elements of primary tumors that have been broken up by extensive partial regression are occasionally mistaken clinically and even histologically for satellites, an error that can be avoided if the characteristic fibrosis and pigmented macrophages in the papillary dermis in these areas of regression are recognized.

Microscopic satellites, defined as noncontiguous nests of tumor in the reticular dermis or fat that are greater than 0.05 mm in diameter, are rare in thin tumors, but Day et al. (14) observed them in 88 of 161 melanomas (55 percent) thicker than 1.51 mm. Studying primarily the reexcision specimens, we found satellites in 22 percent of tumors thicker than 2.25 mm (13). These data suggest that pathologists examining wide excision specimens should "breadloaf" them to search for satellites, particularly when the primary tumor is thick, because such satellites are associated with a greater risk of subsequent local recurrence (15) and are highly correlated with nodal metastasis (16). Survey sections taken from within the specimen are more likely to yield positive findings than the more usual multiple sections of the specimen margins, which are hardly ever positive in a wide (1 cm or more) excision.

In-transit metastases differ from satellites only in their location, beyond 5 cm of the primary tumor. Like satellites, they are believed to be true metastases, probably tumor emboli that become arrested in lymphatics and proliferate to form a mass lesion that is usually recognized in follow-up (figs. 11-4, 11-5). Roses et al. (17) found in-transit metastases in 12 of 282 clinical stage I melanomas (4.3 percent) thicker than 1 mm. We found in-transit metastases in 6 of 109 primary melanoma cases, all in the 27 tumors thicker than 2 mm, where the incidence was 24 percent (13). All of our patients with in-transit metastases, and 76 percent of those in Roses' series, subsequently developed disseminated disease.

Satellites and in-transit metastases are morphologically similar to one another, and likely represent examples of locoregional lymphatic spread. By their nature, confined to the local region of the primary tumor, satellites are likely to be discovered during definitive therapy (biopsy or reexcision) of the primary tumor. In-transit metastases often constitute the first expression of metastasis in follow-up, and they are highly correlated with risk for more distant spread, either to lymph nodes or to viscera (18). Satellites and in-transit metastases may present in slightly different ways depending on their location in the skin or subcutis, but generally are observed clinically as a firm to hard, slightly colored (often purple), painless, freely mobile mass. Some lesions, especially the larger ones, may be painful and appear inflamed. Extensive permeation of dermal lymphatics also mimics an inflammatory condition, and has been reported as *inflammatory melanoma*, similar to the much more common analogous inflammatory carcinoma of the breast (19).

DERMAL AND SUBCUTANEOUS METASTASES

Dermal and *subcutaneous metastases* (satellites, in-transit, or nonregional metastases) are similar in their cytology and histologic configuration to metastases in lymph nodes or viscera (fig. 11-6). The cell type is usually epithelioid, probably since this is the most common cell type of primary melanomas. Often, a spindle cell melanoma metastasizes true to type, especially in desmoplastic and neurotropic melanomas (20), tumors where the spindle cell morphology apparently reflects schwannian differentiation. The histologic appearance of such lesions is similar to that described in the sections relating to these lesions.

Occasionally, a dermal metastasis is mimicked by local persistence or recurrence of a primary melanoma in which the more superficial component was removed by previous biopsy or attempted excision. When a dermal deposit of melanoma is detected in a patient whose primary melanoma was not established previously, it is incumbent upon the pathologist to obtain a clinical history of such an event and to carefully search for evidence of superficial scarring at a histologic level.

It has been recently reported that rare primary melanomas arise de novo within the dermis, producing a pattern that mimics a dermal metastasis. Although few cases have been studied, such "primary dermal melanomas" are believed to have a more favorable prognosis than other forms of primary melanoma, and certainly a better outcome than would be predicted for a dermal metastasis. Thus, in situations where a suspected solitary dermal metastasis is encountered and there is no evidence of a conventional primary lesion, no history of previous attempted removal, and no evidence of superficial scarring, this possibility must be considered (21,22).

LYMPH NODE METASTASES: ELECTIVE AND SELECTIVE LYMPHADENECTOMY

Malignant melanoma commonly metastasizes to the regional lymph nodes, and involvement of lymph nodes by metastatic melanoma is associated with a significantly worse prognosis. There is a substantial number of survivors of metastatic disease in regional lymph nodes, however, as discussed in following sections.

Clinical Features. Although less common than before in the present age of sentinel

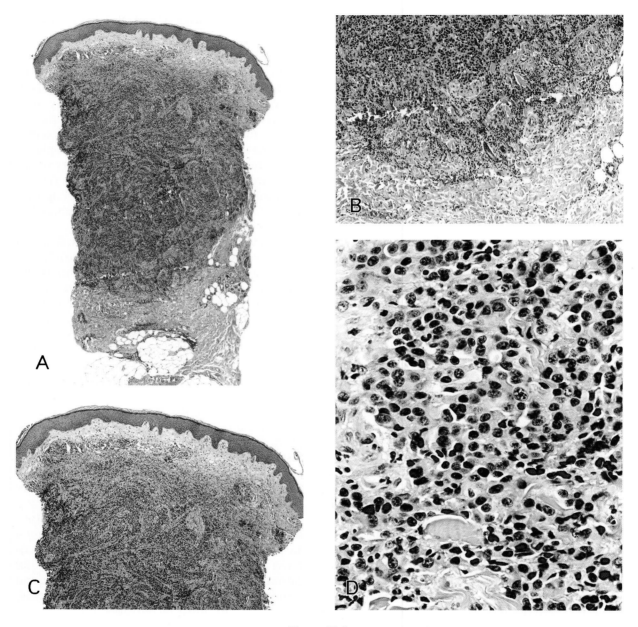

Figure 11-5

METASTATIC MALIGNANT MELANOMA IN DERMIS

A–C: This punch biopsy shows a tumor in the reticular dermis.

D: Higher magnification shows uniformly atypical cells infiltrating the dermis, with little or no evidence of maturation to the base.

lymphadenectomy, clinically evident metastatic disease may be discovered in the regional lymph nodes, by either patients or clinicians, as a usually painless firm mass. Sometimes, there is associated tenderness and calor, suggesting the possibility of an inflammatory process, but

in a patient with a mass who has a history of a primary melanoma, especially a tumorigenic one, metastatic disease must be presumed present until proven otherwise.

Typically, the diagnosis is confirmed with a fine needle aspiration biopsy (FNAB) or a lymph

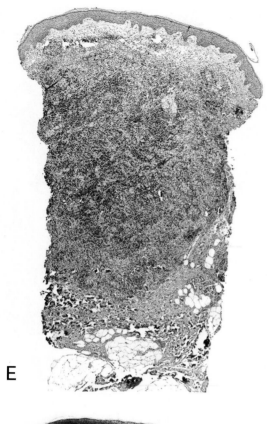

E

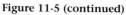

Figure 11-5 (continued)

E,F: A Melan-A stain is focally positive. Staining for Phospho-Erk (pErk) was also done. This member of the MAP kinase pathway indicates that the pathway is constitutively activated in this neoplasm.

G,H: pErk staining is also present in the overlying epithelium. Mitotic figures are usually readily detectable, although not in this example.

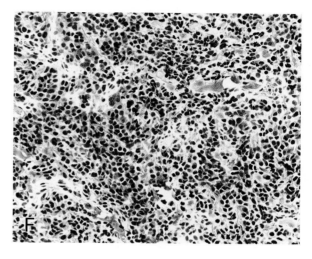

F

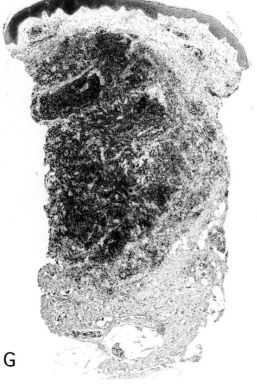

G

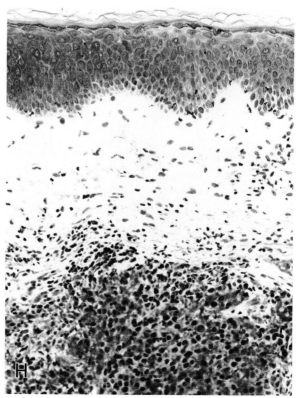

H

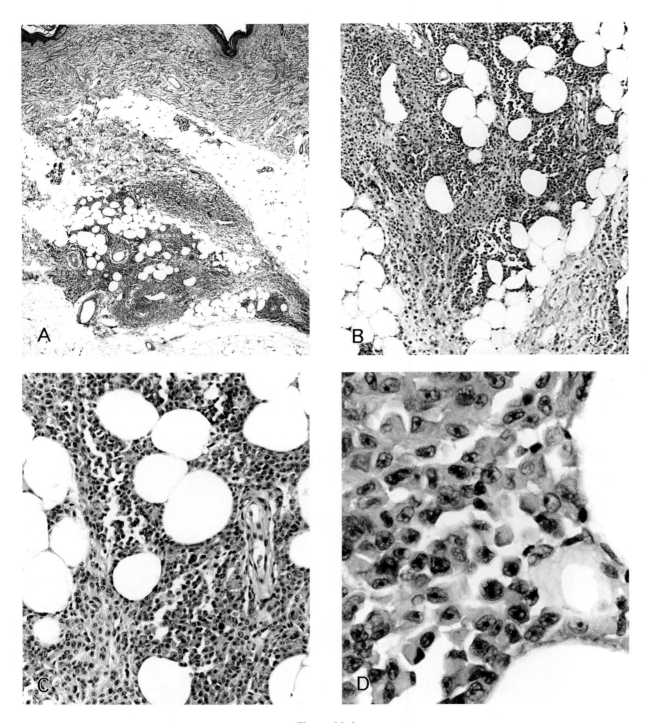

Figure 11-6

METASTATIC MALIGNANT MELANOMA IN SUBCUTIS

A: The tumor is in the subcutaneous tissue, honeycombing the fat.

B: Uniformly atypical cells infiltrate among fat cells.

C,D: Tumor cells infiltrate adipose tissue. The lesional cells in this case have a rhabdoid phenotype, with eosinophilic cytoplasm compressing the nucleus. Immunohistochemical studies would be necessary to identify this lesion as melanoma if there is no confirming history.

node biopsy, following which a "completion" or "therapeutic" lymph node dissection is done. The extent of such a therapeutic dissection when analyzed by quartiles of the number of nodes removed is an independent factor in overall survival, especially in patients with involvement of multiple lymph nodes. Therefore, it is important to document the number of positive and negative nodes removed (23).

Subclinical metastatic disease may be discovered in one of two ways: either through an elective lymph node dissection (ELND), or through a selective lymphadenectomy or sentinel lymph node dissection (SLND). ELND is performed in patients with clinically negative nodes to detect subclinical metastases that might spread beyond the lymph node basin. This procedure affects survival only if, at the time of the procedure, the patient does not already have established micrometastatic disease beyond the lymph node basin. Alternatively, it is possible that lymph node metastatic disease serves primarily as a marker for tumors that have the capacity for spread beyond the lymph nodes, and have already done so in a proportion of the cases. While some retrospective studies demonstrated apparent benefit from the ELND (23–26), other retrospective (27) and prospective studies (28) found no benefit, except perhaps in certain subsets (26). These differences are no doubt due to unstudied variables such as unwitting selection biases.

Whether ELND improves survival or not, the procedure has the disadvantage that only those patients whose lymph nodes are positive can derive any benefit from it. The SLND was developed to identify, by less invasive procedures, the subset of patients with positive nodes so that the expense and morbidity of full node clearance can be limited to those patients who are likely to have positive nodes. In this procedure, a blue dye and a radiolabel are injected into the skin at the primary site. The first lymph node to receive the label is designated the sentinel node, which is also the first node to receive metastatic cells. If the sentinel node is negative, the remainder of the node basin is also negative, with a high degree of certainty. If the sentinel node is positive, full clearance is done with the intent of removing tumor in the hope of improving survival (29). This procedure is

diagnostically and prognostically accurate and thus widely accepted.

An interim analysis of survival data from a multicenter randomized trial of wide excision alone versus wide excision plus lymphatic mapping and selective lymphadenectomy has recently been published (30,31). Improved survival was demonstrated in the subset of patients with positive nodes, although the overall melanoma-specific survival was the same between the two groups, discussed in more detail in the next section.

Microscopic Findings. In a bulky lymph node deposit, FNAB analysis or lymph node biopsy is usually diagnostic, and there are no adverse prognostic effects of the biopsy procedure (32). The lesional cells have abundant cytoplasm, usually epithelioid or cuboidal in configuration, which may contain melanin pigment. There may be an admixture of lymphocytes and melanophages. The nuclei are large and ovoid, often with prominent nucleoli and intranuclear "inclusions," which are actually invaginations of cytoplasm into the nucleus. If pigment and other classic features are absent, the cytomorphologic features of melanoma can be extremely variable, and can mimic other poorly differentiated neoplasms. Baloch and colleagues (33) described 10 cases of metastatic melanoma with distinct, cohesive papillary tissue fragments observed in FNAB specimens. These papillary fragments exhibited a central fibrovascular core with attached tumor cells, in a background of single scattered malignant cells, macrophages, and focal necrosis. Similar papillary structures may be seen in biopsy specimens as well, where they represent pseudopapillary structures formed by extensive necrosis, with preservation of viable tumor cells around blood vessels.

Common in metastatic melanomas in lymph nodes and elsewhere is a spindle cell component, and even in the absence of other more diagnostic fractures, the combination of spindle and epithelioid morphology in a lymph node metastasis should suggest the possibility of melanoma. In other cases, the cells are highly pleomorphic, mimicking a pleomorphic carcinoma or sarcoma. The combination of apparent epithelial and sarcomatous differentiation in a single neoplasm should suggest the possibility of melanoma. Some lesions are entirely comprised of spindle cells, raising the possibility of a spindle cell sarcoma such as a peripheral nerve sheath tumor, leiomyosarcoma, or fibrosarcoma. Immunohistochemical studies, including S-100 protein, HMB45 antigen, Melan-A, leukocyte common antigen, polyvalent keratin, factor VIII, desmin, smooth muscle actin, and HHF35, or electron microscopy may be performed to confirm the diagnosis of melanoma and rule out other competing possibilities.

SELECTIVE LYMPHADENECTOMY: SENTINEL LYMPH NODE BIOPSY

The pathologist's role in the process of selective lymphadenectomy (sentinel lymph node sampling) has been comprehensively reviewed by Cochran et al. (34). The sentinel node is the first lymph node on the direct lymphatic drainage path from the primary tumor. This node is immune-modulated by the primary tumor and is the node most likely to contain the earliest metastases (34). Patients with a negative sentinel node are very unlikely to have tumor in the nonsentinel nodes in the same region (29). Accurate assessment of the sentinel node requires careful evaluation of multiple sections that are removed from the areas of the node (the "equator" region) most likely to contain tumor. Sections (often more than one level) are stained with hematoxylin and eosin (H&E) and immunohistochemically with antibodies directed to tumor-associated markers (S-100 protein, HMB45, and Melan-A/MART-1). The question of whether molecular biology techniques such as reverse transcriptase-polymerase chain reaction (RT-PCR) for melanoma markers detect clinically significant additional nodes that contain occult true tumor deposits has been addressed in a randomized trial (35), and although the yield of positive findings appears to be increased, this procedure provides no additional prognostic information beyond standard histopathologic analysis and remains investigational.

In a positive sentinel node biopsy, the deposit of tumor cells is often small, but usually readily evident with routine stains, or with the aid of S-100 protein, HMB45, or Melan-A staining (fig. 10-38). In some cases, the tumor is present as single cells or small clusters. If the nuclear characteristics are those of melanoma, we usually accept the diagnosis of a microscopic metastasis (fig. 11-7).

The prognostic significance of histologic parameters in sentinel nodes was addressed in a recent study (36). Three independent significant parameters predicted a poor prognosis, namely, the presence of infiltration of the sentinal node capsule, a depth of penetration into the node of 2 mm or greater, and the size of the largest tumor deposit of 30 cells or more. In another study, additional nonsentinel node positivity was not observed in patients with submicrometastases (less than 0.1 mm), leading these authors to question the utility of completion lymphadenectomy for such patients (37).

When evaluating a sentinel lymph node biopsy, care must be taken to avoid diagnosing nevus cell rests as micrometastases (fig. 11-7). These rests are commonly detected and are related in some cases to the nevi, including congenital nevi, in the skin drained by the lymph node (38). The nevus cells rests are typically present in the capsule or in the connective tissue of sinusoids, rather than in the parenchyma of the node. They usually lack cytologic atypia and mitoses, are usually HMB45 and Ki-67 negative (39), and may be positive for *p16*, a tumor suppressor gene that is less likely to be expressed in melanoma cells (40). Small deposits of tumor cells must also be differentiated from dendritic cells and from nerve sheath cells, which, like the capsular and trabecular nevus cells, express S-100 protein antigen in their cytoplasm (41).

The optimal technique for sentinel lymph node assessment in patients with melanoma has not been defined. In a recent study, approximately 30 percent of the lymph nodes were positive by molecular analysis (PCR) compared with approximately 20 percent by routine pathologic analysis (42). The disease-free survival rates were 60, 30, and 10 percent, respectively, for patients with pathologic/PCR findings of +/+, +/-, and -/- in their lymph nodes. In another study using immunohistochemistry for three markers (S-100 protein, HMB45, and Melan-A), micrometastases were found in 28 percent of cases and benign nevus inclusions were found in a similar number (43). Melan-A was the most sensitive marker. HMB45 labeled 82 percent of the metastases and 16 percent of the benign nevi. Micrometastases were detected on the first section plane in about half of the patients, with

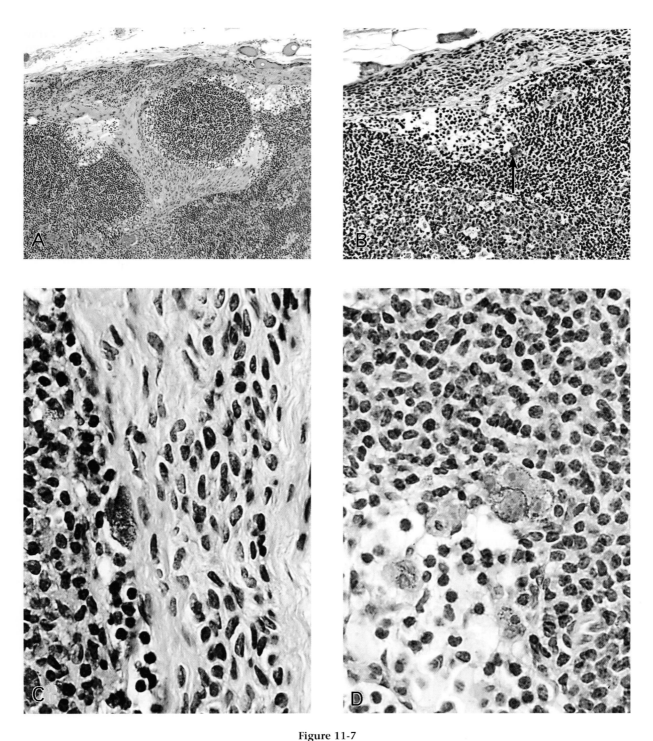

Figure 11-7

CAPSULAR NEVUS AND SUBTLE METASTATIC MELANOMA IN A SENTINEL NODE

A: Nevus cells are in the capsule and in sinusoidal septal fibrous tissue.
B: A few atypical cells stain with Melan-A (arrow).
C: An atypical melanocyte is positive for Melan-A in the peripheral sinus beneath the capsule.
D: A group of atypical melanocytes with nucleoli and cytoplasmic pigment in the parenchyma of the lymph node.

the detection rate increasing with the number of sections. It was concluded that extensive serial sectioning with immunohistochemical analysis substantially increases the histopathologic detection of micrometastases and nevus inclusions to a level approaching that reported for molecular techniques. In a similar recent study, it was concluded that multiple-level sectioning of sentinel nodes and the use of immunohistochemistry detected additional metastases up to the last section plane in melanoma sentinel nodes (44). In this study, one initial 4-mm H&E-stained section was made from each block. When negative, an additional section was done at the first level for immunohistochemistry and four step ribbons were cut at an interval of 250 mm. From these ribbons, one section was stained with H&E, one was used for immunohistochemistry with S-100 protein, and one for HMB45 or Melan-A. Although more levels of sectioning may increase the yield even further, it was considered that this protocol ensures a reasonable workload for the pathologist with an acceptable sensitivity when compared with the published literature.

The need for extreme sensitivity in sentinel lymph node analysis has been questioned in a thoughtful editorial by Wick and Patterson (45). Although it is true, as discussed above, that patients with microscopically positive lymph nodes or with positive molecular findings have a significantly worse prognosis than those with negative nodes (42), the therapeutic implications of this finding are disputed. In a recent large, prospective, multi-institutional study, PCR analysis on sentinel nodes and peripheral blood provided no additional prognostic information beyond standard histopathologic analysis of sentinel nodes (35). It was concluded that RT-PCR remains investigational and should not be used to direct adjuvant therapy at this time. Nevertheless, the publication of interim findings from the Multicenter Selective Lymphadenectomy Trial (31) provided evidence that the sentinel lymph node sampling procedure (based on routine histopathology with immunohistochemistry), followed by completion lymph node dissection for positive cases, significantly improved melanoma survival among patients with nodal metastases, although the melanoma-specific survival rate was similar in the treatment and control groups. The survival

benefit is therefore small overall, and the value of the procedure as a staging exercise has been emphasized. In the present state of knowledge, however, adjuvant therapy for patients with high-risk melanoma provides only modest benefit, and the staging information is therefore of limited value for individual patients except in the context of a therapeutic trial, or when a decision is made prospectively to use adjuvant therapy in the case of a positive result (45,46).

Completion node dissection is usually done for patients with a positive sentinel lymph node biopsy. Trials are underway to determine whether this is necessary in every patient (47). Compared with the practice of ELND, which was formerly common in some centers, SLND with completion dissection offered only to patients with positive sentinel nodes certainly reduces the number of patients exposed to this potential source of morbidity. In addition, the procedure offers the benefit of reducing the incidence of bulky lymph node disease, which is distressing to patients.

SPECIAL STUDIES FOR DIAGNOSIS OF OLIGOMELANOTIC OR AMELANOTIC MELANOMA

Although a lack of pigment (amelanotic melanoma) is rare in primary melanomas, it is not uncommon in metastases. Diagnostic strategies for establishing the diagnosis of a melanocytic tumor in these cases include the demonstration of subtle pigment by close scrutiny or by enhancing stains, and electron microscopy. Today, however, most cases are diagnosed by immunohistochemistry.

Neoplastic Melanin Production

Although immunopathology is now almost routinely used to confirm the diagnosis of a melanocytic neoplasm, melanin pigment in cytologically malignant cells is diagnostic of melanoma or a related lesion, with certain exceptions. Thus, it is important to rule out the phenomenon of pigment transfer from benign melanocytes to the cells of a nonmelanocytic neoplasm. This phenomenon is common, for example, in pigmented basal cell carcinomas, which do not usually cause diagnostic difficulty, but pigmentation is apt to be more confusing if seen in other neoplasms that simulate melanoma, such as in mammary or extramammary Paget disease (48). Other phenotypic attributes, such as keratin or mucin production in such tumors, may help differentiate them from melanomas.

The melanocytes that are found within these pigmented nonmelanocytic neoplasms are benign, dendritic, reactive cells. Ultrastructurally, these melanosomes (except in certain rare pigmented neuroendocrine neoplasms) are mature, stage IV melanized organelles that are generally aggregated in membrane-bound clusters as "compound melanosomes," unlike the immature and often abnormal premelanosomes that are found in most melanomas. The diagnosis is usually easily established by a simple immunohistochemical panel, which may include keratins, carcinoembryonic antigen (CEA), and epithelial membrane antigen (EMA) to label the carcinomas; S-100 protein, HMB45, and Melan-A/MART 1 to label the melanomas; and the use of additional markers such as microphthalmia-associated transcription factor (MITF) (49).

Although most melanomas contain at least some focal demonstrable melanin, this pigment can be missed by the unwary observer, particularly if it is subtly present and is not consciously searched for (as when the diagnosis of melanoma is not considered). In the initial investigation of a tumor that has features suggestive of melanoma but is apparently amelanotic, the first step should be the careful scanning of a number of section planes, taken from different areas of the tumor if it is large. In our experience, pigment, if present, is likely to be found near areas of necrosis. Pigment may occasionally be seen only in benign infiltrating macrophages, and this finding should be ignored if the area of melanophagic pigment is beneath the epidermis where it can potentially be explained by pigmentary incontinence.

Special Stains for Melanin Pigment

Special stains for melanin pigment have two uses: the specific identification of a pigment that is visible in an H&E-stained section and the search for pigment in an apparently amelanotic tumor. Despite the advent of increasingly specific immunopathologic reagents, the demonstration of melanin pigment in a characteristic distribution and lesional background is still the simplest diagnostic tool that is available in every laboratory. Immunopathologic stains and electron microscopy may also be useful in those cases in which the standard stains are negative. If there is a clear history of a primary melanoma, and the other criteria for metastatic melanoma are met (see Table 11-1), it is often appropriate to sign out an amelanotic metastasis descriptively as "malignant epithelial tumor consistent with metastatic melanoma" to avoid the delay and the expense of a series of special investigations. The silver-based stain for melanin granules used in our laboratory is a simple silver nitrate method, usually used in conjunction with permanganate bleaching, to identify a brown pigment as melanin. Other pigments may bleach with permanganate, so that the reaction should not be regarded as absolutely diagnostic of melanin.

More sensitive silver techniques for melanin detection include the Fontana, Grimelius, Sevier-Munger, and Warthin-Starry (pH 3.2) stains (50, 51). The silver stains, with or without bleaching, should not be regarded as absolutely specific, since they will stain other granules in cells, such as neurosecretory granules, and melanosomes may be present in cells that are not those of a melanoma. A pattern of staining frequently seen in melanomas, and virtually diagnostic of melanocytic differentiation, is that of very tiny finely divided dusty granules (which are individual, partially melanized premelanosomes), filling the cytoplasm of a single tumor cell and outlining the dendritic cytoplasm.

An iron stain can rule out hemosiderin pigment, especially in a case where pigment is obvious. This is important, because although it is generally considered that iron pigment is more refractile than melanin, and may differ in color, in our experience, it may be difficult to differentiate between hemosiderin and melanin in certain lesions. This stain also identifies Monsel pigment, which has been the source of error in several of our consultation cases, with unfortunate results for occasional patients who have been overtreated as a result of the overdiagnosis of the depth of invasion. Monsel solution is a styptic ferrous salt commonly used by dermatologists to control bleeding after shave or punch biopsies (52–54). The reaction not only stains collagen brown, but also stimulates a histiocytic response. The histiocytes with brown cytoplasmic pigment are easily mistaken for melanoma cells.

Immunopathology

Immunopathologic techniques are commonly used for the further investigation of an amelanotic tumor whose differential diagnosis includes melanoma. The available antigens include differentiation antigens, like tyrosinase, and structural antigens, such as S-100 protein antigen (55), as well as an emerging group of antigens with relative specificity for melanoma, many of which have been discovered because of their immunogenicity in patients. The most useful of these are those that survive the process of paraffin embedding (56,57). Antigens that can be stained only in frozen sections or that react only in vitro are of little or no use in diagnosis today, but may have a role in the future. This enhanced future role would require changes in the present methods of handling biopsy tissues, including the routine freezing and storing of a portion of the specimen, and perhaps the routine use of short-term tissue cultures for diagnosis. These studies would be more likely to be performed if the markers in question had predictive value in selecting appropriate biologic therapeutic agents that might be developed in the future.

S-100 protein is a calcium-binding protein that is present in a wide variety of neoplasms and benign cells, including melanocytes and their benign and malignant tumors, Schwann cells and their tumors, Langerhans cells and neoplasms, sweat gland cells, and fat cells, to provide an incomplete list. Nakajima et al. (58) found S-100 protein staining in 43 of 47 primary and metastatic malignant melanomas using a peroxidase-antiperoxidase technique in paraffin-embedded sections. Reactivity seems to be inversely proportional to the amount of melanin pigment, a useful property when diagnosing melanoma. Thus, only 4 of 26 "negative to slightly pigmented" melanomas showed "negative to slight reactivity" in their study. This antibody is of no use in discriminating benign from malignant melanocytic lesions, since it reacts with most nevi, and it stains a variety of tumors and normal tissues, including schwannomas, neurofibromas and granular cell tumors, neoplastic Langerhans cells, cartilaginous neoplasms and chordomas, mammary epithelial tumors, and benign and malignant sweat gland tumors (59). A report described S-100 protein reactivity in two lesions convincingly considered to be malignant fibrous histiocytomas on other grounds (60). Because of its low specificity, S-100 protein staining is of diagnostic value for melanoma only in selected cases, where lesions with irrelevant specificities can be ruled out on the basis of other clinicopathologic findings. Using the S-100 protein antibody and a battery of immunohistochemical markers for lymphoma with electron microscopy, Cochran et al. (61) in 1982 were able to substantiate the diagnosis of melanoma in all of 24 patients where the differential diagnosis lay between anaplastic tumor, melanoma, and lymphoma.

HMB45 is another diagnostically useful antibody that is a specific marker of immature, activated, and neoplastic melanocytes. In a study of melanomas and sarcomas composed in part or entirely of epithelioid cells, the antibody stained 17 of 18 melanomas and 5 of 6 clear cell sarcomas, lesions believed to represent melanomas of soft tissue (62). Examples of epithelioid neurofibrosarcoma, epithelioid sarcoma, and epithelioid leiomyosarcoma and synovial sarcoma were all negative. This antibody appears to be highly specific for melanoma and related lesions, although it is less sensitive than S-100 protein. It tends to be negative in spindle cell melanomas, including desmoplastic and neurotropic melanomas, which unfortunately are often the lesions in which diagnostic assistance by immunohistochemistry is most necessary. HMB45 reactivity is said to be optimal in alcohol-based fixatives such as Carnoy solution, although staining is also demonstrated in formalin- and Bouin-fixed material. In these fixatives, protease pretreatment may increase the sensitivity (57). Although HMB45 antigen generally does not stain dermal nevus cells, this antigen is reactive in dermal cells of dysplastic but not common nevi (63). It also may react with the superficial portions of Spitz nevi, and with some nevus variants (e.g., cellular blue nevi).

Intermediate filaments can be observed in melanomas by electron microscopy, and these have been investigated using panels of antibodies against these cytoskeletal proteins. Melanomas, like nonmuscle sarcomas, lymphomas, and solid leukemia, in general contain vimentin filaments (64), but vimentin reactivity is common in tumors and cells of other types and thus is of little or no differential diagnostic value. It is important to establish that a tumor is keratin negative before making a diagnosis of melanoma based on relatively nonspecific stains such as S-100 protein.

In a study of epithelial and melanocytic markers in routinely processed paraffin sections of malignant melanoma, all primary and most metastatic malignant melanomas showed positive staining with anti-S-100 protein, HMB45, and antivimentin (65). Reactivity with polyclonal CEA was observed in 15 (48 percent) of the 31 lesions; 14 of them were metastatic. No lesion was reactive with monoclonal CEA. Significant cytokeratin (CK) staining was evident in only 3 (9.7 percent) lesions (all metastatic), which also stained specifically with anti-CK18. EMA was observed only focally in 2 (6.5 percent) lesions. There was no correlation between staining by epithelial markers of the primary tumors and their metastases. All lesions with CK or EMA staining showed concomitant extensive staining for S-100 protein, HMB45, and vimentin. It was concluded that epithelial marker reactivity is more common in metastases of malignant melanomas and is not correlated to the reactivity of the primary tumors.

In cases where the differential diagnosis includes a histiocytic neoplasm, such as a xanthoma or a histiocytoma, it is important to be aware that many "histiocytic markers" are also reactive with some melanomas. Pernick et al. (66) evaluated primary and metastatic melanomas with common markers used for histiocytes. Melanoma immunoreactivity (more than 5 percent of tumor cells) was as follows: alpha-1-antitrypsin (AAT), 95 percent; CD68/KP1, 86 percent; HAM56, 26 percent; Mac387, 7 percent; and muramidase, 30 percent. AAT and CD68 immunostains were diffusely positive almost as frequently as traditional melanoma markers, although with weaker intensity. HAM56, Mac387, and muramidase were less commonly positive and exhibited focal staining. The authors concluded that, depending on the context, histiocytic markers may not be helpful in differentiating histiocytes and histiocytic tumors from melanomas. Conversely, most melanomas in this differential diagnostic category are likely to be positive with specific melanoma markers, which are negative in histiocytic lesions. In a recent study, all of 15 histiocytic proliferations were negative for Melan-A, tyrosinase, and HMB45 (67).

In the last few years, immunologic techniques have resulted in the production of a wide range of antibodies that, to some extent, react preferentially with malignant tumor cells, but the goal of producing truly "tumor-specific" antigens has been elusive (68–72). Some antibodies that are reactive in paraffin sections seem to have potentially useful reactivity for melanomas, although they cross-react with benign lesions, especially dysplastic nevi (73). Proliferation markers and some other markers, such as transcription factors or adhesion molecules, are currently under review as prognostic and, to some extent, diagnostic reagents. Expression profiling studies now underway may result in the detection of panels of antigens that can be used to characterize lesions, in terms of their differentiation as melanocytic or not, and perhaps also in terms of their biologic potential.

Electron Microscopy

The use of electron microscopy in the diagnosis of a difficult metastatic tumor is hampered by the frequent unavailability of suitably prepared tissue. In a few cases, repeat biopsy of tumors is necessary to obtain tissue for this procedure. Since the diagnostic premelanosomes are resistant to formalin fixation and embedding procedures, useful results can occasionally be obtained from paraffin blocks (74). The sensitivity of electron microscopy depends on the scanning of multiple thin sections for melanosomes, however, and unless the microscopist is able to scan at high magnification for long periods of time, this method may be no more sensitive than a good silver stain.

As a means of increasing the sensitivity of electron microscopy, a silver stain can be used to identify areas in paraffin blocks or thin sections (75), followed by electron microscopic examination of the positive regions of the tumor. In this way, the sensitivity of silver staining is combined with the high specificity of ultrastructural premelanosome identification, although the abnormal premelanosomes that characterize many melanomas may be difficult to distinguish from lysosomes with specificity.

The identification of premelanosomes can be regarded as specific for melanoma only when these structures are seen in an appropriate cell from an appropriate neoplasm. For example, compound melanosomes may be seen in normal and neoplastic keratinocytes and in other epithelial cells because of the phenomenon of pigment transfer from normal melanocytes; similarly, melanosomes have been described in the phagocytic cells of eruptive histiocytomas (76).

Melanin pigment produced by neoplastic cells may be seen in a variety of neuroendocrine neoplasms. A recent review described a case of melanin-producing medullary carcinoma of the thyroid (77), and reviewed reports of pigment synthesis (with melanosome production) in tumors of the adrenal gland and sympathetic ganglia, melanotic schwannoma, pigmented ganglioneuroblastoma, pigmented thymic carcinoid, and clear cell sarcoma. Conditions such as these should be ruled out before an unequivocal diagnosis of melanoma is made in a pigmented neoplasm.

Summary

At present, the workup of a suspected amelanotic epithelioid cell melanoma in our laboratory consists of immunohistochemical staining for S-100 protein antigen, keratin AE1/AE3, and Melan-A or HMB45. In a spindle cell lesion, we add smooth muscle actin and desmin. An S-100 protein-, Melan-A-, or HMB45-positive, keratin-negative lesion with consistent histology is considered diagnostic of melanoma. In these circumstances, we do not consider electron microscopy to be cost-effective, since failure to find diagnostic melanosomes does not change the diagnosis or the management of the patient. Convincing instances of unequivocal keratin reactivity of melanomas have been described (in acetone-fixed frozen sections), so that keratin reactivity, although it remains rare in paraffin sections, can no longer be said to absolutely rule out melanoma (78). In such a case, specific tests such as HMB45 and, especially, electron microscopy, are needed to make the specific diagnosis, especially in unusual circumstances such as the occasional presentation of an amelanotic metastatic melanoma with an unknown primary site. A strongly and diffusely S-100 protein-positive spindle cell tumor is consistent with a spindle cell melanoma, even in the absence of Melan-A or HMB45 reactivity.

REFERENCES

1. Yu LL, Heenan PJ. The morphological features of locally recurrent melanoma and cutaneous metastases of melanoma. Hum Pathol 1999;30:551-555.
2. Griffiths RW, Briggs JC. Incidence of locally metastatic ('recurrent') cutaneous malignant melanoma following conventional wide margin excisional surgery for invasive clinical stage I tumours: importance of maximal primary tumour thickness. Br J Surg 1986;73:349-353.
3. Barr RJ, King DF. The significance of pseudoinclusions within the nuclei of melanocytes of certain neoplasms. In: Ackerman AB, ed. Pathology of malignant melanoma. New York: Masson; 1981:269-272.
4. Busam KJ. Metastatic melanoma to the skin simulating blue nevus. Am J Surg Pathol 1999;23:276-282.
5. King R, Busam K, Rosai J. Metastatic malignant melanoma resembling malignant peripheral nerve sheath tumor: report of 16 cases. Am J Surg Pathol 1999;23:1499-1505.
6. Collina G, Losi L, Taccagni GL, Maiorana A. Myxoid metastases of melanoma: report of three cases and review of the literature. Am J Dermatopathol 1997;19:52-57.
7. Shea CR, Kline MA, Lugo J, McNutt NS. Angiotropic metastatic malignant melanoma. Am J Dermatopathol 1995;17:58-62.
8. Adler MJ, Beckstead J, White CR Jr. Angiomatoid melanoma: a case of metastatic melanoma mimicking a vascular malignancy. Am J Dermatopathol 1997;19:606-609.
9. Koh HK, Sober AJ, Day CL Jr, et al. Prognosis of clinical stage I melanoma patients with positive elective regional node dissection. J Clin Oncol 1986;4:1238-1244.
10. Slingluff CL Jr, Vollmer R, Seigler HF. Stage II malignant melanoma: presentation of a prognostic model and an assessment of specific active immunotherapy in 1,273 patients. J Surg Oncol 1988;39:139-147.
11. Kornberg R, Harris M, Ackerman AB. Epidermotropically metastatic malignant melanoma. Differentiating malignant melanoma metastatic to the epidermis from malignant melanoma primary in the epidermis. Arch Dermatol 1978;114:67-69.
12. Heenan PJ, Clay CD. Epidermotropic metastatic melanoma simulating multiple primary melanomas. Am J Dermatopathol 1991;13:396-402.
13. Elder DE, Guerry D 4th, Heiberger RM, et al. Optimal resection margin for cutaneous malignant melanoma. Plast Reconstr Surg 1983;71:66-72.
14. Day CL Jr, Harrist TJ, Gorstein F, et al. Malignant melanoma. Prognostic significance of "microscopic satellites" in the reticular dermis and subcutaneous fat. Ann Surg 1981;194:108-112.
15. Kelly JW, Sagebiel RW, Calderon W, Murillo L, Dakin RL, Blois MS. The frequency of local recurrence and microsatellites as a guide to reexcision margins for cutaneous malignant melanoma. Ann Surg 1984;200:759-763.
16. Harrist TJ, Rigel DS, Day CL Jr, et al. "Microscopic satellites" are more highly associated with regional lymph node metastases than is primary melanoma thickness. Cancer 1984;53:2183-2187.
17. Roses DF, Harris MN, Rigel D, Carrey Z, Friedman R, Kopf AW. Local and in-transit metastases following definitive excision for primary cutaneous malignant melanoma. Ann Surg 1983;198:65-69.
18. Karakousis CP, Choe KJ, Holyoke ED. Biologic behavior and treatment of intransit metastasis of melanoma. Surg Gynecol Obstet 1980;150:29-32.
19. Haupt HM, Hood AF, Cohen MH. Inflammatory melanoma. J Am Acad Dermatol 1984;10:52-55.
20. Reed RJ, Leonard DD. Neurotropic melanoma. A variant of desmoplastic melanoma. Am J Surg Pathol 1979;3:301-311.
21. Cassarino DS, Cabral ES, Kartha RV, Swetter SM. Primary dermal melanoma: distinct immunohistochemical findings and clinical outcome compared with nodular and metastatic melanoma. Arch Dermatol 2008;144:49-56.
22. Swetter SM, Ecker PM, Johnson DL, Harvell JD. Primary dermal melanoma: a distinct subtype of melanoma. Arch Dermatol 2004;140:99-103.
23. Chan AD, Essner R, Wanek LA, Morton DL. Judging the therapeutic value of lymph node dissections for melanoma. J Am Coll Surg 2000;191:16-22.
24. Balch CM. Surgical management of regional lymph nodes in cutaneous melanoma. J Am Acad Dermatol 1980;3:511-524.
25. Balch CM. The role of elective lymph node dissection in melanoma: rationale, results, and controversies. J Clin Oncol 1988;6:163-172.
26. Balch CM, Soong SJ, Bartolucci AA, et al. Efficacy of an elective regional lymph node dissection of 1 to 4 mm thick melanomas for patients 60 years of age and younger. Ann Surg 1996;224:255-263.
27. Elder DE, Guerry D 4th, VanHorn M, et al. The role of lymph node dissection for clinical stage I malignant melanoma of intermediate thickness (1.51-3.99 mm). Cancer 1985;56:413-418.

28. Veronesi U. Delayed node dissection in stage one malignant melanoma: justification and advantages. Cancer Invest 1987;5:47-53.

29. Morton DL, Wen DR, Wong JH, et al. Technical details of intraoperative lymphatic mapping for early stage melanoma. Arch Surg 1992;127:392-399.

30. Morton DL, Chan AD. The concept of sentinel node localization: how it started. Semin Nucl Med 2000;30:4-10.

31. Morton DL, Thompson JF, Cochran AJ, et al. Sentinel-node biopsy or nodal observation in melanoma. N Engl J Med 2006;355:1307-1317.

32. Kelemen PR, Wanek LA, Morton DL. Lymph node biopsy does not impair survival after therapeutic dissection for palpable melanoma metastases. Ann Surg Oncol 1999;6:139-143.

33. Baloch ZW, Sack MJ, Yu GH, Gupta PK. Papillary formations in metastatic melanoma. Diagn Cytopathol 1999;20:148-151.

34. Cochran AJ, Huang RR, Guo J, Wen DR. Current practice and future directions in pathology and laboratory evaluation of the sentinel node. Ann Surg Oncol 2001;8:13S-17S.

35. Scoggins CR, Ross MI, Reintgen DS, et al. Prospective multi-institutional study of reverse transcriptase polymerase chain reaction for molecular staging of melanoma. J Clin Oncol 2006;24:2849-2857.

36. Satzger I, Volker B, Al GM, Meier A, Kapp A, Gutzmer R. Prognostic significance of histopathological parameters in sentinel nodes of melanoma patients. Histopathology 2007;50:764-772.

37. van Akkooi AC, de Wilt JH, Verhoef C, et al. Clinical relevance of melanoma micrometastases (<0.1 mm) in sentinel nodes: are these nodes to be considered negative? Ann Oncol 2006;17:1578-1585.

38. Holt JB, Sangueza OP, Levine EA, et al. Nodal melanocytic nevi in sentinel lymph nodes. Correlation with melanoma-associated cutaneous nevi. Am J Clin Pathol 2004;121:58-63.

39. Yan S, Brennick JB. False-positive rate of the immunoperoxidase stains for MART1/MelanA in lymph nodes. Am J Surg Pathol 2004;28:596-600.

40. Lohmann CM, Iversen K, Jungbluth AA, Berwick M, Busam KJ. Expression of melanocyte differentiation antigens and ki-67 in nodal nevi and comparison of ki-67 expression with metastatic melanoma. Am J Surg Pathol 2002;26:1351-1357.

41. Starz H. Pathology of the sentinel lymph node in melanoma. Semin Oncol 2004;31:357-362.

42. Romanini A, Manca G, Pellegrino D, et al. Molecular staging of the sentinel lymph node in melanoma patients: correlation with clinical outcome. Ann Oncol 2005;16:1832-1840.

43. Abrahamsen HN, Hamilton-Dutoit SJ, Larsen J, Steiniche T. Sentinel lymph nodes in malignant melanoma: extended histopathologic evaluation improves diagnostic precision. Cancer 2004;100:1683-1691.

44. Gietema HA, Vuylsteke RJ, de Jonge IA, et al. Sentinel lymph node investigation in melanoma: detailed analysis of the yield from step sectioning and immunohistochemistry. J Clin Pathol 2004;57:618-620.

45. Wick MR, Patterson JW. Sentinel lymph node biopsies for cutaneous melanoma. Am J Surg Pathol 2005;29:412-414.

46. Verma S, Quirt I, McCready D, Bak K, Charette M, Iscoe N. Systematic review of systemic adjuvant therapy for patients at high risk for recurrent melanoma. Cancer 2006;106:1431-1442.

47. Essner R. Sentinel lymph node biopsy and melanoma biology. Clin Cancer Res 2006;12:2320s-2325s.

48. Sau P, Solis J, Lupton GP, James WD. Pigmented breast carcinoma. A clinical and histopathologic simulator of malignant melanoma. Arch Dermatol 1989;125:536-539.

49. Granter SR, Weilbaecher KN, Quigley C, Fisher DE. Role for microphthalmia transcription factor in the diagnosis of metastatic malignant melanoma. Appl Immunohistochem Mol Morphol 2002;10:47-51.

50. Palmer AA, Hall BE, Lew M. A comparison of some methods for identifying amelanotic and oligomelanotic melanoma metastases in paraffin sections. Pathology 1985;17:335-339.

51. Warkel RL, Luna LG, Helwig EB. A modified Warthin-Starry procedure at low pH for melanin. Am J Clin Pathol 1980;73:812-815.

52. Olmstead PM, Lund HZ, Leonard DD. Monsel's solution: a histologic nuisance. J Am Acad Dermatol 1980;3:492-498.

53. Duray PH, Livolsi VA. Recurrent dysplastic nevus following shave excision. J Dermatol Surg Oncol 1984;10:811-815.

54. Wood C, Severin GL. Unusual histiocytic reaction to Monsel's solution. Am J Dermatopathol 1980;2:261-264.

55. Moore BW. A soluble protein characteristic of the central nervous system. Biochem Biophys Res Commun 1965;19:739-744.

56. van Duinen SG, Ruiter DJ, Hageman P, et al. Immunohistochemical and histochemical tools in the diagnosis of amelanotic melanoma. Cancer 1984;53:1566-1573.

57. Corwin DJ, Gown AM. Review of selected lineage-dependent antibodies useful in routinely processed tissues. Arch Pathol Lab Med 1989;113:645-652.

58. Nakajima T, Watanabe S, Sato Y, Kameya T, Shimosato Y, Ishihara K. Immunohistochemical demonstration of S100 protein in malignant melanoma and pigmented nevus, and its diagnostic application. Cancer 1982;50:912-918.

59. Nakajima T, Watanabe S, Sato Y, Kameya T, Hirota T, Shimosato Y. An immunoperoxidase study of S-100 protein distribution in normal and neoplastic tissues. Am J Surg Pathol 1982;6:715-727.

60. Abdelatif OM, Khankhanian NK, Crosby JH, Chamberlain CR, Seigler MM, Tom GD. Malignant fibrous histiocytoma and malignant melanoma: the role of immunohistochemistry and electron miocroscopy in the differential diagnosis. Mod Pathol 1989;2:477-485.

61. Cochran AJ, Wen DR, Herschman HR, Gaynor RB. Detection of S-100 protein as an aid to the identification of melanocytic tumors. Int J Cancer 1982;30:295-297.

62. Swanson PE, Wick MR. Clear cell sarcoma. An immunohistochemical analysis of six cases and comparison with other epithelioid neoplasms of soft tissue. Arch Pathol Lab Med 1989;113:55-60.

63. Smoller BR, McNutt NS, Hsu A. HMB-45 staining of dysplastic nevi. Support for a spectrum of progression toward melanoma. Am J Surg Pathol 1989;13:680-684.

64. Ramaekers FC, Puts JJ, Moesker O, Kant A, Vooijs GP, Jap PH. Intermediate filaments in malignant melanomas. Identification and use as marker in surgical pathology. J Clin Invest 1983;71:635-643.

65. Ben-Izhak O, Stark P, Levy R, Bergman R, Lichtig C. Epithelial markers in malignant melanoma. A study of primary lesions and their metastases. Am J Dermatopathol 1994;16:241-246.

66. Pernick NL, DaSilva M, Gangi MD, Crissman J, Adsay V. "Histiocytic markers" in melanoma. Mod Pathol 1999;12:1072-1077.

67. Busam KJ, Granter SR, Iversen K, Jungbluth AA. Immunohistochemical distinction of epithelioid histiocytic proliferations from epithelioid melanocytic nevi. Am J Dermatopathol 2000;22:237-241.

68. Elder DE, Rodeck U, Thurin J, et al. Antigenic profile of tumor progression stages in human melanocytic nevi and melanomas. Cancer Res 1989;49:5091-5096.

69. Brocker EB, Suter L, Bruggen J, Ruiter DJ, Macher E, Sorg C. Phenotypic dynamics of tumor progression in human malignant melanoma. Int J Cancer 1985;36:29-35.

70. Kan Mitchell J, Imam A, Kempf RA, Taylor CR, Mitchell MS. Human monoclonal antibodies directed against melanoma tumor-associated antigens. Cancer Res 1986;46:2490-2496.

71. Brogelli L, Carli P, Reali UM, Pimpinelli N, Moretti S. Antigenic phenotype of radial growth phase melanomas with or without a vertical growth phase portion. Tumori 1988;74:157-162.

72. McGregor BC, McGregor JL, Weiss LM, et al. Presence of cytoadhesins (IIb-IIIa-like glycoproteins) on human metastatic melanomas but not on benign melanocytes. Am J Clin Pathol 1989;92:495-499.

73. Imam A, Mitchell MS, Modlin RL, Taylor CR, Kempf RA, Kan-Mitchell J. Human monoclonal antibodies that distinguish cutaneous malignant melanomas from benign nevi in fixed tissue sections. J Invest Dermatol 1986;86:145-148.

74. Carstens PH, Kuhns JG. Ultrastructural confirmation of malignant melanoma. Ultrastruct Pathol 1981;2:147-149.

75. van Duinen SG, Ruiter DJ, Scheffer E. A staining procedure for melanin in semithin and ultrathin epoxy sections. Histopathology 1983;7:35-48.

76. Umbert IJ, Winkelmann RK. Eruptive histiocytoma. J Am Acad Dermatol 1989;20:958-964.

77. Singh K, Sharma MC, Jain D, Kumar R. Melanotic medullary carcinoma of thyroid—report of a rare case with brief review of literature. Diagn Pathol 2008;3:2-7.

78. Miettinen M, Franssila K. Immunohistochemical spectrum of malignant melanoma. The common presence of keratins. Lab Invest 1989;61:623-628.

12 PROGNOSTIC MODELS FOR MELANOMA

STAGING AND MICROSTAGING OF MALIGNANT MELANOMA

The staging of cancer is a shorthand system of describing the extent of disease. Staging typically includes three major categories of disease: 1) localized to the primary site, 2) regional lymph node metastasis without evident distant disease, and 3) with distant metastasis. Staging systems are of clinical value to the extent that they categorize patients into groups whose prognosis differs significantly, especially when treatment also differs among the groups. Staging can be regarded as an empirical tool that tests the hypothesis that the selected staging categories define populations of patients that are homogeneous with respect to survival (1). In these terms, presently available staging systems are only partially successful.

Stage is a powerful predictor of survival, but many patients are not categorized into clinically useful subsets. Balch and Soong (2) found the 8-year survival rate of 537 patients with malignant melanoma clinically confined to the primary site to be 71 percent, the 3-year survival rate of 82 patients with regional lymph node involvement patients was 37 percent, and none of 16 patients presenting with distant metastatic disease survived beyond 2 years. Although there were highly significant differences among the staging categories, most (85 percent) of the cases presented as localized disease, with an overall survival rate of 71 percent.

To achieve a useful stratification of melanoma patients, they must be further divided into subsets. This subdivision, which has been termed microstaging, is a process that considers various clinical and microscopic attributes of the primary tumor and the host to predict survival of groups of patients that are homogeneous with respect to these attributes. A TNM classification that combines staging and microstaging information into a single system (3) is presently the standard of care and has recently been updated.

In addition, it may be appropriate at times to use prognostic models that have been developed by particular research groups for specific purposes (e.g., estimating the survival probability of individual patients as a means of supporting clinical decisions regarding therapy).

Prognostic models are accurately predictive when applied to large groups of patients (4), but should be used with caution in individual patients. Microstaging of primary tumors by standard techniques retains some predictive power when applied to patients with regional nodal metastases, in whom there are subsets with favorable survival (5–7). Microstaging is most effective, however, when applied to patients with localized tumors in whom the clinically apparent disease is confined to the local site. A fraction of these patients have occult nodal metastases. Indeed, an important potential use of microstaging is to predict the likelihood that nodal metastases are present, information that is used in trials of regional lymphadenectomy and adjuvant therapy (8–11).

The potential for metastasis of a primary melanoma can be assessed using clinical and histologic "prognostic variables" (or "prognostic attributes"). A prognostic variable is an attribute of a primary melanoma that has been statistically associated with survival. Most of the known survival associations have been determined empirically, but the empirical discovery of such associations can suggest relationships of biological interest. For example, the favorable survival association of an attribute such as an infiltrative lymphocytic response at the base of the vertical growth phase (12) can suggest that there is effective host resistance to the tumor.

The variables that are of prognostic value may be determined histologically or clinically, and are entered in a database for correlation with survival. The precision of microstaging depends on the number and power of variables that are considered simultaneously, although a few of these, such as tumor thickness, are sufficiently powerful predictors of survival that it may be sufficient to consider them as single variables for some routine clinical purposes. The application of multivariate analysis to melanoma databases was an important advance in the development of a sophisticated microstaging process (8,13). Multivariate analysis considers a given putative prognostic variable in relation to other variables to determine whether its relationship with survival is "independent." An independent prognostic variable adds explanatory power to the survival function in the presence of other known independent variables. Variables found in a multivariate analysis to be "dependent" presumably derive their association with survival from correlations with other variables, and in part for this reason, the exact variables that enter any given prognostic model differ slightly from one database to another. For example, levels of invasion, ulceration, the location of the lesion, and the sex of the patient are all predictive of survival as single variables, but each of these factors has been found to be dependent in some of the published prognostic models. This fact should not, however, lead to the conclusion that any of these properties is necessarily irrelevant to survival. Because the results of analyses in different databases often differ appreciably, putative prognostic associations should ideally be confirmed by another analytic method, and in another database. Several models have now been described for melanoma that meet at least some of these requirements, and these models are tools for categorizing patients according to expected survival. This categorization has value in clinical decision making, and is of particular importance in the stratification of clinical trials.

Many of the microstaging attributes for melanoma have been discussed in a detailed review by Vollmer (14). The pathology of some of these attributes is considered in the next section. Several of these parameters are incorporated in useful prognostic models developed in several laboratories. Issues relating to melanoma staging and microstaging have been reviewed by Gershenwald et al. (15). Some of the areas at issue include the relevance of level of invasion versus tumor thickness, optimal cutoffs for tumor thickness, importance of ulceration, the grouping of satellites with in-transit metastases,

the inclusion of microsatellites and local recurrences as separate staging criteria, the replacement of the size of nodal mass with the number of positive nodes, the importance of nodal metastases in more than one nodal basin, and the prognostic significance of categories of distant metastases. Issues relating to the staging of primary tumors and their locoregional metastases are discussed in the sections following.

MICROSTAGING ATTRIBUTES (PATHOLOGIC AND CLINICAL)

Phase of Tumor Progression

As discussed above, metastasis is rare in melanomas that are confined to the radial growth phase, i.e., nontumorigenic melanomas. In two studies from the prospectively accrued database of the University of Pennsylvania's Pigmented Lesion Clinic, there were no deaths from these nontumorigenic melanomas, in which the survival rate was estimated as 100 percent, with a confidance interval of 1 percent (16,17). Our extended experience and that of others suggest that there may be a low but definite metastasis rate in these patients of the order of 1 to 2 percent. In a population-based study, the survival rate of patients with vertical growth phase melanoma was 84 percent, compared to 98.2 percent when vertical growth phase was absent (nontumorigenic or microinvasive melanoma) (18). The rare examples of metastasizing nontumorigenic cases may reflect sampling error of small primaries, where a small vertical growth phase could be missed even after multiple sectioning. It is also theoretically possible that a small group of cells, or even a single cell, might in rare instances have metastasized without leaving a residual trace at the primary site. Most of these lesions, in our experience, have either had mitotic activity in the dermis (nontumorigenic but mitogenic melanomas), or have been cases of largely or completely regressed melanomas. Some of these lesions have been found in the region of lymph nodes containing metastatic tumor or have been associated with distant metastases, suggesting that the primary tumor may have regressed after the metastatic event (fig. 12-1). All of these occurrences are rare, given the rarity of metastasis found in association with nontumorigenic melanomas.

428

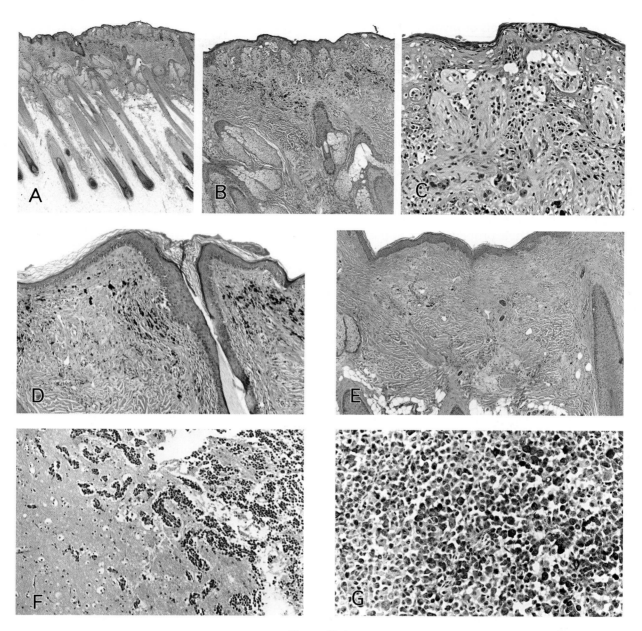

Figure 12-1

EXTENSIVE REGRESSION OF A NONTUMORIGENIC MELANOMA ASSOCIATED WITH BRAIN METASTASES

A: This lesion, from the scalp of a 41-year-old patient, shows a focal area of atypical melanocytic proliferation flanked by large areas of regression.

B: In the area of melanocytic proliferation, there are large atypical epithelioid melanocytes, arranged in confluent nests near the dermal-epidermal junction.

C: Confluent nests and pagetoid proliferation of uniformly atypical epithelioid melanocytes. A few cells are present in the dermis but there is no dermal tumorigenic or mitogenic proliferation.

D: The adjacent papillary dermis is widened with patchy lymphocytes and melanophages, indicative of radial growth phase regression.

E: In another area, there is greater thickening of the papillary dermis with fibrosis, possibly representing regressed tumorigenic melanoma.

F: The patient presented with this brain metastasis, and the pigmented lesion was subsequently discovered on her skin.

G: Melan-A staining highlights the metastatic melanoma in the brain.

Clark Levels of Invasion

Described by Clark in 1967 (19), the characterization of melanomas into five levels of invasion represented the first widely accepted microstaging method for malignant melanoma. The levels of invasion can be viewed as a method of defining a step-wise progression of biologic properties that are associated with the malignant behavior of melanoma cells. The levels of invasion are defined as follows. At level I, melanoma cells are confined to the epidermis (in situ melanoma). The major acquired property that distinguishes level I cells from normal melanocytes is their propensity for apparently inexorable growth, but these cells lack the ability to traverse the basement membrane and are therefore limited to the normal microenvironment of melanocytes, the epidermis (albeit often with "pagetoid" escape upward from the dermal-epidermal junction). In level II invasion, melanoma cells extend from the epidermis into the papillary dermis, but the papillary dermis is not filled or expanded. In general, level I and level II invasion correspond to in situ and microinvasive radial growth phase, respectively, although a few small vertical growth phase micronodules do not fill the papillary dermis, and thus meet the criteria for level II invasion (e.g., those defined as tumorigenic as a consequence of exceeding in size any junctional nest). In our experience, about 90 percent of level II melanomas are in the radial growth phase. The biologic property that distinguishes most level II melanomas from level I is their ability to traverse the basement membrane and invade the dermis. However, the cells are nontumorigenic in most cases, suggesting that they have the capacity to invade and survive in the papillary dermis, but not to proliferate there.

Level III invasion, in contrast, represents a true tumor in the vast majority of cases, with a vertical growth phase nodule that fills and expands the papillary dermis (fig. 12-2). This ability to form an expansile tumor nodule appears to represent a qualitatively new property acquired by the evolving neoplastic cells. Level III melanomas, with only rare exceptions, should be classified as having entered the vertical growth phase, and expansion and filling of the papillary dermis are important criteria for recognition of vertical growth phase disease. Polypoid melano-

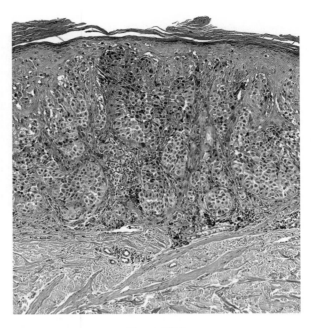

Figure 12-2

MALIGNANT MELANOMA, CLARK LEVEL III

Tumor cells fill and expand the papillary dermis without infiltrating the reticular dermis.

mas, which may greatly expand the papillary dermis but not fill it, are classified as level III tumors by definition.

Level IV invasion constitutes infiltration of tumor cells among reticular dermis collagen fibers (fig. 12-3). Since the papillary dermis represents a microenvironment that is specialized to support the epithelium (the normal epidermis and adnexa), while the "leathery" reticular dermis is less hospitable, the progression to level IV invasion perhaps reflects properties of the melanoma cells that are of significance in terms of tissue infiltration and invasion, and thus of the potential for metastasis. For example, the cells may acquire receptors or growth factors that alter their relationship with their stroma. Some observers have divided level IV invasion into two subcategories (a and b), representing invasion of the superficial reticular dermis and deep reticular dermis, respectively (20). In this regard, it is also important to note that many level III melanomas have areas where several cells appear to show early involvement of the most superficial reticular dermis. There is a tendency to report such lesions as showing superficial level IV involvement. In Clark's original

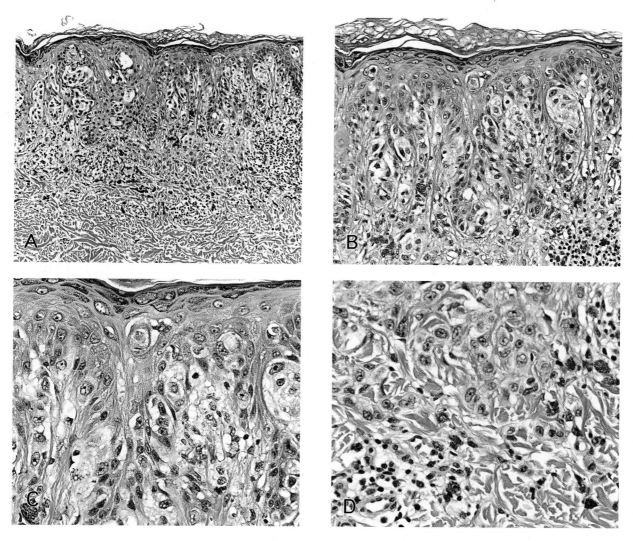

Figure 12-3

MALIGNANT MELANOMA, SUPERFICIAL SPREADING TYPE, WITH "THIN" CLARK LEVEL IV INVASION

A: There is extensive pagetoid proliferation of uniformly atypical melanocytes in the epidermis. Slightly to the right of center, somewhat smaller, uniformly atypical epithelioid cells infiltrate the dermis.
B: The uniformly atypical cells infiltrate reticular dermis collagen fibers.
C: Higher magnification of the uniformly atypical cells in the epidermis.
D: Smaller but uniformly atypical melanocytes infiltrate reticular dermis collagen fibers at the base.

descriptions, however, involvement of the superficial reticular dermis by only one to several cells was not regarded as constituting true level IV disease. This is particularly important in view of the present policy of some centers to perform sentinel lymph node sampling for primary melanomas that are less than 1 mm in measured depth but that show level IV microstaging.

Level V invasion represents infiltration of tumor cells from the reticular dermis into the subcutaneous fat. This may be the only stage in the hierarchy of levels that represents a quantitative rather than qualitative change in the properties of the tumor cells.

The level of invasion is highly associated with survival when considered as a single variable. In one population-based study, which may avoid referral and other biases that could be associated with findings from specialized clinic populations, the survival rate of patients with level II melanoma was 98.8 percent; level III, 92.5 percent; level IV, 76.7 percent; and level V, 75 percent (18). These 5-year survival rates are considerably better than the longer survival data from most specialized clinic databases. For example, in the Penn Pigmented Lesion Group, the 8-year survival rate for patients with level II melanomas was 96.3 percent, compared with 76.1 percent, 60.7 percent, and 38.5 percent for levels II, IV, and V, respectively (19).

The survival association of levels appears to be explained by other variables in many multivariable analyses. These results vary among databases, however. For example, level IV invasion was found to be negatively associated with survival in a series of thin melanomas, suggesting that levels were synergistic with thickness as predictors of survival in that particular dataset (21). In another analysis, level of invasion was one of four independent prognostic variables, along with thickness, ulceration, and mitotic rate (22), and in a study of 1,469 Danish cases, the independent variables included levels of invasion, gender of the patient, lesional location, mitotic rate, tumor cell type (spindle versus other), and lymphocytic response, in addition to thickness (20). These findings, as well as those from other studies, suggest that staging melanomas by level may continue to provide useful prognostic information (23,24). Indeed, melanoma level was used in the 2001 version of the American Joint Committee on Cancer (AJCC) staging system to subdivide stage I tumors, as discussed in detail later in this chapter (25). Further, as described above, an understanding of the levels of invasion is of descriptive value in the concept of tumor progression in melanomas.

Breslow Tumor Thickness

First introduced as a means of microstaging melanomas by Breslow in 1970 (26), the evaluation of tumor thickness by micrometer measurement from the top of the granular layer to the deepest tumor cell soon came to be recognized as the single strongest prognostic variable for melanoma apparently confined to the primary site. Over the last few years, its use as a single variable has appropriately supplanted that of levels of invasion, as several studies have indicated that the levels add little information to that gained by thickness measurement in large series of melanoma cases. Nevertheless, levels have been identified as independent variables (in addition to thickness and other attributes) in several studies (20–23,27), as discussed above.

In his original publications, Breslow identified a group of melanomas thinner than 0.76 mm that rarely metastasized, and the good prognosis of this group of patients has been repeatedly confirmed since. In our experience, the 8-year survival rate of patients with melanomas thinner than 0.76 mm is about 98 percent. Among these thin melanomas, most are in the radial growth phase, but about 15 percent show early vertical growth phase, and it is in this category of thin tumors with vertical growth phase that some potential for metastasis exists. In our experience, the metastasis rate is approximately 10 percent for patients with vertical growth phase melanomas thinner than 0.76 mm.

Breslow also identified a group of tumors in the range of 0.76 to 1.50 mm that appeared to benefit from elective lymph node dissection, but he later attributed this apparent benefit to surgical selection bias (28). Some subsequent retrospective studies tended to suggest that elective lymph node dissection might increase survival for patients with melanomas in the thickness range of 1.50 to 3.99 mm. This remains controversial. A survival benefit was not seen in two earlier, prospective randomized studies, while the results of retrospective multivariable studies have been conflicting (8,29). A large, randomized trial only suggested benefit in subgroups identified retrospectively (30). Nevertheless, the thickness ranges mentioned above remain in common use as "breakpoints" delineating categories of patients at increasing risk. In such a scheme, low-risk patients are those with tumors less than 0.76 mm in greatest thickness, patients with tumors 0.76 to 1.50 mm are designated low-intermediate risk, those with tumors 1.50 to 3.99 mm are at high-intermediate risk, and those with tumors thicker than 4.00 mm are at very high risk for recurrence. In several recent studies, different breakpoints have been used. In the population-based study of Barnhill et al. (18), the 5-year survival rate of patients with melanomas less than 0.76 mm in thickness was 97.9 percent; for those with tumors of 0.76 to 1.69 mm, it was 91.7 percent; for those of 1.7 to 3.6 mm, it was 72.8 percent; and for those over 3.6 mm, it was

57.5 percent. In the Penn Pigmented Lesion Group, the corresponding 10-year survival rates were 96 percent, 83 percent, 59 percent, and 29 percent, respectively (31).

The breakpoints of 1, 2, and 4 mm have been selected by the AJCC for use in the TNM classification (32). There is controversy as to the most appropriate breakpoints, and as to whether risk in fact increases in the step-wise fashion implied by these intervals (33,34). Although fairly good evidence in favor of a linear progression has been presented (35), the categorization of cases into thickness intervals of the sort mentioned above is in general more convenient than the use of a linear function.

While the pathologic evaluation of thickness may seem straightforward, there are some potential difficulties. By definition, thickness is measured from the top of the granular layer to the deepest invasive tumor cell. This means that a tumor with marked epidermal hyperplasia may be measured as quite "thick" when the invasive tumor, in fact, consists only of a few cells in the dermis. In this circumstance, it is appropriate to add a note to the pathology report mentioning that the prognosis may be better than that which would have been expected by thickness alone. The presence of ulceration also creates some difficulties in determining thickness. By convention in an ulcerated neoplasm, the thickness should be measured from the ulcer bed (the surface of the ulcer) to the deepest invasive tumor cell. It is possible that the significance of ulceration as a prognostic variable in some databases results from the "downstaging" of the tumor in terms of its thickness, since such tumors presumably were thicker prior to the occurrence of the ulceration.

The phenomenon of tumor spread downward in the basal epithelium of skin appendages, a common feature in melanomas, also creates difficulties in choosing the deepest tumor cell for evaluation of thickness (see fig. 9-27). When cells are in the epithelium of skin appendages they are not invasive and thus can be ignored because thickness measurements, by definition, are based on invasive tumor. When tumor cells invade outward from a skin appendage into the adventitial dermis which surrounds the appendage and is a continuation of the papillary dermis, they may represent the equivalent of level II or III invasion, depending upon whether or not the adventitial dermis is filled and expanded. We do not measure the depth of the melanoma from the surface to these invasive tumor cells in the adventitial dermis, preferring to choose an area of the neoplasm where invasive cells extend directly from the surface epidermis. Rarely, melanoma cells invade the reticular dermis directly from a site of periadnexal adventitial spread, resulting in a focus of reticular dermal invasion that is deeper than where the lesion more conventionally invades directly from the overlying epidermis. While measurement of this deeper focus may be provided as a worse scenario, in addition to the more conventional measurement, it should be emphasized that the biologic and prognostic significance of such foci has not as yet been fully determined. Microscopic satellites in the reticular dermis have been used as the point of thickness measurement by some observers (36), but we prefer to measure the deepest invasive contiguous tumor cell, while commenting on the presence of microscopic satellites in the reticular dermis, or fat, as the case may be. Finally, the thickness cannot be determined in tangentially sectioned or curetted melanomas. The subject of tumor thickness and its relationship to other prognostic variables was the subject of an extensive review (37).

In a theoretical model of tumor growth, Smolle (38) demonstrated that time was the most important factor contributing to tumor thickness. Other important factors in his study were tumor cell motility, particularly when stimulated by stromal elements, a lower rate of tumor cell loss, and pronounced proliferation associated with high numbers of cell cycle generations in the tumor cells. He considered that these findings were in agreement with experimental data indicating that metastatic capacity may depend on increased motility, stroma-induced motility stimulation, evasion from the host immune system, and genetic instability made manifest during cell cycling.

Dermal Mitotic Rate

The analysis of mitotic rate, like that of thickness, is a simple quantitative determination that can be done by any pathologist using simple equipment. The possibility that mitotic rate correlates with tumor doubling time and thus with prognosis is an obvious hypothesis, and the prognostic significance of mitotic rate was recognized by Cochran in an early prognostic model (39). Schmoeckel and Braun-Falco (40) and others also used mitotic rate to generate a prognostic index based on the product of mitotic rate and thickness. While some substantial studies have failed to establish an independent relationship between mitotic rate and survival (41,42), it is our opinion that mitotic rate is among the strongest of predictive variables when it is determined in the vertical growth phase. Mitoses in the epidermal component of the radial growth phase are irrelevant to prognosis (though they are of diagnostic value), and the lack of separation of these phases of tumor progression in many studies may account for the discrepancies in reported results.

We record mitotic rate as the number of mitoses per square millimeter of vertical growth phase tumor. In effect, because mitoses define the presence of a vertical growth phase, the presence of one may infer the other, although a tumorigenic vertical growth phase, especially when small, may commonly have a mitotic rate of zero. We endeavor to identify the most mitotically active area of the tumor, and then count mitoses over at least 1 mm^2, which represents about 3 to 4 high-power fields in most modern wide-field 40X objectives. In a small dermal component with one or a few mitoses, we count as many fields as possible, and then extrapolate the result to a rate per square millimeter. In such cases, a comment should be added to the effect that such an extrapolation may not be as reliable as one made in a larger tumor, with more observations (mitoses). The exact area of a high-power field should be determined for each microscope using a millimeter scale on the stage to determine the diameter of the field, and the standard formula to determine the area of the circle (i.e., πr^2).

We, like others, have found mitotic rate to be highly predictive of survival (12,18,22,43–46). In a population-based study, the mitotic rate was the only independent predictive attribute in addition to thickness. The survival rate was 98.7 percent for patients with a mitotic rate of 0, 85.1 percent when the mitotic rate was 0.1 to 6.0, and 68.2 percent when the rate was over 6 mitoses/mm^2 (18).

Mitotic rate in our practice is determined only in the vertical growth phase, and is categorized as absent, low (fewer than 6/mm^2), or high (6 or greater). As is also the case with thickness measurements, there is a strong dose-response relationship between mitotic rate and survival, in that the survival becomes progressively worse as the mitotic rate increases. Biologically, it is certainly reasonable to suppose that tumors with a higher proliferative fraction, as judged by the presence of more numerous mitoses, may be more aggressive neoplasms, a hypothesis that has been confirmed by flow cytometric studies of proliferative indices in melanomas (47).

Tumor-Infiltrating Lymphocytes and Other Immunocompetent Cells in the Vertical Growth Phase

The host inflammatory response to melanoma is a diagnostically important microscopic feature, but the interpretation of its relationship to survival poses considerable complexities. To understand the relationship, it is important to consider the radial and vertical growth phases separately. In the radial growth phase, a brisk host response is commonly present, and this may result in the appearance of areas of partial regression, which may correlate at the clinical level with the impression of the patient that the melanoma is "breaking up" and "going away," a belief that may in some cases delay presentation to a physician. This phenomenon of regression is discussed in the next section.

A host response also exists to the vertical growth phase, although it is generally less than that to the radial growth phase. We characterize the host response to the vertical growth phase as either infiltrative (tumor-infiltrating lymphocytes [TILs]), or noninfiltrative (noninfiltrating lymphocytes [NILs]) (fig. 12-4). In the infiltrative pattern, lymphocytes extend among tumor cells, often rosetting around individual cells and sometimes associated with observable degeneration of the tumor cells so surrounded (fig. 12-5). In the noninfiltrative pattern, lymphocytes do not extend among individual tumor cells, but rather infiltrate the dermis that abuts the tumor. We have found infiltrating, but not noninfiltrating, lymphocytes in the vertical growth phase to be significantly associated with survival. Indeed, this "TIL" response was second only to

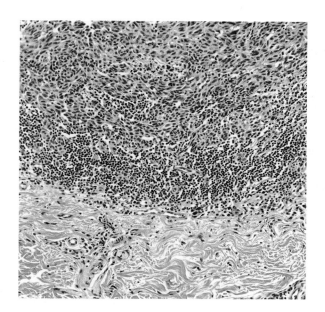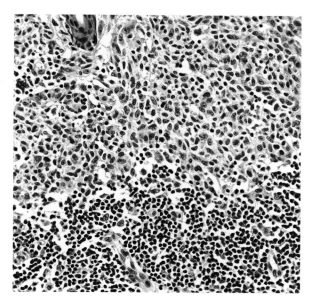

Figure 12-4

**MALIGNANT MELANOMA, TUMORIGENIC VERTICAL GROWTH PHASE,
WITH BRISK TUMOR-INFILTRATING LYMPHOCYTES**

Left: As seen in figure 8-32, tumor-infiltrating lymphocytes, present among lesional cells, extend across the base of the lesion.
Right: The lymphocytes are among and in contact with the melanoma cells.

mitotic rate in predictive power as judged by the survival odds ratio in a prognostic study to be discussed later (12). In addition, in two recent studies, it has been found that the TIL response in the primary tumor, along with Breslow thickness and other attributes, was predictive of the presence of a positive sentinel node (48,49). The TIL response is characterized as brisk (a dense continuous band of lymphocytes among tumor cells across the entire base or throughout the tumor), nonbrisk (a discontinuous band or focal collection of lymphocytes among tumor cells at the base or within the tumor), or absent (fig. 12-6). There is a strong dose-response relationship between the TIL grade and survival (see Survival Models for Melanoma Patients).

It is of considerable biologic interest that NILs and lymphocytes in the radial growth phase, whether infiltrating or not, appear to have no association with survival, either positive or negative (12,45).

In one study, the immunocompetent cells in primary melanomas included natural killer (NK) cells, macrophages, and granulocytes; T cells constituted only 5 to 10 percent of the infiltrate, and B cells less than 5 percent (50). The T cells

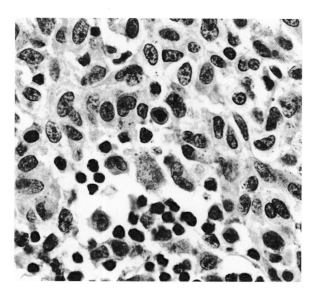

Figure 12-5

TUMOR-INFILTRATING LYMPHOCYTES

This field shows lymphocytes "satelliting" around degenerating tumor cells.

may be of greatest significance, as it has been shown that T cells with cytotoxic granules are present among the infiltrating cell population

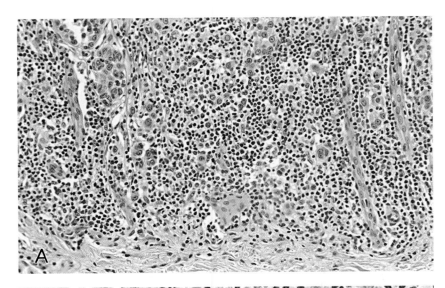

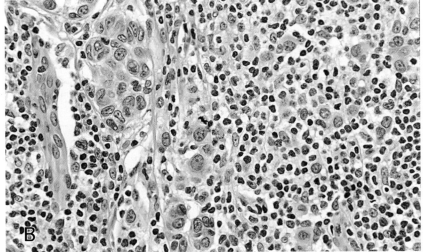

Figure 12-6

BRISK VERSUS NONBRISK TUMOR-INFILTRATING LYMPHOCYTES

A: The lymphocytes are present among the tumor cells and extend across the entire base of the lesion.

B: Tumor-infiltrating lymphocytes are among tumor cells.

C: In another area, the host response was absent, therefore qualifying the lymphocytic response as nonbrisk overall.

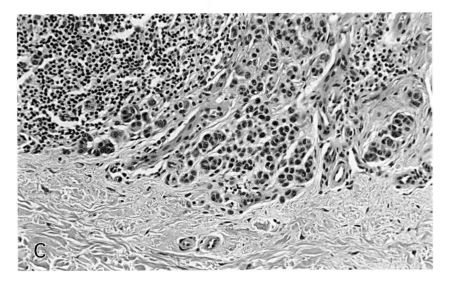

(51). In general tumor biology, TILs have been found to correlate with survival in some tumors, such as colorectal carcinomas and some breast carcinomas; in many other neoplasms, however, the presence of TILs does not correlate with survival, or may even be a negative factor (50). In melanoma, several studies have demonstrated a favorable association of increasing TILs with survival (12,52–54); however, not all studies have confirmed the association (18). In one study, image analysis was used to determine that increased lymphocytic infiltrates within the tumor and subjacent to its base significantly correlated with delayed time to metastasis and longer survival period. The size of the lymphocytic infiltrate at the tumor base in relation to tumor area is of prognostic value: the larger the ratio, the greater the time interval from metastasis to death (54). In a formal study, it was recently demonstrated that the reproducible categorization of TIL can be easily taught, and can be applied with an acceptable level of reproducibility in routine diagnostic practice (55).

Some of the antigens that are recognized by TILs have been identified in ex vivo studies (see later sections), but most of these have not been studied for their correlation with the host response in situ. A recent study addressed this question for the melanoma-associated antigen (MAGE) family, which consists of a number of antigens recognized by cytotoxic T lymphocytes (56). Positive immunostaining for MAGE was associated with a brisk TIL response involving the vertical growth phase. Because, as discussed above, TILs in melanoma are associated with longer survival, these findings suggest a potential role for MAGE as a prognostic marker.

Tumor-Infiltrating Lymphocytes in the Radial Growth Phase

A host response, consisting of lymphocytes and histiocytes, often with diffuse fibroplasia in the papillary dermis, is often present in the radial growth phase. The lymphocytic response may extend among the tumor cells (TILs), or be present adjacent to them but not among them (NILs). No relation with survival is detected among tumors with differing degrees of infiltrating or noninfiltrating lymphocytic response in the radial growth phase, in contrast to the vertical growth phase where a brisk TIL response is associated with improved survival (12). The

T lymphocytes in the radial growth phase are about equally divided among CD4- and CD8-positive cells. In the radial and vertical growth phase compartments, there is a significant population of T-cell restricted intracellular antigen (TIA)-1-positive cytotoxic T cells ("killer" T cells) (51). Other immunocompetent cells have not been studied in detail in the radial growth phase host response. TIL responses to the radial growth phase of melanoma must be separated from true regression, which does correlate with prognosis (see below).

Radial Growth Phase Regression

Probably as a consequence of lesional cell destruction by cytotoxic T cells, it is common for localized areas of partial disappearance to occur in melanoma lesions. These areas are almost always confined to the radial growth phase compartment, although a similar phenomenon is, rarely, apparent in the vertical growth phase, and even in metastases. This may be noticed by patients who feel that the melanoma is breaking up and going away. Unfortunately, the disappearance is often not complete. Paradoxically, the presence of partial regression has been found in several studies to correlate with metastasis of thin melanomas (57–61), or with worsened prognosis in tumorigenic melanomas (see fig. 12-1) (12). Other studies have failed to confirm these findings, and the matter is still at issue (62–65).

In our experience, regression is present in about a third of the metastasizing thin melanomas we have seen, but a vertical growth phase is usually also present (with only rare exceptions). It is possible that regression plays a permissive role in the development of vertical growth phase, perhaps by obliterating radial growth phase cells while allowing the growth of vertical growth phase cells that lack the antigens recognized by the host response. Alternatively (and perhaps more likely), a small tumorigenic or mitogenic component was present in the area of regression before it regressed. In any case, in our experience, regression is the only attribute of the radial growth phase that has a significant (negative) correlation with survival (12).

Regression in the radial growth phase is defined by us as a local area within a melanoma where there is fibroplasia and usually a lymphocytic infiltrate, often with melanophages and

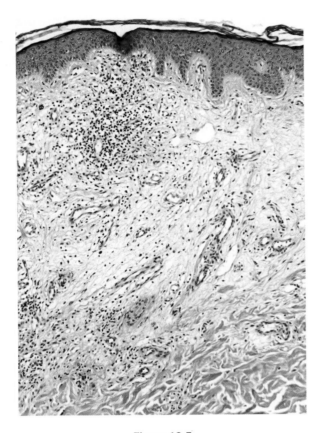

Figure 12-7

RADIAL GROWTH PHASE REGRESSION

The papillary dermis is widened with diffuse fibroplasia and an admixture of inflammatory cells, which often include melanophages. There is no melanoma present in this area of "locally complete" regression; however, melanoma is likely to be present in adjacent skin.

prominent vessels, with absence of melanoma in both the epidermis and the dermis (fig. 12-7). Adjacent to this area of "regressive fibroplasia" (on one side or the other, or on both sides), there is usually melanoma present in either the epidermis, dermis, or both. This phenomenon may be termed "locally complete" regression. Frequently, diffuse eosinophilic fibroplasia indistinguishable from regressive fibroplasia is observed in the presence of melanoma cells in the overlying epidermis. This finding, which we interpret as a stromal response to the tumor, is not considered to represent locally complete regression. Conversely, occasional examples of putative complete disappearance of a melanoma ("globally complete regression") are observed.

In these cases, there is no residual diagnostic melanoma and the diagnosis is necessarily inferential, but may be supported by a convincing clinical history of an evolving and then regressing lesion, consistent with a primary melanoma. Unfortunately, a few of these "globally" or "completely" regressed melanomas have been found, concurrently or in follow-up, to be associated with regional lymph node or distant metastases, which presumably occurred before the complete regression of the primary lesion.

Kang et al. (66) have provided a detailed description and definition of three phases of regression. Early regression is a "zone of papillary dermis and epidermis within a recognizable melanoma, characterized by dense infiltrates of lymphocytes disrupting/replacing nests of melanoma cells within the papillary dermis and possibly the epidermis as compared to adjoining zones of tumors; degenerating melanoma cells may or may not be recognizable. There is no recognizable fibrosis." Intermediate regression, in addition to the above, is characterized by "reduction (loss) in the amount of tumor (a disruption in the continuity of the tumor) or absence of tumor in the papillary dermis and possibly the epidermis, and replacement by varying admixtures of lymphoid cells and increased fibrous tissue (as compared to normal papillary dermis) in this zone. Variable telangiectasia and melanophages may be present." In late regression, in addition to the above, there is "marked reduction" or "loss" of tumor in the zone of regression, and there is "replacement and expansion of the papillary dermis by extensive fibrosis (usually dense and horizontally disposed)" as well as variable telangiectasia, lymphocytes, melanophages, and effacement of the epidermis. Our own definition more or less corresponds to that of the above late regression when there is loss of tumor in the area of regression (locally complete regression).

Using the definitions of Kang et al., studies showed that interobserver reproducibility was good (90 percent or better) between two observers for the presence or absence of regression, but agreement rates fell and the patterns were often mixed for the subdivisions described above. The reproducibility of the classification of regression has been studied by others, sometimes with poor results, indicating the importance of a detailed definition of regression agreed upon by the participants prior to the study (66,67).

Ulceration

The association of ulceration of a primary melanoma with unfavorable survival has been reviewed in several large databases (22,68,69). In one study, ulcers greater than 3 mm in diameter were prognostically significant, while smaller ulcers had no survival associations (70). Similar importance was attached to ulcer width in another study (41), but this parameter is not considered in the recent AJCC staging system (32). As noted above, it is possible that an ulcer might serve to "downstage" a melanoma by resulting in a spuriously low thickness measurement. In the population-based study of Barnhill et al. (18), the survival rates for patients with and without ulceration were 91.6 percent and 66.2 percent, respectively. A working group recently defined an ulcer as a local full-thickness loss of continuity of the epithelium, with evidence of a host response such as fibrin deposition, inflammation, granulation tissue, or fibrosis, and with thinning, effacement, or reactive hyperplasia of the adjacent epithelium at the periphery of the ulcer (71) (see fig. 9-38). Erosions that lack evidence of a response may represent a biopsy artifact. A prior shave biopsy may exactly resemble an ulcer as defined above, but should not be so classified in prognostic models.

Microscopic Satellites

In some analyses, the presence of microscopic satellites is an independent adverse prognostic variable. Satellites are discrete foci of tumor in the connective tissue discontinuous from the main tumor, and are considered to most likely represent locoregional metastases (70). In older and some current literature, satellites were distinguished from in-transit metastases by an arbitrary cutoff limit of 5 cm from the primary tumor. The recent AJCC staging scheme, however, merged satellite metastases and in-transit metastases into a single staging entity that is grouped as stage III disease (32).

In some studies, satellites are not independent variables (12), perhaps because they are relatively uncommon, so that the studies cannot observe a survival effect. In a matched pair study designed to focus on this question, satellites were significantly associated with a worse outcome (72). In a population-based study, the survival rates of patients without (n = 512) and with (n = 18) satellites were 90 percent and 66.7 percent, respectively (18). In our experience, satellites appear to be associated with an increased risk for local recurrence, even after a formal wide excision has been done. It must be emphasized, however, that microscopic satellites are rare, and their hypothetical presence does not justify wide excisions designed to "capture" melanoma cells in the process of spreading from their primary site. Metastases that develop after complete excision of a primary melanoma that does not recur locally must be the consequence of spread from the primary site prior to the excision.

Vascular Invasion

Vascular invasion is closely related to satellites, as most satellites presumably occur as a result of angiolymphatic invasion. It is generally not possible to distinguish between vascular and lymphatic invasion (fig. 12-8). Definite or "true" angiolymphatic invasion is rarely observed in primary melanomas, which may, at least in part, explain its failure to have independent significance in most multivariable studies. In a population-based study, the survival rates of patients without (n = 533) and with (n = 7) angiolymphatic invasion were 89.1 percent and 42.9 percent, respectively (18). It seems likely that angiolymphatic invasion, when present, is likely to be associated with a poor prognosis.

Borgstein et al. (73) studied a series of 258 patients, recording lymphatic invasion either as tumor cell aggregates in an endothelial-lined space at the primary site or in afferent lymphatics of a sentinel lymph node specimen. They considered microscopic satellites as "unequivocal" evidence of lymphatic invasion. Unequivocal lymphatic invasion was observed in 14 of the patients (5.4 percent, 6 of whom had satellites); 13 (93 percent) of these 14 patients subsequently developed in-transit metastases. In 244 of 258 patients (94.6 percent), there were no signs of lymphatic invasion, and only 4 patients (1.6 percent) had a locoregional recurrence (p <.001). It was concluded that lymphatic invasion is an important prognostic parameter that should be considered in the stratification of trials.

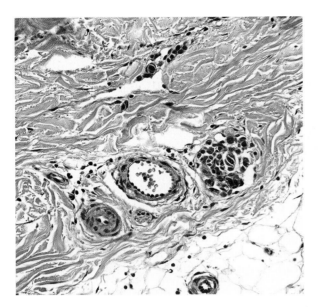
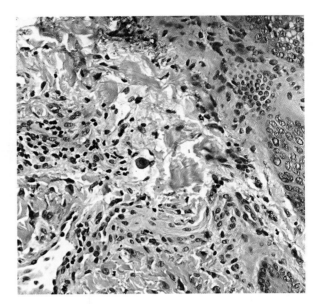

Figure 12-8

MALIGNANT MELANOMA WITH ANGIOLYMPHATIC INVASION

Left: Tumor cells are present in two separate endothelial-lined channels.
Right: In another example, a single cell is present in an endothelial-lined channel.

In another important study, "definite" vascular invasion was defined as the presence of tumor cells within blood or lymphatic vessels; while in "uncertain" or "mural" vascular invasion melanoma cells were present immediately adjacent to the endothelium (fig. 12-9) (74,75). The presence of either type of vascular involvement was associated with a significantly increased risk of relapse and death. In a multivariate analysis, vascular involvement was the second most important factor (after tumor thickness) for predicting survival. If confirmed, this study will expand the definition of vascular invasion. A similar phenomenon has also been described as "extravascular migratory metastasis" by Barnhill and Lugassy (76).

Morphometric Attributes

Nuclear morphometry has been used in an effort to correlate nuclear parameters with survival. In one study comparing tumor thickness, DNA index as determined by flow cytometry, and volume-weighted nuclear volume measured stereologically, only the latter was a significant predictor of prognosis in a multivariable analysis (77). The number of cases in the study was small, however. In a case-control study, 24 thin metastasizing melanomas were compared with 48 matched nonmetastasiz-ing cases by morphometric assessment of nuclear area, shape and density, nucleolar area, analysis of DNA content, and expression of proliferating cell nuclear antigen (PCNA) (78). Multivariable analysis showed significant differences between metastasizing and nonmetastasizing melanomas with regard to the nuclear correlation coefficient ($p = 0.005$), standard deviation of nuclear shape ($p = 0.017$), and nuclear density ($p = 0.030$), indicating that thin melanomas with pleomorphic and possibly densely packed nuclei are associated with recurrence. The other attributes studied were not significant.

Age, Sex, and Anatomic Location

Demographic or clinical factors that are associated with survival in melanoma patients include age, anatomic site, sex, and stage. The effect of age is the least consistent, but some studies have found a better prognosis for younger patients (41,43). This may be particularly true for melanomas that develop in infancy and childhood, although larger studies are needed before definitive statements can be made. In addition, despite a higher rate of sentinel node metastasis, patients under 30 years of age do not have a worse survival, due to their having a more

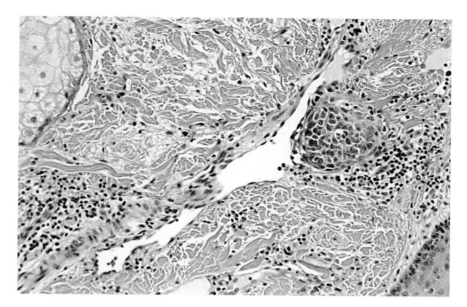

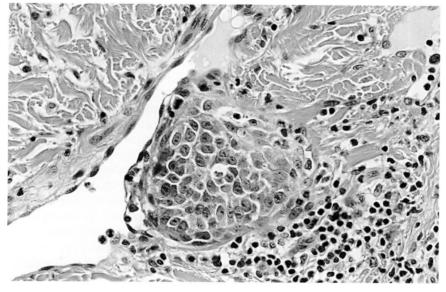

Figure 12-9

"UNCERTAIN" OR "MURAL" VASCULAR INVASION

The presence of tumor cells undermining endothelial cells, as here, has been associated with impaired survival.

favorable clinicopathologic profile (79). The superior survival of female patients, and of patients whose melanomas are on the limbs compared to the trunk, has been demonstrated in most multivariable studies (31,52,80), but interactions among these variables often complicate the interpretation of the findings (81,82).

Lymph Node Metastases

Stage is perhaps the most important single prognostic factor, and the prognostic models discussed in this chapter have demonstrated most of their predictive capacities in patients with clinically localized tumors (AJCC stages I and II). Stage III, defined as regional lymph node metastasis, is associated with a dramatic deterioration of prognosis, which has been estimated overall as a 40 percent reduction in the 5-year survival rate (83). Regional lymph node metastases may be discovered at the time of primary tumor diagnosis or at a later time, or they may occur without an identifiable primary lesion. According to the findings from the University of Alabama database, the prognosis for each patient group is about the same, if measured from the time of discovery of the metastasis

(84). The characteristics of the primary retain some reduced significance in some subsets of patients with regional lymph node metastases, particularly when the extent of nodal disease is limited, for example, to less than 20 percent of the total nodes removed (5). The number of involved nodes is highly predictive of prognosis. Patients with one microscopically positive node have a 5-year survival rate of about 70 percent if there is no ulceration in the primary tumor, or 50 percent if ulceration is present. The survival rate for patients with nonulcerated tumors is about 60 percent with two to three nodes microscopically involved and 27 percent with three or more nodes involved. For ulcerated tumors, the survival rates are 50 percent and 37 percent, respectively (84).

SURVIVAL MODELS FOR MELANOMA PATIENTS

Many groups have developed prognostic models for melanoma in an effort to provide accurate predictions of survival probability and thus to assist in formulating a basis for clinical decision making. Because the models are derived from the study of cases in populations, they necessarily have limited accuracy when applied to the individual patient, especially when applied outside the group originally used for model building. Nevertheless, the models provide information of value when considering the extent of primary therapy, the use of adjuvant therapy with differing degrees of toxicity, and the frequency and extent of follow-up, as well as in the patient's personal planning. As discussed above, Clark and Breslow introduced very powerful single variables, namely, levels of invasion (19,85) and tumor thickness (26,86), that successively revolutionized the field of prognostication for melanoma. However, the introduction of extensive multivariable modeling of a large clinicopathologic database by Day et al. (13,27,33,45,71,87–100) allowed for the effect of these attributes to be considered in relation to each other and to other clinical and statistical attributes. These seminal studies are of interest to this day, and have provided a basis for additional modeling efforts that aim to address a range of issues from individualized prognosis to stratification for clinical trials.

Among the many available prognostic models, the best developed, which we consider to have potential value in clinical practice and research, are those of Clark et al. (12), Soong (101), and Cochran et al. (41). Differences in study design, as well as other variables peculiar to the databases, no doubt explain the variation in the attributes that have been considered to be independently associated with survival in these and other similar studies (27,91,94). Soong, for example, found thickness, ulceration, surgical treatment (elective node dissection), anatomic site, and pathologic stage to be independently associated with survival in a Cox model, while Clark et al. found ulceration, treatment, and pathologic stage to be dependent while mitotic rate, tumor-infiltrating lymphocytes, and the gender of the patient were independent variables. The level of invasion was a dependent variable in both of the above studies, but was found to be significant in a study confined to intermediate thickness melanomas (27), as well as in several other recent studies that were mentioned above (20–22). Cochran et al. found five variables that were linked to survival: gender, site of primary, age relative to 60 years, Breslow thickness, and presence and width of ulceration. Mitotic rate and "intratumoral inflammation" were not independently significant. Some of these differences in prognostic attributes may be explained by the fact that most studies have not distinguished radial growth phase melanomas, with their near perfect freedom from metastasis, from the vertical growth phase cases among which there is considerable survival variation. Although other differences in study design could be invoked to explain some of the variance, differences in referral pattern of cases and random variation in outcome among the databases must also exist, suggesting that no one model can be considered to be definitive. Survival rates in the one available detailed population-based study appear to be superior to those in most referral center–based studies, again suggesting the possibility of referral or other local bias (18).

In considering prognostic models, prognostication for individual melanoma patients is still highly imperfect in a "n of 1" setting (i.e., for the individual patient). Even for patients who may have an excellent predicted probability of survival, a small percentage will, in fact, develop metastatic disease and die from their melanoma. Conversely, patients with the most high-risk tumors, as judged by prognostic modeling, still may survive their disease. Just as the low-risk AJCC stage I tumors with Breslow thickness of 1 mm or less account for an increasing proportion of new melanoma cases, a corresponding increase in deaths will occur for melanoma in the future judged to be "low-risk" by current "state-of-the-art" prognostic modeling. This consideration provides an impetus, and an opportunity, to refine these prognostic models so as to recognize subsets of cases at different levels of risk.

PROGNOSTIC MODELS FOR SURVIVAL IN PATIENTS WITH LOCALIZED MELANOMA

In this section, we consider several models that are based on robust clinical datasets and rigorous statistical analyses, and that provide a format suitable for pathologists and clinicians to conveniently estimate prognosis for individual patients, based on readily determinable clinico-pathologic attributes.

Soong Multivariate Prognostic Model

Soong et al. (24,102) developed generalized multivariate prognostic models to address survival, either immediately following a diagnosis of melanoma or after a disease-free interval. The model was based on 4,568 patients of the University of Alabama at Birmingham and the Sydney Melanoma Unit. Four clinical factors (age, sex, lesion location, and initial surgical treatment), and four pathologic attributes (thickness, level of invasion, ulceration, and growth pattern) were evaluated. The Cox proportional model was used (103). Six dominant factors were identified: thickness, ulceration, location, level of invasion, and sex (all $p = 0.002$ or less). Age was of borderline significance ($p = 0.049$). When further analyses were done in tumor thickness subsets, surgical treatment proved significant in certain subgroups. A prognostic model was then determined for each thickness subgroup. The predicted 5- and 10-year survival rates were presented in a convenient tabular form and are reproduced in Table 12-1.

According to this model, the inclusion of certain attributes depends on their relationship to others, so that not all attributes are involved in the prediction of survival for each case. Also, the survival rates have been adjusted for the effects of surgical treatment in those subgroups where such treatment is a significant factor. Now that sentinel node biopsy is an almost universal procedure, this model should be more widely applicable than it might have been in an era when there were wide disparities in policies relating to elective lymph node dissection (see later section).

Soong et al. (24,102) also developed models for prediction of survival during follow-up. At 5 years of follow-up, the thickness and location of the lesion were significant, while at 10 years only thickness was significant (Table 12-2). The diminishing number of attributes could reflect the diminishing power of the model as the number of observations decreases with the length of follow-up.

Other prognostic models for subsets of cases, and a potentially useful clinical staging system, have been presented by Soong and Weiss in a detailed summary of their work (24).

Cochran Individualized Prognostic Model

Cochran et al. (41) studied 1,042 patients who were a subset of the John Wayne Cancer Institute Melanoma Database, UCLA and St John's Hospital, Santa Monica. The patients were first divided into an estimation set and a test set. The Cox proportional hazards model was used in a stepwise manner to choose variables in a multivariable setting. The resulting model was then applied to the test set to confirm or reject the importance of the selected variables. Then, data were combined from the two halves of the study for the generation of a final model. In addition, a similar analysis was carried out using a tree-structured censored survival regression model, which according to the authors gave the same conclusion as the Cox model. Variables considered included most of the standard attributes, however, growth phase (presence or absence of vertical growth phase), and therefore also TIL in this growth phase, were not considered, a major difference from the Clark model. Survival was found to be related to five variables: gender, site of primary, age relative to 60 years, and presence and width of ulceration. The probability of survival is calculated for an individual patient using a two-step approach. The survival-linked variables are multiplied us-

Table 12-1

PREDICTED 5- AND 10-YEAR SURVIVAL RATES FOR PATIENTS WITH LOCALIZED MELANOMA[a]

Tumor Thickness (mm)	Anatomic Site	Ulceration	Clark Level	Sex	5-Year Survival Rate (%)	10-Year Survival Rate (%)
<0.76	Extremity		II		99	97
	Extremity		Other		97	94
	Axial		II		96	92
	Axial		Other		91	84
0.76–1.49	Extremity	No	II		98	97
	Extremity	No	Other		93	89
	Extremity	Yes	II		94	91
	Extremity	Yes	Other		82	72
	Axial	No	II		95	93
	Axial	No	Other		85	77
	Axial	Yes	II		88	81
	Axial	Yes	Other		64	49
1.50–2.49	Extremity	No			86	81
	Extremity	Yes			76	69
	Axial	No			76	67
	Axial	Yes			61	49
2.50–3.99	Extremity	No		Female	80	72
	Extremity	No		Male	73	62
	Extremity	Yes		Female	74	64
	Extremity	Yes		Male	64	51
	Axial	No		Female	73	63
	Axial	No		Male	63	51
	Axial	Yes		Female	65	52
	Axial	Yes		Male	53	39
4.00–7.99		No	II/III		80	73
		No	IV/V		68	58
		Yes	II/III		67	57
		Yes	IV/V		51	38
>8.00					43	25

[a]Modified from table 3-3 from Soong SJ, Weiss HL. Predicting outcome in patients with localized melanoma. In: Balch CM, Houghton AN, Sober AJ, Soong SJ, eds. Cutaneous melanoma. St. Louis, Quality Medical Publishing, Inc., 1998:55.

ing the coefficients listed in Table 12-3, which are then converted into survival probability using conversion factors for either 3-, 5-, or 10-year survival rate, raised to the power of the survival variable (Table 12-4).

The probability can be calculated using a hand calculator or a simple computer spreadsheet. According to the authors, the techniques provided "highly accurate" predictions for individual patients in the validation set. To this date, however, this model has not been tested in a dataset completely different than that used to build the model.

Similar tables were developed for the likelihood of recurrence. The significant variables for recurrence (disease-free survival) were anatomic site, melanoma subtype, Breslow thickness, and presence and width of ulceration. In this model, the relative risk scores for various mela-

Table 12-2

ESTIMATED PROBABILITIES OF MELANOMA DEATH WITHIN THE NEXT 5 YEARS IF A PATIENT IS FREE OF DISEASE 5 YEARS AFTER DIAGNOSIS OF LOCALIZED MELANOMA[a]

Tumor Thickness (mm)	Anatomic Site	No. of Patients	Probability of Melanoma Death Within 5 Years
<1.5	Extremity	846	2%
	Axial	582	5%
>1.5		631	9%

[a]Modified from table 3-6 from Soong SJ, Weiss HL. Predicting outcome in patients with localized melanoma. In: Balch CM, Houghton AN, Sober AJ, Soong SJ, eds. Cutaneous melanoma. St. Louis, Quality Medical Publishing, Inc., 1998:56.

noma subtypes were: 1.7 (most likely to recur) for nodular and acral-lentiginous melanomas, 1.4 for lentigo maligna melanoma, 1.2 for un-

Table 12-3

**CALCULATION OF RISK SCORE
FOR DEATH FROM MELANOMA[a]**

Gender	Risk Score[b]	Age	Risk Score
Male	1.8	60+ years	3.3
Female	1	<60 years	1

Breslow Thickness (mm)		Ulceration (mm)	
6+	1.75	5+	4.2
2 to 6	3.8	2 to 5	2.6
1 to 2	2	0 to 2	1.6
0 to 1	1	0	1

Site	
Head/trunk	1.75
Extremity	1

[a]Modified from Table 4 from Cochran AJ, Elashoff D, Morton DL, Elashoff R. Individualized prognosis for melanoma patients. Hum Pathol 2000;31:329.
[b]The risk score is obtained by multiplying the weighted factors, i.e., gender factor x age factor x Breslow factor x ulceration factor x site factor = risk score.

Table 12-4

CALCULATION OF PROBABILITY OF SURVIVAL[a]

Survival Probability At:	Risk Score[b]
3 years	0.987
5 years	0.975
10 years	0.960

[a]Data from reference 41.
[b]The risk score is obtained by multiplying the weighted factors, i.e., gender factor x age factor x Breslow factor x ulceration factor x site factor = risk score.

classifiable, and 1.0 for superficial spreading melanoma. Considering the anatomic site, the score was 2.1 for head/trunk versus extremities. Thickness and ulceration width were correlated in a dose-response pattern similar to that in Table 12–3 for survival.

Clark Progression-Based Survival Model (Model Predicting Survival in Stage I Melanoma Based on Tumor Progression)

Since survival is 100 percent in radial growth phase melanomas irrespective of thickness or any other risk factor, Clark et al. (12) considered that models for prediction of survival should be based first on the phase of tumor progression, followed by further characterization of the factors associated with survival in vertical growth phase (tumorigenic) cases, i.e., those melanomas that have potential competence for metastasis but that exhibit substantial variance in the probability of metastasis. The probability of metastasis is almost zero in some vertical growth phase cases, while other cases are at extremely high risk. Thickness explains some but not all of this variance. This group studied 484 patients, all of whom had been followed for 8 years or until death by the Pigmented Lesion Group at the University of Pennsylvania. The model was developed in a test group of 386 patients, and

validated in a group of 98 patients whose cases had not been used for building the model.

The survival rate for 122 patients with no vertical growth phase (radial growth phase only) was 100 +/- 1 percent. A logistic regression model for 8-year survival of the 264 patients with vertical growth phase melanomas in clinical stage I characterized six variables as independent predictors of survival. In order of relative predictive weight for favorable survival, the six independent variables were: relatively low mitotic rate (0 or fewer than $6/mm^2$), presence of brisk or moderate TILs, thickness of less than 1.7 mm, location on extremity skin excluding volar/subungual skin, female sex, and absence of regression in the radial growth phase. The odds ratios for the predictors of survival, indicative of the relative risk associated with each factor, are shown in Table 12-5. The small survival odds effect for thickness compared to other series is probably explained by the fact that much of the predictive power of thickness in early studies derived from the excellent survival of patients with "thin" melanomas. The good survival of these patients, however, is likely due to more than 90 percent of them being nontumorigenic radial growth phase melanomas which are almost incapable of metastasis. This model differs from previous models like that of Soong (101) and Cochran et al. (41) in that it was developed only on vertical growth phase tumors. The output from the logistic regression analysis provides an estimate of survival probabilities, presented in a simple tabular format (Tables 12-5 and 12-6).

The Clark survival model is applied as a two-step procedure by first identifying cases of pure radial growth phase melanoma. For these cases, the predicted survival is 100 ± 1 percent. Then, the prognosis for tumorigenic

445

Table 12-5

ODDS RATIOS FOR INDEPENDENT PREDICTORS OF SURVIVAL[a]

Prognostic Variable	Categories	Adjusted Odds Ratio[b]
Mitotic rate	0.0/mm^2	11.69
	0.1-6.0/mm^2	3.49
	>6.0/mm^2	1.00
TILs[c]	brisk	11.31
	nonbrisk	3.51
	absent	1.00
Thickness	<1.7 mm	4.04
	>1.7 mm	1.00
Anatomic site	extremities	3.80
	axial/subvol	1.00
Sex	female	2.92
	male	1.00
Regression	absent	2.79
	present	1.00

[a]Data from Table 4 from reference 12.
[b]The adjusted odds ratio expresses the likelihood of death, compared to a patient whose tumor lacks the attribute under consideration, all other attributes being held constant. For example, a patient whose melanoma has a mitotic rate higher than 6 is almost 12 times as likely to die than a patient whose tumor has no mitoses, all other variables being equal.
[c]TILs = tumor-infiltrating lymphocytes.

cases is obtained from the probability formula, expressed in tabular form. The model generates a survival probability at 8 years with confidence intervals (Table 12-6). For example, a 52-year-old man with a nodular melanoma of the thigh that was 3.99 mm thick, having a mitotic rate of 3.6, nonbrisk TILs, and no regression, had a survival probability of 0.86 (range, 0.69 to 0.94), and was in fact alive at 13.2 years after therapy. A 47-year-old man had a superficial spreading melanoma of the abdomen that was 0.76 mm thick, with a mitotic rate of 13.6, absent TILs, and regression in the radial phase. His predicted survival probability was 0.16 (range, 0.06 to 0.37), and he died 18.8 months after therapy. The predicted survival probabilities of the two patients illustrated above in a model based on thickness alone were 0.32 and 0.88, respectively. When the model was applied to the validation sample of 98 cases, 89 percent of the outcomes were correctly predicted.

In an independent external study, Pritchard and Woosley (105) validated this model using a database of 55 patients from a different geographic location (North Carolina) and observed virtually identical accuracy of predicting 8-year survival for patients with radial growth phase

Table 12-6

PROBABILITIES OF 8-YEAR SURVIVAL FOR VERTICAL GROWTH PHASE (AJCC[a] I OR II)[b]

Mitoses Thickness (< or >1.7 mm)	TILs[c]	Regression	Female Arm, Leg <1.7	>1.7	Female Axial, Subvol <1.7	>1.7	Male Arm, Leg <1.7	>1.7	Male Axial, Subvol <1.7	>1.7
0.0/mm^2	Brisk	Absent	1.0	.99	1.0	.98	1.0	.98	.99	.95
		Present	1.0	.99	.99	.95	.99	.96	.96	.86
	Nonbrisk	Absent	1.0	.98	.98	.94	.99	.95	.96	.84
		Present	.99	.95	.96	.85	.97	.88	.89	.66
	Absent	Absent	.99	.94	.95	.82	.96	.85	.86	.60
		Present	.96	.86	.87	.61	.89	.67	.69	.35
0.1–6.0/mm^2	Brisk	Absent	1.0	.98	.98	.94	.99	.95	.95	.84
		Present	.99	.95	.96	.84	.97	.87	.88	.65
	Nonbrisk	Absent	.99	.95	.95	.82	.96	.86	.87	.61
		Present	.96	.86	.87	.62	.90	.68	.70	.36
	Absent	Absent	.95	.83	.84	.57	.87	.63	.65	.31
		Present	.88	.64	.66	.32	.71	.38	.40	.14
>6.0/mm^2	Brisk	Absent	.99	.94	.95	.81	.96	.85	.86	.60
		Present	.96	.85	.86	.61	.89	.67	.68	.35
	Nonbrisk	Absent	.95	.84	.84	.57	.88	.63	.65	.31
		Present	.88	.64	.66	.32	.72	.38	.40	.14
	Absent	Absent	.85	.59	.61	.28	.67	.33	.34	.12
		Present	.68	.34	.35	.12	.42	.15	.16	.04

[a]AJCC = American Joint Committee on Cancer.
[b]Data from Tables 6 and 7 from reference 12.
[c]TILs = tumor-infiltrating lymphocytes; axial/subvol includes head, neck, trunk, and volar and subungual locations.

(100 percent) and vertical growth phase (85.1 percent) melanomas (104). In a subsequent study using the same dataset, the model was compared to a simple thickness model (101). While there was a suggestion of a modest improvement for the multiple variable model, the difference was not statistically significant in this small study of 55 cases (105). It seems likely that the multivariate model provides useful information beyond that supplied by the currently used simple thickness model based on cutoff points; still, additional studies of larger datasets from multiple centers are needed to better define the role of such detailed prognostic modeling programs for planning therapy and for conducting clinical trials (12).

In another evaluation of the model in a different database of 259 patients, Tuthill et al. (106) found that TILs, primary site, and thickness had independent predictive value. Using the Clark logistic regression prediction model, 8-year survival was predicted in 72.9 percent of 166 patients and melanoma-specific mortality in 43 percent of 74 patients. The combined or overall accuracy of the model was only 64 percent. This dataset was a group of patients who were to be randomized into a clinical trial and did not include patients with melanomas of Breslow thickness under 0.76, and therefore is not directly comparable. Nevertheless, these data indicate the need for independent confirmation, and also illustrate the fact that the accuracy of any model is best in the dataset in which it was developed, or a very similar dataset (107).

Gimotty et al. (107) have pointed out that the percent of patients correctly predicted by a model depends on the "case mix" of a cohort. To demonstrate this interrelationship, these authors identified a new validation cohort from their database based on the original eligibility criteria for the Clark model. This new cohort included 691 patients with primary melanoma who also had complete data on all variables in the model (approximately 46 percent of those seen between 1980 and 1990). In this validation cohort, 40 percent of patients had thin lesions, less than 0.75mm. For the 511 of these patients with lesions with vertical growth phase, predicted probabilities were computed using the original Clark model. It was found that 84 percent of the patients were correctly classi-

fied, exactly as found with the original model. When the Tuthill thickness eligibility criterion was then applied, removing all patients in the new validation cohort whose lesion thickness was less than or equal to 0.75 mm (322 patients with vertical growth phase lesions), the proportion of patients correctly predicted decreased to 76 percent.

Because many centers do not routinely report attributes such as growth phase/tumorigenicity, mitotic rate, TIL, and so on, Schuchter et al. (31) used the Penn Pigmented Lesion Clinic database to develop a model for survival prediction using attributes likely to be readily available to the clinician and present in most pathology reports (Table 12-7). The model was based on 488 patients followed for more than 10 years. Four variables were found to be independently related to survival: lesion thickness (odds ratio 50.8), site of melanoma (4.4), patient age (3.0), and patient sex (2.0).

Use of the model in a validation sample not used for model building resulted in a reduction to 50 percent in erroneous predictions. In an external validation study using a population-based cohort with 5 years of follow-up, it was concluded that a similar model developed for 5 years of follow-up was generalizable to the Connecticut tumor registry population, and that a simpler single variable model based on thickness cutoff points could be used with a small loss of accuracy (108). In this dataset, death from melanoma was not associated with lesion location, patient age, or patient sex, and it is possible that these attributes may play a greater role in the causes of death between 5 and 10 years. A simple table can be used to estimate prognosis for individual patients according to the Schuchter model.

TNM Staging System for Melanoma

The tumor-node-metastasis (TNM) system of tumor staging considers factors related to the primary tumor, to regional lymph nodes (and other regional soft tissues), and to distant metastases in a classification system that is associated with the probability of survival. The factors considered in the primary tumor (T) category include some of the microstaging attributes discussed above. Thus, the TNM classification combines staging and microstaging information

Table 12-7

PROBABILITIES OF 10-YEAR SURVIVAL IN PATIENTS WITH LOCALIZED PRIMARY CUTANEOUS MELANOMA[a]

Variable	Extremity Location		Axial Location	
	Female Patients	Male Patients	Female Patients	Male Patients
Thickness <0.76 mm				
Age ≤60	.99	.98	.97	.94
Age >60	.98	.96	.92	.84
Thickness 0.76–1.69 mm				
Age ≤60	.96	.93	.86	.75
Age >60	.90	.81	.67	.50
Thickness 1.70–3.60 mm				
Age ≤60	.89	.80	.65	.48
Age >60	.73	.57	.38	.24
Thickness >3.60 mm				
Age ≤60	.74	.58	.39	.24
Age >60	.48	.32	.18	.10

[a]Data from reference 31.

in a single format. In the current system (109), the T attributes are classified pathologically after excision of the melanoma (pT), as described below (25,110). The TNM model therefore considers pathologic attributes of the primary tumor, but staging for metastases is defined in part clinically. Lymph node metastases, for example, are defined in terms of the number of lymph nodes involved as well as volume (coded as "micrometastasis" if lymph node metastasis has been diagnosed at sentinel node biopsy or at elective lymphadenectomy, or as "macrometastasis" if clinically positive and pathologically confirmed by therapeutic lymphadenectomy) (25,110). Among macrometastases, the size of the nodes is no longer used in staging, based on evidence that the number of nodes but not their size is significant prognostically (111–116). In other prognostic models, it has been demonstrated that microstaging of the primary tumor retains prognostic significance in melanoma patients who are clinically negative but pathologically positive for metastases to regional nodes (5,7,117), and this was also reflected in the 2009 AJCC staging system, where ulceration of the primary tumor retains significance in some patients with nodal metastases.

The recently updated version (2009) of the TNM categories is presented in Table 12-8 and the final stage groupings are in Table 12-9 (110). Clinical staging includes microstaging of the primary melanoma and clinical/radiologic evaluation for metastases. By convention, clinical staging should be used after complete excision of the primary melanoma, with clinical assessment for regional and distant metastases. Pathologic staging includes microstaging of the primary melanoma and pathologic information about the regional lymph nodes after partial or complete lymphadenectomy. Patients with pathologic stage 0 or stage 1A do not require pathologic evaluation of their lymph nodes.

The TNM staging system differs from previously used, simple, primarily clinical staging systems (localized, regional, and metastatic disease) in that pathologic attributes of the primary neoplasm (microstaging attributes) are considered in the definition of the first three stage groups. Tumors in stage groups I and II are nonmetastatic, and stage III may or may not be associated with metastasis (Table 12-9). Stage IV is always metastatic. Since these stages are different from those defined in other staging systems, it is necessary that the system in use should be clearly specified when staging is used as a basis for therapy or prognosis.

The AJCC Melanoma Staging Committee has listed the following guidelines that it used to determine the criteria to be used in the TNM classification and the stage groupings (25). First, the staging system should be practical, reproducible, and applicable to the diverse needs of all medical disciplines. Second, the criteria should accurately reflect the biology of melanoma based on consistent outcome results of patients treated at multiple institutions from

Table 12-8

MELANOMA TNM CLASSIFICATION[a]

T Classification

	Thickness	Ulceration Status
T1	≤1.0 mm	a: without ulceration and mitosis <1/mm^2 b: with ulceration or mitoses >1/mm^2
T2	1.01–2.0 mm	a: without ulceration b: with ulceration
T3	2.01–4.0 mm	a: without ulceration b: with ulceration
T4	>4.0 mm	a: without ulceration b: with ulceration

N Classification

No. of Metastatic Nodes		Nodal Metastatic Mass
N1	1 node	a: micrometastasis[b] b: macrometastasis[c]
N2	2–3 nodes	a: micrometastasis[b] b: macrometastasis[c] c: in-transit met(s)/satellite(s) without metastatic nodes
N3	4 or more metastatic nodes, or matted nodes, or in-transit met(s)/satellite(s) with metastatic node(s)	

M Classification

	Site	Serum Lactate Dehydrogenase
M1a	Distant skin, subcutaneous, or nodal metastases	Normal
M1b	Lung metastases	Normal
M1c	All other visceral metastases Any distant metastasis	Normal Elevated

[a]Modified from Table 1 from Balch CM, Gershenwald JE, Soong SJ, et al. Final version of the American Joint Committee on Cancer staging system for cutaneous melanoma. J Clin Oncol 2009;27:6199-6206.
[b]Micrometastases are diagnosed after sentinel or elective lymphadenectomy.
[c]Macrometastases are defined as clinically detectable nodal metastases confirmed by therapeutic lymphadenectomy or when nodal metastasis exhibits gross extracapsular extension.

Table 12-9

STAGE GROUPINGS FOR CUTANEOUS MELANOMA[a]

0	Clinical Staging[b]			Pathologic Staging[c]		
	T	N	M	T	N	M
0	Tis	N0	M0	Tis	N0	M0
IA	T1a	N0	M0	T1a	N0	M0
IB	T1b	N0	M0	T1b	N0	M0
	T2a	N0	M0	T2a	N0	M0
IIA	T2b	N0	M0	T2b	N0	M0
	T3a	N0	M0	T3a	N0	M0
IIB	T3b	N0	M0	T3b	N0	M0
	T4a	N0	M0	T4a	N0	M0
IIC	T4b	N0	M0	T4b	N0	M0
III	Any T	N1 N2 N3	M0			
IIIA				T1-4a	N1a	M0
				T1-4a	N2a	M0
IIIB				T1-4b	N1a	M0
				T1-4b	N2a	M0
				T1-4a	N1b	M0
				T1-4a	N2b	M0
				T1-4a/b	N2c	M0
IIIC				T1-4b	N1b	M0
				T1-4b	N2b	M0
				Any T	N3	M0
IV	Any T	Any N	Any M1	Any T	Any N	Any M1

[a]Modified from Table 2 from Balch CM, Gershenwald JE, Soong SJ, et al. Final version of the American Joint Committee on Cancer staging system for cutaneous melanoma. J Clin Oncol 2009;27:6199-6206.
[b]Clinical staging includes microstaging of the primary melanoma and clinical/radiologic evaluation of metastases by convention; it should be used after complete excision of the primary melanoma with clinical assessment for regional and distant metastases.
[c]Pathologic staging includes microstaging of the primary melanoma and pathologic information about the regional lymph nodes after partial or complete lymphadenectomy; pathologic stage 0 or stage 1A patients are the exception: they do not require pathologic evaluation of their lymph nodes.

multiple countries. Third, the criteria used should be evidence-based and reflect the dominant prognostic factors consistently identified in Cox multivariate regression analyses. Fourth, the criteria should be relevant to current clinical practice and regularly incorporated in clinical trials. Fifth, the required data should be sufficiently easy for tumor registrars to identify in medical records to code staging information.

The staging system is primarily based on survival studies performed at collaborating institutions. Survival rates for 27,639 patients from the new AJCC database are shown in Table 12-10 (110).

As can be seen in Table 12-8, in the present classification, mitotic rate (or in fact "mitogenicity"—the presence or absence of any mitoses) has replaced Clark level IV as a stage modifier for defining AJCC stage Ib melanomas. Ulceration remains in use as a stage modifier. The survival rates of patients with ulcerated melanomas are similar to those for patients in the next AJCC thickness category. For example, the 5-year survival rate is 79 percent for patients with a T3a nonulcerated melanoma and 8 percent for

Table 12-10

SURVIVAL RATES FOR MELANOMA BY T CATEGORIES[a]

T Category	Thickness	Number of Patients	10-Year Survival Rate
T1	<1 mm	11,841	92%
T2	1–2 mm	8,046	80%
T3	2–4 mm	5,291	63%
T4	>4 mm	2,461	50%

[a]Modified from Table 3 from Balch CM, Gershenwald JE, Soong SJ, et al. Final version of the American Joint Committee on Cancer staging system for cutaneous melanoma. J Clin Oncol 2009;27:6199-6206.

those with a T2b ulcerated melanoma, and accordingly both are classified as stage IIA (Table 12-9) (110). The effects of ulceration and mitogenicity are similar to one another in thin melanomas. For example, the 10-year survival rate is 95 percent for those with nonulcerated and nonmitogenic T1 melanomas, and drops to 88 percent if any mitoses are present. Ulcerated T1 melanomas are associated with mitogenicity in 78 percent of patients, while the 10-year survival rate is the same regardless of whether the tumor is mitogenic or not (85 versus 87 percent) (110). Mitogenicity adds little to prediction in thicker melanomas, although mitotic rate has been useful in different models as reviewed previously (12). Survival rates by T category are presented in Table 12-10.

The determination of mitogenicity will be discussed in forthcoming staging manuals and the concept is discussed elsewhere in this volume. For the purposes of AJCC staging, it is recommended that the tumor should first be scanned to identify the "hot spot" where mitoses are most numerous, and then the number of mitoses in one square millimeter of tumor should be recorded. This requires calibration of microscopes by determining (using a ruler or preferably a stage micrometer) the radius of a high-power field and using the formula for the area of a circle for determining the area of the field. A square millimeter will represent about 3 to 5 high-power fields in most microscopes. If the determined area is not close (within 10 percent) to a whole square millimeter, a correction factor may be applied, but if this is done, the resulting number should then be rounded

to the nearest whole number. The practice of recording mitoses as "<1/mm^2" when no mitoses are seen should be discontinued, and the rate should be recorded as zero. In our opinion and that of others with whom we have discussed this issue, it is not appropriate to exhaustively section tumors to rule out a rare mitosis for at least two reasons: first, the prognostic value of mitogenicity has been established in studies of thousands of cases that were routinely processed at dozens of referring institutions. To radically change the manner of determining mitotic rate would therefore change the underlying data on which these conclusions have been drawn, with unpredictable results; second, with the advent of targeted therapy, it is important, in our view, to preserve as much tissue as possible in the blocks of tumor for possible future use in genotyping or other predictive studies that may be needed to determine optimal therapy for patients who have developed metastatic disease.

With regard to advanced disease, there are few changes in the revised AJCC classification. In the case of sentinel lymph node metastasis detection, it is stated that immunohistochemical detection of nodal metastases is acceptable, with no lower limit of size to designate N+ disease (110). The possible existence of a lower limit of size (such as submicroscopic micrometastases <0.1 mm) is the subject of ongoing clinical trials. In addition, in our opinion, the pathologist should be convinced that the immunohistochemically positive cells are melanoma cells and not nevus cells, Schwann cells, or some artifact.

Penn Models for Survival Prediction in Thin (AJCC Stage I) Melanoma

Gimotty et al. (118) from the University of Pennsylvania Pigmented Lesion Group evaluated factors associated with prognosis in 887 patients with thin primary melanoma (AJCC stage I) by Cartesian Regression Tree (CART) analysis. They demonstrated interactions among mitotic rate, tumorigenicity (radial or vertical growth phase), and gender, useful in predicting survival in these patients. The overall prognosis for this group of patients is for a 92 percent 10-year survival rate (110). As demonstrated in the model, however, based on these simple attributes, subsets of patients at risk of metastasis ranged from 0.5

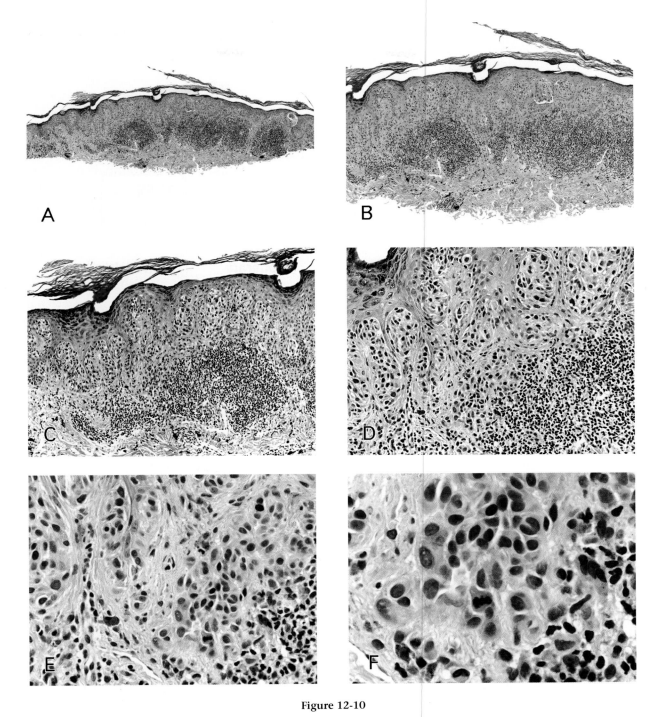

Figure 12-10

MALIGNANT MELANOMA, SUPERFICIAL SPREADING TYPE, MITOGENIC BUT NONTUMORIGENIC

A,B: Scanning magnification shows a broad lesion with irregular thickening and thinning of the epidermis, and a brisk perivascular to focally band-like lymphocytic infiltrate in the papillary dermis.

C,D: High magnification shows a cluster of cells in the dermis, not larger than the largest clusters in the epidermis, consistent with invasive but nontumorigenic melanoma.

E,F: The single mitosis present in this invasive cluster is consistent with mitogenic but nontumorigenic invasive vertical growth phase melanoma.

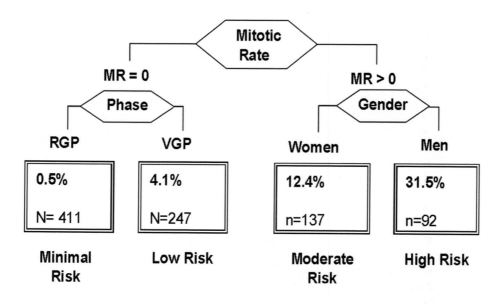

Figure 12-11

METASTASIS-FREE SURVIVAL IN THIN MELANOMAS (N = 887)

(Figure 2 from Gimotty PA, Guerry D 4th, Ming ME, et al. Thin primary cutaneous malignant melanoma: a prognostic tree for 10-year metastasis is more accurate than American Joint Committee on Cancer staging. J Clin Oncol 2004;22:3673.)

percent to 31.5 percent. It was demonstrated by Receiver operating curve (ROC) analysis that survival prediction using this model was more accurate for patients with thin melanoma than the 2002 AJCC model itself. Although tumorigenicity is usually required for metastasis, we have observed metastasis in mitogenic but nontumorigenic melanomas (illustrated in fig. 12-10), and the presence of dermal mitoses has also been associated with risk for sentinel lymph positivity in thin melanomas (119). These considerations demonstrate that recognition of tumorigenicity and mitogenicity in thin melanomas can have significant clinical implications. Patients whose melanomas have these attributes may be considered for staging by selective lymphadenectomy. On the other hand, the model also clearly identifies a group of patients whose risk is so low that sentinel node sampling is clearly inappropriate (fig. 12-11). The model may be informative for clinical use, but has not been confirmed in another database.

Recognizing that tumor mitotic rate is not universally available in pathology reports, the Penn group recently used data from 26,291 patients with thin melanomas from the United States population-based Surveillance, Epidemiology, and End Results (SEER) cancer registry to develop a model which was then validated using 2,389 patients seen by the University of Pennsylvania's Pigmented Lesion Group (PLG). In the SEER-based classification tree, which included lesion thickness, anatomic level, ulceration, and site, and patient sex and age, 10-year survival rates ranged from 89.1 percent to 99.0 percent. Prognostication and related clinical decision making in the majority of patients with melanoma can be improved now using this validated, SEER-based classification.

A new PLG-based tree was also developed which identified survival groups using tumor level, tumor cell mitotic rate, and patient sex, and had better discrimination, with survival rates ranging from 83.4 percent to 100.0 percent (120). This new model requires validation in another data set before it can be used in practice.

The survival rates for the validated model are shown in Table 12-11. This model is evidence based and peer reviewed, and can be used for prognostication and therapy. It should be noted, in comparison with Table 12-10, that the survival rates, in general, are considerably better than

Table 12-11

EXPANDED 2002 AJCC CLASSIFICATION FOR THIN MELANOMAS (<1 MM)[a]

Category	Number of Cases	Survival Rate[b]
Not Ulcerated		
Level II, thickness <0.78 mm, age <60	10,648	99.0
Level II, thickness <0.78 mm, age >60	5,258	97.5
Level III, thickness <0.78 mm, other sites	4,169	96.8
Level III, thickness <0.78 mm, head and neck	664	92.1
Level II/III, thickness >0.78 mm, women	1,397	95.6
Level II/III, thickness >0.78 mm, men	1,608	90.6
Level IV/V	2,213	91.4
Ulcerated		
Level II/III	215	88.9
Level IV/V	119	69.8

[a]Data from figure 1 from refence 119.
[b]SEER database 10-year survival rate.

those in the current prognostic table for patients with stage IA. This difference is likely due to selection bias in the latter series, compared to the population-based SEER data. Conversely, when both of the modifying factors for stage I, Clark level IV, and ulceration are present, the prognosis for these patients is significantly worse than that for AJCC stage IB patients, which is based on the presence of either one of these two risk factors. These patients might, therefore, be considered for additional therapeutic options.

The new PLG model resembles that in the earlier publication (118), with level of invasion serving as a surrogate for growth phase, and requires validation in another dataset before it can be uncritically used. However, this model adds weight to the considerable body of evidence which suggests that mitotic rate, or mitogenicity in thin melanomas, is a significant prognostic variable that has been added to the next iteration of the AJCC/UICC staging system.

SURVIVAL IN PATIENTS WITH LYMPH NODE METASTATIC MELANOMA

The survival rates for patients with metastatic melanoma are somewhat variable, but generally poor. For some patients with limited nodal disease (stage IIIA), the 10-year survival rate is above 50 percent, but when distant metastasis is present (stage IV), the prognosis is uniformly dismal (25). As previously noted, it is of interest that, despite a higher rate of sentinel lymph node metastasis, patients under 30 years of age do not have a worse survival rate because they have a more favorable clinicopathologic profile (79). Therefore, the discovery of lymph node metastases, especially when confined to a single node, should not be regarded as a death sentence.

SURVIVAL IN PATIENTS WITH DISTANT METASTATIC MELANOMA

Barth et al. (121) undertook a retrospective analysis of data for 1,521 patients with AJCC stage IV melanoma treated by the staff of the John Wayne Cancer Institute. The median survival period for these 1,521 patients was 7.5 months; the estimated 5-year survival rate was 6 percent. Three independent variables significantly predicted survival: initial site of metastases, disease-free interval before distant metastases, and stage of disease preceding distant metastases. Patients were divided into three distinct prognostic groups based on the initial site of metastases: cutaneous, nodal, or gastrointestinal metastases (median survival of 12.5 months; estimated 5-year survival rate 14 percent); pulmonary metastases (8.3 months, 4 percent); and metastases to the liver, brain, or bone (4.4 months, 3 percent). There was no significant change in the survival rate of patients with AJCC stage IV melanoma during the 22-year review period. The development of targeted therapy for melanoma will hopefully result in improvement of these grim statistics in the near future.

SURGICAL PATHOLOGY REPORT FOR PRIMARY MELANOMA

Pathology reports should include information essential for the optimal management of a primary melanoma by clinicians. In addition, other information, such as histogenetic type and precursor lesions, may be provided for clinicopathologic and epidemiologic correlation, as these may affect the future management of the patient and advice to the patient's family. Barnhill and Mihm (122), and Cochran et al. (36) have presented their recommendations for a pathology report. Based on these and our own

Table 12-12

PATHOLOGY REPORT FOR PRIMARY MELANOMA

Patient and Gross Pathology Information

Specimen identification data:	name, age, medical record number
How the specimen was received:	fresh, type of fixative
Exact anatomic site of the tumor:	typically provided by surgeon
Type of surgical procedure:	excision, reexcision, incision, punch or shave biopsy
Gross dimensions of specimen:	length, diameter, and thickness
Gross dimensions of lesion:	lesion diameter, diameter of any nodule
Gross description of lesion:	border, color, elevation, ulceration, scale/crust
Description of background skin:	color pigmentation, other lesions if any

Essential Microscopic Information

Diagnosis of primary melanoma:	
Breslow thickness:	
Clark level of invasion:	I, II, III, IV, V
Ulceration:	presence or absence and width
Adequacy of surgical margins:	a statement as to completeness of excision; if not adequate or doubtful, a measurement of margin width may be provided, especially in a biopsy

If present, desmoplastic vertical growth phase, neurotropism, extensive radial growth phase regression, dermal mitotic activity ("mitogenicity"), vascular/lymphatic invasion, microscopic satellites.

Additional Information That Has Epidemiologic and/or Prognostic Significance in Some Databases

Phase of progression:	tumorigenic (vertical growth phase) or nontumorigenic (radial growth phase)
Radial growth phase and type:	SSM, LMM, ALM, MLM[a] or pagetoid, lentiginous, mixed
Dermal mitotic rate:	measured per square millimeter in the vertical growth phase
Tumor-infiltrating lymphocytes:	absent, nonbrisk, brisk
Associated nevus/precursor:	compound, dysplastic, congenital pattern nevus, lentigo

[a]SSM = superficial spreading melanoma; LLM = lentigo maligna melanoma; ALM = acral-lentiginous melanoma; MLM = mucinous-lentiginous melanoma.

practice, a useful pathology report is presented in Table 12-12. As Cochran et al. have written: "The recommendations are intended as suggestions, and adherence to them is completely voluntary. In special clinical circumstances, the recommendations may not be applicable. The recommendations are intended as an educational resource rather than a mandate." While therapeutic recommendations may be offered in a pathology report, the surgical and medical management of the melanoma is the responsibility of the patients' treating physicians, and the provision of therapeutic recommendations is not a standard of care for pathologists.

REFERENCES

1. Elder DE. Prognostic guides to melanoma. In: Mackie RM, ed. Clinics in oncology, Vol 3. London: Saunders; 1984:457-476.
2. Balch CM, Soong SJ. Characteristics of melanoma that predict the risk of metastasis. In: Costanzi J, ed. Malignant melanoma I. London: Martinus Nijhoff; 1983:117-150.
3. Greene FL, Balch CM, Page DL, et al. AJCC cancer staging manual. New York: Springer; 2002.
4. Soong SJ. A computerized mathematical model and scoring system for predicting outcome in melanoma patients. In: Balch CM, Milton GW, eds. Cutaneous melanoma. Clinical management and treatment results worldwide. Philadelphia: Lippincott; 1985:353-367.
5. Day CL Jr, Sober AJ, Lew RA, et al. Malignant melanoma patients with positive nodes and relatively good prognoses: microstaging retains prognostic significance in clinical stage I melanoma patients with metastases to regional nodes. Cancer 1981;47:955-962.
6. Callery C, Cochran AJ, Roe DJ, et al. Factors prognostic for survival in patients with malignant melanoma spread to the regional lymph nodes. Ann Surg 1982;196:69-75.
7. Cochran AJ, Lana AM, Wen DR. Histomorphometry in the assessment of prognosis in stage II malignant melanoma. Am J Surg Pathol 1989;13:600-604.
8. Elder DE, Guerry DI, VanHorn M, et al. The role of lymph node dissection for clinical stage I malignant melanoma of intermediate thickness (1.51-3.99 mm). Cancer 1985;56:413-418.
9. Mraz-Gernhard S, Sagebiel RW, Kashani-Sabet M, Miller JR, Leong SP. Prediction of sentinel lymph node micrometastasis by histological features in primary cutaneous malignant melanoma. Arch Dermatol 1998;134:983-987.
10. Karakousis GC, Gimotty PA, Botbyl JD, et al. Predictors of regional nodal disease in patients with thin melanomas. Ann Surg Oncol 2006;13:533-541.
11. Kesmodel SB, Karakousis GC, Botbyl JD, et al. Mitotic rate as a predictor of sentinel lymph node positivity in patients with thin melanomas. Ann Surg Oncol 2005;12:449-458.
12. Clark WH Jr, Elder DE, Guerry DI, et al. Model predicting survival in stage I melanoma based on tumor progression. JNCI 1989;81:1893-1904.
13. Lew RA, Day CL Jr, Harrist TJ, Wood WC, Mihm MC Jr. Multivariate analysis. Some guidelines for physicians. JAMA 1983;249:641-643.
14. Vollmer RT. Malignant melanoma. A multivariate analysis of prognostic factors. Pathol Annu 1989;24:383-407.
15. Gershenwald JE, Buzaid AC, Ross MI. Classification and staging of melanoma. Clin Lab Med 2000;20:785-815.
16. Elder DE, Guerry D 4th, Epstein MN, et al. Invasive malignant melanomas lacking competence for metastasis. Am J Dermatopathol 1984;6:55-61.
17. Guerry D 4th, Synnestvedt M, Elder DE, Schultz D. Lessons from tumor progression: the invasive radial growth phase of melanoma is common, incapable of metastasis, and indolent. J Invest Dermatol 1993;100:342S-345S.
18. Barnhill RL, Fine JA, Roush GC, Berwick M. Predicting five-year outcome for patients with cutaneous melanoma in a population-based study. Cancer 1996;78:427-432.
19. Clark WH Jr. A classification of malignant melanoma in man correlated with histogenesis and biologic behavior. In: Montagna W, Hu F, eds. Advances in the biology of the skin, Vol. VIII. New York: Pergamon Press; 1967:621-647.
20. Sondergaard K, Schou G. Therapeutic and clinico-pathological factors in the survival of 1,469 patients with primary cutaneous malignant melanoma in clinical stage I. A multivariate regression analysis. Virchows Arch [A] 1985;408:249-258.
21. Kelly JW, Sagebiel RW, Clyman S, Blois MS. Thin level IV malignant melanoma. A subset in which level is the major prognostic indicator. Ann Surg 1985;202:98-103.
22. Ronan SG, Han MC, Das Gupta TK. Histologic prognostic indicators in cutaneous malignant melanoma. Semin Oncol 1988;15:558-565.
23. Marghoob AA, Koenig K, Bittencourt FV, Kopf AW, Bart RS. Breslow thickness and Clark level in melanoma: support for including level in pathology reports and in American Joint Committee on Cancer Staging [see comments]. Cancer 2000;88:589-595.
24. Soong SJ, Weiss HL. Predicting outcome in patients with localized melanoma. In: Balch CM, Houghton AN, Sober AJ, Soong SJ, eds. Cutaneous melanoma. St. Louis, Quality Medical Publishing, Inc., 1998:51-64.
25. Balch CM, Buzaid AC, Soong SJ, et al. Cutaneous melanoma. Final version of the American Joint Committee on Cancer staging system for cutaneous melanoma. J Clin Oncol 2001;19:3635-3648.

26. Breslow A. Thickness, cross-sectional areas and depth of invasion in the prognosis of cutaneous melanoma. Ann Surg 1970;172:902-908.

27. Day CL Jr, Mihm MC Jr, Sober AJ, et al. Prognostic factors for melanoma patients with lesions 0.76 - 1.69 mm in thickness. An appraisal of "thin" level IV lesions. Ann Surg 1982;195:30-34.

28. Breslow A. Tumor thickness, level of invasion and node dissection in stage I cutaneous melanoma. Ann Surg 1975;182:572-575.

29. Balch CM. The role of elective lymph node dissection in melanoma: rationale, results, and controversies. J Clin Oncol 1988;6:163-172.

30. Balch CM, Soong S, Ross MI, et al. Long-term results of a multi-institutional randomized trial comparing prognostic factors and surgical results for intermediate thickness melanomas (1.0 to 4.0 mm). Intergroup Melanoma Surgical Trial [see comments]. Ann Surg Oncol 2000;7:87-97.

31. Schuchter L, Schultz DJ, Synnestvedt M, et al. A prognostic model for predicting 10-year survival in patients with primary melanoma. Ann Intern Med 1996;125:369-375.

32. Balch CM, Buzaid AC, Atkins MB, et al. A new American Joint Committee on Cancer staging system for cutaneous melanoma. Cancer 2000;88:1484-1491.

33. Day CL Jr, Lew RA, Mihm MC Jr, et al. The natural break points for primary-tumor thickness in clinical stage I melanoma [letter]. N Engl J Med 1981;305:1155.

34. Balch CM, Soong SJ, Shaw HM, Milton GW. An analysis of prognostic factors in 4000 patients with cutaneous melanoma. Cutaneous melanoma. In: Balch CM, Milton GW, Shaw HM, Soong SJ, eds. Clinical management and treatment results worldwide. Philadelphia: Lippincott; 1985:321-352.

35. Vollmer RT, Seigler HF. Using a continuous transformation of the Breslow thickness for prognosis in cutaneous melanoma. Am J Clin Pathol 2001;115:205-212.

36. Cochran AJ, Bailly C, Cook M, et al. Recommendations for the reporting of tissues removed as part of the surgical treatment of cutaneous melanoma. Association of Directors of Anatomic and Surgical Pathology. Hum Pathol 1997;28:1123-1125.

37. Kopf AW, Welkovich B, Frankel RE, et al. Thickness of malignant melanoma: global analysis of related factors. J Dermatol Surg Oncol 1987;13:345-390, 401-420.

38. Smolle J. Biological significance of tumor thickness. Theoretical considerations based on computer simulation. Am J Dermatopathol 1995;17:281-286.

39. Cochran AJ. Method of assessing prognosis in patients with malignant melanoma. Lancet 1968;2:1062-1064.

40. Schmoeckel C, Braun-Falco O. Prognostic index in maligant melanoma. Arch Dermatol 1978;114:871-873.

41. Cochran AJ, Elashoff D, Morton DL, Elashoff R. Individualized prognosis for melanoma patients. Hum Pathol 2000;31:327-331.

42. Attis MG, Vollmer RT. Mitotic rate in melanoma: a reexamination. Am J Clin Pathol 2007;127:380-384.

43. Duncan LM, Deeds J, Cronin FE, et al. Melastatin expression and prognosis in cutaneous malignant melanoma. J Clin Oncol 2001;19:568-576.

44. Massi D, Borgognoni L, Franchi A, Martini L, Reali UM, Santucci M. Thick cutaneous malignant melanoma: a reappraisal of prognostic factors. Melanoma Res 2000;10:153-164.

45. Karjalainen JM, Eskelinen MJ, Nordling S, Lipponen PK, Alhava EM, Kosma VM. Mitotic rate and S-phase fraction as prognostic factors in stage I cutaneous malignant melanoma. Br J Cancer 1998;77:1917-1925.

46. Sondergaard K, Schou G. Survival with primary cutaneous malignant melanoma, evaluated from 2012 cases. A multivariate regression analysis. Virchows Arch A Pathol Anat Histopathol 1985;406:179-195.

47. Merkel DE, McGuire WL. Ploidy, proliferative activity and prognosis. DNA flow cytometry of solid tumors. Cancer 1990;65:1194-1205.

48. Kruper LL, Spitz FR, Czerniecki BJ, et al. Predicting sentinel node status in AJCC stage I/II primary cutaneous melanoma. Cancer 2006;107:2436-2445.

49. Taylor RC, Patel A, Panageas KS, Busam KJ, Brady MS. Tumor-infiltrating lymphocytes predict sentinel lymph node positivity in patients with cutaneous melanoma. J Clin Oncol 2007;25:869-875.

50. Bodey B, Bodey B Jr, Siegel SE, Kaiser HE. Controversies on the prognostic significance of tumor infiltrating leukocytes in solid human tumors. Anticancer Res 2000;20:1759-1768.

51. Lyle S, Salhany KE, Elder DE. TIA-1 positive tumor-infiltrating lymphocytes in nevi and melanomas. Mod Pathol 2000;13:52-55.

52. Clemente CG, Mihm MC Jr, Bufalino R, Zurrida S, Collini P, Cascinelli N. Prognostic value of tumor infiltrating lymphocytes in the vertical growth phase of primary cutaneous melanoma. Cancer 1996;77:1303-1310.

53. Mihm MC Jr, Clemente CG, Cascinelli N. Tumor infiltrating lymphocytes in lymph node melanoma metastases: a histopathologic prognostic indicator and an expression of local immune response. Lab Invest 1996;74:43-47.

54. Pastorfide GC, Kibbi AG, de Roa AL, et al. Image analysis of stage 1 melanoma (1.00-2.50 mm): lymphocytic infiltrates related to metastasis and survival. J Cutan Pathol 1992;19:390-397.

55. Busam KJ, Antonescu CR, Marghoob AA, et al. Histologic classification of tumor-infiltrating lymphocytes in primary cutaneous malignant melanoma. A study of interobserver agreement. Am J Clin Pathol 2001;115:856-860.

56. Busam KJ, Iversen K, Berwick M, Spagnoli GC, Old LJ, Jungbluth AA. Immunoreactivity with the anti-MAGE antibody 57B in malignant melanoma: frequency of expression and correlation with prognostic parameters. Mod Pathol 2000;13:459-465.

57. Kornstein MJ, Brooks JS, Elder DE. Immunoperoxidase localization of lymphocyte subsets in the host response to melanoma and nevi. Cancer Res 1983;43:2749-2753.

58. Massi D, Franchi A, Borgognoni L, Reali UM, Santucci M. Thin cutaneous malignant melanomas (< or =1.5 mm): identification of risk factors indicative of progression. Cancer 1999;85:1067-1076.

59. Taran JM, Heenan PJ. Clinical and histologic features of level 2 cutaneous malignant melanoma associated with metastasis. Cancer 2001;91:1822-1825.

60. Gromet MA, Epstein WL, Blois MS. The regressing thin malignant melanoma: a distinctive lesion with metastatic potential. Cancer 1978;42:2282-2292.

61. Ronan SG, Eng AM, Briele HA, Shioura NN, Das Gupta TK. Thin malignant melanomas with regression and metastases. Arch Dermatol 1987;123:1326-1330.

62. McLean DI, Lew RA, Sober AJ, Mihm MC Jr, Fitzpatrick TB. On the prognostic importance of white depressed areas in the primary lesion of superficial spreading melanoma. Cancer 1979;43:157-161.

63. Cochran AJ, Diehl V, Stjernsward J. Regression of primary malignant melanoma associated with a good prognosis despite metastasis to lymph nodes. Rev Eur Etud Clin Biol 1970;15:969-972.

64. McGovern VJ, Shaw HM, Milton GW. Prognosis in patients with thin malignant melanoma: influence of regression. Histopathology 1983;7:673-680.

65. Kelly JW, Sagebiel RW, Blois MS. Regression in malignant melanoma. A histologic feature without independent prognostic significance. Cancer 1985;56:2287-2291.

66. Kang S, Barnhill RL, Mihm MC Jr, Sober AJ. Histologic regression in malignant melanoma: an interobserver concordance study. J Cutan Pathol 1993;20:126-129.

67. Corona R, Mele A, Amini M, et al. Interobserver variability on the histopathologic diagnosis of cutaneous melanoma and other pigmented skin lesions. J Clin Oncol 1996;14:1218-1223.

68. Balch CM, Soong SJ, Murad TM, Ingalls AL, Maddox WA. A multifactorial analysis of melanoma. II. Prognostic factors in patients with stage I (localized) melanoma. Surgery 1979;86:343-351.

69. Shaw HM, Balch CM, Soong SJ, Milton GW, McCarthy WH. Prognostic histopathological factors in malignant melanoma. Pathology 1985;17:271-274.

70. Day CL Jr, Harrist TJ, Gorstein F, et al. Malignant melanoma. Prognostic significance of "microscopic satellites" in the reticular dermis and subcutaneous fat. Ann Surg 1981;194:108-112.

71. Spatz A, Cook MG, Elder DE, Piepkorn M, Ruiter DJ, Barnhill RL. Interobserver reproducibility of ulceration assessment in primary cutaneous melanomas. Eur J Cancer 2003;39:1861-1865.

72. León P, Daly JM, Synnestvedt M, Schultz DJ, Elder DE, Clark WH Jr. The prognostic implications of microscopic satellites in patients with clinical stage I melanoma. Arch Surg 1991;126:1461-1468.

73. Borgstein PJ, Meijer S, Van Diest PJ. Are locoregional cutaneous metastases in melanoma predictable? Ann Surg Oncol 1999;6:315-321.

74. Kashani-Sabet M, Sagebiel RW, Ferreira CM, Nosrati M, Miller JR 3rd. Tumor vascularity in the prognostic assessment of primary cutaneous melanoma. J Clin Oncol 2002;20:1826-1831.

75. Kashani-Sabet M, Sagebiel RW, Ferreira CM, Nosrati M, Miller JR 3rd. Vascular involvement in the prognosis of primary cutaneous melanoma. Arch Dermatol 2001;137:1169-1173.

76. Barnhill RL, Lugassy C. Angiotropic malignant melanoma and extravascular migratory metastasis: description of 36 cases with emphasis on a new mechanism of tumour spread. Pathology 2004;36:485-490.

77. Sorensen FB, Kristensen IB, Grymer F, Jakobsen A. DNA level, tumor thickness, and stereological estimates of nuclear volume in stage I cutaneous malignant melanomas. A comparative study with analysis of prognostic impact. Am J Dermatopathol 1991;13:11-19.

78. Bjornhagen V, Mansson-Brahme E, Lindholm J, Mattsson A, Auer G. Morphometric, DNA and PCNA in thin malignant melanomas. Med Oncol Tumor Pharmacother 1993;10:87-94.

79. Chagpar RB, Ross MI, Reintgen DS, et al. Factors associated with improved survival among young adult melanoma patients despite a greater incidence of sentinel lymph node metastasis. J Surg Res 2007;143:164-168.

80. Aitchison TC, Sirel JM, Watt DC, MacKie RM. Prognostic trees to aid prognosis in patients with cutaneous malignant melanoma. Scottish Melanoma Group. BMJ 1995;311:1536-1539.

81. Miller JG, Mac Neil S. Gender and cutaneous melanoma. Br J Dermatol 1997;136:657-665.

82. Dabrowska DM, Elashoff RM, Ho W, Morton DL. Identifying predictive factors in melanoma progression. Oncol Rep 1998;5:569-575.

83. Reintgen DS, Albertini J, Miliotes G. The accurate staging and modern day treatment of malignant melanoma. Cancer Res Ther Control 2001;4:183.

84. Stadelmann WK, Rapaport DP, Soong SJ, Reintgen DS, Buzaid AC, Balch CM. Prognostic clinical and pathologic features. In: Balch CM, Houghton AN, Sober AJ, Soong SJ, eds. Cutaneous melanoma. St Louis: Quality Medical Pub. Inc.; 1998:11-36.

85. Clark WH Jr, From L, Bernardino EA, Mihm MC Jr. The histogenesis and biologic behavior of primary human malignant melanomas of the skin. Cancer Res 1969;29:705-727.

86. Breslow A. Prognosis in cutaneous melanoma: tumor thickness as a guide to treatment. Pathol Annu 1980;15:1-22.

87. Day CL Jr, Sober AJ, Fitzpatrick TB, Mihm MC Jr. Prognosis in malignant melanoma. J Am Acad Dermatol 1980;3:525-526.

88. Day CL Jr, Sober AJ, Kopf AW, et al. A prognostic model for clinical stage I melanoma of the lower extremity. Location on foot as independent risk factor for recurrent disease. Surgery 1981;89:599-603.

89. Day CL Jr, Sober AJ, Kopf AW, et al. A prognostic model for clinical stage I melanoma of the trunk Location near the midline is not an independent risk factor for recurrent disease. Am J Surg 1981;142:247-251.

90. Day CL Jr, Sober AJ, Kopf AW, et al. A prognostic model for clinical stage I melanoma of the upper extremity. The importance of anatomic subsites in predicting recurrent disease. Ann Surg 1981;193:436-440.

91. Day CL Jr, Mihm MC Jr, Lew RA, et al. Prognostic factors for patients with clinical stage I melanoma of intermediate thickness (1.51 - 3.39 mm). A conceptual model for tumor growth and metastasis. Ann Surg 1982;195:35-43.

92. Day CL Jr, Harrist TJ, Lew RA, Mihm MC Jr. Classification of malignant melanomas according to the histologic morphology of melanoma nodules. J Dermatol Surg Oncol 1982;8:874-875, 900.

93. Day CL Jr, Mihm MC Jr, Sober AJ, Fitzpatrick TB, Malt RA. Narrower margins for clinical stage I malignant melanoma. N Engl J Med 1982;306:479-482.

94. Day CL Jr, Lew RA, Mihm MC Jr, et al. A multivariate analysis of prognostic factors for melanoma patients with lesions greater than or equal to 3.65 mm in thickness. The importance of revealing alternative Cox models. Ann Surg 1982;195:44-49.

95. Day CL Jr, Mihm MC Jr, Lew RA, Kopf AW, Sober AJ, Fitzpatrick TB. Cutaneous malignant melanoma: prognostic guidelines for physicians and patients. CA Cancer J Clin 1982;32:113-122.

96. Day CL Jr. Subsite concept for metastases in clinical stage I melanoma. Lancet 1982;2:154.

97. Day CL Jr, Lew RA, Sober AJ. Malignant melanoma prognostic factors 1: use of photography. J Dermatol Surg Oncol 1983;9:364-367.

98. Day CL Jr, Mihm MC Jr, Sober AJ, et al. Predictors of late deaths among patients with clinical stage I melanoma who have not had bony or visceral metastases within the first 5 years after diagnosis. J Am Acad Dermatol 1983;8:864-868.

99. Day CL Jr, Lew RA. Malignant melanoma prognostic factors 3: surgical margins. J Dermatol Surg Oncol 1983;9:797-801.

100. Day CL Jr, Lew RA. Malignant melanoma prognostic factors 2: the subsite concept. J Dermatol Surg Oncol 1983;9:525-526.

101. Soong SJ. A computerized mathematical model and scoring system for predicting outcome in melanoma patients. In: Balch CM, Milton GW, Shaw HM, Soong SJ, eds. Cutaneous melanoma. Clinical management and treatment results worldwide. Philadelphia: J.B.Lippincott; 1985:353-367.

102. Soong SJ, Shaw HM, Balch CM, McCarthy WH, Urist MM, Lee JY. Predicting survival and recurrence in localized melanoma: a multivariate approach. World J Surg 1992;16:191-195.

103. Cox DR. Regression models and life tables. J R Stat 1972;B34:184.

104. Szymik B, Woosley JT. Further validation of the prognostic model for stage I malignant melanoma based on tumor progression. J Cutan Pathol 1993;20:50-53.

105. Pritchard ML, Woosley JT. Comparison of two prognostic models predicting survival in patients with malignant melanoma. Hum Pathol 1995;26:1028-1031.

106. Tuthill RJ, Unger JM, Liu PY, Flaherty LE, Sondak VK. Risk assessment in localized primary cutaneous melanoma: a Southwest Oncology Group study evaluating nine factors and a test of the Clark logistic regression prediction model. Am J Clin Pathol 2002;118:504-511.

107. Gimotty PA, Guerry D, Elder DE. Validation of prognostic models for melanoma. Am J Clin Pathol 2002;118:489-491.

108. Margolis DJ, Halpern AC, Rebbeck T, et al. Validation of a melanoma prognostic model. Arch Dermatol 1998;134:1597-1601.

109. Edge SB. AJCC cancer staging manual, 7th ed. American Joint Committee on Cancer. New York: Springer; 2010.

110. Balch CM, Gershenwald JE, Soong SJ, et al. Final version of 2009 AJCC melanoma staging and classification. J Clin Oncol 2009;27:6199-6206.

111. Kretschmer L, Neumann C, Preusser KP, Marsch WC. Superficial inguinal and radical ilioinguinal lymph node dissection in patients with palpable melanoma metastases to the groin—an analysis of survival and local recurrence. Acta Oncol 2001;40:72-78.

112. Hughes TM, A'Hern RP, Thomas JM. Prognosis and surgical management of patients with palpable inguinal lymph node metastases from melanoma. Br J Surg 2000;87:892-901.

113. Kretschmer L, Preusser KP, Marsch WC, Neumann C. Prognostic factors of overall survival in patients with delayed lymph node dissection for cutaneous malignant melanoma. Melanoma Res 2000;10:483-489.

114. Messaris GE, Konstadoulakis MM, Ricaniadis N, Leandros E, Androulakis G, Karakousis PC. Prognostic variables for patients with stage III malignant melanoma. Eur J Surg 2000;166:233-239.

115. Mann GB, Coit DG. Does the extent of operation influence the prognosis in patients with melanoma metastatic to inguinal nodes? [see comments]. Ann Surg Oncol 1999;6:263-271.

116. Strobbe LJ, Jonk A, Hart AA, Nieweg OE, Kroon BB. Positive iliac and obturator nodes in melanoma: survival and prognostic factors [see comments]. Ann Surg Oncol 1999;6:255-262.

117. Balch CM, Soong SJ, Murad TM, Ingalls AL, Maddox WA. A multifactorial analysis of melanoma: III. Prognostic factors in melanoma patients with lymph node metastases (stage II). Ann Surg 1981;193:377-388.

118. Gimotty PA, Guerry D 4th, Ming ME, et al. Thin primary cutaneous malignant melanoma: a prognostic tree for 10-year metastasis is more accurate than American Joint Committee on Cancer staging. J Clin Oncol 2004;22:3668-3676.

119. Sondak VK, Taylor JM, Sabel MS, et al. Mitotic rate and younger age are predictors of sentinel lymph node positivity: lessons learned from the generation of a probabilistic model. Ann Surg Oncol 2004;11:247-258.

120. Gimotty PA, Elder DE, Fraker DL, et al. Identification of high-risk patients among those diagnosed with thin cutaneous melanomas. J Clin Oncol 2007;25:1129-1134.

121. Barth A, Wanek LA, Morton DL. Prognostic factors in 1,521 melanoma patients with distant metastases. J Am Coll Surg 1995;181:193-201.

122. Barnhill RL, Mihm MC Jr. Histopathology and precursor lesions, 3rd ed. In: Balch CM, Houghton AN, Sober AJ, Soong SJ, eds. Cutaneous melanoma. St Louis: Quality Medical Pub.; 1998:103-133.

Index*

*In a series of numbers, those in boldface indicate the main discussion of the entity.